Female Urinary Incontinence

女性尿失禁

[美] Anne P. Cameron　原著
马　乐　陈　娟　主审
张春莲　王忠民　主译

中国科学技术出版社
·北　京·

图书在版编目（CIP）数据

女性尿失禁 / (美) 安妮 · P. 卡梅伦 (Anne P. Cameron) 原著 ; 张春莲 , 王忠民主译 . — 北京 : 中国科学技术出版社 , 2024.7

ISBN 978-7-5236-0667-4

Ⅰ. ①女… Ⅱ. ①安… ②张… ③王… Ⅲ. ①女性—尿失禁—诊疗 Ⅳ. ① R694

中国国家版本馆 CIP 数据核字 (2024) 第 082957 号

著作权合同登记号：01-2023-6273

First published in English under the title

Female Urinary Incontinence

edited by Anne P. Cameron

策划编辑 靳 婷 延 锦

责任编辑 靳 婷

文字编辑 张 龙

装帧设计 佳木水轩

责任印制 徐 飞

出　　版 中国科学技术出版社

发　　行 中国科学技术出版社有限公司

地　　址 北京市海淀区中关村南大街 16 号

邮　　编 100081

发行电话 010-62173865

传　　真 010-62179148

网　　址 http://www.cspbooks.com.cn

开　　本 889mm × 1194mm 1/16

字　　数 521 千字

印　　张 19.5

版　　次 2024 年 7 月第 1 版

印　　次 2024 年 7 月第 1 次印刷

印　　刷 北京盛通印刷股份有限公司

书　　号 ISBN 978-7-5236-0667-4/R · 3254

定　　价 258.00 元

译者名单

主　审　马　乐　首都医科大学附属北京妇产医院
　　　　陈　娟　北京协和医院

主　译　张春莲　湖北省十堰市太和医院（湖北医药学院附属医院）
　　　　王忠民　大连市妇女儿童医疗中心

副主译　张逸群　湖北省十堰市太和医院（湖北医药学院附属医院）
　　　　鲁选文　湖北省十堰市太和医院（湖北医药学院附属医院）
　　　　张娟娟　湖北省十堰市太和医院（湖北医药学院附属医院）
　　　　方彩云　湖北省十堰市太和医院（湖北医药学院附属医院）
　　　　刘雪琴　湖北省十堰市太和医院（湖北医药学院附属医院）
　　　　杜士明　湖北省十堰市太和医院（湖北医药学院附属医院）
　　　　朱维培　苏州大学附属第二医院
　　　　肖斌梅　中南大学湘雅医院
　　　　辛德梅　清华大学附属垂杨柳医院
　　　　韩燕华　中山大学附属中山人民医院

译　者（以姓氏笔画为序）
　　　　王彦淞　湖北省十堰市太和医院（湖北医药学院附属医院）
　　　　王高法　湖北省十堰市太和医院（湖北医药学院附属医院）
　　　　王婷婷　湖北省十堰市太和医院（湖北医药学院附属医院）
　　　　邓春雷　湖北省十堰市太和医院（湖北医药学院附属医院）
　　　　付义霞　湖北省十堰市太和医院（湖北医药学院附属医院）
　　　　吕跃峰　湖北省十堰市太和医院（湖北医药学院附属医院）
　　　　朱辉英　中山大学附属中山人民医院
　　　　任松森　湖北省十堰市太和医院（湖北医药学院附属医院）
　　　　刘丽娜　清华大学附属垂杨柳医院
　　　　刘利芬　苏州大学附属第二医院
　　　　杨　洋　湖北省十堰市太和医院（湖北医药学院附属医院）
　　　　杨丰美　湖北省十堰市太和医院（湖北医药学院附属医院）
　　　　吴建淮　首都医科大学附属北京妇产医院
　　　　吴意光　首都医科大学附属北京妇产医院
　　　　冷小飞　湖北省十堰市太和医院（湖北医药学院附属医院）
　　　　张志军　湖北省十堰市太和医院（湖北医药学院附属医院）
　　　　张宏明　欧亚迪斯公司学术部
　　　　张晶晶　湖北省十堰市太和医院（湖北医药学院附属医院）

林甜甜　中山大学附属中山人民医院
罗全慧　湖北省十堰市太和医院（湖北医药学院附属医院）
郑　蓉　湖北省十堰市太和医院（湖北医药学院附属医院）
赵　琳　湖北省十堰市太和医院（湖北医药学院附属医院）
赵　锐　湖北省十堰市太和医院（湖北医药学院附属医院）
胡　雪　湖北省十堰市太和医院（湖北医药学院附属医院）
钟　诚　领汇医疗科技有限公司学术部
秋　忠　青海省黄南州人民医院
俞亚平　中南大学湘雅医院
洪　开　湖北省十堰市太和医院（湖北医药学院附属医院）
贺　敏　湖北省十堰市太和医院（湖北医药学院附属医院）
高　珊　大连市妇女儿童医疗中心
郭娅迪　首都医科大学宣武医院
黄润强　湖北省十堰市太和医院（湖北医药学院附属医院）
曹　梅　湖北省十堰市太和医院（湖北医药学院附属医院）
曹　琳　湖北省十堰市太和医院（湖北医药学院附属医院）
曹晓静　首都医科大学电力教学医院
龚坤雪　湖北省十堰市太和医院（湖北医药学院附属医院）
崔　瑜　湖北省十堰市太和医院（湖北医药学院附属医院）
崔明华　湖北省十堰市太和医院（湖北医药学院附属医院）
程　萍　湖北省十堰市太和医院（湖北医药学院附属医院）
鲁军体　湖北省十堰市太和医院（湖北医药学院附属医院）
曾康康　湖北省十堰市太和医院（湖北医药学院附属医院）
鄢金柱　湖北省十堰市太和医院（湖北医药学院附属医院）
蒲晓丽　湖北省十堰市太和医院（湖北医药学院附属医院）

内容提要

本书引进自 Springer 出版社，是一部全面介绍女性尿失禁的实用著作。全书共六篇 27 章，主要从女性尿失禁的诊断与病因、保守疗法、急迫性尿失禁的药物和手术治疗、女性压力性尿失禁的手术治疗、尿失禁的其他因素和原因，以及特殊人群的尿失禁等方面进行了阐述。全书内容实用，阐释简明，图文并茂，可作为广大泌尿科医生、妇科医生的案头必备指南。

译者前言

我们很荣幸能够为您带来这部 *Female Urinary Incontinence* 的中文译本。

1999 年北京妇产医院引进开展了国内第一例 TVT 手术，这是一个女性尿失禁防治工作方面的标志性事件；随后女性尿失禁临床诊疗逐步推广开来，并拓展为全面的女性盆底功能障碍疾病综合防治；盆底学科及女性泌尿外科正在发展成为一门独立的临床亚学科。

虽然我们在女性尿失禁及盆底疾病防治方面已经取得了巨大的进步及发展，但我国幅员辽阔，人口众多，人口老年化发展迅速，所以防治女性尿失禁及盆底功能障碍疾病是临床面临的艰巨社会职责，因此迫切需要像 *Female Urinary Incontinence* 这样的专著来了解国际女性尿失禁防治的动态，以作为临床工作中重要的参考。

Female Urinary Incontinence 作为美国泌尿外科女医师协会主席、密歇根大学泌尿外科学系 Anne P. Cameron 教授的一部力作，汇聚了美、英、澳 50 余位全部由女性专家组成的作者团队，这是一部旨在帮助女性了解和处理尿失禁问题的重要著作。尿失禁是一种常见但往往被忽视的健康问题，它会对女性的生活质量和心理健康产生重大影响。我们希望通过本书提供有关尿失禁的全面信息，帮助女性更好地理解这一问题，并找到适合自己的解决方案。

本书的作者是一群在尿失禁领域经验丰富的专家，她深入研究了尿失禁的各种类型、原因和治疗方法。她以简洁明了的语言，结合丰富的临床案例和最新的研究成果，向读者介绍了尿失禁的病理机制、诊断方法和治疗选择。无论您是正在经历尿失禁问题，或是对这一话题感兴趣，本书都将为您提供宝贵的知识和实用的建议。

在翻译本书的过程中，我深深感受到自己对女性健康的关注和责任。我希望通过将本书引入国内读者的视野，能够为更多的女性提供帮助和支持。尿失禁是一个敏感的话题，很多女性因为羞于启齿而忍受了很多不必要的困扰和痛苦。我希望这本书能够打破沉默，让更多的女性意识到，尿失禁是可以被理解和解决的，她们不必孤单面对这个问题。

最后，我们要感谢所有为本书付出努力的人，包括原书的作者、出版商和编辑团队！

我们还要感谢参与中文版翻译的来自全国各地的专家、医生及出版社编辑的辛勤工作！特别感谢太和医院妇产科团队，他们在女性尿失禁及盆底疾病防治方面积累丰富经验，他们为本书的翻译工作提供了大量的学术指导与支持！

大家的辛勤工作使得这本书能够问世，并且为读者提供了一份宝贵的资源。我们也要感谢您，亲爱的读者，因为您的阅读和支持是我们翻译本书的动力。

希望本书能够对您有所帮助，带给您新的认识和启示。让我们一起努力，为女性的健康和福祉做出贡献！

马　乐　张春莲

原书前言

女性尿失禁对女性的生活质量和整体健康有重大影响。大小便失禁会使女性面临尿路感染的风险，并限制她们的日常生活，如工作、锻炼和亲密关系。同时，额外支出的卫生棉和其他卫生保健用品，甚至需要药物和手术治疗，均会增加她们对经济压力的焦虑。

可惜的是，尽管大多数女性都想解决尿失禁的问题，但女性尿失禁的话题在专业的医疗随访过程中却很少被讨论。值得关注的是，在过去的 5 年里，女性尿失禁的诊断和治疗均有了显著的革新及进展。不少新疗法进入临床实践，包括 β_3 受体激动药的使用，以经皮胫神经刺激为代表的微创治疗，甚至传统的生物网片材料及手术方式都有了显著的改进，大量新疗法进入临床试验阶段。

本书将对包括病因学、解剖学、诊断学（包括对尿流动力学的深入探讨）、治疗方案（从保守治疗到复杂手术）及未来发展趋势等进行全面详细的介绍。文中介绍了一些关于女性尿失禁的指南和专家共识，如美国泌尿学会（AUA）和女性盆底医学和泌尿生殖道重建学会（SUFU）关于压力性尿失禁和膀胱过度活动症的指南，这些指南将作为治疗方案制订的重要参考依据。在本书中，我们还将重点关注大龄儿童、老年人，以及复杂尿路重建后的女性和变性女性等特殊人群的尿失禁问题。同时，我们还将在书中对以往指南或综述中被忽视的尿失禁少见原因，如瘘管和尿道憩室等问题进行相关介绍，以期能够更全面地阐述女性尿失禁的相关问题。

本书将根据以下脉络来为各位阐述女性尿失禁的相关问题。第一篇介绍女性尿失禁的病因及诊断标准，其中包括尿失禁的诊疗成本分析、详细的诊断流程及标准。同时，还着重参考了尿流动力学相关章节的专业内容。在开篇的章节将为读者提供详细的可视化示例。随后对膀胱和尿道 / 盆底解剖及功能进行详细介绍和讲解，对过往的治疗历史进行系统回顾，阐述解剖结构及功能的改变与治疗效果的相关性。

第二篇重点讲述了女性尿失禁保守治疗的相关内容，主要包括患者与医务人员如何沟通配合进行行为矫正及盆底功能康复锻炼。

第三篇从药物治疗、微创治疗一直到复杂手术治疗等方面详细介绍。其中，我们还专门用一章的篇幅来着重介绍以往较少有文献报道的有关治疗失败的管理策略。

第四篇重点关注压力性尿失禁的治疗与研究进展，如微创治疗及包括生物网片在内的侵入性手术治疗，其中特别用一章的篇幅来介绍手术治疗的相关并发症和疗效不佳的问题，因为这是一个极具争议的话题。

我们知道，许多其他盆底功能问题也可导致尿失禁，尽管它们通常不会在女性尿失禁的相关著作中被专题讨论。但我们考虑到其他盆底功能异常在尿失禁的鉴别诊断中具有相当的重要性，因此，我们在第五篇加入了关于盆底脏器脱垂与女性尿失禁的相关内容，复杂尿路重建（如原位新膀胱术和性别重置术）后的尿失禁诊断和处理原则，以及更为罕见的情况（如瘘管）引起的尿失禁内容。

第六篇重点关注了尿失禁的特殊人群，她们应该有不同的治疗模式和注意事项，如儿科患者、老年人、神经源性下尿路功能障碍的女性。在此部分，我们还专门介绍了关于大便失禁与尿失禁的相关内容，因为很少有医生学者可以同时解决这两个问题。在本书的最后部分，我们还对女性尿失禁的探索性治疗与研究进展进行了介绍，以期开阔读者的视野，促进女性尿失禁诊疗水平的发展。

本书作为一部全面系统阐述女性尿失禁问题的专业著作，本书对初级保健提供者、妇科医生、泌尿科医生、医学生及从事女性盆腔医学与重建外科（FPMRS）的医生，均有裨益。同时，本书还为患者及医务人员提供了有价值的讲义和治疗流程，可以作为临床护理工作者的参考工具。

鉴于本书讨论的主题是女性大小便失禁的问题，并且女性医务人员在女性盆腔医学和重建外科手术领域迅速崛起。作为女性泌尿外科协会、女性盆底医学和泌尿生殖道重建学会的会员，我知道很多优秀的女性并且和她们建立了良好的联系，她们都是本领域专家并参与了本书的编写工作。本书的作者团队由来自全球各地的女性泌尿外科专家组成，她们每个人都根据其专业特色参与了相关章节的编写工作。

真诚推荐初级保健提供者、泌尿科医生、妇科医生、女性泌尿科医生、儿科泌尿科医生、泌尿妇科医生、功能性胃肠病学家、基础和转化医学家、准备从事以上领域工作的医学生、泌尿科和妇科住院医生和研究人员等阅读本书。

目 录

第一篇 女性尿失禁的诊断与病因

第二篇 保守疗法

第三篇 急迫性尿失禁的药物和手术治疗

第四篇 女性压力性尿失禁的手术治疗

第五篇　尿失禁的其他因素和原因

第六篇　特殊人群的尿失禁

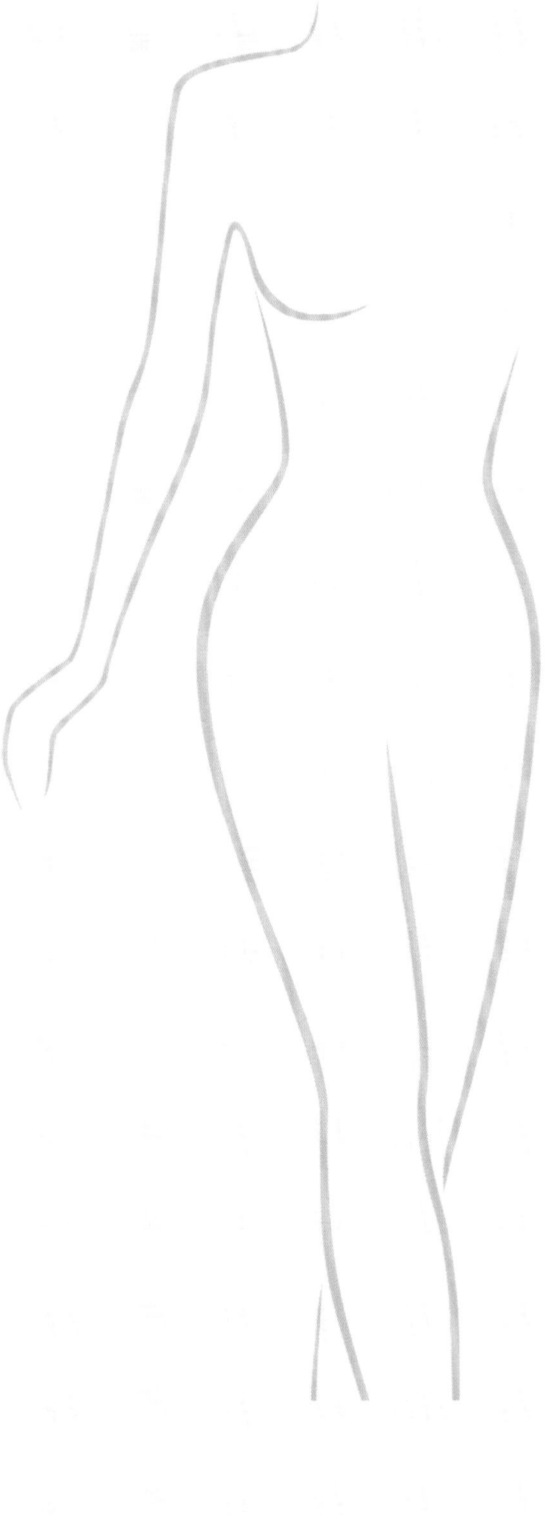

第一篇 女性尿失禁的诊断与病因

Diagnosis and Etiology of Incontinence in Women

第 1 章　女性尿失禁的流行病学、定义和经济花费

Epidemiology, Definitions, and Cost of Incontinence in Women

Cynthia S. Fok　Rachael Gotlieb　Nissrine Nakib　著

盆底疾病在女性中很常见。盆底障碍包括盆腔器官脱垂、尿失禁、肛门失禁。本章主要阐述了尿失禁（UI）的流行病学，重点讨论 5 方面内容：①尿失禁的定义；②尿失禁发生率；③尿失禁危险因素；④尿失禁症状及类型；⑤女性尿失禁的社会差异。

一、女性尿失禁的定义

尿失禁的定义为不自主的排尿，是困扰女性群体的一种常见症状。尿失禁的表现方式有很多，病因也有很多，描述和定义尿失禁症状及类型可以帮助对患者进行评估和治疗。

2010 年，国际妇科泌尿协会（IUGA）和国际尿控学会（ICS）组建了一个联合工作组，定义了女性盆底功能障碍的术语。该文件提供了一些关于女性尿失禁的术语[1]。表 1–1 列出了不同类型尿失禁定义的摘要。

功能性尿失禁是一种与独立生理或病理过程相关的不自觉排尿，因此一些造成尿失禁的原因可能是可逆的。通过“DIAPPERS”记忆口诀，可以了解功能性尿失禁的常见原因[2]。

- D：药物（如乙二醇）。
- I：感染（如尿路感染）。
- A：萎缩（如更年期）。
- P：心理障碍（如谵妄、抑郁、痴呆）。
- P：药理学（如利尿药、麻醉药、镇静药）。
- E：内分泌疾病（如高血糖、高钙血症）。
- R：限制流动性。
- S：大便嵌塞。

膀胱过度活动症（OAB），虽然本身不是一种疾病，但在讨论尿失禁时，经常被认为是一种引起疾病的条件。膀胱过度活动症是指在无尿路感染或其他明显病理情况下的尿急，常合并尿频、夜尿，伴或不伴急迫性尿失禁（UUI）[1]。

二、尿失禁发生率

在讨论尿失禁的比率时，我们首先必须定义患病率和发病率。患病率的定义是在特定时间内某一特定人群中的所有病例除以该人群中有患病风险的人数。发病率是一段时间内人群中的新病例数除以这段时间纳入观察的总人数。

表 1–1　尿失禁的定义

尿失禁种类	定　义
压力性尿失禁	在体力活动、打喷嚏或咳嗽时不自觉排尿
急迫性尿失禁	与尿急有关的不自觉排尿
体位性尿失禁	与体位的改变有关的不自觉排尿
夜遗尿	睡眠时发生的不自觉排尿
混合性尿失禁	与尿急、体力消耗、喷嚏或咳嗽有关的不自觉排尿
连续性尿失禁	持续的不自觉排尿
不自觉尿失禁	无意识的排尿
性交时尿失禁	性交时发生不自觉排尿
功能性尿失禁	与独立生理或病理过程有关的不自觉排尿

女性尿失禁很常见。在后续的数据描述中，我们将主要关注尿失禁在美国的患病率。文献中报道的尿失禁患病率因为问题的提问方式和人群的不同通常是一个变量。在一大型流行病学研究中显示，所有类型尿失禁的患病率为 5%～64%。请参阅表 1-2 列出的关于女性尿失禁的大型流行病学研究摘要。

（一）不同年龄段尿失禁的发生率

尿失禁发生率随年龄的增长而增加。团体健康合作组织发现，30—39 岁女性中 28% 存在尿失禁，而 80—90 岁的女性中 55% 存在尿失禁。在 30—39 岁的女性中，45% 存在压力性尿失禁（SUI），10% 存在急迫性尿失禁，41% 存在混合性尿失禁（MUI），8% 存在严重尿失禁。与此相反，80—90 岁的女性只有 16% 存在压力性尿失禁，其余的急迫性尿失禁 20%、混合性尿失禁 53%、严重尿失禁 33%[7]。护士健康研究显示，随着年龄的增加，压力性尿失禁的发生率降低，急迫性尿失禁的发生率却逐渐增加[9]。虽然 EPIC 研究不是一项以美国成年人为基础的研究，但它是一项来自加拿大、德国、意大利、瑞典和英国 18 岁及以上成年人的研究，这项研究也证明了女性尿失禁与年龄有密切关系。39 岁及以下女性的发生率为 7.3%，40—59 岁女性的发生率为 13.7%，60 岁以上女性的发生率为 19.3%[13]。

表 1-2　大型女性尿失禁流行病学研究综述

研　究	按类型划分的尿失禁发生率	总尿失禁数据
女性健康倡议 *n*=23 296 例 50—79 岁绝经后女性	• SUI：51% • UUI：49% • MUI：14%	报道过的最高发生率显示，64% 的女性报道有过 UI[3]
美国国家健康和营养调查（2005—2016 年） 对 20 岁及以上美国女性进行横断面调查 2001—2004 年队列 *n*=4229 2005—2016 年队列 *n*=15 003	• SUI：26% • UUI：10% • MUI：16%	• 49.6% 报道有 UI[4] • 53% 报道任何 UI[5] • 2005—2016 年队列中 30% 报道有中度至重度尿失禁，较 2005—2010 年队列的 17.1% 有所增加[5, 6]
团体健康合作 *n*=3536 例 30—90 岁的女性	• SUI：14% • UUI：5% • MUI：21%	45% 的尿失禁被定义为“至少每月发生任何量的渗漏”[7]
护士健康研究 女性注册护士（1976 年登记的 30—55 岁女性）。尿失水问题于 1996 年首次提出。2000—2002 年，该队列中新的尿失水发生率[9]	• SUI：2% • UUI：0.7% • MUI：0.9%	• 34.1% 的人在过去 12 个月内每月至少有 1 次漏尿[8] • 9.2% 的人在过去 12 个月，至少每月发生 UI • 27.6% 的人在前 12 个月有新的 UI 发生[9]
40 岁及以上成人下尿路症状流行病学[10] *n*=15 861 例女性	• SUI：31.8% • UUI：24.4%	
Kaiser Permanente 节制相关风险流行病学研究（KP CARES）[11] 25—84 岁女性	SUI：15%	
Kaiser 机构尿失禁生殖风险研究（RRISK）[12] 40—69 岁女性		28.6% 的人每周至少发生 1 次尿失禁

SUI. 压力性尿失禁；UUI. 急迫性尿失禁；MUI. 混合性尿失禁；UI. 尿失禁

NHANES 队列研究显示，压力性尿失禁在40—59 岁的女性中最常见（32%），但急迫性尿失禁和混合性尿失禁在 60 岁以上的女性中发生率较高（分别为 19% 和 25%）。此外，40 岁以下的女性不太可能被尿失禁症状所困扰，年龄较大的女性更可能出现中度或严重 / 非常严重的症状[5]。健康、衰老和身体组成研究显示，21% 的 70—79 岁女性至少每周发生尿失禁。在这个队列研究中，急迫性尿失禁的发生率与压力性尿失禁相似（急迫性尿失禁为 42%，压力性尿失禁为 40%）[14]。

（二）不同种族或民族尿失禁的发生率

2001—2004 年 NHANES 的数据显示，在控制年龄、胎次、体重指数和不同种族 / 民族尿失禁发生率活动水平的情况下，美国白种人女性和墨西哥裔女性发生压力性尿失禁的概率约是非洲裔女性的 2.5 倍[4]。2005—2016 年 NHANES 再次报道，非西班牙裔黑种人女性急迫性尿失禁发生率最高，为 18%；其他群体为 9%。同时，该组压力性尿失禁发生率最低，为 16%；其他组为 28%[5]。

Kaiser 组织关于尿失禁生殖风险的研究中也指出，美国非洲裔和亚洲裔女性可能比白种人女性尿失禁的发生率低[10]。研究还表明，白种人女性（41%）比非洲裔女性（31%）或拉丁裔女性（30%）尿失禁发生率高，拉丁裔女性（9%）比非洲裔女性（14%）或白种人女性（15%）混合性尿失禁的发生率低[15]。尿失禁发生率的差异，会随着女性年龄的增长而持续变化。健康、衰老和身体成分研究显示，70—79 岁的白种人女性，每周发生尿失禁的可能性是非洲裔女性的 2 倍（27% vs. 14%）[14]。

2002—2004 年尿失禁发生率的研究（EPI）表明，在美国密歇根州东南部，非洲裔女性尿失禁的总体发生率为 14.6%，而白种人女性为 33.1%。虽然两组漏尿的次数没有差异，但美国非洲裔女性的漏尿量明显更高。白种人女性尿失禁中约一半（50.1%）为几滴漏尿，而非洲裔女性尿失禁中约一半（50.6%）的情况为尿湿内裤或衬垫。此外，两组在压力性尿失禁和急迫性尿失禁发生率上存在差异，但混合性尿失禁的发生率并没有差异。约 39.2% 的白种人女性有压力性尿失禁，非洲裔女性中压力性尿失禁为 25%；相比之下，非洲裔女性有 23.8% 为急迫性尿失禁，但白种人女性中只有 11%[16]。

西班牙老年流行病学研究（Hispanic EPESE）显示，美国 15% 的墨西哥裔女性在过去一个月内有尿失禁症状。那些存在尿失禁的人群倾向于年龄较大、接受正规教育较少，文化适应率较高的人群。同时，日常生活方式、既往使用雌激素、既往妊娠史和多次分娩也对女性尿失禁产生影响。在此尿失禁人群中，混合性尿失禁最常见（41.8%），其次是急迫性尿失禁（33.1%），再次是压力性尿失禁（10%）[17]。

Huang 等报道，70% 的亚洲裔女性在过去 12 个月中有尿失禁症状。约 27% 报道每日存在症状，38% 报道每周存在症状。在尿失禁患者中，压力性尿失禁（27%）和急迫性尿失禁（25%）的患者数量相当[18]。

三、尿失禁的危险因素

有多种危险因素可能使女性发生尿失禁。风险因素如年龄、种族与民族、妊娠和分娩史、家族史、体育活动、吸烟和肥胖等通常都与尿失禁有关。同时尿失禁也与盆底障碍有关，包括脱垂，肠易激综合征，既往盆腔手术包括子宫切除术，神经系统疾病包括多发性硬化症、帕金森病、痴呆和其他疾病（如糖尿病和尿路感染）。

（一）年龄

综上所述，年龄增长是女性尿失禁的一个公认且不可改变的危险因素。年龄与各类型尿失禁发生率增高有关。老年女性中尿失禁报道人数更多、尿失禁症状更重，同时存在急迫性或混合性尿失禁[5, 7]。

（二）产次和分娩方式

Blomquist 等对母亲分娩后结局（MOAD）中

获得的相关数据进行了研究，该研究为一项对2008年10月到2013年12月的产妇纵向队列研究。调查者从一家社区医院5～10年的就诊人群中招募，从他们第一次分娩（指数出生）起每年随访，持续达9年。后续工作于2017年4月结束。1528例入组病例（剖宫产组778例，顺产组565例，手术顺产组185例），初产年龄中位数为30.6岁，其中经产1092例（72%）（总计2887次分娩），中位年龄为38.3岁。在自然分娩组，压力性尿失禁15年累积发生率为34.3%（95%CI 29.9%～38.6%），膀胱过度活动症15年累积发生率为21.8%（95%CI 17.8%～25.7%）。与自然阴道分娩相比，剖宫产分娩中发生压力性尿失禁和膀胱过度活动症的风险显著降低[19]。

（三）家族史

女性尿失禁包括压力性尿失禁、急迫性尿失禁和混合性尿失禁，表现为家庭聚集性。基于对丹麦登记的双胞胎人口研究表明，急迫性尿失禁和混合性尿失禁有显著的遗传倾向[20]。此外，瑞典的双胞胎研究显示，压力性尿失禁存在很强的遗传风险[21]。已经有人提出急迫性尿失禁[22]和压力性尿失禁[23]的基因位点。

盆底疾病网（Pelvic Floor Disorders Network）发表了一项全基因组关联研究（GWAS），对2241例急迫性尿失禁病例和来自女性健康倡议的776例对照组进行了研究，确定了6个与急迫性尿失禁相关的位点[24]。Penney等利用护士健康研究（NHS）进行了一项GWAS，以确定与尿失禁风险相关的遗传变异[25]。他们在染色体8q23.3和1p32.2两个位点上发现了8个与尿失禁显著相关的单核苷酸多态性（SNP）。对于尿失禁亚型，没有SNP能达到全基因组意义。该GWAS为尿失禁的遗传关联提供了初步证据，值得进一步研究。

（四）体力活动

高强度运动与尿失禁风险增加相关，这种联系甚至见于年轻未生育女性中。参加高强度运动的未分娩女性尿失禁发生率为38.6%，而不参加高强度运动的女性则为19.9%，这可能是运动强度增加导致，运动本身不是病因，所以不建议女性完全不进行运动[26]。

（五）吸烟

护士健康Ⅱ研究（NHS Ⅱ）中指出，吸烟可能使频繁或严重漏尿分别增加20%和34%[27]。其他研究也显示了类似的结果。SWAN研究报道称，与从不吸烟的人相比，当前吸烟者中，中重度尿失禁的风险增加了38%[28]。挪威的一项尿失禁流行病学（EPINCONT）研究显示，在27 936例年龄为20—64岁的女性中，吸烟者发生严重尿失禁的风险比从不吸烟者高40%[29]。有几个原因可以解释该现象：①吸烟使相关胶原蛋白生成减少，从而削弱盆底支撑结构和韧带；②吸烟者的咳嗽症状直接影响尿道括约肌。吸烟相关的其他合并症包括血管疾病、哮喘和慢性阻塞性肺疾病（COPD），对膀胱和尿道功能也有其他直接和间接影响[30]。考虑到对尿控的负面影响和多种健康风险，建议所有吸烟的女性戒烟。

（六）盆腔手术

盆腔手术对盆底有不同程度的影响。大多数流行病学研究使用既往子宫切除术作为既往盆腔手术的替代。尿失禁与既往子宫切除术没有明确的关系。团体健康合作组织发现，子宫切除术史与尿失禁［优势比（OR）为1.33，P=0.004］及严重尿失禁（OR=1.55，P=0.002）的概率增加相关[7]。这与护士健康研究形成对比，该研究未发现子宫切除术史与尿失禁存在关系[9]。

（七）相关疾病

一些疾病可能增加尿失禁的风险。

1. 肥胖

众所周知，肥胖会增加尿失禁的风险[31]。体重指数≥30kg/m^{2}即可被定义为肥胖，世界卫生组织（WHO）估计，全世界超重和肥胖的成年人分别为19亿人和6亿人[32]。在病因学上，3个（译著注：原书似有误，已修改）与肥胖相关可增加尿失禁风险的因素有：①腹部脂肪增加，导致膀胱内压力增加；②尿道运动过度和腹部压力增加，引起逼尿肌不稳定；③椎间盘突出，影响膀胱神经支配[33]。尿流动力学研究支持这些观点，他们发现体重减轻会导致膀胱内压力降低和膀胱容量增加。在 Bulbuller 等的一项研究中，120 例接受腹腔镜胃袖状切除术（LSG）的肥胖女性被要求在术前和术后 6 个月填写国际尿失禁咨询问卷（ICIQ-UI-SF）和尿失禁影响问卷（IIQ-7）[34]。他们发现 120 例患者中，72 例（60%）术前存在尿失禁，72 例患者尿失禁类型占比为急迫性尿失禁 23 例（31.95%）、压力性尿失禁 18 例（25%）、混合性尿失禁 31 例（43.05%）。术后 6 个月，超重减重率为 70.33%（SD=14.84%）。对于 3 种尿失禁亚型来说，术后 6 个月的 ICIQ-UI-SF 和 IIQ-7 评分均较术前显著下降（$P<0.05$）。术前、术后 ICIQ-UI-SF 问卷评分，急迫性尿失禁分别为 8.76 和 2.64；压力性尿失禁为 8.77 和 2.57；混合性尿失禁为 10.58 和 3.74。IIQ-7 问卷得分，急迫性尿失禁分别为 6.73 和 2.53；压力性尿失禁为 7.10 和 2.27；混合性尿失禁为 7.68 和 3.16。因此，可以告知超重或肥胖的女性，减肥可以改善急迫性尿失禁或压力性尿失禁症状，并鼓励女性为减重而努力。

2. 便秘

一项包含 16 项 35 629 例参与者和 6054 例尿失禁患者的观察研究性 Meta 分析发现，便秘与女性尿失禁风险显著相关，OR=2.46（95%CI 1.79～3.38）。然而，还需要进一步进行前瞻性研究来明确其因果关系[35]。由于便秘本身就是一个麻烦的问题，所以向女性建议调节粪便硬度有一定益处。

3. 盆腔疼痛

基于我们的临床观察发现，盆底肌肉疼痛（PFMP）与“刺激性”排尿症状有显著相关性。然而，Meister 等的一项研究分析了盆底肌肉疼痛与尿频、急迫性尿失禁的关系，在控制绝经后状态后似乎没有相关性[36]。他们认为，需要更多的尿窘迫指数问卷进行进一步研究，包括额外的刺激症状，可能有利于更好地发现其相关性。

4. 慢性呼吸系统疾病

女性患慢性肺部疾病（CLD）已被证明与尿失禁有关，这种情况在老年女性中更为明显，与同龄的无慢性疾病的女性相比，这也意味着更多的痛苦。Button 等的一项前瞻性研究观察了囊性纤维化（CF，n=38）、慢性阻塞性肺疾病（COPD，n=27）的女性和 69 例没有慢性肺部疾病的健康女性[37]。所有三组中的大多数女性均报道了尿失禁发作（CF 为 71%，COPD 为 70%，健康女性为 55%）。与同年龄的健康对照组相比，囊性纤维化女性报道的尿失禁事件更多，其中压力性尿失禁更常见。此外，患有慢性肝病的女性其患尿失禁的可能性是健康女性的 2 倍。

5. 糖尿病

团体健康合作组织发现糖尿病不是尿失禁的危险因素，但却是严重尿失禁的危险因素（OR=1.83，P=0.01）[7]。

糖尿病与尿失禁相关的病理生理学显示，疾病导致逼尿肌过度活动，从而增加尿失禁的风险[38]。

四、尿失禁的经济花费

尿失禁对女性个人和社会而言，成本都是高昂的，可分为直接成本和间接成本。直接成本是指与疾病的管理或治疗直接相关的成本，如使用自我护理产品（如尿失禁垫）、医疗护理（如诊断、治疗、检测、物理治疗）、药物费用及尿失禁相关并发症的治疗（如皮肤破裂、跌倒伤）。间接成本是指与寻求护理和治疗相关的劳动力损失和工资损失。除了经济成本之外，一些女性可能还经历着因尿失禁引起的疼痛、痛苦和生活质量下降。

（一）不同程度的尿失禁

尿失禁是一种常见且昂贵的疾病。据报道，美国每年因尿失禁所花费的费用高达 195 亿美元。其中，每年 42 亿美元用于社区居住的成年人，53 亿美元用于收容机构的老年人[39]。2004 年，美国在女性尿失禁方面的支出估计超过 2.06 亿美元，2013 年增加到 2.46 亿美元[40]。美国紧急尿失禁的全国成本在2007年一度达到65.9美元，预计到2020年将上升到826亿美元[41]。据估计，2015年美国成人尿失禁的市场规模将达到72亿美元，这一情况促使许多新的、可重复使用的尿失禁产品的开发和销售[42]。

尿失禁诊断研究（DAISy）小组在2006年的报道中称，患有严重尿失禁的女性每年可能需要支付900美元的日常护理费用，其中包括尿失禁用品、卫生纸、纸巾和洗衣费用。这意味着对所有尿失禁女性而言，每年494.12美元的护理费用尤其重要，因为调查中报道的大多数女性年收入不到10万美元，53%的人低于4万美元[43]。

Kaiser组织在尿失禁的生殖风险研究中发现，女性平均每年为尿失禁支付超过250美元的自付费用。随着尿失禁的严重程度从中度到重度，每周费用为0.93～7.82美元，而混合性尿失禁、尿失禁严重、体重指数较高、非洲裔女性的费用更高[44]。

1. 压力性尿失禁

关于压力性尿失禁的非手术治疗，一项成本－效果分析，比较了盆底治疗、一次性尿失禁卫生棉条、自适应子宫托或特定的尿失禁子宫托。研究发现最具成本效益的非手术治疗是盆底治疗[45]。

尿失禁治疗网络（UITN）针对压力性尿失禁手术疗效（SISTEr）试验，观察了女性压力性尿失禁自我管理的成本，发现女性每年在压力性尿失禁管理上花费约750美元。他们还发现，女性每月愿意支付118～132美元来完全消除症状。家庭收入高或尿失禁次数多的女性愿意花费更多[46]。此外，SISTEr试验显示，在压力性尿失禁手术后2年，自我管理费用平均降低了72%（每个女性每年减少625美元）[47]。

2. 急迫性尿失禁

在行为矫正和盆底治疗后，可应用抗胆碱能类药物和β受体激动药治疗急迫性尿失禁，其中包括多种药物，甚至包括一些无商标的药物。一项基于医疗保险受益人药物费用的研究表明，2000—2015年，女性每年平均花费约168美元在购买药物上[48]。

一项研究对急迫性尿失禁的药物费用与经皮胫神经刺激（PTNS）、膀胱内肉毒杆菌毒素注射和骶神经调节在24个月内的费用进行了比较。在这一时间内，开始服药和继续服药的患者费用平均为1787美元。接受经皮胫神经刺激治疗的患者平均费用上升到6626美元，接受米拉贝隆/抗毒蕈碱联合治疗的患者为7032美元，接受肉毒杆菌毒素治疗的患者为10 183美元，接受骶神经调节治疗的患者为39 952美元[49]。

ROSETTA显示，为期2年的研究显示，接受骶神经调节的人均累积费用为35 680美元，而膀胱内注射肉毒杆菌毒素的人均累积费用为7460美元[50]。

五、女性盆底疾病的社会差异

阅读关于女性盆底障碍的文献发现其存在社会差异，受年龄、种族/民族、社会及经济地位和居住地点等因素影响，女性在知识、卫生保健获取和寻求卫生保健行为方面存在差异，这些差异可能会影响女性盆底疾病相关文献的普遍适用性。

目前的文献显示，女性盆底疾病（包括尿失禁）在知识、求医行为和治疗方面存在差异。

几项研究表明，女性对尿失禁危险因素和治疗方案的认识存在种族差异。对美国康涅狄格社区居住的成年女性关于盆腔器官脱垂和尿失禁知识问卷的反应分析显示，非洲裔女性明显不太可能认识到分娩是尿失禁的危险因素。非白种人女性对尿失禁的危险因素、预防策略和治疗方案的了解程度也明显偏低[51]。

美国女性健康研究（SWAN）没有发现种族/民族、社会经济和教育状况的不同是阻止中年女性寻求尿失禁治疗的因素。在这项研究中，症状持续时间和定期医疗护理是与寻求治疗更显著相关的因素[52]。

2005—2016年NHANES数据的分析表明，社会经济地位越低，描述有急迫性尿失禁症状女性的概率越高[53]。

一项回顾性研究统计了美国某城市三级护理中心盆底治疗就诊率的结果显示，与那些非拉丁裔女性相比，拉丁裔女性不太容易开始或完成盆底治疗[54]。

一项对2001—2010年医疗保险受益人中观察骶骨神经调节使用情况的研究发现，在此期间那些接受植入的更有可能是65岁以下、生活在美国西部以外地区的白种人女性[55]。

Anger等研究发现，女性医保受益人在压力性尿失禁的诊断、接受吊带手术的可能性、吊带手术术后并发症等方面存在种族差异。1999—2001年的研究显示，白种人女性比非白种人女性更容易被诊断为压力性尿失禁。在这个研究中，白种人女性和拉丁裔女性比非洲裔或亚洲裔女性更有可能接受吊带手术；然而，非白种人女性在吊带手术后发生术后并发症的可能性是白种人女性的2倍。在悬吊手术后的第1年，非白种人女性比白种人女性更容易出现非泌尿系统并发症、盆腔器官脱垂和泌尿系统阻塞。这种趋势在急迫性尿失禁的诊断或重复尿失禁手术中也可见，但没有达到统计学意义[56]。斯坦福大学研究了2005—2011年接受门诊尿道吊带手术女性的并发症发生率。这项研究发现，在手术后的前30天内非洲裔美国人更可能出现至少有1次计划外就诊[57]。

总结

尿失禁是女性的常见问题。尿失禁发生率受很多因素的影响，其中包括年龄、种族/民族、家族史和其他合并症。对每个女性来说，尿失禁的社会成本可能是不同的，但总体社会成本非常高。健康方面的差异影响到对尿失禁女性的治疗和护理。

参考文献

[1] Haylen BT, de Ridder D, Freeman RM, Swift SE, Berghmans B, Lee J, et al. An International Urogynecological Association (IUGA)/International Continence Society (ICS) joint report on the terminology for female pelvic floor dysfunction. Neurourol Urodyn. 2010;29(1):4–20.

[2] Demaagd GA, Davenport TC. Management of urinary incontinence. P T. 2012;37(6):345–61H.

[3] Hendrix SL, Cochrane BB, Nygaard IE, Handa VL, Barnabei VM, Iglesia C, et al. Effects of estrogen with and without progestin on urinary incontinence. JAMA. 2005;293(8):935–48.

[4] Dooley Y, Kenton K, Cao G, Luke A, Durazo-Arvizu R, Kramer H, et al. Urinary incontinence prevalence: results from the National Health and Nutrition Examination Survey. J Urol. 2008;179(2):656–61.

[5] Lee UJ, Feinstein L, Ward JB, Kirkali Z, Martinez-Miller EE, Matlaga BR, et al. Prevalence of urinary incontinence among a nationally representative sample of women, 2005–2016: findings from the urologic diseases in America Project. J Urol. 2021;205(6):1718–24.

[6] Wu JM, Vaughan CP, Goode PS, Redden DT, Burgio KL, Richter HE, et al. Prevalence and trends of symptomatic pelvic floor disorders in U.S. women. Obstet Gynecol. 2014;123(1):141–8.

[7] Melville JL, Katon W, Delaney K, Newton K. Urinary incontinence in US women: a population-based study. Arch Intern Med. 2005;165(5):537–42.

[8] Grodstein F, Fretts R, Lifford K, Resnick N, Curhan G. Association of age, race, and obstetric history with urinary symptoms among women in the Nurses' Health Study. Am J Obstet Gynecol. 2003;189(2):428–34.

[9] Lifford KL, Townsend MK, Curhan GC, Resnick NM, Grodstein F. The epidemiology of urinary incontinence in older women: incidence, progression, and remission. J Am Geriatr Soc. 2008;56(7):1191–8.

[10] Coyne KS, Sexton CC, Thompson CL, Milsom I, Irwin D, Kopp ZS, et al. The prevalence of lower urinary tract symptoms (LUTS) in the USA, the UK and Sweden: results from the Epidemiology of LUTS (EpiLUTS) study. BJU Int. 2009;104(3):352–60.

[11] Lukacz ES, Lawrence JM, Contreras R, Nager CW, Luber KM. Parity, mode of delivery, and pelvic floor disorders. Obstet Gynecol. 2006;107(6):1253–60.

[12] Rortveit G, Subak LL, Thom DH, Creasman JM, Vittinghoff E, Van Den Eeden SK, et al. Urinary incontinence, fecal incontinence and pelvic organ prolapse in a population-based, racially diverse cohort: prevalence and risk factors. Female Pelvic Med Reconstr Surg. 2010;16(5):278–83.

[13] Irwin D, Milson I, Hunskaar S, Reilly K, Kopp Z, Herschorn S, Coyne K, Kelleher C, Hampel C, Artibani W, Abrams P. Population-based survey of urinary incontinence, overactive bladder, and other lower urinary tract symptoms in five countries: results of the EPIC Study. Eur Urol. 2006;50:1306–15.

[14] Jackson RA, Vittinghoff E, Kanaya AM, Miles TP, Resnick HE, Kritchevsky SB, et al. Urinary incontinence in elderly women: findings from the Health, Aging, and Body Composition Study. Obstet Gynecol. 2004;104(2):301–7.

[15] Sze EH, Jones WP, Ferguson JL, Barker CD, Dolezal JM. Prevalence of urinary incontinence symptoms among black, white, and Hispanic women. Obstet Gynecol. 2002;99(4):572–5.

[16] Fenner DE, Trowbridge ER, Patel DA, Patel DL, Fultz NH, Miller JM, et al. Establishing the prevalence of incontinence study: racial differences in women's patterns of urinary incontinence. J Urol. 2008;179(4):1455–60.

[17] Espino DV, Palmer RF, Miles TP, Mouton CP, Lichtenstein MJ, Markides KP. Prevalence and severity of urinary incontinence in elderly Mexican-American women. J Am Geriatr Soc. 2003;51(11):1580–6.

[18] Huang AJ, Thom DH, Kanaya AM, Wassel-Fyr CL, Van den Eeden SK, Ragins AI, et al. Urinary incontinence and pelvic floor dysfunction in Asian-American women. Am J Obstet Gynecol. 2006;195(5):1331–7.

[19] Blomquist JL, Muñoz A, Carroll M, Handa VL. Association of delivery mode with pelvic floor disorders after childbirth. JAMA. 2018;320(23):2438–47.

[20] Rohr G, Kragstrup J, Gaist D, Christensen K. Genetic and

environmental influences on urinary incontinence: a Danish population-based twin study of middle-aged and elderly women. Acta Obstet Gynecol Scand. 2004;83(10):978–82.
[21] Wennberg AL, Altman D, Lundholm C, Klint A, Iliadou A, Peeker R, et al. Genetic influences are important for most but not all lower urinary tract symptoms: a population-based survey in a cohort of adult Swedish twins. Eur Urol. 2011;59(6):1032–8.
[22] Norton P, Milsom I. Genetics and the lower urinary tract. Neurourol Urodyn. 2010;29(4):609–11.
[23] McKenzie P, Rohozinski J, Badlani G. Genetic influences on stress urinary incontinence. Curr Opin Urol. 2010;20(4):291–5.
[24] Richter HE, Whitehead N, Arya L, Ridgeway B, Allen-Brady K, Norton P, et al. Genetic contributions to urgency urinary incontinence in women. J Urol. 2015;193(6):2020–7.
[25] Penney KL, Townsend MK, Turman C, Glass K, Staller K, Kraft P, et al. Genome-wide association study for urinary and fecal incontinence in women. J Urol. 2020;203(5):978–83.
[26] Almousa S, Bandin van Loon A. The prevalence of urinary incontinence in nulliparous adolescent and middle-aged women and the associated risk factors: a systematic review. Maturitas. 2018;107:78–83.
[27] Danforth KN, Townsend MK, Lifford K, Curhan GC, Resnick NM, Grodstein F. Risk factors for urinary incontinence among middle-aged women. Am J Obstet Gynecol. 2006;194(2):339–45.
[28] Sampselle CM, Harlow SD, Skurnick J, Brubaker L, Bondarenko I. Urinary incontinence predictors and life impact in ethnically diverse perimenopausal women. Obstet Gynecol. 2002;100(6):1230–8.
[29] Hannestad YS, Rortveit G, Daltveit AK, Hunskaar S. Are smoking and other lifestyle factors associated with female urinary incontinence? The Norwegian EPINCONT Study. BJOG. 2003;110(3):247–54.
[30] Bump RC, McClish DK. Cigarette smoking and urinary incontinence in women. Am J Obstet Gynecol. 1992;167(5):1213–8.
[31] Dumoulin C, Hunter KF, Moore K, Bradley CS, Burgio KL, Hagen S, et al. Conservative management for female urinary incontinence and pelvic organ prolapse review 2013: summary of the 5th International Consultation on Incontinence. Neurourol Urodyn. 2016;35(1):15–20.
[32] Subak LL, Richter HE, Hunskaar S. Obesity and urinary incontinence: epidemiology and clinical research update. J Urol. 2009;182(6 Suppl):S2–7.
[33] Cummings JM, Rodning CB. Urinary stress incontinence among obese women: review of pathophysiology therapy. Int Urogynecol J Pelvic Floor Dysfunct. 2000;11(1):41–4.
[34] Bulbuller N, Habibi M, Yuksel M, Ozener O, Oruc MT, Oner OZ, et al. Effects of bariatric surgery on urinary incontinence. Ther Clin Risk Manag. 2017;13:95–100.
[35] Lian WQ, Li FJ, Huang HX, Zheng YQ, Chen LH. Constipation and risk of urinary incontinence in women: a meta-analysis. Int Urogynecol J. 2019;30(10):1629–34.
[36] Meister MR, Sutcliffe S, Badu A, Ghetti C, Lowder JL. Pelvic floor myofascial pain severity and pelvic floor disorder symptom bother: is there a correlation? Am J Obstet Gynecol. 2019;221(3):235.e1–e15.
[37] Button BM, Holland AE, Sherburn MS, Chase J, Wilson JW, Burge AT. Prevalence, impact and specialised treatment of urinary incontinence in women with chronic lung disease. Physiotherapy. 2019;105(1):114–9.
[38] Mokdad AH, Bowman BA, Ford ES, Vinicor F, Marks JS, Koplan JP. The continuing epidemics of obesity and diabetes in the United States. JAMA. 2001;286(10):1195–200.
[39] Hu TW, Wagner TH, Bentkover JD, Leblanc K, Zhou SZ, Hunt T. Costs of urinary incontinence and overactive bladder in the United States: a comparative study. Urology. 2004;63(3):461–5.
[40] Feinstein L, Matlaga B. In: Services UDoHaH, editor. Urologic diseases in America. National Institutes of Health: US Government Printing Office; 2018. p.14.
[41] Coyne KS, Wein A, Nicholson S, Kvasz M, Chen CI, Milsom I. Economic burden of urgency urinary incontinence in the United States: a systematic review. J Manag Care Pharm. 2014;20(2):130–40.
[42] Alam PA, Huang JC, Clark BA, Burkett LS, Richter LA. A cost analysis of icon reusable underwear versus disposable pads for mild to moderate urinary incontinence. Female Pelvic Med Reconstr Surg. 2020;26(9):575–9.
[43] Subak LL, Brown JS, Kraus SR, Brubaker L, Lin F, Richter HE, et al. The "costs" of urinary incontinence for women. Obstet Gynecol. 2006;107(4):908–16.
[44] Subak L, Van Den Eeden S, Thom D, Creasman JM, Brown JS, for the Reproductive Risks for Incontinence Study at Kaiser (RRISK) Research Group. Urinary incontinence in women: direct costs of routine care. Am J Obstet Gynecol. 2007;197(6):596.e1–9.
[45] Simpson AN, Garbens A, Dossa F, Coyte PC, Baxter NN, McDermott CD. A cost-utility analysis of nonsurgical treatments for stress urinary incontinence in women. Female Pelvic Med Reconstr Surg. 2019;25(1):49–55.
[46] Subak LL, Brubaker L, Chai TC, Creasman JM, Diokno AC, Goode PS, et al. High costs of urinary incontinence among women electing surgery to treat stress incontinence. Obstet Gynecol. 2008;111(4):899–907.
[47] Subak LL, Goode PS, Brubaker L, Kusek JW, Schembri M, Lukacz ES, et al. Urinary incontinence management costs are reduced following Burch or sling surgery for stress incontinence. Am J Obstet Gynecol. 2014;211(2):171.e1–7.
[48] Kinlaw AC, Jonsson Funk M, Conover MM, Pate V, Markland AD, Wu JM. Impact of new medications and $4 generic programs on overactive bladder treatment among older adults in the United States, 2000–2015. Med Care. 2018;56(2):162–70.
[49] Kraus SR, Shiozawa A, Szabo SM, Qian C, Rogula B, Hairston J. Treatment patterns and costs among patients with OAB treated with combination oral therapy, sacral nerve stimulation, percutaneous tibial nerve stimulation, or onabotulinumtoxinA in the United States. Neurourol Urodyn. 2020;39(8):2206–22.
[50] Harvie HS, Amundsen CL, Neuwahl SJ, Honeycutt AA, Lukacz ES, Sung VW, et al. Cost-effectiveness of sacral neuromodulation versus onabotulinumtoxinA for refractory urgency urinary incontinence: results of the ROSETTA randomized trial. J Urol. 2020;203(5):969–77.
[51] Mandimika CL, Murk W, Mcpencow AM, Lake AG, Miller D, Connell KA, et al. Racial disparities in knowledge of pelvic floor disorders among community-dwelling women. Female Pelvic Med Reconstr Surg. 2015;21(5):287–92.
[52] Waetjen LE, Xing G, Johnson WO, Melnikow J, Gold EB, (SWAN) SoWsHAtN. Factors associated with seeking treatment for urinary incontinence during the menopausal transition. Obstet Gynecol. 2015;125(5):1071–9.
[53] Lee JA, Johns TS, Melamed ML, Tellechea L, Laudano M, Stern JM, et al. Associations between socioeconomic status and urge urinary incontinence: an analysis of NHANES 2005 to 2016. J Urol. 2020;203(2):379–84.
[54] Shannon MB, Genereux M, Brincat C, Adams W, Brubaker L, Mueller ER, et al. Attendance at prescribed pelvic floor physical therapy in a diverse, urban urogynecology population. PM R. 2018;10(6):601–6.
[55] Laudano MA, Seklehner S, Sandhu J, Reynolds WS, Garrett KA, Milsom JW, et al. Disparities in the use of sacral neuromodulation among Medicare beneficiaries. J Urol. 2015;194(2):449–53.
[56] Anger JT, Rodríguez LV, Wang Q, Chen E, Pashos CL, Litwin MS. Racial disparities in the surgical management of stress incontinence among female Medicare beneficiaries. J Urol. 2007;177(5):1846–50.
[57] Dallas KB, Sohlberg EM, Elliott CS, Rogo-Gupta L, Enemchukwu E. Racial and socioeconomic disparities in short-term urethral sling surgical outcomes. Urology. 2017;110:70–5

第2章 女性尿失禁的解剖学与生理学
Anatomy and Physiology of Female Urinary Incontinence

Felicity Reeves Tamsin Greenwell 著

缩略语

POD	pouch of Douglas	道格拉斯窝
POP	pelvic organ prolapse	盆腔器官脱垂
PUJ	pelvi-ureteric junction	盆腔－输尿管交界处
SUI	stress urinary incontinence	压力性尿失禁
TVT	tension free vaginal tape	无张力性阴道悬吊术
VUJ	vesico-ureteric junction	膀胱－输尿管交界处

学习目标

- 描述女性骨盆和会阴的正常解剖
- 描述排尿的正常生理并关注相关病理及影响
- 描述盆腔器官之间的相互关系
- 列出女性骨盆的血液及神经供应和淋巴回流
- 了解解剖学与泌尿系病因在女性尿失禁的临床相关性
- 将这些知识应用到临床实践中去评估和管理女性尿失禁患者

准确的认识和理解泌尿生殖道下段和女性骨盆的正常解剖及生理非常重要。这些知识支撑了诊断、鉴别诊断、制订管理计划，以及影响女性泌尿生殖系统和盆底导致尿失禁的条件。McGuire发现并不是所有的压力性尿失禁都与尿道支持障碍（过度活跃性失禁）有关，并从尿流动力学方面描述了漏尿点压力，用来帮助鉴别运动过度和固有括约肌缺陷[1]。他关于过度活跃性压力性尿失禁女性中尿道膀胱角丧失的研究也有助于理解这种分化。测量咳嗽时的尿道内压力和腹部压力有助于了解过度活跃性压力性尿失禁，其引起尿失禁的机制是尿道膀胱角失去正常结构，升高的腹腔内压力转移到尿道和膀胱，从而导致漏尿[2]。女性的尿失禁可能表现为压力性和（或）急迫性，持续存在的瘘管，先天性输尿管异位或溢流。病因可分为解剖学病因、神经学病因、特发性病因、医源性病因［手术后和（或）放疗后］和产科病因。Petros的积分理论包含了Delancey等的吊床理论，其解释了引起女性尿失禁的多因素原因[3]。完整的理论陈述如下“脱垂和大多数盆底症状，如尿道压力漏、急迫漏、肠道异常、膀胱排空，主要是由于阴道及其支持韧带的松弛”[3]。韧带的力量依赖于雌激素，绝经后女性可能遭受激素替代疗法导致的韧带松弛。此外，妊娠期激素的变化也非常重要。从妊娠 3 个月开始，激素的变化会影响胶原蛋白产生的类型和数量，从而导致韧带逐渐松弛和无力。虽然妊娠期的激素变化会在产后消失，但韧带的薄弱和松弛仍然存在。由于盆底肌肉与骨盆韧带相互连接，骨盆韧带的松弛也会对肌肉的力量和连接产生不利影响，并可能导致排尿或排便失禁[3]。子宫作为盆腔中心锚定点的重要性同样也不可低估，子宫切除术后失去这种中心支持往往导致盆底无力，继而发展为尿失禁或盆腔器官脱垂。会阴体虽然只有 4cm，但在阴道后端和直肠之间提供力量和中心支撑。阴道分娩时，会阴体通常被拉伸和削弱。虽然剖腹产消除了阴道分娩对盆底肌肉骨骼的拉伸和创伤，但导致妊娠期和分娩后结缔组织虚弱的激素变化依然存在，并仍然会影响控制能力和盆底支持功能。与无症状的女性相比，存在压力性尿失禁的女性中最大尿道闭合压力降低 42%[4]。

本章主要介绍了女性排尿的生理学、骨盆和韧带、骨盆侧壁、会阴、骨盆底、下尿路和生殖器官、子宫支撑水平、血液供给、淋巴管和骨盆的神经供给。对排尿的控制依赖于上述结构之间完整而协调的相互关系。应强调导致尿失禁的解剖和（或）生理病理的临床相关性，以帮助理解病理生理学和处理。

一、定义

- 会阴是骨盆下方的菱形区域。女性的尿道、阴道、直肠和肛门都通过它到达末端。
- 骨盆是一种盆状的骨结构，位于腹部下方，会阴和下肢上方，连接脊柱和下肢。盆腔器官、肌肉、神经、淋巴和血管都包含在其中。
- 盆底肌是由直接支持盆腔器官和间接支持腹部器官的 4 种主要肌肉组成的漏斗状肌层。直肠、阴道和尿道从其中穿过，并且盆底肌肉可以帮助其控制各自的功能。同时盆底组织将盆腔和会阴分开。
- 会阴浅隙是尿生殖膈下筋膜以上、会阴浅筋膜（Colle 筋膜）以下的空间。它包括坐海绵体肌、球海绵肌和会阴浅横肌。
- 会阴深隙是在盆底深筋膜以上，尿生殖膈上筋膜以下的空间。它包括会阴深横肌和尿道膜部括约肌。
- 改良唇脂肪垫皮瓣法（MMLFPF）是在 Martius 所描述的球海绵体肌法基础上的一种间断性方法。它选取来自大阴唇内的脂肪组织，以血管蒂为蒂，用于阴道和尿道手术后促进愈合和改善局部组织质量。
- 瘘管是两个上皮表面之间的异常连接，常见于阴道和膀胱之间，即膀胱阴道瘘。
- 压力性尿失禁（SUI）分类（由 Blaivas 和 Olsson 定义）是基于影像尿流动力学检查（VUDS）的发现，并可通过膀胱颈在休息时和咳嗽时与耻骨联合下缘（IMPS）的位置关系进行评估。
  - 0 型：有压力性尿失禁病史，但影像尿流动力学检查未显示压力性尿失禁。
  - Ⅰ型：咳嗽或受压时膀胱颈下降<2cm。静息状态下膀胱颈位置正常。
  - Ⅱa 型：咳嗽或受压时膀胱颈下降>2cm，静息状态下膀胱颈位置正常。
  - Ⅱb 型：膀胱颈静息位置异常低（低于耻骨联合下缘水平），咳嗽或受压时表现为压力性尿失禁。
  - Ⅲ型：膀胱颈在正常静息状态处于膀胱颈开放状态，静息状态下即存在压力性尿失禁（固有括约肌缺乏）[5]。

（一）排尿的生理学

正常排尿的定义是在无梗阻的情况下，在正常时间内自主持续地收缩逼尿肌，从而使膀胱完全排空[6]。在排尿过程中（即在逼尿肌压力上升时），通过主动松弛尿道，尿道压力会下降从而使排尿协调。

正常膀胱以低压储存尿液，在合适情况下可自主排空尿液。这涉及自主神经系统和高级控制中心之间复杂而微妙的相互作用。

在储尿期，胸腰椎交感神经兴奋刺激去甲肾上腺素释放神经递质，通过 β_3 受体介导引起逼尿肌舒张，通过 α_1 受体介导协调膀胱颈收缩。

在排尿期，起源于脊髓 $S_{2\sim4}$ 节段的节前副交感神经引起逼尿肌收缩，随后通过激活 M3 毒蕈碱通道（一个 G 蛋白耦联受体，导致钙离子及钙调蛋白相互作用增加，进而增加肌球蛋白轻链激酶）使节后副交感神经神经元释放乙酰胆碱。副交感神经受到刺激后，还通过释放一氧化氮来降低尿道括约肌张力。

阴部神经受 Onuf 核（位于骶髓前角）的体细胞神经支配，通过以乙酰胆碱为神经递质的烟碱受体刺激尿道括约肌收缩。

在更高控制层，脑桥排尿中枢负责协调排尿，当膀胱充盈时，通过膀胱内的牵张受体接收信号，并通过副交感神经系统向膀胱发送刺激信号，通过躯体系统向尿道外括约肌发送抑制信号，以刺激协调排尿。脑桥排尿中心还接收来自前额叶皮质、丘脑、脑桥和延髓的信号。

在神经系统疾病中，如脑血管意外［脑中风（CVA）或卒中］影响额叶皮质，由于脱抑制和无法克服排尿需求并控制排尿至合适时机，可能发生社交失禁。在脊髓病变中，症状取决于病变水平，如果远端自主脊髓保持完整，可发生反射性排尿。而完全性脊髓损伤则可导致排尿失调，从而导致逼尿肌括约肌协同失调，使膀胱收缩对抗尿道括约肌收缩，导致膀胱压力持续升高，并出现因输尿管引流受损和膀胱内高压力传递至肾脏而导致肾衰竭的风险。其他神经系统疾病如多发性硬化和帕金森病也可出现一系列的膀胱和肠道功能障碍，但最常见的是与神经源性逼尿肌过度活动相关的急迫性尿失禁。逼尿肌过度活动是膀胱充盈期逼尿肌收缩的尿流动力学表现，与急迫感和（或）急迫性尿失禁症状相关。当逼尿肌压力大于尿道括约肌张力和压力时，就会出现漏尿。

（二）骨盆和骨盆韧带

1922 年，Bonney 首先提出关于压力性尿失禁原因的假设（即尿道和膀胱颈支撑的丧失）[7]。众所周知盆腔器官需要物理支持，子宫为韧带提供锚定点的重要性已被反复强调。妊娠期和绝经后的激素变化对韧带胶原蛋白的组成和强度产生不利影响，降低了肌肉收缩对韧带的作用。骨盆的骨性尺寸也可能影响控尿，据报道存在压力性尿失禁症状的女性的耻骨下角比同龄正常女性的宽 2.3°～3°[8]。

1. 骨盆的骨性结构

女性骨盆的骨质较男性骨盆轻而薄（图 2–1 和图 2–2）。融合的髋骨：坐骨、髂骨和耻骨构成髋臼和骨盆前外侧骨，而骶骨和尾骨构成骨性骨盆的后侧面（图 2–1 和图 2–2）。与男性骨盆相比，女性骨盆的耻骨弓角度更宽，骶骨曲线更浅，从而产生更大的骨盆入口和出口，方便阴道分娩。临床检查阴道和会阴时，可以触诊到髂骨、耻骨结节和坐骨结节。

站立时，骨盆入口向前倾斜，以耻骨联合上缘、耻骨嵴后缘、髂骨弓线、骶骨翼的前缘，还有骶岬为界（图 2–1）。盆腔出口边界为尾骨尖、坐骨结节和骶结节韧带、耻骨下支和耻骨联合下缘。5 节融合椎骨形成骶骨，其中包含 8 个椎间孔（每侧 4 个），用于连接成对的骶神经（S_1、S_2、S_3 和 S_4）。

耻骨联合是通向外生殖器的一个关节软骨，同时是 2 块耻骨的连接关节。每块耻骨的上支形成了闭孔的外侧面，而闭孔的内侧面则是由耻骨下支和坐骨联合的坐骨支形成。

骨性骨盆分为大骨盆（或称“假骨盆”，因为它是腹腔的一部分）和小骨盆（或真骨盆）。大骨盆前部不完全，外侧以髂骨为界，后方以骶骨基部为界。小骨盆（真）包含盆腔入口，位于盆腔边缘后方。后方以骶骨和尾骨为界，前方以髂骨内表面和坐骨前外侧和耻骨联合为界。

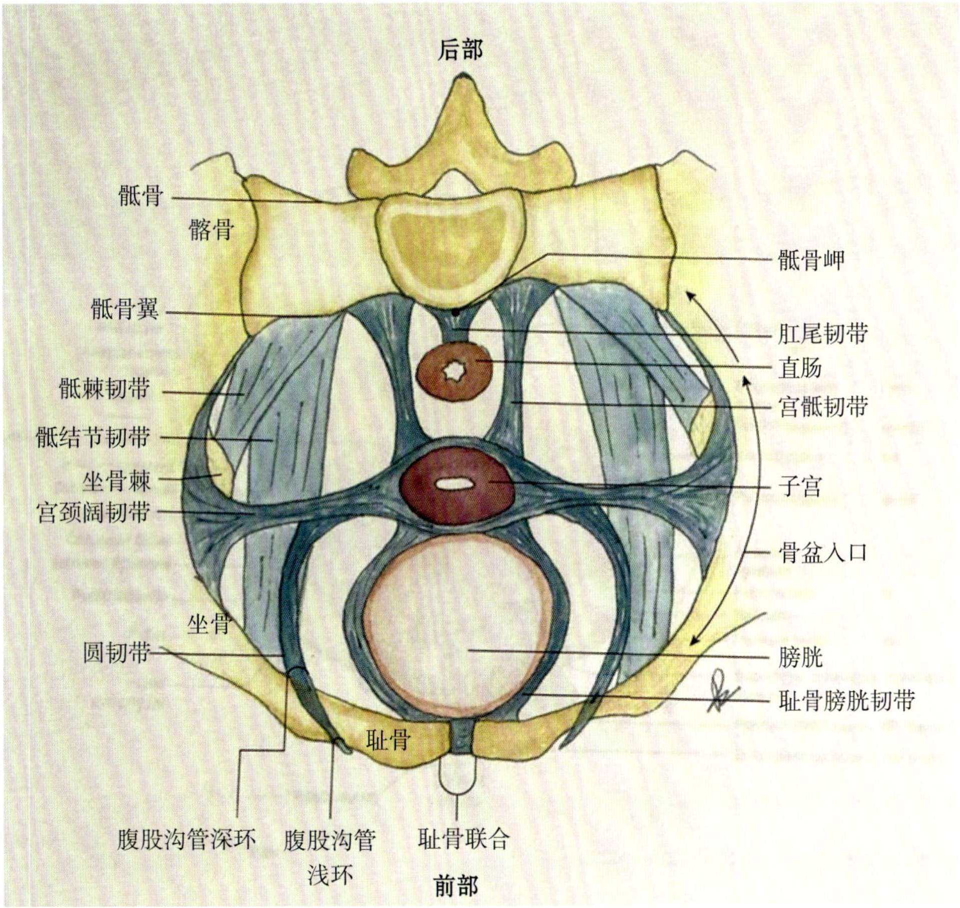

▲ 图 2-1 骨盆和韧带横断面观

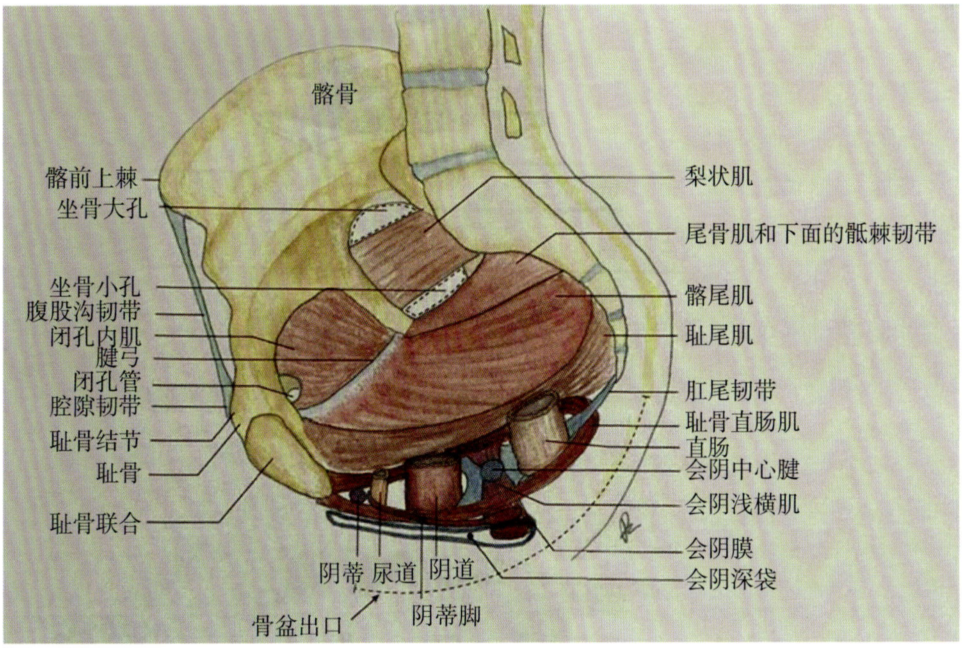

▲ 图 2-2 （医学角度）左半骨盆切除后矢状面观，为了展示相对关系已将肛提肌和骨盆器官切除

2. 骨盆韧带

韧带是一种结缔组织，它将骨头连接在一起，形成关节连接或支持内部器官。骨盆韧带包括以下6个（图2–1至图2–4）。

- 骶棘韧带在两侧连接骶骨和坐骨棘。
- 骶结节韧带连接骶骨和坐骨结节。
- 腹股沟韧带（Poupar 韧带）从两侧髂前上棘延伸至耻骨结节，标志着从骨盆到下肢的过渡。
- 腔隙韧带呈月牙形从腹股沟内侧韧带延伸至两侧的耻骨结节。
- 骶髂韧带分为前后两个部分从骶骨延伸到髂骨穿过两侧的骶髂关节。
- 闭孔韧带自两侧从闭孔膜上方穿过。

这些韧带的胶原结缔组织会对雌激素和孕激素的变化做出反应。雌激素维持韧带胶原蛋白的强度，因此在绝经后的女性中韧带强度较弱。由于先天性结缔组织虚弱和胶原蛋白紊乱[3]，未生育女性也可见韧带无力（虽然不太常见）。子宫切除术及其他造成中心物理支持结构丧失的手术也可能会减少主韧带和宫骶韧带的血液供应，从而导致缺血改变，引起韧带无力。

坐骨大切口和小切口在坐骨的后部被坐骨棘隔开。骶结节和骶棘韧带穿过这些缺口形成坐骨大孔和小孔。骶棘韧带可经阴道触诊触及，在治疗阴道脱垂的骶棘固定手术中通常将阴道壁与骶棘韧带缝合以提供支撑（图2–4）。

盆筋膜腱弓是一条坚固的结缔组织带，它将坐骨棘上方的坐骨连接到耻骨下部。

3. 骨盆孔

坐骨大切迹是骨盆后方的一个切迹，位于髂后上棘下方，坐骨棘上方，这个切迹和骶棘及骶结节韧带形成坐骨大孔。所有的神经血管结构进出骨盆都必须通过它（其内包含梨状肌）。臀上神经（来自骶神经丛的 L_4～S_1 神经根）和血管从骨盆通过坐骨大孔进入梨状肌上方的臀区。臀下神经（来自骶神经丛 L_5～S_2 神经根）及血管、坐骨神经（来自 L_4～S_3 神经根）、股后皮神经（来自 $S_{1\sim3}$ 神经根）、股方肌神经（来自 L_4～S_1 神经根）从骨盆出发，经梨状肌下方的坐骨大孔进入臀区或下肢（图2–2），通往闭孔内肌的神经（来自神经根 L_5～S_2）、阴部神经（来自神经根 $S_{2\sim4}$）和阴部内血管也通过坐骨大孔进出骨盆，在坐骨棘水平处环绕骶棘韧带，经坐骨小孔进入会阴。

坐骨小切迹是骨盆后侧坐骨棘下方的一个小切迹（图2–2）。与骶棘韧带和骶结节韧带交叉形成坐骨小孔。其内包含闭孔内肌肌腱，是会阴的进出点。通往闭孔内肌的神经（由 L_5～S_2 神经根）与阴部内血管及阴部神经（由 $S_{2\sim4}$ 神经根）经坐骨小孔进入会阴。

阴部神经在梨状肌和尾骨肌之间（图2–2和图2–4），经坐骨大孔进入骨盆，然后绕过骶棘韧带，经坐骨小孔进入会阴。它于坐骨直肠窝外侧壁沿阴部内动静脉向前行 Alcock 管（阴部管）。这个管道是一层增厚的闭孔内筋膜鞘。在进入 Alcock 管之前或进入 Alcock 管时，阴部神经分支发出直肠下神经（来自神经根 $S_{2\sim4}$）（图2–4）。然后在会阴膜后缘分支进入会阴神经和阴蒂背神经。会阴神经分支形成浅（皮）和深（肌）会阴神经，支配会阴浅、深隙、下阴道和阴唇的横纹肌。阴蒂的背神经受感觉神经支配，对保证正常的性功能至关重要（图2–4）。

阴部神经和阴部内血管是主要的会阴部神经血管供应（在女性会阴部分有进一步的描述）。阴部神经支配尿道外横纹（自主）括约肌，阴部神经损伤可导致阴唇和阴蒂感觉丧失、大便和尿失禁。阴部神经在阴道分娩和职业自行车运动中尤其容易受损。在分娩过程中，如果需要缓解疼痛，可在坐骨棘区域进行阴部神经阻滞和经阴道局部麻醉注射。

闭孔神经（来自 $L_{2\sim4}$ 神经根）和血管通过位于闭孔内侧的闭孔管从骨盆进入大腿内侧腔室。25% 的人有副闭孔神经（神经根 L_3 和 L_4），其通过闭孔的中外侧离开骨盆。闭孔在进行经尿道中段吊带手术治疗压力性尿失禁中是套管针通过的位置。在穿刺闭孔膜时应注意尽量向内侧穿刺，避开闭孔神经、闭孔血管和闭孔副神经。闭孔神

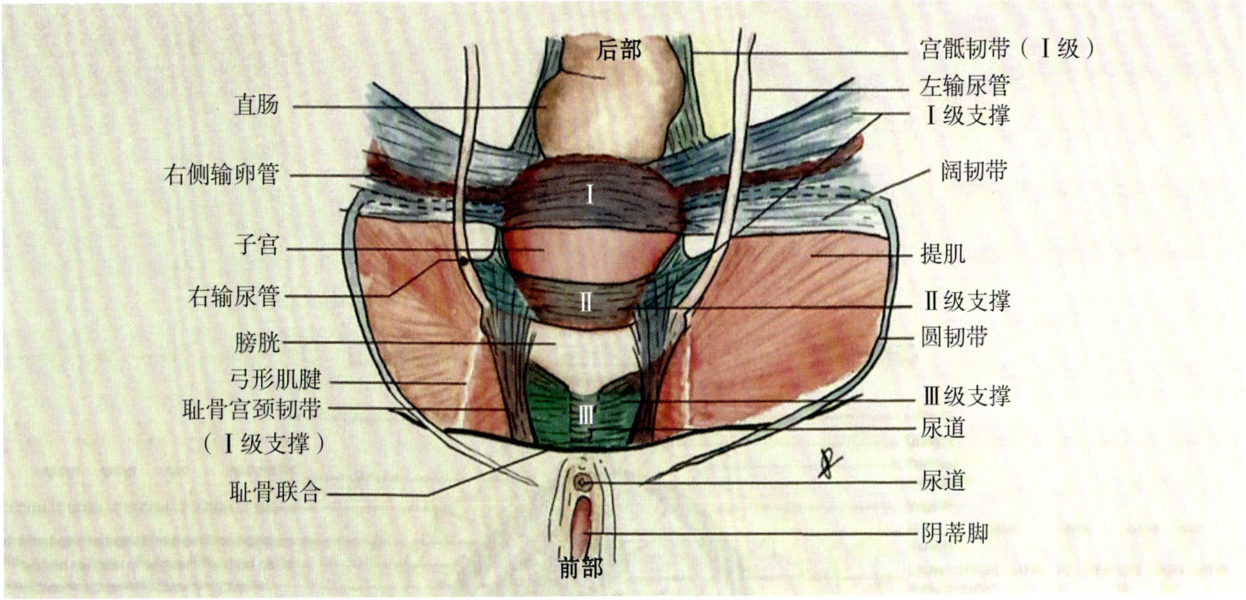

▲ 图 2-3　盆腔横切面以显示阴道和子宫的三级支持结构

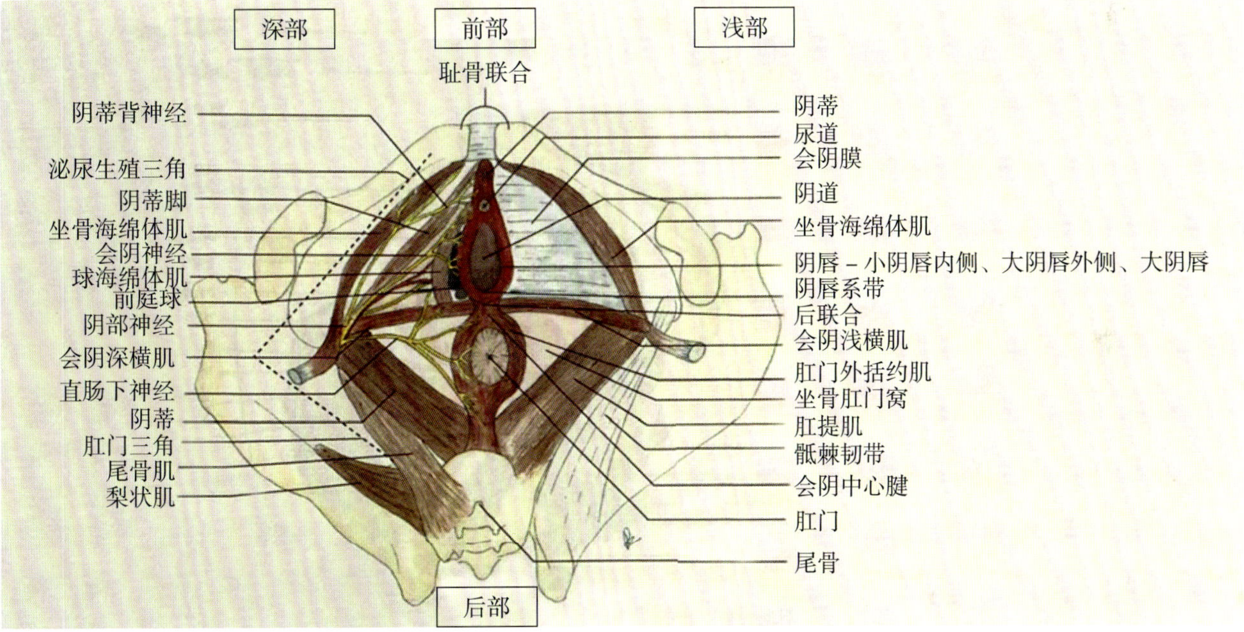

▲ 图 2-4　女性盆腔深部（左）和浅部（右）结构横断面图示

经在经内窥镜膀胱肿瘤切除术中也有意外受刺激的风险，特别是侧壁肿瘤的手术中。刺激会导致突发的强烈大腿内收反应（闭孔踢），有可能导致膀胱意外穿孔。

（三）骨盆侧壁

1. 骨盆侧壁肌肉（表 2-1）

耻骨的主体和分支连同耻骨联合形成骨盆前壁，闭孔内肌和坐骨小孔构成骨盆外侧壁，骶骨、髂骨和骶髂关节构成骨盆后壁。位于后侧的梨状肌通过坐骨大孔离开骨盆附着于股骨，骶神经丛和髂内血管穿过梨状肌内侧。梨状肌起源于骶骨前表面和髂骨的臀表面终止于股骨大转子，充当延伸髋关节的外旋肌和固定髋关节的外展肌，由梨状肌神经支配（骶神经丛 $S_{1\sim2}$）。闭孔内肌起

表 2-1 骨盆底及骨盆壁肌肉

肌 肉	起 点	终 点	功 能	神 经	血管及淋巴
闭孔内肌	闭孔膜、同侧耻骨下支和坐骨	股骨大转子内侧表面	髋关节旋外	闭孔内神经、L_5、S_1	臀上动脉
梨状肌	骶骨	股骨大转子内侧上缘	髋关节旋外	L_5、S_1、S_2	臀上动脉、臀下动脉、阴部动脉及相应的静脉
肛提肌	• 坐骨棘 • 耻骨体 • 闭孔筋膜内弓	• 会阴体，会阴膜 • 肛门尾骨体 • 阴道壁、直肠壁和肛管壁	• 支持盆腔器官，肛肠交界处和阴道的括约肌 • 对抗腹部压力的增加	阴部神经（$S_{2\sim4}$）、S_4	• 臀下动脉、膀胱下动脉、阴部动脉 • 相应的静脉和淋巴管
尾骨肌	• 坐骨棘 • 骶棘韧带	下骶骨和尾骨	• 骨盆器官支持 • 尾骨因子	S_4、S_5	膀胱下动脉、臀下动脉和阴部动脉，以及相应的静脉和淋巴管

源于闭孔膜的内（骨盆）面和邻近的耻骨上支下缘，终止于股骨大转子，其肌腱从会阴发出通过坐骨小孔进入大腿。它是伸展髋关节的外旋肌和固定髋关节的外展肌。其神经分部是从神经到闭孔内肌（神经根 L_5、S_1、S_2）。尾骨肌起源于坐骨棘终止于下骶骨和尾骨。它的作用是支持盆腔器官和弯曲尾骨。其神经支配来自 S_4 和 S_5 的前根。

盆腔内筋膜覆盖盆腔侧壁的内部。它形成了一层强有力的筋膜覆盖在梨状肌和闭孔内肌上。筋膜内部是骨盆血管，外部是脊神经。骶神经丛位于梨状肌之上（在神经供应部分有更详细的讨论）。

2. 盆底

盆底（也称盆腔膈）是盆腔的漏斗状肌底。由肛提肌（神经供应为 S_4 前根及阴部神经 S_2、S_3 和 S_4 支）、尾骨肌（神经供应为 S_3、S_4 前根）、会阴膜、会阴深隙内的会阴深横肌组成。

3. 盆膈肌肉（图 2-2 和图 2-4）

盆膈形成盆腔底部和会阴顶部。它由前面的肛提肌和后面的尾骨肌组成。肛提肌由 3 部分组成：①耻骨直肠肌，U 形的肌肉吊带，起源于耻骨，穿过肛肠连接处，重新插入耻骨；②耻尾肌，起源于耻骨内部，插入尾骨；③髂尾肌，起源于闭孔筋膜的腱弓，插入尾骨。

盆膈近端与耻骨体、闭孔筋膜的腱弓和坐骨棘相连。远端与会阴体（中线纤维肌缝）、肛门尾骨体、尾骨、肛尾韧带、阴道壁、直肠壁和肛管壁相连。肛提肌的作用主要是支撑和稳定盆腔器官（默认是腹部器官），起到一个次要的括约肌作用，维持肛门直肠交界处的角度及阴道近端和尿道相对于阴道中端和尿道远端的角度。这个作用在腹部压力增加的时候尤为重要，如在阴道分娩或排便中受到拉扯时。

会阴体是位于肛门直肠会阴后三角和泌尿生殖会阴前三角交界处的锥体中线纤维肌结构（见会阴切面），为骨盆底和会阴的肌肉和支撑提供了一个中心连接。对会阴体的损害，特别是阴道分娩，可能会导致盆腔器官脱垂（POP）、尿失禁和粪便失禁。骨盆韧带只能在短时间内提供独立的骨盆器官支持。盆腔器官的长期支持作用依赖于盆腔肌肉组织和韧带附着之间的相互作用。

肛提肌被一层坚韧的筋膜覆盖——盆内筋膜由一组网状的胶原纤维组成，其中穿插着弹性蛋白、平滑肌细胞和血管，与腹壁的腹横筋膜相连。盆内筋膜位于肛提肌的正上方，与坐骨棘、腱弓、回肠耻骨韧带（库珀韧带）和弓状线（从骶岬到耻骨上耻骨梳线的连线）相连。

将子宫与盆腔侧壁相连的盆内筋膜区域是宫旁组织。宫旁组织的中间层在子宫颈水平处收缩，形成主韧带和宫骶韧带。盆内筋膜继续向下形成一个薄板，将阴道近端与盆腔侧壁连接在一起——阴道旁组织[9]。DeLancey 描述了子宫 – 阴道支撑的 3 个水平[1]。

Ⅰ级支撑是来自宫旁组织的顶端支持，由主韧带、宫骶韧带、耻骨宫颈韧带和悬吊子宫颈和阴道上缘到盆腔壁的宫旁组织组成。

Ⅱ级支撑是阴道旁组织的水平支持，将阴道中部与骨盆侧壁直接悬吊并固定，并在后方与肛提肌相连。耻骨宫颈筋膜支持膀胱，并与盆内筋膜和阴道前壁融合。阴道后壁与盆内筋膜融合以支持直肠，有助于预防阴道后壁脱垂。

Ⅲ级支撑是由阴道远端与肛提肌外侧、尿道前方和会阴体后方的连接组成。会阴体与骨盆两侧的会阴膜横向连接，帮助支持和稳定阴道远端[9]。

骨盆筋膜与腹膜后筋膜相连形成三层：盆内筋膜代表外层；中间层含有脂肪层及脂肪层的神经血管成分，其需要特定的活动才能接近盆腔器官；骨盆筋膜中间层凝聚形成很强的韧带附着，以支持盆腔器官。这些韧带包括膀胱后侧韧带、宫骶韧带和主韧带。骨盆筋膜的内层位于腹膜深处，覆盖膀胱穹窿和直肠前部。尿道和阴道在泌尿生殖孔处通过肛提肌，其为盆腔隔膜前段最薄弱的区域，然后通过会阴深隙进入会阴（图 2–2、图 2–4 和图 2–5）。泌尿生殖间隙的前方由肛提肌和耻骨支撑，后方由肛门外括约肌和会阴体支撑[9]。静息状态的肛提肌在正常情况下，通过拉动尿道、阴道和直肠朝向耻骨，来维持泌尿生殖间隙的闭合。如果肛提肌损伤无力（如阴道分娩后），就不能再以这种方式关闭泌尿生殖间隙，支撑筋膜的结缔组织最终失效，引起脱垂和（或）尿 / 大便失禁[9]。

（四）子宫支持（图 2–1 和图 2–3）

子宫的支撑作用不仅需要足够强大从而维持子宫的位置，而且还需要具有妊娠期扩张的能力。子宫的支撑作用存在几个水平，子宫切除术和破坏支撑后有阴道穹窿脱垂的风险。结缔组织包围盆腔所有器官，在某些区域，结缔组织密度增加以形成额外的纤维肌肉韧带从而增加支撑能力。这些结缔组织与腹壁的腹膜外部分连接，但是在坐骨直肠窝下方被肛提肌和骨盆筋膜分开。

阔韧带是一层双层的腹膜（折叠成一层），覆盖在子宫体的外侧，使子宫与骨盆侧壁相连。输卵管位于阔韧带褶皱的上缘。阔韧带是女性盆腔器官的保护层。在阔韧带之间是卵巢悬韧带、子宫圆韧带、子宫和卵巢的血管及淋巴。卵巢悬韧带在子宫和输卵管的连接处连接卵巢的内侧和子宫。其内部走行着卵巢血管和淋巴。

子宫圆韧带是卵巢韧带的延续，在卵巢、子宫至盆腔边缘走行，自腹股沟韧带中点进入腹股沟管深环，穿过腹股沟管，止于大阴唇皮下组织，是胚胎时期女性引带的残留。

对子宫的支撑作用主要来自 3 组韧带：主韧带、耻骨宫颈韧带和宫骶韧带。主韧带（宫颈横韧带）为扇形纤维肌韧带，从子宫颈和阴道穹窿延伸至骨盆侧壁，其位于阔韧带的下段为子宫颈提供横向支撑。宫骶韧带从子宫颈两侧向后延伸至骶骨中部，筋膜覆盖在梨状肌上。它提供向后的张力，行直肠检查时可在直肠两侧触及，当站立时，其位置是垂直的。耻骨宫颈韧带连接在耻骨联合与子宫颈和膀胱的前方。从侧面看，膀胱由盆脏筋膜支撑。

（五）会阴

会阴位于骨盆下方，被连接两侧坐骨结节前端的横线分割成 2 个不等的三角形。肛门三角较大，尿生殖三角较小。肛门三角包含肛门，而尿生殖三角包含女性的外生殖器（图 2–4 和框 2–1）。

框 2-1　女性会阴肌肉（图 2-4）

女性尿生殖三角的肌肉均受阴部神经会阴支（S_2、S_3 和 S_4）支配，其血液供应来自髂内动脉前分支的阴部内动脉

- 会阴浅横肌位于尿生殖膈下筋膜的下方（或表面），起自两侧的坐骨结节向内走行插入会阴体并起到支撑作用
- 会阴深横肌位于尿生殖膈下筋膜上方（或深层），起自坐骨结节及其分支并汇合于中心腱，为会阴体提供额外的支撑
- 球海绵肌起到阴道括约肌的作用，支持阴蒂（阴蒂背动脉分支）的勃起，起自女性会阴体插入前庭球的筋膜和海绵体脚的腱膜
- 坐骨海绵体肌起自坐骨结节及其分支并向前延伸，环绕阴蒂体并插入阴蒂海绵体上方的腱膜，对阴蒂的勃起有作用
- 尿道括约肌起于耻骨弓，环绕尿道周围，使尿道自主收缩

1. 会阴深隙，会阴膜，会阴体（图 2-2 和图 2-4）

会阴深隙（DPP）位于盆底下方，会阴膜上方。阴道和尿道穿过会阴深隙。会阴深隙包含支撑和关闭尿道的肌肉，即肛门外括约肌、尿道阴道括约肌（其包围和支撑尿道和阴道），以及尿道膜部括约肌。紧挨着会阴深隙的是会阴膜，一个三角形的增厚筋膜，在处女膜水平覆盖尿生殖三角，并附着于耻骨弓的外侧。会阴膜是骨盆底部的重要支撑结构，其上有一个裂孔，尿道和阴道通过它进入会阴。会阴膜还为外生殖器和会阴浅隙（SPP）表面的肌肉提供附着。会阴膜将尿道、阴道和会阴体与坐骨耻骨分支相连[9]。会阴膜在坐骨结节之间的连线处有一个后游离边缘。会阴体（PB）在这个后游离边缘的中间。会阴深横肌是一对小肌肉，起源于坐骨结节（会阴膜上方），在会阴深隙内水平走行，插入会阴体。其作用是稳定会阴体（框 2-1）。会阴体位于尿生殖三角和肛门三角的交界处，是骨盆底和会阴许多肌肉的插入部位，因此是一个重要的骨盆底和会阴支撑结构。阴道分娩会对会阴体和相关支撑造成损害导致松弛继而导致盆腔器官脱垂。

2. 会阴浅隙（图 2-2、图 2-4 和图 2-5）

会阴浅隙位于会阴膜下，会阴浅筋膜（Colles 筋膜）上。其内包括会阴浅横肌、球海绵体肌和坐骨海绵体肌。会阴浅横肌是一成对的小肌肉，起自女性会阴体附着于前庭球的筋膜和海绵体脚的腱膜。其作用是稳定会阴体（框 2-1），它们的神经供应来自会阴神经深支（神经根 S_2、S_3 和 S_4）。球海绵体肌是一成对的小肌肉，起源于会阴体，向前延伸覆盖前庭球，止于阴蒂脚表面的腱膜。它们的神经供应来自阴部神经的会阴支（神经根 S_2、S_3 和 S_4），其作用是帮助阴蒂勃起、性高潮时收缩和闭合阴道。坐骨海绵体肌是一对起源于坐骨和耻骨下支下方的小肌肉，它向下向前延伸，覆盖阴蒂脚，最终插入附着在阴蒂下表面的腱膜和前庭球上。其神经支配来自阴部神经的会阴支（神经根 S_2、S_3 和 S_4），功能是帮助阴蒂勃起，并在性高潮时稳定阴道。

会阴浅隙也包含阴蒂的两个海绵体（其包含勃起组织）。海绵体脚起源于该区域并与耻骨弓相连。它的远端游离端向前及内侧走行，融合形成阴蒂体。前庭球含有额外的勃起组织，位于阴道开口周围。它们附着在会阴膜上，并被球海绵体肌覆盖。前庭球位于尿道开口处前面的中线上，在前方汇合形成阴蒂头。阴蒂的脚部由坐骨海绵体肌覆盖。前庭大腺位于前庭球的后方。

3. 女性外生殖器特征（图 2-4）

从前到后，女性会阴包括阴阜、阴蒂和阴蒂包皮、尿道外口、阴道口、阴道后联合（或阴唇系带）、会阴和会阴体，以及后部的肛门。阴道前壁与尿道的关系非常密切。阴道后壁经会阴体与直肠分开。阴道口也被称为阴道前庭，在没有性交或使用过卫生棉条的女性中，阴道口可能被阴道处女膜的薄膜部分堵塞。成对的无毛小阴唇包围着阴蒂，并包围着阴道前庭。成对的大阴唇（内部无毛，外部有毛）从侧面环绕小阴唇，并在前面与阴阜融合。大阴唇内部有一深脂肪垫，它由阴部内动脉后外侧和阴部外动脉前内侧供血。这

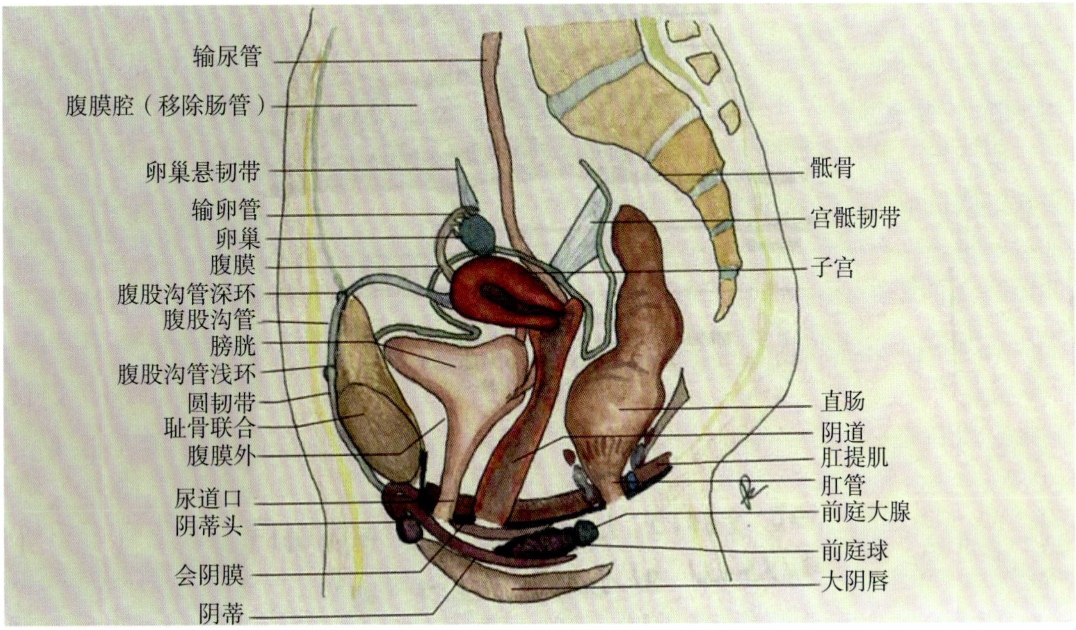

▲ 图 2-5　女性盆腔和下腹部矢状切面

种双血供使唇脂肪垫可作为血管瓣被用于膀胱阴道瘘闭合术中（如改良的唇间隔脂肪垫皮瓣手术），它被放置在闭合的膀胱和阴道之间进行供血。

4. 坐骨肛门窝（图 2-4）

坐骨肛门窝是位于肛门三角区皮肤与盆腔隔膜之间的一个大的筋膜排列空间，其中充满脂肪和松散的结缔组织。坐骨肛门窝位于肛管和尾骨尖之间的肛尾韧带上方，其外侧与坐骨和闭孔肌相连，内侧与肛管相连，后方与骶结节韧带和臀大肌相连，前方与尿生殖膈底（会阴深隙的纤维肌结构）相连。

（六）女性骨盆器官

1. 生殖器官

(1) 子宫和宫颈：子宫是一个壁厚呈梨形的器官，主要由平滑肌构成，其位于膀胱后方直肠前方的骨盆中。子宫有由 3 部分组成：子宫底、子宫体和子宫颈。子宫底位于子宫体的上方，子宫体形成该器官的上 2/3。输卵管与子宫底的上外侧相连，与子宫腔相通。覆盖子宫的腹膜形成外侧的阔韧带。输卵管系膜覆盖输卵管并使其呈悬空状态。子宫最低的 1/3 是子宫颈，是子宫最窄的部分。子宫颈内口与子宫腔相连，宫颈外口通往阴道上部。子宫颈的阴道部分在阴道穹窿内。宫颈管由柱状上皮构成，在阴道中由柱状上皮转化为复层鳞状上皮。宫颈管和邻近的过渡区是宫颈涂片筛检癌前病变和恶性病变的地方。

覆盖子宫底、子宫后部和直肠前部的腹膜形成一个被称为道格拉斯窝的区域（rectouterine pouch）。腹腔内的任何炎症，如阑尾炎、卵巢囊肿破裂或输卵管卵巢脓肿，都会导致液体聚集在道格拉斯窝内。腹膜覆盖在子宫体的前部和膀胱上部的部分形成膀胱子宫陷凹。子宫动脉在离子宫颈很近的地方从输尿管上方穿过圆韧带。由于这种密切的解剖关系，在子宫切除术时存在远端输尿管损伤的危险。耻骨宫颈韧带、主韧带和宫骶韧带支撑宫颈和子宫的位置。

(2) 输卵管：输卵管长约 10cm，分为 3 部分。外侧的漏斗部为卷曲在两侧卵巢顶部的毛状部分，中间是扩张的壶腹部，内侧狭窄的峡部连接输卵管与子宫和宫腔。输卵管允许卵子从卵巢进入子宫进行繁殖。受精通常发生在输卵管内，而着床通常发生在子宫内。如果着床发生在输卵管内，随之而来的异位妊娠可能会导致输卵管破裂伴出血并危及生命。

(3) 卵巢：双侧卵巢分别位于两侧骨盆外侧的卵巢窝内，闭孔神经、髂内、髂外血管与卵巢距离较近，行卵巢切除术时应注意不要损伤这些结构。卵巢通过卵巢系膜与阔韧带相连，通过与圆韧带相连的卵巢悬韧带与子宫相连。圆韧带起源于子宫侧面的宫旁组织，向外通过腹股沟管内环离开骨盆到达大阴唇和阴阜的皮下组织。

2. 下尿路器官

(1) 膀胱：膀胱是一个空心的梨形器官，主要由平滑肌组成。膀胱在低压状态下储存尿液而不发生泄漏，并可以自主排空。膀胱上部有一个圆顶、两个侧壁、一个前壁和一个基底。脐尿管是胎儿尿囊的残存结构，起源于膀胱前壁的顶端，并在脐正中韧带内走行到达脐部。膀胱基部通过盆腔筋膜与宫颈上段和阴道紧密相连。对于曾经做过盆腔手术或放射治疗的患者来说，这是一个很常见的瘘管形成部位。受影响的患者可能出现持续性尿失禁，表现为尿液不断从膀胱流到阴道。

膀胱壁由四层组成：外膜的脂肪层、逼尿肌、固有层（结缔组织）、内尿路上皮（移行尿路上皮细胞）。三角区是膀胱后壁上靠近膀胱颈的一个三角形扁平区域。其上外侧缘由输尿管口界定，输尿管口之间有输尿管间脊。输尿管通过斜行的壁内隧道进入膀胱，它可以防止尿液通过输尿管回流到肾脏。如果该抗反流通道缺乏，将发生膀胱输尿管反流（VUR），导致输尿管、肾盂和肾盏不同程度的扩张（积水）。如果膀胱输尿管反流伴随尿路感染或膀胱高压，将导致肾盂肾炎和（或）肾功能丧失。膀胱颈平滑肌与尿道平滑肌相连，在生理上作为一个自主括约肌起作用。这种自主括约肌有助于在膀胱充盈时保持上尿道和膀胱颈的闭合。膀胱和膀胱颈由盆内筋膜向后支撑。Retzius 耻骨后间隙以前腹横筋膜和后腹膜为界。脐尿管在脐正中韧带内穿过此区域。脐尿管是胎儿尿囊的残存结构，胎儿尿囊为胎儿在子宫时通过脐带将尿液从膀胱排出的组织。脐尿管畸形形成的囊肿极少发展为恶性肿瘤，主要表现为脐带分泌物。脐尿管可用于辅助分离膀胱，通常在膀胱切除术中被识别、移动、结扎和分割。

腹膜覆盖直肠的前外侧和膀胱的后壁、穹窿和前壁的上部。随着膀胱的膨胀和增大，覆盖膀胱上部的腹膜和腹膜内内容物（如肠管）被不断增大的膀胱穹窿顶挤压。对于一个没有做过腹部手术或没有腹膜破裂的患者，这是一个可以直接进入膀胱的腹膜腔自由空间。经耻骨联合的上缘触诊显露的膀胱可达两指宽，可直接进行膀胱抽吸或对无法行尿道导尿的急性尿潴留患者行经皮耻骨上导管置入膀胱引流，再或者对特定尿失禁的患者进行治疗。

(2) 尿道（图 2–2、图 2–4、图 2–6 和图 2–7）：女性尿道的长度约为 3.5cm。尿道是一个中空的管状结构，最内层的尿路上皮内有丰富的黏膜下血管丛，被平滑横纹肌纤维所包围。尿道平滑肌由内纵层和外环层组成，可通过无意识的自主收缩辅助尿道闭合。尿道外括约肌在尿道中点环绕尿道，由两种类型的肌纤维组成，一种为慢缩肌纤维，其持续活跃并且不易疲劳，以便在长时间内保持尿道的张力和收缩，另一种为快缩肌纤维，其位于括约肌复合体的近端部分受自主肌（横纹肌）控制。尿道外括约肌产生尿道壁张力和加压，有助于维持排尿自制。横纹肌最宽的区域在尿道中间的 1/3 处，大部分横纹肌位于尿道前部，呈马蹄形或 Ω 形。括约肌纤维的远端插入耻骨弓下的阴道壁，并与会阴膜融合。女性的尿节制依赖于括约肌的质量。尿道后方有大量结缔组织和呈马蹄形的条纹括约肌。尿道内的节制是通过尿道腔（主动和被动）的接合、来自尿道壁的外部压力、控制来自腹部压力变化的能力、神经血管刺激以及筋膜和韧带的支持来实现的。条纹状尿道外括约肌贡献了 1/3 的尿道静息张力[9]。耻骨尿道韧带从尿道近端延伸至耻骨，止于耻骨联合用于辅助支撑尿道。由于韧带损伤、结缔组织无力或尿道外括约肌缺损而导致的尿道（和膀胱颈）过度活动，可导致压力性尿失禁（咳嗽、打喷嚏或用力时漏尿）。尿道同时有骨盆内筋膜和骨盆底肌肉的额外

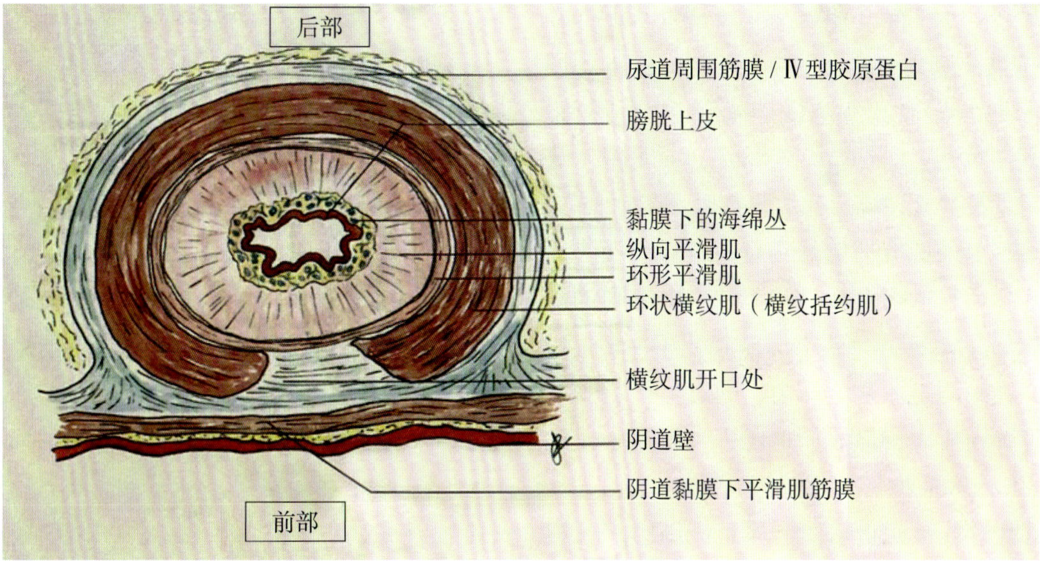

▲ 图 2-6　女性尿道横截面

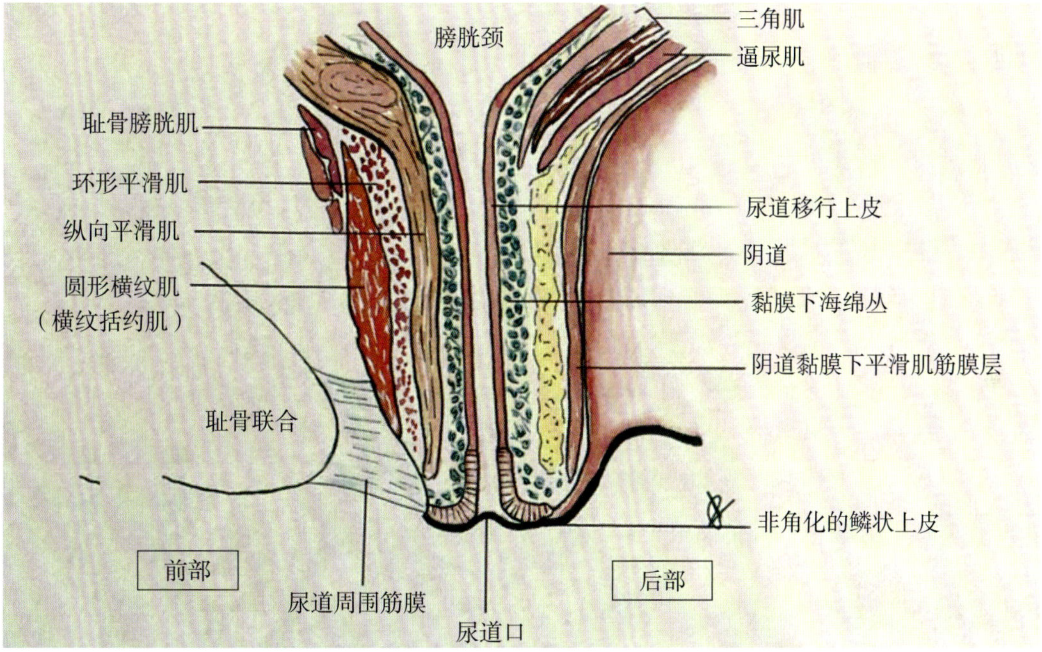

▲ 图 2-7　女性尿道冠状面

支撑。在对尿道支撑的贡献方面，Rud 报道称横纹肌贡献了 33%，血管贡献了 28%，其余 39% 的支撑来自肌肉和结缔组织[10]。一旦年龄超过25岁，横纹肌细胞会逐年减少，它导致进行性的括约肌功能障碍，每 10 年最大尿道闭合压力（MUCP）将下降约 15%[11]。在低龄人群中，阴道分娩、括约肌功能障碍和尿道支撑问题对压力性尿失禁的影响更大。血管丛的作用目前仍不清楚，然而其作用是突出的，可能有助于封闭尿道。尿道的支撑似乎不像先前所认为的与尿失禁有关[1]。有多个主要位于尿道远端和中段 1/3 处的黏膜下腺与尿道憩室重合。在透视检查中，与看起来保持在一个更固定的位置的远端尿道相比，近端尿道和膀胱颈被视为可活动的[12]。

尿道闭合压力是膀胱内压力与尿道内压力的差值。当尿道内压高于膀胱内压时，尿液留存于膀胱中。自 1967 年 Toews、Brown 和 Wickham（1969）描述了利用带侧孔的导尿管沿尿道的不同长度测量压力起，就开始有关于尿道压力的测量。导管位置传感器（Harrison 和 Constable 发明）于 1970 年问世，其允许连续读数并叠加。在此之前，在 1948 年，压力是用垂直压力计（Bors 发明）测量的，然后是气球技术其只能测量一个有限的长度。1972 年，Malvern 和 Edwards 描述了一种机械型截断装置来测量尿道内压力。通过这个装置可以记录膀胱内压力、最大尿道压力（尿道中段）、尿道长度、最大括约肌压力[13]。

尿道既有连接阴道前壁和尿道周围组织至腱弓的筋膜支撑，也有连接尿道周组织至肛提肌内侧缘的肌肉支撑[9]。这种支撑能维持膀胱颈的水平，同时允许其在排尿期的动态运动。当腹部压力增加时（如咳嗽），尿道的支持组织可以让尿道被压在阴道前壁上，以促进尿道与阴道的贴合和控尿。肌肉和（或）韧带哪里出现薄弱，哪里就可能会出现压力性尿失禁。

治疗压力性尿失禁手术的目的是通过悬吊阴道外侧组织至耻骨上支的髂耻韧带（Burch 阴道悬吊）来抬高膀胱颈，或者在尿道中段下放置天然组织或合成吊带，使其穿过耻骨后或闭孔形成尿道后支撑，为尿道和（或）膀胱颈提供支持。

(3) 输尿管（图 2–3 和图 2–5）：了解输尿管的结构非常重要，从而避免其在盆腔手术中无意损伤。输尿管为中空管状结构，长约 25cm。它们起源于漏斗状肾盂，并沿位于腰椎横突线上的腰大肌走行，向下延伸至膀胱。在走行过程中，输尿管穿过生殖股神经，当其穿过靠近子宫颈外侧边界的圆韧带时，远端的子宫动脉从其上穿行（桥下流水是一个很好的解剖学标志），同时在左侧骨盆其在乙状结肠动脉旁穿过。在髂总动脉分叉处经骨盆入口进入骨盆，沿骨盆侧壁走行经壁内隧道进入膀胱内，以输尿管口为出口。输尿管通过蠕动（或丸状）肌肉运动将尿液顺行移至膀胱。输尿管最窄的地方分别是盆腔 – 输尿管交界处（PUJ）、盆腔边缘、膀胱 – 输尿管交界处（VUJ）。这些地方也是输尿管结石梗阻最常见的部位。

3. 其他盆腔脏器

直肠和肛门（图 2–1、图 2–2、图 2–4 和图 2–5）：直肠是大肠的倒数第二部分，位于骶骨前方，其远端有一个可扩张的部分，叫作壶腹，允许暂时储存肠内容物（粪便），直到有合适时机排便。直肠从 S_3 椎体平面开始，与上面的乙状结肠和下面的肛管相连。直肠有两个曲折，分别是耻骨直肠肌形成的骶骨曲和肛门直肠曲，这有助于控制粪便的储存。直肠的血供来自直肠上动脉、中动脉和下动脉（分别是肠系膜下动脉、髂内动脉和阴部内动脉的分支）。直肠的静脉引流是通过与动脉相对应的静脉提供。上 1/3 的直肠在其前部和外侧被腹膜覆盖，中部直肠仅有前部被腹膜覆盖，而下 1/3 直肠在腹膜水平以下，不被任何腹膜覆盖。腹膜在直肠和子宫之间形成直肠凹陷（道格拉斯窝）。

直肠壶腹在盆腔底部肌肉内于耻骨直肠肌水平处（肛肠交界处）形成肛管。肛管长约 4cm，位于会阴部的肛门三角内。休息时，它是空的，由肛门内括约肌控制排便和排气。肛门内括约肌由不随意的环形平滑肌组成，肛门外括约肌则由横纹肌组成。肛门括约肌的肌肉或神经损伤可导致大便失禁。损伤可能是由于盆腔放疗、神经系统疾病（如糖尿病、多发性硬化症或脊髓损伤等），以及阴道分娩引起。肛门黏膜形成纵向折叠，称为肛柱，并向远端合并在梳状线形成一圈围绕肛管的肛门瓣。梳状线位于肛门尾骨膜的水平。其以上的动脉供应来自直肠上动脉（与中间吻合），以下来自直肠下动脉（与中间吻合）。在梳状线以下，肛管由非角化的鳞状上皮（肛梳）构成，其远端止于齿状线（白线），并在肛门外口过渡到真正的皮肤。

（七）盆底的血液供应（图 2–8）

1. 动脉

髂总动脉起源于 T_{10} 水平的腹主动脉分支。每条髂总动脉长约 3cm，几乎在骶髂关节处分叉（在

L_5/S_1 水平处）立刻分为髂内动脉和髂外动脉。女性骨盆和会阴均由髂内动脉供应。盆腔静脉系统完全流入髂内静脉（图 2-8）。

2. 髂内动脉

髂内动脉分为前支和后支，后支进一步分支成 3 条动脉：髂腰动脉、骶外侧动脉和臀上动脉。髂腰动脉是后支的第一支，向上走行到骶髂关节，负责髂肌、腰大肌、腰方肌和马尾的血供（马尾包括腰骶神经根，以及脊髓后部终止于 L_1/L_2 的尾神经）。骶外侧动脉是后支的第二支，走行于梨状肌的表面，负责梨状肌和椎管血供。臀上动脉是后支的第三支，向后延伸通过坐骨大孔出骨盆，在梨状肌上方负责臀肌区域肌肉的血供。

髂内动脉的前支按起源顺序排列有以下 7 个分支。

- 闭塞性脐动脉，其近端可能发自膀胱上动脉，远端闭塞，位于脐内侧韧带内，并不总是呈闭塞状态。
- 膀胱上动脉为膀胱上缘供血。
- 阴道动脉，相当于男性的膀胱下动脉，为阴道、膀胱的下半部分和直肠供血。

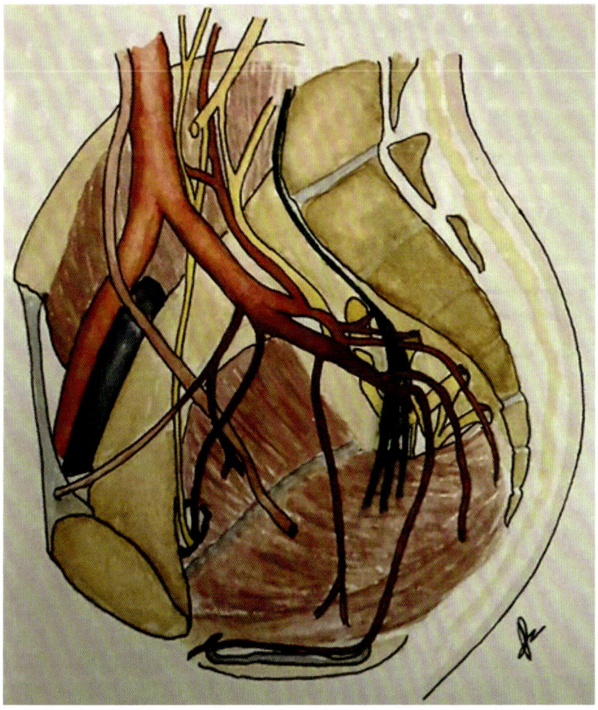

▲ 图 2-8　女性右侧骨盆切除盆腔器官后矢状面观，显示骨盆神经血管走行

- 闭孔动脉在盆腔侧壁向前向下延伸，为髂骨和股骨头供血。
- 直肠中动脉与直肠血管广泛吻合，为直肠、直肠上动脉和直肠下动脉供血。
- 阴部内动脉从坐骨大孔穿过骨盆，绕过骶棘韧带通过坐骨小孔进入会阴，并支配会阴的所有结构的血供。
- 子宫动脉在肛提肌表面走行，在阔韧带远端跨越输尿管，为子宫供血，也为阴道和卵巢供血。

3. 骨盆和会阴特定结构和器官的动脉血液供应

(1) 卵巢：卵巢（性腺）动脉起源于腹主动脉 L_1 水平，位于肾动脉下方，在骨盆边缘跨过髂外血管进入卵巢悬韧带，在阔韧带处延伸并在子宫外壁内侧与子宫动脉吻合，为子宫和输卵管提供分支血供。

(2) 阴道：阴道的上部由子宫动脉供血，而阴道的其余部分的血供由直肠中动脉和阴部动脉提供。

(3) 尿道：尿道由阴部内动脉供血。

(4) 直肠和肛门：直肠血供来自直肠上动脉（肠系膜下动脉的延续）、直肠中动脉（髂动脉的直肠前分支）和直肠下动脉（阴部内动脉的分支）。肛管接收直肠下血管的供应，直肠下血管由此演变为浅表血管供应肛门外括约肌和肛周皮肤。

（八）静脉

髂内静脉收集从盆腔器官、盆腔壁、会阴部、外生殖器，以及下肢和臀部回流的静脉血。髂内静脉于骨盆的坐骨大切迹水平处形成，经骨盆边缘出骨盆，并与每侧的髂外静脉（引流下肢静脉）汇合，成为髂总静脉，再与之相连形成下腔静脉。髂内静脉位于腰大肌上髂内动脉的后方。除髂腰动脉和脐动脉外，骨盆静脉与髂内动脉的其他分支是成对存在的。

直肠和子宫周围存在静脉丛，与骶外侧静

脉一起流入髂内静脉。静脉丛相互连接，环绕盆腔器官。直肠静脉丛是一个门体静脉系统的交流区。其他交流区分别位于是食管远端和脐部。在慢性肝功能障碍等引起的门静脉高压中，门静脉高压会导致吻合处侧支血管的受压。继而导致静脉扩张，临床上可出现食管或直肠静脉曲张出血。水母头现象就是脐周围皮肤下扩张的静脉丛。

阴蒂通过一条深部的背部静脉引流，这条静脉在耻骨弓状韧带和会阴膜之间进入骨盆，并与膀胱静脉丛相连。阴蒂皮肤的静脉引流则是经阴部外静脉进入大隐静脉。

卵巢静脉起源于阔韧带内的蔓状神经丛。两侧各有 2 条卵巢静脉，最终合并成 1 条静脉并顺着腹膜后的卵巢动脉走行。左侧卵巢（性腺）静脉首先引流进入左肾静脉然后流入下腔静脉。右侧卵巢静脉直接流入下腔静脉。肾脏肿瘤可能延伸至肾静脉，尤其是左侧，并进入下腔静脉，导致在横断面成像中看到卵巢静脉曲张，这一情况取决于扩散程度和（或）唇静脉的曲张程度。

（九）骨盆神经丛 & 骨盆和会阴的神经支配

1. 骶神经丛，尾椎神经丛和躯体神经

骶神经丛由来自 L_4、L_5 和 S_1、S_2、S_3、S_4 前支的运动神经和感觉神经组成。骶神经丛位于梨状肌表面被筋膜覆盖。骶交感神经干有 4 个神经节（起源于脊髓 T_{10}～L_2 段），在尾骨前缘形成不等数量神经节。神经的功能是协调控制排尿、排便和性高潮。骶神经丛的分支包括坐骨神经、下肢的臀神经和阴部神经。其他分支包括盆底，臀肌的运动神经，大腿部的皮肤感觉神经。躯体神经是周围神经系统的一部分，并控制骨骼随意肌的运动。盆腔内脏神经携带来自交感神经系统和副交感神经系统的纤维。盆腔内脏神经对其他所有内脏神经来说是独特的，只有盆腔内脏神经携带交感纤维。

尾神经丛主要由 S_5、尾神经和部分 S_4 组成，为尾骨区的皮神经提供支持。

2. 下尿路神经支配：内脏神经丛

下尿路由躯体神经、副交感神经和交感神经支配。其功能由高级和局部脊髓中枢协调，控制排尿和存尿的调节，以及适时的排尿。

胸腰段脊髓（T_{10}～L_2）产生交感神经，其在 L_3～S_1 椎前侧形成上下腹丛。交感神经兴奋可引起尿道和膀胱底部平滑肌收缩，抑制副交感神经对逼尿肌收缩的作用，从而利于尿液的储存。这使得膀胱可以在低压力下储存尿液。交感神经纤维也控制生殖道的平滑肌收缩（尤其是射精），男性的尿道内括约肌，以及男性和女性的肛门内括约肌。上腹下神经丛在 S_1 处分叉，形成左右下腹部神经。2 条下腹部神经进入骨盆并向外侧移动形成椎前神经丛，承载交感神经、副交感神经和传入神经纤维。

下腹部神经与携带副交感神经（$S_{2\sim4}$）的盆腔内脏神经连接，在直肠两侧的腹膜后间隙形成双侧的下腹下神经丛。然后进一步形成 3 个神经丛：直肠神经丛、子宫阴道神经丛和膀胱神经丛。阴蒂的勃起组织是由下腹丛的末端分支控制，它进入并穿过会阴深隙。

骶脊髓（$S_{2\sim4}$ 节段）产生副交感神经，副交感神经在盆腔神经中走行，当其受到刺激时，会引起逼尿肌收缩以促进排尿。这一协调中心被称为脊髓排尿中心。膀胱功能的主要控制中心是脑干的脑桥排尿中心。副交感神经同时还可以刺激勃起和调节肠神经系统。

直肠的交感神经由腹下神经支配，副交感神经由盆腔内脏神经支配。来自骶髓（Onuf 的核）的体神经进入阴部神经（S_2、S_3 和 S_4），其支配尿道横纹括约肌，在受到刺激时可引起括约肌收缩。

肛提肌由骶神经直接纤维支配，该神经纤维来自 S_4 和阴部神经的分支。尾骨肌由 S_4 和 S_5 支配。梨状肌的神经支配来源于 S_1 和 S_2 神经根的腹侧支。

3. 其他重要的神经

(1) 阴部神经（图 2-4 和图 2-9）：坐骨肛门窝的外侧壁包含来自于 S_2、S_3 和 S_4 神经根的阴部神经。阴部神经从骨盆出发经坐骨大孔进入臀区。

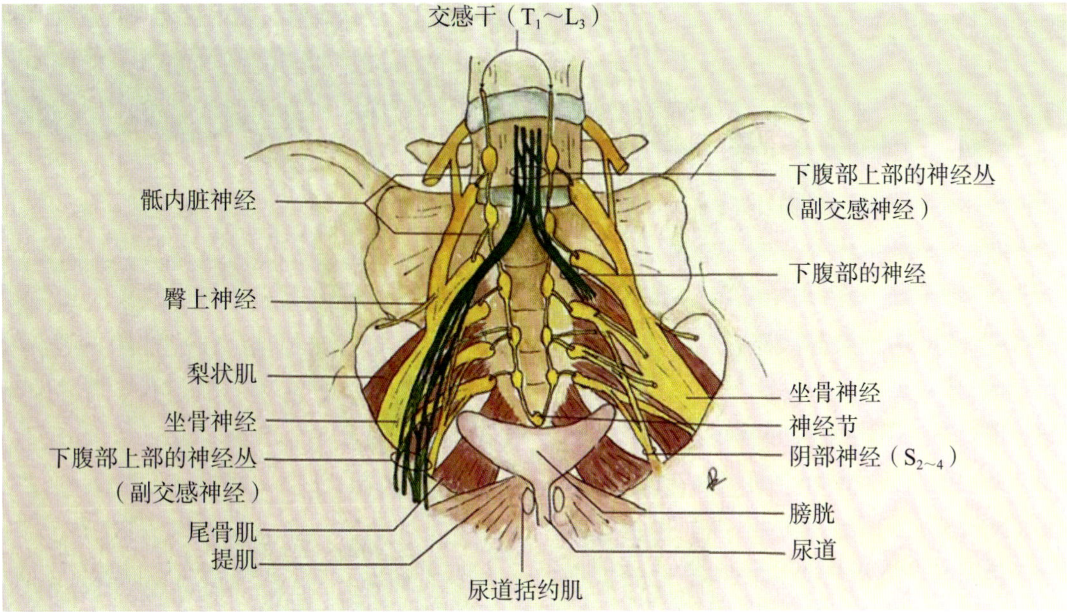

▲ 图 2-9　骶骨前盆神经，冠状面观

然后在坐骨棘处的骶棘韧带周围弯曲通过坐骨小孔进入会阴。一旦进入会阴，阴部神经就进入会阴管（Alcock 管），其为闭孔内筋膜的凝聚形成，并在阴道管内沿的坐骨直肠窝的外侧向前移动。出阴部管时，阴部神经的分支成为直肠下神经，它支配肛周皮肤和肛门外括约肌。在会阴膜的后缘，阴部神经分裂形成会阴神经，为外阴提供感觉神经，为肛提肌和会阴浅横肌提供运动神经（主要来自 S_3 和 S_4 神经纤维），还有一个分支即阴蒂背神经，支配阴蒂。

(2) 闭孔神经：闭孔神经（来自 $L_{2\sim4}$ 神经根）是腰丛的一个分支，自腰肌发出，沿盆腔侧壁由闭孔上外侧边界进入闭孔管，控制大腿内侧的内收肌。

(3) 感觉神经：从阴阜和阴唇的感觉纤维通过生殖股神经和髂腹股沟神经返回 L_1。会阴部的感觉神经通过坐骨小神经经股后皮神经到达 S_1、S_2 和 S_3。感觉传入神经对于检测膀胱壁内的疼痛、温度和拉伸感很重要。

（十）女性骨盆淋巴

了解所有骨盆的淋巴引流部位是很重要的，特别是与感染和恶性肿瘤有关的器官的淋巴引流。盆腔脏器的淋巴引流主要是向髂内外淋巴结引流，同时也有其他淋巴系统参与。髂淋巴经髂总淋巴结、腹主动脉旁淋巴结或腰椎淋巴结引流至胸导管。胸导管位于 T_{12} 节段处，向上延伸到颈部，并在左锁骨下静脉和左颈内静脉连接处流入静脉系统。左边的胸导管引流身体大部分的淋巴，除了引流到淋巴管的右侧胸部、右手臂、头部和颈部的淋巴。右侧淋巴管在右侧锁骨下静脉与右侧颈内静脉交界处汇入静脉系统。淋巴结病或淋巴结切除术可导致远端淋巴水肿，其最常见于四肢。

1. 尿道

膀胱淋巴引流到髂内和髂外淋巴结。根治性膀胱（尿路上皮）癌的淋巴结切除术中需要切除这些淋巴结和血管，切除这些淋巴结后将引起开放的淋巴管泄漏，可导致淋巴囊肿的形成。

尿道淋巴引流到髂内淋巴结和腹股沟浅淋巴结。原发性尿道癌是非常罕见的，但是对于有排尿阻塞症状和尿道“木质”感的女性患者，紧急活检是必要的。根治性手术应包括腹股沟淋巴结切除和髂淋巴结切除。

2. 生殖器官

子宫和输卵管的淋巴引流进入髂内、外淋巴结和骶淋巴结。阴道的下 1/3 及外阴和尿道的淋巴引流到腹股沟浅淋巴结，而上 2/3 流入髂外淋巴结和髂内淋巴结。

卵巢淋巴引流进入腹主动脉旁的区域淋巴结，其是卵巢的胚胎学起源。这意味着卵巢肿瘤的淋巴结转移在临床上很难被发现，除非巨大且明显才能在腹部发现。

在阴唇内侧的阴户和会阴的淋巴系统折叠向上引流到阴阜，腹股沟浅淋巴结和股淋巴结。

3. 直肠和肛门

直肠的淋巴引流跟随血管回到环绕肠系膜下血管起源的主动脉前淋巴结。下肛管的淋巴引流随阴道和尿道引流至腹股沟浅淋巴结。其余直肠的淋巴引流至肠系膜下淋巴结、髂内淋巴结（直肠中动脉）、直肠旁淋巴结和主动脉前淋巴结。

二、总结

本章的目的是讨论正常女性骨盆的解剖和生理学，以及导致尿失禁和（或）脱垂的可能因素。这将为了解这些疾病的诊断打下良好的基础，有助于指导临床检查和调查，并找到突出的手术标志。本章的学习有助于理解本书的其余部分。

三、关键信息

盆腔器官由肌肉和韧带支撑。任何薄弱都可能导致盆腔器官脱垂或压力性尿失禁。妊娠和顺产对盆腔解剖有显著影响。病史可以发现尿失禁的可能原因，其中包括症状、持续时间、既往手术和（或）治疗，如伴随彻底检查的放疗。对于持续尿失禁的患者，应考虑溢尿、先天性异位输尿管和泌尿道瘘管。

肛提肌由 3 块肌肉组成，骨盆器官的主要血供来自髂内动脉。

致谢：感谢 Suzanne Biers 女士的贡献。

延伸阅读

[1] Gray's anatomy for students
[2] Gynaecology by 10 teachers
[3] Oxford handbook of clinical urology
[4] Oxford textbook of urological surgery
[5] Whats's new in the functional anatomy of pelvic organ prolapse? John O. L. Delancey. Curr Opin Obstet Gynecol. 2016;28(5):420–9

参考文献

[1] Delancey JO. Why do women have stress urinary incontinence? Neurourol Urodyn. 2010;29(Suppl 1):S13–7.
[2] Enhorning G. Simultaneous recording of intravesical and intra-urethral pressure. A study on urethral closure in normal and stress incontinent women. Acta Chir Scand Suppl. 1961;Suppl 276:1–68.
[3] Petros P. The integral system. Cent Eur J Urol. 2011;64(3):110–9.
[4] DeLancey JO, Trowbridge ER, Miller JM, Morgan DM, Guire K, Fenner DE, et al. Stress urinary incontinence: relative importance of urethral support and urethral closure pressure. J Urol. 2008;179(6):2286–90; discussion 90
[5] Blaivas JG, Olsson CA. Stress incontinence: classification and surgical approach. J Urol. 1988;139(4):727–31.
[6] Abrams P, Cardozo L, Fall M, Griffiths D, Rosier P, Ulmsten U, et al. The standardisation of terminology in lower urinary tract function: report from the standardisation sub-committee of the International Continence Society. Urology. 2003;61(1):37–49.
[7] Bonney V. On diurnal incontinence of urine in women. J Obstet Gynaecol Br Emp. 1923;30:358–65.
[8] Berger MB, Doumouchtsis SK, DeLancey JO. Bony pelvis dimensions in women with and without stress urinary incontinence. Neurourol Urodyn. 2013;32(1):37–42.
[9] Wei JT, De Lancey JO. Functional anatomy of the pelvic floor and lower urinary tract. Clin Obstet Gynecol. 2004;47(1):3–17.
[10] Rud T, Andersson KE, Asmussen M, Hunting A, Ulmsten U. Factors maintaining the intraurethral pressure in women. Investig Urol. 1980;17(4):343–7.
[11] Rud T. Urethral pressure profile in continent women from childhood to old age. Acta Obstet Gynecol Scand. 1980;59(4):331–5.
[12] Muellner SR. The physiology of micturition. J Urol. 1951;65(5):805–13.
[13] Edwards L, Malvern J. The urethral pressure profile: theoretical considerations and clinical application. Br J Urol. 1974;46(3):325–35.

第 3 章　女性尿失禁的诊断
Diagnosis of Urinary Incontinence in Women

Elizabeth Dray　Haritha Pavuluri　著

尿失禁是女性中广泛流行的疾病，可对患者的生活质量产生负面影响，并造成显著的社会和个人经济负担[8]。一名有症状的女性平均每年将花费 750 美元用于处置尿失禁[20]。通过治疗患者的尿失禁可以大幅度减轻这一负担[21]。为了进行有效治疗，临床医生必须首先进行准确诊断。本章我们将回顾女性尿失禁的鉴别诊断，什么样的病史和体格检查结果可以帮助区分这些病因，以及可以加强这些数据的无创伤性检测。最后，我将确定何时进一步采取有创的或资源密集型的研究，以表述尿失禁。

一、鉴别诊断

确定尿失禁原因的第一步建立在确定感知的潮湿实际上是尿液。非尿液因素造成的潮湿包括生理性或病理性的阴道分泌物，以及肛周液或渗出液。正常阴道分泌物的数量和质量在女性之间可能有很大差异。阴道分泌物增加可由感染或恶性肿瘤引起，如需区分来源，可进行阴道清洁度检测、性病检测和阴道镜检查。有些人可能会对正常的分泌物感到痛苦，一旦排除了感染性或其他病理病因，就可以通过健康教育解除担忧。在既往有盆腔手术、放疗或恶性肿瘤的情况下，可形成腹膜阴道瘘，导致腹腔液体从阴道持续流出。极少数情况下，患者也可能在输卵管和阴道之间产生瘘管。也应提高警惕腹水或使用腹膜透析是非尿液性持续渗漏液体的原因。

在终身尿失禁特别是长期持续的尿失禁发病因素中，控尿机制之外的异位输尿管和其他先天解剖结构的异常应该被考虑在内。

在患者的病情检查中，应始终考虑一过性尿失禁的原因。一过性尿失禁的原因可以通过助记器（谵妄、感染、萎缩性阴道炎、心理性、药物性、尿量过多、活动受限、粪便阻塞）来记录[14]。将与尿失禁发作时其他健康事件或新药物特异性相关的病史是做出此类诊断不可或缺的一部分。通常，这些疾病不需要泌尿科干预，而是进行推断、推理和专业的交流（如转诊到内分泌科、便秘等）。功能性尿失禁虽然不总是短暂性的，但却是泌尿科医生很容易过度治疗患者的首要情况。功能性尿失禁是指个体具有正常排尿功能，但当进入洗手间时控尿能力下降，可能会出现的尿失禁。此外，典型潜在合并症的第二种表现，如痴呆或帕金森病。针对这类患者的“治疗”可能很简单，如为患者提供床边马桶或让他们进行物理治疗以改善活动能力。

尿失禁应分为急迫性尿失禁（UUI）、压力性尿失禁（SUI）和混合性尿失禁（MUI）。充盈性尿失禁是指膀胱过度充盈时存在尿失禁[3]。持续性尿漏、性交后尿失禁和排尿后滴漏本身并不是尿失禁的表现形式，而是尿急或急迫性尿失禁、尿潴留或解剖异常（如泌尿瘘管或尿道痉挛 / 狭窄）的表现。所有形式的尿失禁都需要病史采集之外的评估，并且在许多专家看来，在患者接受侵入性治疗前应直接观察渗漏的情况。

二、病史和体格检查

当评估一名女性尿失禁患者时，采集完整的病史至关重要。既往病史应包括手术史（特别是既往盆腔、产科或背部手术史）、病史（神经系统疾病、内分泌功能障碍、结缔组织疾病、放疗、外伤），以及妇产科病史（包括产次、绝经前或绝经后状态）。此外，目前使用的药物，以及先前有关尿失禁的药物治疗，都应采集。外源性激素、拟交感神经药、交感神经药、抗胆碱药和利尿药都可能导致尿失禁的症状。在采集尿失禁现病史时，可以通过询问患者是否伴随咳嗽 / 打喷嚏的动作、紧迫性，或者两者兼有来主观地描述尿失禁。如果答案是两者兼而有之，应该问患者哪个对他们更麻烦。应尝试评估患者渗漏的严重程度和频率，这可以通过患者每天使用的卫生巾或内裤的数量，以及由于尿失禁而换衣服的次数来确定。此外，询问内裤或卫生巾的尿液饱和度很重要，因为一些患者可能会因受到相对少量的尿液溢出而困扰，即使没有饱和，也会频繁地更换卫生巾或内裤。应评估白天和夜间的排尿频率，以及是否伴随排尿困难、盆腔疼痛、尿路感染和血尿。应评估患者的下尿路梗阻症状（用力、主观不完全排空、尿流不畅）、胃肠道症状（即粪便失禁或便秘）和脱垂主诉，因为盆底疾病经常共存[9]。应询问患者神经系统症状，特别是年轻女性如果出现新发急迫性尿失禁，因为尿失禁可能是神经系统疾病（如多发性硬化症）的预兆。最后，评估尿失禁对患者生活质量的影响非常重要。在绝大多数情况下，尿失禁不会危及生命，只有在对患者造成困扰时，才应进行干预。

患者尿失禁的特征也可以使用各种经过验证的问卷进行评估。常用的指标包括泌尿生殖系统疾病清单简表（UDI-6）、尿失禁影响问卷简表（IIQ-7）、尿失禁国际咨询问卷简表（ICIQ-SF）、KING 氏健康问卷（KHQ）、全球患者严重程度量表（PGI-S）和密歇根州尿失禁症状指数（M-ISI）。这些问卷评估压力性尿失禁、急迫性尿失禁、严重程度和生活质量，似乎大多数相关性很强[10]。除了尿失禁的症状外，还可以使用盆底损伤列表（PFDI）评估脱垂和结肠直肠症状。

单凭病史在评估尿失禁方面并不完全可靠，要进行一定的体格检查，如评估年龄、体重和身体虚弱程度，这些与尿失禁相关的因素都要被评估，因为这些可能作为患者是否能进行手术的依据[24]。腹部检查可以提供重要的信息，如是否存在切口、耻骨上肿胀或十分柔软。每例接受尿失禁初步评估的患者都应进行盆腔检查，其中包括评估外生殖器（包括雌激素状态）、尿道、子宫和附件，以及是否存在盆腔器官脱垂（POP）。此外，仰卧式咳嗽压力试验（CST）是诊断女性压力性尿失禁的金标准。这是在患者以截石位且膀胱充盈到舒适程度的情况下进行的，如果伴随咳嗽或 Valsalva 动作出现尿失禁则认为是阳性；如果仰卧位不能确定是否出现尿失禁，则可以站立位重复测试。仰卧式咳嗽压力试验阳性与经尿流动力学检查证明的压力性尿失禁相关性＞90%[6]。还可以在休息时评估尿道位置和活动性，并在用力和咳嗽时评估尿道的过度活动。超过 30° 的移动性通常被认为是异常的。这种可以通过“Q-tip 测试”来辅助（只有在体格检查不确定时才需要），在进行 Valsalva 动作之前将润滑过的 Q-tip 棉签放置在尿道中。虽然存在尿道过度活动可能有助于确定患者是否适合进行特定的手术干预（如尿道悬吊术），但在诊断压力性尿失禁方面似乎没有任何显著的预测价值[5]。应使用分离式窥镜检查对盆腔器官脱垂进行评估，并使用标准化且可重复的分类技术［如 Baden-Walker 或盆腔器官脱垂定量（POP-Q）系统］进行文档记录。如果有已知或疑似神经系统疾病病史，可进行简短的神经系统检查，以评估直肠括约肌张力及是否存在球海绵体反射（表 3-1）。

三、无创检测

可以使用多种无创检查来获取更多信息并排除尿失禁的潜在原因。尿液分析通常是在尿失禁患者中进行的第一项实验室检查。尿液分析异常，

表 3-1 现有症状的历史、过去的病史、体格检查和诊断检测的常见结果

	压力性尿失禁	急迫性尿失禁	充盈性尿失禁	功能性尿失禁	长期 / 解剖性尿失禁	混合性尿失禁
现病史	咳嗽，打喷嚏，活动，大笑时漏尿	如厕前突然急迫感后伴随漏尿，夜尿症，无意识	两者的混合症状（SUI 和 UUI+ 尿道阻塞性症状）	认知或身体上的损害，无法独立生活	持续泄漏	两者的混合症状（SUI 和 UUI）
体格检查 / 诊断试验	• 仰卧咳嗽压力测试阳性 • 尿道高活动性（Q-tip 测试）	• 漏尿量多，漏尿速度快，由于膀胱充盈触发的尿失禁 • 偶尔由咳嗽引起（压力测试）	触诊或 PVR 时发现膀胱充盈	不能活动或独立生活能力下降	• 卫生棉条测试异常 • 尿道溃破 • 经过阴道漏尿 • 盆腔影像显示异位输尿管	• 仰卧位压力测试阳性 • 漏尿量多，漏尿速度快的尿失禁
过去的病史	• 孕产次数多 • 肥胖	• 神经系统疾病 • 反复发作膀胱炎 • 盆腔放疗	• 吊带手术史，神经系统疾病 • 尿道器械使用 • 抗胆碱药物治疗	• 痴呆 • 不能活动 • 精神疾病	• 既往盆腔手术、创伤、辐射或恶性肿瘤 • 慢性留置导尿管 • 童年尿失禁	• 孕产次数多 • 肥胖 • 年龄

SUI. 压力性尿失禁；UUI. 急迫性尿失禁；PVR. 残余尿量

如存在血液、葡萄糖或白细胞酯酶（LE），可提示尿失禁的继发性原因。如果发现不明原因的血尿（高倍镜视野≥3 个红细胞），应进行膀胱镜检查（AUA 血尿指南）。如果尚未诊断出糖尿病，则应立即进行内分泌或内科转诊，以进行糖尿病检查；如果这是已知的共病，则应与社区医院就血糖控制进行沟通。如果发现白细胞酯酶（LE）或亚硝酸盐，应进行尿培养，因为尿路感染可能是患者尿失禁的来源或症状加重的因素。

应获得排尿后残余尿量（PVR），以排除膀胱排空不完全，并用于评估干预措施（如尿路解痉药或吊带手术）是否适当。残余尿量可通过无创超声或无菌插入导尿管导出获得，这两种方式被认为等效[22]。残余尿量升高没有通用的定义。然而，绝大多数女性的 PVR＜100ml[22]。虽然在没有高风险特征的无症状个体中，PVR≥300ml 是可以接受的，但根据定义，尿失禁是一种症状[18]。因此，作者建议在 PVR＞100ml 时，在不可逆的干预之前，需要进行更具创伤性的病情检查。

膀胱排尿日记或排尿频率体积图是显示尿失禁特征和提示患者不适应的行为的有用方法。这些可以保持记录 24～72h。患者报告的尿频、夜尿和尿失禁存在显著的记忆偏差，患者往往高估其症状的严重程度[19]。排尿日记提供了液体过多的客观证据或膀胱刺激性消耗，能够让临床医生向患者提供个体化的干预治疗项目。

对于尿垫称重测试的作用是有争议的，主要用于学术背景的研究。20h 尿垫试验比 1h 尿垫试验更具临床相关性，虽然定义各不相同，但如果在此期间尿丢失量＞1.3g，通常被认为是阳性[2]。然而，应该注意的是，研究表明，在自我报告的“自控”和“失禁”组中，垫重量试验之间的差异很小[15]。尿失禁的严重程度更常用的替代指标是每天的尿垫，用于检查尿失禁严重程度的一个更常用的替代方法是统计每天使用的尿垫数，这可以通过患者病史进行评估。重要的是要表述出尿垫的饱和度，因为即使尿垫相对干燥时，个体每次排尿时都可能更换他们的尿垫。

染料检测是评估渗漏的另一种有用的检测方法，特别是在确定渗漏是否为与尿液相对应得其他液体或确定瘘管部位方面。为了确定尿液是否是潮湿的来源，患者可以服用 200mg 口服吡啶

（Pyridium），并戴上几个小时的尿垫。如果液体是尿液，则是橙色的；汗液、腹膜液或阴道分泌物将保持无色。寻找瘘管时，插入卫生棉条，并在膀胱内滴注染料，如亚甲蓝。卫生棉条近端染色提示膀胱阴道瘘，远端染色可能表明尿道渗漏。如果担心输尿管阴道瘘，则进行双染料试验。在这种情况下，膀胱中充满亚甲蓝溶液，伴随着口服吡啶。卫生棉条的橙色染色是输尿管阴道瘘的特征，蓝色染色可能继发于膀胱阴道瘘或尿道失禁[17]。

影像学检查在评估女性尿失禁中的作用有限。如果临床怀疑尿道憩室或异位输尿管，盆腔 MRI 是一种敏感的、不过成本过高的明确诊断手段。肾脏超声检查对于诊断肾盂积水具有敏感性和特异性，如果存在上尿路恶性病变的高风险特征，应进行肾超声检查。如果担心这是导致患者尿失禁的因素，经阴道或经阴道超声检查可能有助于可见先前用于盆底重建的网片[16]。

四、高级测试

当患者尿失禁的病因不能搞清楚时，可以考虑两种先进的检查方法：膀胱镜检查和尿流动力学检查（UDS）。但对于无并发症的压力性尿失禁或急迫性尿失禁患者，以及 AUA 指南内提及的 Gormley OAB Kobashi SUI 患者的初始病情检查并不适用。然而，在许多情况下，为了安全且彻底地评估更复杂的病例，可能需要一种或两种方法。

膀胱镜检查的作用是直接观察患者的膀胱和尿道，从而排除可能导致或加重患者的病理症状。虽然常规膀胱镜检查对于大多数患者来说并不会影响结果，但是很明显，膀胱镜检查对于患者的检查是一个常识性的辅助手段。例如，一个终身吸烟者伴有急性尿失禁和排尿困难，尿培养阴性，应该接受膀胱镜检查，以排除膀胱癌作为其刺激性下尿路症状的原因。此外，对于先前做过阴道补片手术的尿失禁患者（特别是有复发性尿路感染病史的患者），应该做膀胱镜检查以排除网片排异侵蚀。如果患者符合血尿的诊断标准（AUA 指南诊断血尿），也应进行膀胱镜检查和适当的上尿路成像。

多通道尿流动力学检查（UDS）用于研究膀胱储存和排空（如膀胱测量），评估充盈期间膀胱的压力和容积、排尿期间膀胱的压力和尿流率，以及对压力 – 流量的研究。多通道尿流动力学检查与尿流测定法和简单膀胱测定不同在于其客观地测量膀胱压力。通常，多通道尿流动力学检查是同时通过电极片或针电极测量尿道括约肌和骨盆底肌肉的肌电图（EMG）。在尿失禁的研究中，首要目标是鉴定急迫性尿失禁和压力性尿失禁。重要的是要记住，一方面，膀胱顺应性降低或不完全膀胱排空也可能导致漏尿，在为检查尿失禁而进行的研究中，主要目标通常是识别尿急或压力性尿失禁；另一方面，顺应性降低或膀胱排空不完全也可能导致渗漏。急迫性尿失禁常与尿流动力学检查造成的逼尿肌过度活动（DO）有关。逼尿肌过度活动是对膀胱充盈过程中逼尿肌无意识收缩的尿流动力学检查观察，可能伴有尿失禁，也可能不伴有尿失禁。在已知神经系统疾病中，这被称为神经源性逼尿肌过度活动[1]。此外，多达 50% 的急迫性尿失禁患者可能没有尿流动力学检查造成的逼尿肌过度活动，约 15% 的没有急迫性尿失禁的患者可有“试验诱发”的逼尿肌过度活动[23]。尿流动力学检查结果并不比令人信服的病史更重要。压力性尿失禁的定义取决于在尿流动力学检查中的漏尿点压力（ALPP）。腹部漏尿点压力是在没有逼尿肌收缩的情况下由于腹压升高而发生尿漏的预确定性膀胱内疾病一种膀胱内压力，在没有逼尿肌收缩的情况下，由于腹部压力增加而导致尿液漏尿[1]。没有压力性尿失禁的患者在任何腹压下都没有尿失禁，因此没有腹部漏尿点压力。较低的腹部漏尿点压力与压力性尿失禁严重程度恶化有关。根据惯例，低于 60cmH_2O 的腹部漏尿点压力被认为是内在括约肌缺陷的表现。然而，这并没有考虑到是否存在尿道高活动性的检查，因此应该谨慎解读[11]（表 3–2）。

做尿流动力学检查的患者选择的时机仍然是一个有争议的话题。许多专家以前主张在有创伤性的或不可逆性的治疗之前进行常规尿流动力学检查。这随着 VALUE 试验的发表而改变，这是一项大型的、多中心的随机对照试验，结果显示在放置吊带之前接受尿流动力学检查的无并发症压力性尿失禁女性与没有接受尿流动力学检查的女性之间的结果没有差异[13]。最近一项数据分析表明在进行三线治疗膀胱过度活动症（OAB）之前做尿流动力学检查没有明显的益处，同时对于压力性尿失禁也没有强有力的数据[4]。大多数专家赞同在以下情况需要做尿流动力学检查：进行侵入性介入抗失禁或脱垂手术治疗之前、严重的尿失禁、不明确的尿失禁症状、残余尿量升高或显著的梗阻症状、神经性下尿路功能障碍、咳嗽压力测试中无法引发压力性尿失禁和单纯性膀胱炎[7]。

总结

至少 1/4 的女性患有某种程度的尿失禁[12]。所有泌尿外科医生和妇科医生都应该擅长评估这些情况。检查应包括考虑非泌尿系统潮湿的来源和暂时性尿失禁的原因，以及评估之前的盆腔放疗、手术、妇科或产科病史。尿失禁的特点应该是确定症状持续时间、刺激、加重因素、严重程度，以及并存的梗阻症状。所有的患者都应该接受盆腔和腹部检查，至少应进行尿液分析和残余尿量评估。影像学检查和更具侵入性的诊断检查应该在个体化的基础上进行。

表 3-2 国际控尿协会界定的关于尿流动力学检查的调查结果

	ICS 定义	
逼尿肌过度活动	膀胱测压过程中逼尿肌的阶段性收缩 膀胱造影波形图	
神经源性逼尿肌过度活动	在患有临床相关的神经系统疾病患者中膀胱测压时出现逼尿肌阶段性收缩 膀胱造影波形图	
顺应性降低存储功能障碍（RCSD）	膀胱测压过程中逼尿肌压力的非阶段性升高 容量 / 顺应性降低	
充盈感减弱	充盈膀胱期间感觉减弱	
逼尿肌漏尿点压力（DLPP）	在没有逼尿肌收缩或腹压增高的情况下发生漏尿的最低压力 ＞40cmH$_2$O 的女性导致发病风险增加	
漏尿点腹压（ALPP）	在固定膀胱容积（200～300ml）时导致尿漏的腹内压力	
	Valsalva 漏尿点压（VLPP）	严重：＜60cmH$_2$O 中等：60～90cmH$_2$O 轻微：＞90cmH$_2$O
	咳嗽漏尿点压（CLPP）	

ICS. 国际尿控制学会
引自 McGuire EJ, Woodside JR, Borden TA, et al. Prognostic value of urodynamic testing in myelodysplastic patients. *J Urol*. 1981; 126:205–9

参考文献

[1] Abrams P, Cardozo L, Fall M, Griffiths D, Rosier P, Ulmsten U, van Kerrebroeck P, Victor A, Wein A. Standardisation Sub-committee of the International Continence Society. The standardisation of terminology of lower urinary tract function: report from the Standardisation Subcommittee of the International Continence Society. Neurourol Urodyn. 2002;21(2):167–78. https://doi.org/10.1002/nau.10052. PMID: 11857671.

[2] Al Afraa T, Mahfouz W, Campeau L, Corcos J. Normal lower urinary tract assessment in women: I. Uroflowmetry and post-void residual, pad tests, and bladder diaries. Int Urogynecol J. 2012;23(6):681–5. https://doi.org/10.1007/s00192–011– 1568– z. Epub 2011 Sep 21. Review. PubMed PMID: 21935667.

[3] D'Ancona C, Haylen B, Oelke M, Abranches-Monteiro L, Arnold E, Goldman H, Hamid R, Homma Y, Marcelissen T, Rademakers K, Schizas A, Singla A, Soto I, Tse V, de Wachter S, Herschorn S; Standardisation Steering Committee ICS and the ICS Working Group on Terminology for Male Lower Urinary Tract & Pelvic Floor Symptoms and Dysfunction. The International Continence Society (ICS) report on the terminology for adult male lower urinary tract and pelvic floor symptoms and dysfunction. Neurourol Urodyn. 2019;38(2):433–77. https://doi.org/10.1002/nau.23897. Epub 2019 Jan 25. PMID: 30681183.

[4] Glass D, Lin FC, Khan AA, Van Kuiken M, Drain A, Siev M, Peyronett B, Rosenblum N, Brucker BM, Nitti VW. Impact of preoperative urodynamics on women undergoing pelvic organ prolapse surgery. Int Urogynecol J. 2020;31(8):1663–8. https://doi.org/10.1007/ s00192–019–04084–8. Epub 2019 Aug 27. PMID: 31456030.

[5] Holroyd-Leduc JM, Tannenbaum C, Thorpe KE, Straus SE. What type of urinary incontinence does this woman have? JAMA. 2008;299(12):1446–56. https://doi.org/10.1001/ jama.299.12.1446. Review. PubMed PMID: 18364487.

[6] Hsu TH, Rackley RR, Appell RA. The supine stress test: a simple method to detect intrinsic urethral sphincter dysfunction. J Urol. 1999;162(2):460–3. https://doi.org/10.1016/ s0022–5347(05)68589–8. PubMed PMID: 10411057.

[7] Kobashi KC, Albo ME, Dmochowski RR, Ginsberg DA, Goldman HB, Gomelsky A, Kraus SR, Sandhu JS, Shepler T, Treadwell JR, Vasavada S, Lemack GE. Surgical treatment of female stress urinary incontinence: AUA/SUFU guideline. J Urol. 2017;198(4):875–83. https://doi.org/10.1016/j.juro.2017.06.061. Epub 2017 Jun 15. PubMed PMID: 28625508.

[8] Krhut J, Gärtner M, Mokris J, Horcicka L, Svabik K, Zachoval R, Martan A, Zvara P. Effect of severity of urinary incontinence on quality of life in women. Neurourol Urodyn. 2018;37(6):1925–30. https://doi.org/10.1002/nau.23568. Epub 2018 Mar 31. PubMed PMID: 29603780.

[9] Lawrence JM, Lukacz ES, Nager CW, Hsu JW, Luber KM. Prevalence and co-occurrence of pelvic floor disorders in community-dwelling women. Obstet Gynecol. 2008;111(3):678–85. https://doi.org/10.1097/ AOG.0b013e3181660c1b. PubMed PMID: 18310371.

[10] Malik RD, Hess DS, Christie A, Carmel ME, Zimmern PE. Domain comparison between 6 validated questionnaires administered to women with urinary incontinence. Urology. 2019;132:75–80. https://doi.org/10.1016/j.urology.2019.07.008. Epub 2019 Jul 13. PubMed PMID: 31310769.

[11] McGuire EJ, Fitzpatrick CC, Wan J, Bloom D, Sanvordenker J, Ritchey M, Gormley EA. Clinical assessment of urethral sphincter function. J Urol. 1993;150(5 Pt 1):1452–4. https://doi.org/10.1016/ s0022–5347(17)35806–8. PubMed PMID: 8411422.

[12] Minassian VA, Drutz HP, Al-Badr A. Urinary incontinence as a worldwide problem. Int J Gynaecol Obstet. 2003;82(3):327–38. https://doi.org/10.1016/s0020–7292(03)00220–0. Review. PubMed PMID: 14499979.

[13] Nager CW, Brubaker L, Daneshgari F, Litman HJ, Dandreo KJ, Sirls L, Lemack GE, Richter HE, Leng W, Norton P, Kraus SR, Chai TC, Chang D, Amundsen CL, Stoddard AM, Tennstedt SL. Design of the Value of Urodynamic Evaluation (ValUE) trial: a non-inferiority randomized trial of preoperative urodynamic investigations. Contemp Clin Trials. 2009;30(6):531–9. https://doi.org/10.1016/ j.cct.2009.07.001. Epub 2009 Jul 25. PubMed PMID: 19635587; PubMed Central PMCID: PMC3057197.

[14] Resnick NM. Urinary incontinence in the elderly. Medical Grand Rounds 1984;3:281–90.

[15] Ryhammer AM, Laurberg S, Djurhuus JC, Hermann AP. No relationship between subjective assessment of urinary incontinence and pad test weight gain in a random population sample of menopausal women. J Urol. 1998;159(3):800–3. PubMed PMID: 9474152.

[16] Staack A, Vitale J, Ragavendra N, Rodríguez LV. Translabial ultrasonography for evaluation of synthetic mesh in the vagina. Urology. 2014;83(1):68–74. https://doi.org/10.1016/j.urology. 2013.09.004. Epub 2013 Nov 12. PubMed PMID: 24231215.

[17] Stamatakos M, Sargedi C, Stasinou T, Kontzoglou K. Vesicovaginal fistula: diagnosis and management. Indian J Surg. 2014;76(2):131–6. https://doi.org/10.1007/s12262–012– 0787– y. Epub 2012 Dec 14. Review. PubMed PMID: 24891778; PubMed Central PMCID: PMC4039689.

[18] Stoffel JT, Peterson AC, Sandhu JS, Suskind AM, Wei JT, Lightner DJ. AUA White Paper on Nonneurogenic Chronic Urinary Retention: Consensus Definition, Treatment Algorithm, and Outcome End Points. J Urol. 2017;198(1):153–60. https://doi.org/10.1016/ j.juro.2017.01.075. Epub 2017 Feb 3. PMID: 28163030.

[19] Stav K, Dwyer PL, Rosamilia A. Women overestimate daytime urinary frequency: the importance of the bladder diary. J Urol. 2009;181(5):2176–80. https://doi.org/10.1016/j. juro.2009.01.042. Epub 2009 Mar 17. PubMed PMID: 19296975.

[20] Subak LL, Brubaker L, Chai TC, et al. High costs of urinary incontinence among women electing surgery to treat stress incontinence. Obstet Gynecol. 2008;111(4):899–907. https:// doi.org/10.1097/AOG.0b013e31816a1e12.

[21] Subak LL, Goode PS, Brubaker L, Kusek JW, Schembri M, Lukacz ES, Kraus SR, Chai TC, Norton P, Tennstedt SL. Urinary incontinence management costs are reduced following Burch or sling surgery for stress incontinence. Am J Obstet Gynecol. 2014;211(2):171.e1–7. https:// doi.org/10.1016/j.ajog.2014.03.012. Epub 2014 Mar 11. PubMed PMID: 24631433; PubMed Central PMCID: PMC4349353.

[22] Tseng LH, Liang CC, Chang YL, Lee SJ, Lloyd LK, Chen CK. Postvoid residual urine in women with stress incontinence. Neurourol Urodyn. 2008;27(1):48–51. https://doi. org/10.1002/nau.20463. PMID: 17563112.

[23] van Waalwijk van Doorn ES, Meier AH, Ambergen AW, Janknegt RA. Ambulatory urodynamics: extramural testing of the lower and upper urinary tract by Holter monitoring of cystometrogram, uroflowmetry, and renal pelvic pressures. Urol Clin North Am. 1996;23(3):345–71. https://doi.org/10.1016/s0094–0143(05)70317–7. Review. PubMed PMID: 8701551.

[24] Whitcomb EL, Lukacz ES, Lawrence JM, Nager CW, Luber KM. Prevalence and degree of bother from pelvic floor disorders in obese women. Int Urogynecol J Pelvic Floor Dysfunct. 2009;20(3):289–94. https://doi.org/10.1007/s00192–008– 0765– x. Epub 2008 Nov 11. PubMed PMID: 19002365; PubMed Central PMCID: PMC4943873.

第4章 女性尿失禁的尿流动力学检查

Urodynamic Testing of Female Incontinence

Anne P. Cameron 著

一、尿流动力学原理

尿流动力学检查（UDS）是从事与尿失禁相关的医护人员能够更准确的诊断女性泌尿系症状的重要工具之一。尿流动力学检查并不能取代详细的问诊及常规检查，在没有临床背景的情况下，孤立的尿流动力学检查结果很难进行临床诊断。在有了基本临床评估但诊断并不十分明确的情况下，应用尿流动力学检查可以更加明确患者的病因，以及分析其病理生理过程。

确定一名患者是否需要进行尿流动力学检查，可以用一个简单公式来进行评估：诊断过程中的不确定性概率乘后续治疗方案的风险概率等于需要尿流动力学检查概率。

诊断的不确定性 × 后续治疗方案的风险概率 =
需要尿动力检查概率

例如，如果患者既往有混合性尿失禁史（压力性尿失禁与急迫性尿失禁的不确定性很高），并且患者选择了盆底康复治疗（后续治疗的风险为0%，因为盆底康复训练既适用于压力性尿失禁又适用于急迫性尿失禁），那么需要做尿流动力学检查的概率就为0%（高 ×0=0）。另一个例子就是，一名患者在吊带手术后出现尿潴留，并持续数月，但在吊带前没有其他下尿路症状且残余尿量很低。在这种情况下，即使手术的风险很高，但诊断的不确定性为0%（0× 高 =0），同样不需要在术前进行尿流动力学检查。

在女性压力性尿失禁患者的诊治过程中，我们对该类患者是否有进行尿流动力学检查的必要进行了评估。评估实验[1]将无并发症的压力性尿失禁患者随机分组，在手术前进行尿流动力学检查和标准临床评估。尿流动力学检查对患者的治疗方案及手术结果并没有影响。因此，在这类患者中，尿流动力学检查并不是必需的。通过后续对尿流动力学检查趋势的统计，自评估实验的研究结论发表以来，术前的尿流动力学检查有所下降[2]。对5%有混合性尿失禁患者的评估显示，术前的尿流动力学检查并未改变术后再次干预的风险。评估实验进一步表明，临床治疗方案可以在没有尿流动力学检查的情况下完成，但要具有效的病史、查体及无创辅助检查[3]。

在更复杂的尿失禁患者群体中我们也进行了尿流动力学效果的评估，这个患者群体中没有一例单纯的压力性尿失禁患者。在285例患者中，有43%的患者因为尿流动力学检查而改变了治疗方案，35%的患者改变了手术计划[4]。其中大多数患者采用了影像尿流动力学检查，影像尿流动力学检查对290.5%患者的诊断有帮助。

还有一些研究，希望通过尿流动力学检查来评估其他类型尿失禁患者在术后的预后效果，Nobrega等对99例骶神经调节术后的逼尿肌过度活动（DO）患者使用尿流动力学检查进行了评估，不幸的是，没能发现任何尿流动力学检查参数能够预测骶神经调节的分期手术是否可以成功[5]。同样的，对于那些进行肉毒杆菌毒素注射的逼尿肌过度活动患者，注射前进行尿流动力学检查并不能预测肉毒杆菌毒素的治疗效果[6]。然而，对于一系列男性患者，尿流动力学检查结果显示膀胱出口梗阻系数较高（伴有残余尿量较多）的确可以预测出需要自行导尿的尿潴留风险较高[7]。

然而，尿流动力学检查通常是泌尿外科的诊断基础，对许多泌尿外科的临床诊断必不可少，如评估神经源性下尿路功能障碍（NGLUTD），以及对膀胱出口梗阻与逼尿肌收缩无力进行鉴别。美国泌尿外科学会（AUA）指南针对尿流动力学检查做出了相应的指导，女性压力性尿失禁（SUI）和膀胱过度活动症（OAB）指南都指出，尿流动力学检查不应该用于无并发症患者的初步检查，但建议将其用于诊断复杂的下尿路症状患者[8, 9]。在本章中，我们对尿流动力学检查均遵循国际尿控协会（ICS）的尿流动力学质量控制标准（GUP）及尿流动力学技术规范[10]。

二、尿动力的替代选择

有几种非侵入式的无创检查可以很好地取代尿流动力学检查中有创的压力流率测定，同样也可以很好的获得对下尿路功能障碍诊断的目的。利用膀胱容量测定仪（超声）或导尿法了解膀胱残余尿量（PVR）是一种非常有效的筛查方法，是评估膀胱是否完全排空的有效手段。当残余尿量非常高或与患者平时的残余尿量值做对比时，这个数值就非常有意义，如一名患者在尿失禁手术前残余尿量为0ml，但术后有了200ml的残余尿量。目前，残余尿量没有明确的正常值[11]；但我们有一个好的经验就是，当一个人随着年龄增长，他的逼尿肌收缩预期就会减弱，如果他的残余尿量小于他的实际年龄，那么他的残余尿量就是完全正常的。残余尿量的测量方法需要具体说明，因为任何一种测量方法都会有造成假阴性或假阳性的可能。例如，超声方法造成假阳性的例子包括腹水、腹膜透析、妊娠或卵巢囊肿，这些都容易造成膀胱外的液体测量错误；而如果膀胱探头未对准膀胱的正确位置，以及导尿时导尿管未完全插入膀胱或过早从膀胱拔出，则可能导致假阴性。

尿流率测定（单纯尿流率）用来测量排尿的速度，以“ml/s”为单位，当尿流率测定与残余尿量测定相结合时，可提供有效的排尿功能障碍的临床信息。尿流率测定应在隐私的环境下让患者进行正常的生理排尿，并且患者的检测应在日常的排尿体位进行。尿流率测定是ICS规定的标准尿流动力学检查中的一个项目[10]，应该在其他检查前进行，以便得到未插尿流动力测压管情况下测得自由尿流率及残余尿结果。患者应该在憋尿的情况下进行尿流率测定，最好在快憋不住时（急尿感情况下）在进行检测。影响尿流率测定的一个重要因素是患者经常在膀胱未憋足的情况下就进行排尿，这往往会导致排尿量过低（＜150ml）。＜150ml尿量的尿流率测定数值会偏低，从而影响尿流率测定结果。而学者们制订的反应最大尿流率与排尿量之间关系的尿流率列线图也将这种排尿量过低的尿流率排除。相反的，如果由于过度憋尿造成膀胱扩张，致使检测前排尿等待时间过长，尿流率测定结果也会异常[10]。

尿流率测定的主要参数包括最大流量（Q_{max}）、平均流量（Q_{ave}）及排尿量。女性的正常尿流率测定值因排尿量不同而有很大差异，这与男性不同，男性的尿流率会随着年龄的增长而降低[12]。实际上，关于女性尿流率正常值的统计数据很少，这点与男性不同，因为男性的尿流率已被广泛用于诊断前列腺梗阻引起的膀胱出口梗阻（BOO），具有明确的正常值[13]。女性以非常高的尿流率（甚至＞30ml/s的高流率）进行排尿，曲线呈挂钟形，排尿时间比男性短。女性平均尿流率（Q_{ave}）为17～24ml/s，在正常女性中，最大尿流率（Q_{max}）为23～33ml/s，排尿量为250～550ml，残余尿通常＜15ml[12]。曲线可表现为挂钟形（正常）、扁平状（尿流率低）、后半部出现峰值的方盒状（有阻塞的可能）、高流率模式（该模式对于女性患者正常）和逼尿肌无力模式(使用腹压排尿，呈锯齿状)（图4-1）。

排尿日记是能够为膀胱功能提供非常重要生理信息的非检测项目。排尿日记可以避免患者在检查室进行检查时产生的尴尬、身体不适，以及非自然膀胱充盈造成的对诊断数据的影响。排尿日记大多记录患者液体摄入量、排尿量、尿急程度、尿失禁的发生情况等内容。这些内容由患者在白天及夜间客观记录，膀胱容量的数据也比在检查环境下测得的数据更真实。这些结果也可以帮助患者根据自身状况制订饮水计划[14]，并可用于测量夜间多尿指数，这对于诊断夜尿症的原因至关重要。

尿垫实验是测量一段时间内漏尿量的简单方法，它通过秤重被漏尿浸湿的尿垫重量减去该尿垫使用前的重量来计算漏尿量。在非月经期女性中，尿垫净增加主要是尿液，但汗液和阴道分泌物也会增加尿垫的重量。

短时尿垫实验可以通过在 15min 内喝 500ml 液体，然后在办公室佩戴尿垫 1h 完成多项规定的体育活动（如步行和爬楼梯）来完成。任何超过 1g 的漏尿量都被认为是尿失禁阳性。长期尿垫实验包括收集所有 24～48h 佩戴的尿垫。在 24h 内净增加 8g 或在任何单个尿垫上净增加 2g 被认为是尿失禁[12]。

有一种简单的膀胱容积压力测定的方法，被称为“眼球式尿动力”（eyeball urodynamics）。首先放置导尿管测量患者的残余尿量，然后使用注射器通过导尿管向膀胱灌注无菌生理盐水，并记录灌注量，在此期间，患者任何忽然产生的急尿感，都可以被记录为逼尿肌过度活动（DO）。随着灌注量的增加，患者的憋尿感逐步增加，这时要将患者产生尿意感的灌注量记录。患者膀胱感觉的记录点，与标准尿流动力学检测时一样，应包括初始尿意感（FD）、正常尿意感（ND）及最大膀胱容量（CC）。当膀胱感觉记录完成，拔出导尿管，并嘱患者仰卧位进行咳嗽或实施 Valsalva 加压实验，并观察是否产生漏尿，如果未出现漏尿

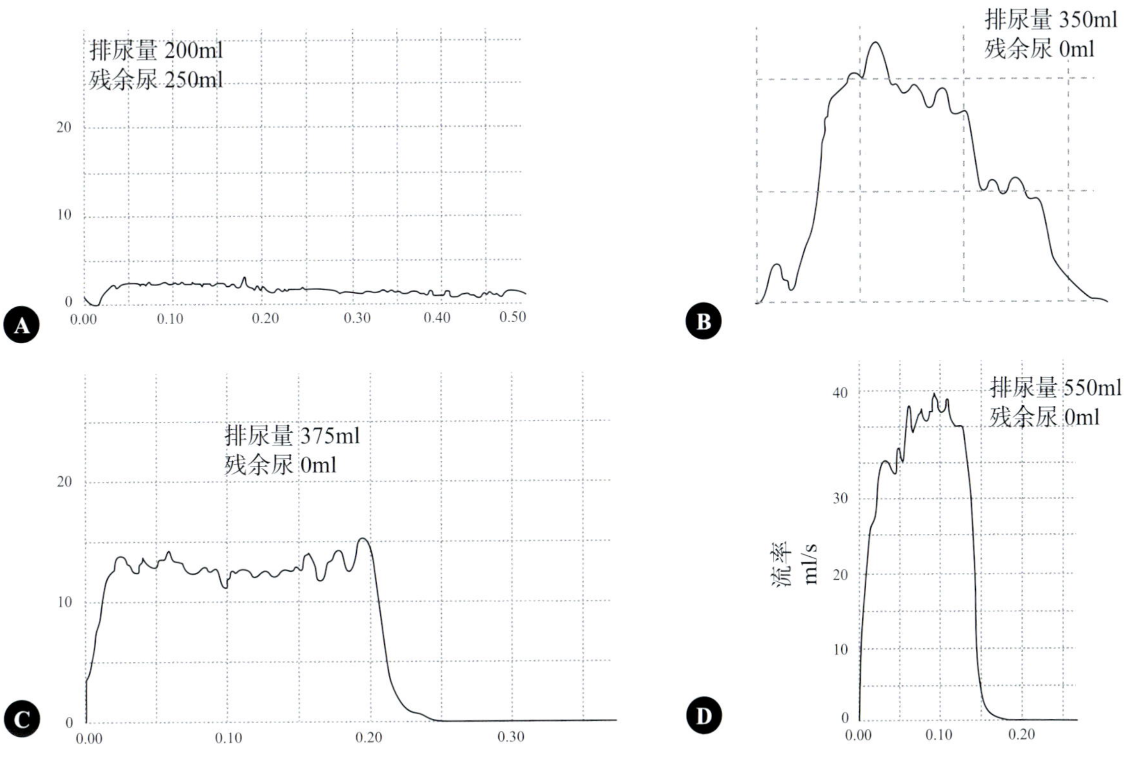

▲ 图 4-1 **A 至 C. 来自同一女性患者不同时期的尿流率曲线，尿道狭窄，最大尿流率为 3ml/s（A），狭窄扩张后正常，最大尿流率为 22ml/s（B），狭窄复发后 1 年，最大尿流率为 15ml/s，后半部出现峰值的方盒状（C）。D. 女性压力性尿失禁的高尿流率模式，最大尿流率为 45ml/s**

（呈阴性），可让患者起身垫上尿垫，并进行增加腹压的动作（如跳跃或蹲下）或咳嗽，最终确定患者是否漏尿。这项检查相比标准尿流动力学检测的优势在于时间更短，并且患者不需要带着连接到尿流动力学检测设备上的测压管，可以方便重复的检测，以便更好地让患者再现症状。这项检查非常适合需要反复增加腹压动作才会出现漏尿的可疑压力性尿失禁患者。对于想要评估是否具有隐匿性压力性尿失禁的脱垂患者，这也是一种理想的检测方法，因为在脱垂改善和未改善的情况下，都可以进行。如果该检测显示在准备脱垂手术的患者中存在压力性尿失禁，那么就为我们在进行盆腔器官脱垂修复手术期是否进行悬吊手术提供了依据；如果该检测不能证明脱垂手术的患者存在压力性尿失禁，但却被临床高度怀疑存在压力性尿失禁，那么可选择进行尿流动力学检查[15]。这种简单的膀胱容积压力测定方法不能提供任何关于排尿期逼尿肌压力的信息或关于逼尿肌过度活动的可靠信息，但非常适合诊断压力性尿失禁。

三、尿流动力学检查的解读

如果要进行尿流动力学检查，您首先需要了解几个问题。如果实际操作尿流动力学检查的技术人员知道面临的问题，则可以最好地优化尿流动力学检查报告。一般来说，大多数尿流动力学检查要了解以下一个或多个问题[16]。

- 受试者是压力性尿失禁、急迫性尿失禁，还是两种都存在？
- 受试者在接受尿失禁手术或其他手术后，是否有压力性尿失禁、急迫性尿失禁或膀胱出口梗阻？
- 在患有神经源性下尿路功能障碍的患者中，她们的泌尿系统是否安全（是否存在输尿管反流、是否存在膀胱顺应性差、膀胱容量是否正常、是否具有逼尿肌过度活动）？
- 对于残余尿量多的患者，是否是逼尿肌收缩力减弱、排尿功能障碍或梗阻造成的？

如果对上述问题中的一个或多个有针对性进行尿流动力学检查，将会使解读数据变得更加容易，技术人员也可以更有针对性地制订尿流动力学检查具体方案。例如，对于有失禁问题但在尿流动力学检查期间没有漏尿的女性，技术人员可以让其进行更多的 Valsalva 和咳嗽动作，或者让其将检测体位改为站立位，以尝试引发漏尿；对于有尿潴留的患者，您可以将膀胱灌注到更高的容量，最大限度地引发排尿机会。这种简单的诊断架构使尿流动力学检查的结果变得更有针对性，因为您的检查目的是围绕着相关的临床问题，并允许您潜在地忽略可能只是为了尿流动力学检查报告标准化才产生的数据。例如，对尿失禁的患者进行压力流率测定时，如果检测前残余尿量正常，我们就不必关心她在测定期是否完全排空了膀胱。

四、尿流动力学检查前的准备及抗生素使用

尿流动力学检查的准备工作其实很简单。患者应该充分饮水，服用所有处方药物，并在检测当天正常饮食。询问患者是否有尿路感染的体征和症状，并至少在检查当天进行尿常规分析以筛查尿路感染。许多研究对尿路感染的定义各不相同，但最好的定义是尿路感染阳性 / 试纸阳性加上提示尿路感染的症状和尿液培养阳性[17]。采用试纸进行尿液分析是最简单的，因此使用最广泛[18]。血液、白细胞酯酶、亚硝酸盐和蛋白质的试纸阴性有 98% 的预测价值[19]。然而，有下尿路功能障碍（LUTS）的女性在试纸上出现白细胞酯酶或亚硝酸盐阳性的情况并不少见。尿液培养需要实验室评估，结果不会在当天公布。因此，在这种情况下（如果可能的话）可以使用尿液显微镜来评估菌尿。在这些情况下，症状评估是至关重要的，因为单独的菌尿不是尿流动力学检查的禁忌证。无症状的尿培养阳性只是菌尿，而不是尿路感染，不需要治疗，也不会改变尿流动力学检查的结果。如果根据试纸或显微镜检查怀疑是菌尿，那么检

查可以继续进行，但要预防性使用抗生素[18]。如果一个女性确实表现出尿路感染的症状，而且试纸呈阳性，她很可能有尿路感染。因此，应该进行尿液培养，并推迟尿流动力学检查，直到她的尿液指标正常[18]。

2017 年发布了尿流动力学检查防止过度使用抗生素最佳做法的政策声明。根据现有证据，泌尿生殖系统解剖正常且无危险因素的女性在进行尿流动力学检查时不需要使用抗生素来预防尿路感染。有很大比例需要尿流动力学检查的患者是声明中所包括的，在该人群中避免使用抗生素可以帮助我们更好管理抗生素的使用，并避免过度使用这些药物及产生不良反应。当检查后尿路感染的风险增加，或者如果他们发生尿路感染，且他们的身体状况会导致更严重的并发症时，推荐使用抗生素，这类患者包括神经源性下尿路功能障碍、膀胱出口梗阻或排尿后残余尿量升高、年龄超过 70 岁、目前存在菌尿（根据试纸结果或怀疑）、免疫抑制 / 使用皮质类固醇药物和免疫缺陷，以及需要长期导尿的患者和那些最近做过关节置入手术的患者。

抗生素的选择应取决于该地区抗生素药物的管理规定。一般来说，单剂量或双倍剂量的甲氧苄啶磺胺甲噁唑是首选。其他需要考虑的因素包括患者对抗生素的过敏性和耐受性，以及先前的尿液培养，尤其是那些有复发性尿路感染或已知菌尿的女性，先前的尿液培养可以指导抗生素的选择。有关抗生素和需要抗生素的风险因素见表 4–1，该表可作为参考指南添加在尿流动力学检查知情同意书中[18]。

尿流动力学检查的其他风险包括测压管插入造成的尿道损伤，可以通过良好的技术和经验将其降至最低；排尿困难，可根据需要用吡啶姆或对乙酰氨基酚 / 布洛芬治疗；有尿潴留风险的患者可能出现短暂的尿潴留；对患者身体或情绪上感到不适，可以通过医护疏导帮助缓解。

对于准备进行尿流动力学检查的患者，如果在情绪上或身体上感到焦虑或不适，会影响尿流动力学检查结果的真实性。在高度焦虑的状态下，排尿更困难，患者对检查的配合度也会受到影响。在一个更关注患者感受的测试中，对 314 例患者的经历进行了调查，50.7% 的患者认为这项检查在情绪上或身体上都没有不舒服，55% 的患者认为检查体验比预期要好，37% 的患者认为检查正如预期那样。然而，29% 的患者感到不舒服，而插入测压管的部位是最不舒服的部位，12% 的患者认为情绪不适是最不舒服的部分，而其中焦虑是最常见的情绪不适（27%），其次是尴尬（18%）。感到身体不适较少的患者是那些年龄较大和存在神经系统疾病的患者[20]。在一项随机试验中，患

表 4–1 尿流动力学检查后尿路感染的风险因素及抗生素的使用

尿流动力学检查前后的抗生素治疗		
是	**否**	**根据安全性和有效性选择的抗生素**
• 神经源性下尿路功能障碍 • 排尿后残余尿量升高 • 无症状菌尿 • 免疫低下 • 长期导尿患者 • 任何形式的留置导管 • 需间歇性导尿患者 • 超过 70 岁 • 关节置入手术<2 年	• 患者无泌尿生殖系统异常 • 糖尿病 • 有泌尿生殖手术史 • 近期住院患者 • 复发性尿路感染史（非当前） • 绝经后女性 • 营养不良 / 肥胖 • 心脏瓣膜疾病 • 置入销、板或螺钉	• 口服复方甲氧苄啶磺胺甲噁唑 • 口服头孢氨苄 500mg、口服阿莫西林 / 克拉维酸 875mg • 口服左氧氟沙星 500mg、口服环丙沙星 500mg、肌内注射庆大霉素 80mg

者的感受对于利用音乐或视频来减缓疼痛和焦虑的干预手段与常规护理手段相比并没有太大差别[21]，检查的感受与对执行检查人员技术能力的信心和对患者隐私的保护有关[22]。

五、系统性解释尿流动力学检查

有许多关于尿流动力学检查标准的参考文献都讨论了尿流动力学检查过程的细微差别[10, 23–25]，这些内容超出了本章的范围，但也是能够顺利完成尿流动力学检查的必要阅读。像其他复杂的诊断研究一样，有一个系统的标准方法来进行尿流动力学检查对于质量控制和确保检测过程不被遗漏是很重要的。

膀胱容积压力测定主要是在膀胱灌注的过程中进行腹压及膀胱压的测量。膀胱容积压力测定的过程以灌注到患者憋不住尿或最大膀胱容量出现漏尿而结束[10]。应指定灌注的溶液和速度。有两种需要考虑的膀胱灌注速度。一种是通过体重（kg）除以 4 估算的最大生理泌尿速度，通常为 20～30ml/min。另一种为了检查的便捷，是尿流动力学检查的灌注速度，比生理的泌尿速度更快。患者在测试期间继续分泌尿液（高达 25% 的体积）。因此，尿流动力学检查的膀胱容量是实际灌注量加上自然分泌的尿液量。在女性中，可以使用直肠测压管或在阴道放置测压管测量腹压，在不适感或患者可接受度方面两者没有差异。但是，阴道放置导管会经常感应不到压力或掉出[10]，所以不太可靠。

膀胱容积压力测定过程需要关注的参数有一个容易记忆的“4C”记忆法：容量（capacity）、顺应性（compliance）、收缩（contractions）、咳嗽（coughs）。此外，还有一个“2S”记忆法：感觉（sensation）、括约肌功能（sphincter function），接下来是压力流率测定部分。

压力流率测定是在患者出现排尿后立即开始，并在逼尿肌压力恢复到压力基线或患者认为排尿完成时结束。需要注意的是，压力流率测定记录的各项参数是患者的自主排尿的参数，而不是由失禁 / 逼尿肌过度活动造成漏尿时产生的参数。压力流率应关注的参数包括以“ml/s”为单位的最大尿流率（Q_{max}）和最大流率下的逼尿肌压力（$PdetQ_{max}$），以及在逼尿肌压力升高的排尿过程中发生的任何腹压升高、尿流率曲线的形状和括约肌开放的情况，即低电位肌电图（EMG）。在压力流率检测的曲线图中，通常 x 轴表示时间，y 轴表示压力流率的数值。压力流率曲线的形状可以是平滑的弧线，也可以是扁平状或波动的曲线[26]。有关尿流动力学测定的具体示例，请参见表 4–2 和图 4–2。

六、尿流动力学诊断

实际上，只有少数诊断可以通过尿流动力学检查的压力流率完成，其中包括压力性尿失禁、逼尿肌过度活动、逼尿肌收缩力减弱 / 膀胱容量减退、膀胱出口梗阻（功能性或解剖性）和膀胱顺应性差。在检查期间增加影像功能可以增加诊断信息，但通常不需要，除非提示解剖异常。在尿流动力学检查分析过程中，如果将上面可能的诊断列表牢记在心，会简化对尿流动力学检查的理解。

七、压力性尿失禁

压力性尿失禁是指喷嚏、咳嗽、大笑或运动等腹部压力增高的情况下出现不自主的尿液自尿道口漏出[27]。压力性尿失禁的尿流动力学检查表现为，在咳嗽及 Valsalva 动作期间，在没有逼尿肌收缩的情况下出现漏尿。在膀胱容量测定期间，当膀胱灌注至 200ml 时，嘱患者行 Valsalva 动作及 3 个渐进性增强的咳嗽，如果没有在逼尿肌过度活动的情况下出现漏尿，则为压力性尿失禁。记录不同情况下出现漏尿时的压力值，咳嗽时出现漏尿的压力值记为咳嗽漏尿点（CLPP），Valsalva 动作出现的漏尿压力值记为 Valsalva 漏尿点（VLPP）。其中，漏尿时被记录的最低压力值为腹压漏尿点（ALPP）。目前还没有一种被普遍接受的漏尿点压力正常值，有些漏尿点压力是记录的腹压数值

表 4-2　尿流动力检查阅读指南

分　类		检测指标	单　位	正常值
膀胱容积压力测定	膀胱容量	最大膀胱容量（MCC）	ml，精确到 10ml 以内	女性接近 500ml
	膀胱顺应性	容量差 / 压力差	ml/cmH_2O	＞20ml/cmH_2O 与上尿路有关，但通常数值更高
	膀胱收缩	在膀胱容积压力测定期间存在逼尿肌过度活动［也可以被视为原发性纤维肌痛综合征（PFS）的附加收缩］	检测期间存在或不存在（s），逼尿肌压力的波幅（cmH_2O），并且需要标注是否存在漏尿	不存在
	咳嗽	进行 Valsalva 漏尿点（VLPP）压力及咳嗽漏尿点（CLPP）压力测定，这两项统称为腹压漏尿点（ALPP）	cmH_2O	不存在
	感觉	记录 • 在膀胱灌注期间出现的初始尿意感（FSF） • 初始排尿欲（FDV） • 强烈排尿欲（SDV）和任何出现的急迫排尿意	ml	• 没有特定的正常值，但各感觉应被标识为正常、缺失、减少或增加 • 预期初始尿意感为膀胱容量的 30%，初始排尿欲为 60%
	括约肌功能	肌电图的电位是否会随着括约肌收缩而上升	在肛周用两片表面电极测量肌电图	肌电图的电位应该随着括约肌收缩而上升
压力流率	$PdetQ_{max}$	最大尿流率时的逼尿肌压力	cmH_2O	在女性中会更低，在正常女性中可能是 0
	Q_{max}	最大尿流率	ml/s	能在女性中很高，没有正常上限
	应力	腹压或膀胱压升高	存在 / 不存在	排尿过程中腹压升高并不总是被视为排尿症状，因为有些人通过腹部收缩来增加排尿，与排尿习惯有关
	括约肌开放度	肌电图记录		排尿时肌电图电位应该下降

（Pabd），还有一些则使用膀胱压力的数值（Pves）。咳嗽漏尿点的压力值往往高于 Valsalva 动作[28]，咳嗽漏尿点或 Valsalva 漏尿点的压力值取自观察到患者漏尿的瞬间。咳嗽是很短暂的，所以很难精准捕捉到漏尿瞬间的压力值。在检测中观察到，这两个值随着膀胱容量的增加而下降，而那些尿失禁更严重的女性往往有较低的腹压漏尿点[28]。如果临床高度怀疑 压力性尿失禁但在检测过程中并未有发现患者漏尿，则应将患者膀胱灌注至最大膀胱容量再重复操作（图 4-3），并可让患者进行额外的动作以便诱发漏尿，如从坐位变为站立位，或者让患者跳跃，最好采用患者日常产生漏尿的动作。

在使用尿流动力学检查诊断压力性尿失禁时，由于要置入测压管，因此可能会影响诊断结果，尽管测压管的管径很细（7F），而且大多数压力性尿失禁患者（>90%）在置管的情况下也出现漏尿，但也会有在体格检查中有压力性尿失禁症状的患者在行尿流动力学检查时并未出现漏尿，而在取出导管后这些患者就会出现压力性尿失禁。有压力性尿失禁但在行尿流动力学检查时没有出现漏尿，但拔管后出现压力性尿失禁的患者比例高达 50%[29]。这些患者并没有非常高的漏尿点压力，在本研究中，Valsalva 漏尿点的平均压力仅为 67cmH_2O. 因此，如果患者具有压力性尿失禁病史或临床检查中发现具有压力性尿失禁，而尿流动力学检查中并未展现出该症状，应取出导管重复检查。为了避免测压过程反复使用新的测压管，可以完成排尿部分的检测，然后重新充盈膀胱后移除测压管以进行漏尿实验[9]。应注意患者检测体位；如果一个只会站着漏尿的患者，仰卧位不会漏尿，坐着也不会漏尿，因此，应在她日常漏尿的体位重复操作。

固有尿道括约肌缺失（ISD）在临床上对尿失禁手术前的诊断非常重要，它会使手术的成功率降低，特别是对于经闭孔合成吊带术[30]。这可以通过最大尿道闭合压来诊断，由于不同的测量技术和不同的参考值，很难给出一个统一的诊断标准值，具体取决于所使用的导管类型[30]。因此，腹压漏尿点更常用于诊断 ISD。ISD 最常以 ALPP <60cmH_2O 的临界值被诊断为 ISD[30]，但最近对 ISD 的定义已经演变成一种不精确的主观诊断。国际尿控协会现在将 ISD 笼统的定义为一种“非常弱的尿道闭合机制”[31]。

八、逼尿肌过度活动

逼尿肌过度活动被定义为在膀胱充盈过程中逼尿肌压力的非自愿升高，无论是自发的还是被诱发刺激的。诱发性动作包括超过生理泌尿速度的膀胱充盈、改变姿势、咳嗽、大笑或洗手 / 流水

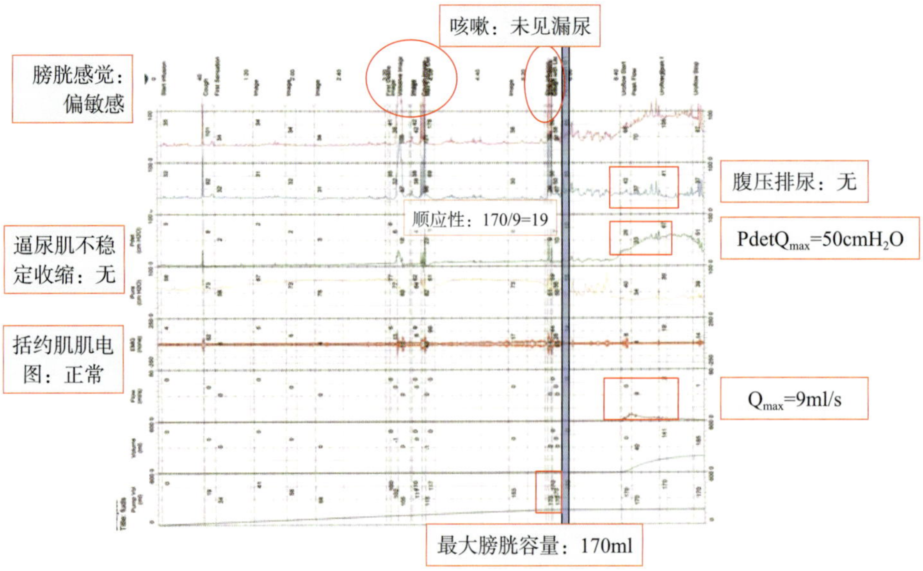

◀ 图 4-2 尿流动力学检查解读，吊带术后新发排尿困难

诊断：膀胱容量减小，顺应性接近正常，无逼尿肌过度活动，无压力性尿失禁，急尿感提前，咳嗽时见括约肌收缩，并且排尿期括约肌放松。当尿流率 9ml/s 时，PdetQ$_{max}$ 为 50cmH_2O，尿流动力学检查显示膀胱出口梗阻，并且影像显示尿道有尿液积聚（图 4-8B）

声。逼尿肌过度活动可能伴有急尿感，或者患者可能无意识地收缩逼尿肌（图 4–4）。

逼尿肌压升高表示膀胱收缩，会产生漏尿。目前没有逼尿肌压最小阈值可诊断为逼尿肌过度活动（低压的逼尿肌过动示例见图 4–6），但是逼尿肌的收缩幅度越大，持续时间越长则表明症状越严重，并且预示着其为神经源性下尿路功能障碍（NGLUTD）[32]。在没有神经系统疾病的患者中，逼尿肌过度活动被认为是特发性的，而在有这些病史的患者中，逼尿肌过度活动则被认为是神经源性的[31]。这两种情况没有明显差别，尿流动力学检查不能用于诊断神经系统疾病。“后收缩”是指在尿流率结束后持续或新的逼尿肌压力升高[10]，这种情况也可诊断为逼尿肌过度活动。还有一种“咳嗽相关逼尿肌过度活动”现象，这是在咳嗽动作后立即发生出现了逼尿肌过度活动，经常被患者误认为是压力性尿失禁，但在尿流动力学检查中可以明显看出是逼尿肌过度活动[10]（图 4–5）。

可能容易与逼尿肌过度活动混淆的常见伪影是检测过程中直肠穹窿收缩或气体通过直肠，这

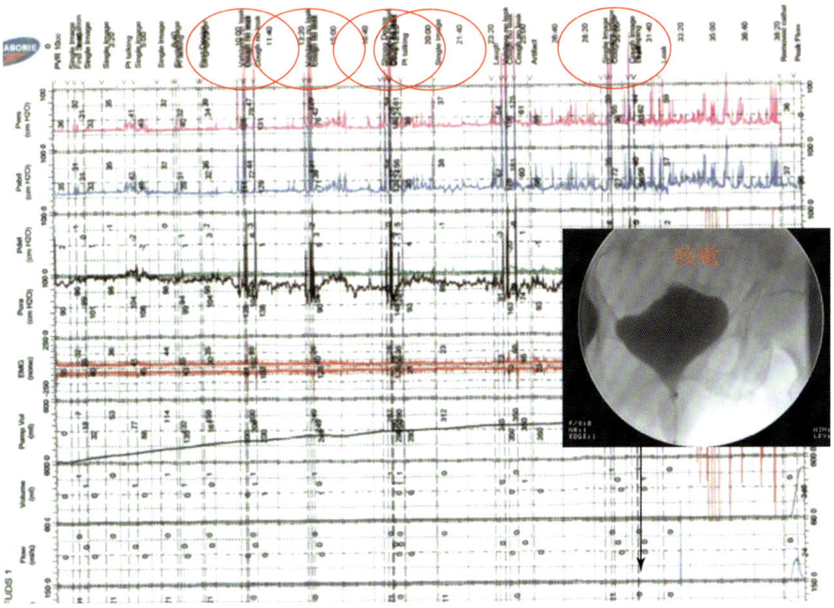

◀ 图 4–3　压力性尿失禁：1 位女性患者在膀胱镜检查中未发现有压力性尿失禁，因此进行了尿流动力学检查，在膀胱灌注至 200ml 时，行腹压漏尿点测量，未出现漏尿，因此，继续将膀胱分别灌注至 250ml、300ml 及 390ml 时，分别重复进行腹压漏尿点测量，尿流率没有记录到任何轻微漏尿（黑箭），但在灌注量 390ml 时，嘱患者咳嗽，同步影像发现患者出现漏尿

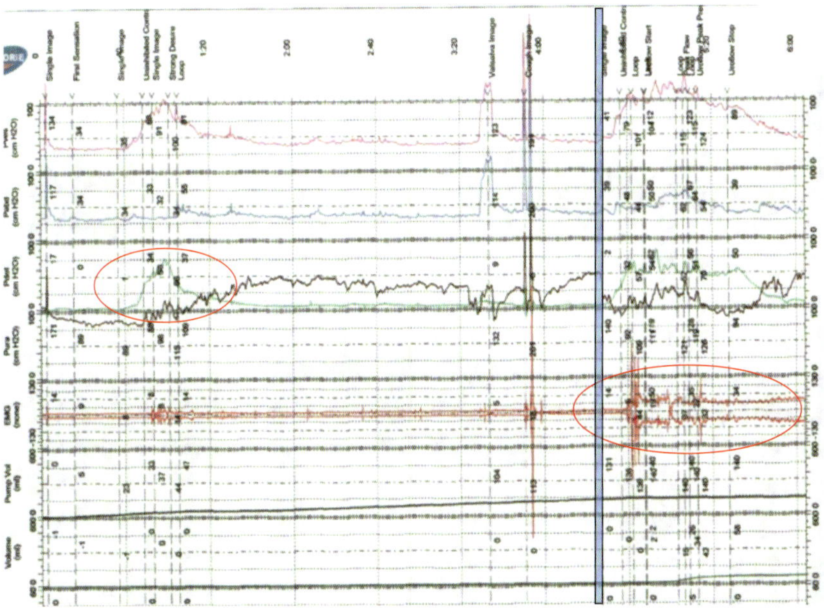

◀ 图 4–4　逼尿肌过度活动兼功能性梗阻：1 位有尿失禁及盆底疼痛的患者。在膀胱充盈至 38ml 时，逼尿肌收缩力高达 80cmH_2O，没有压力性尿失禁，膀胱容量至 131ml 伴有排尿疼痛，PdetQ_{max} 为 56cmH_2O，有梗阻症状，肌电图排尿期明显矛盾收缩（图 4–8E 为其膀胱的顶部旋转外观）

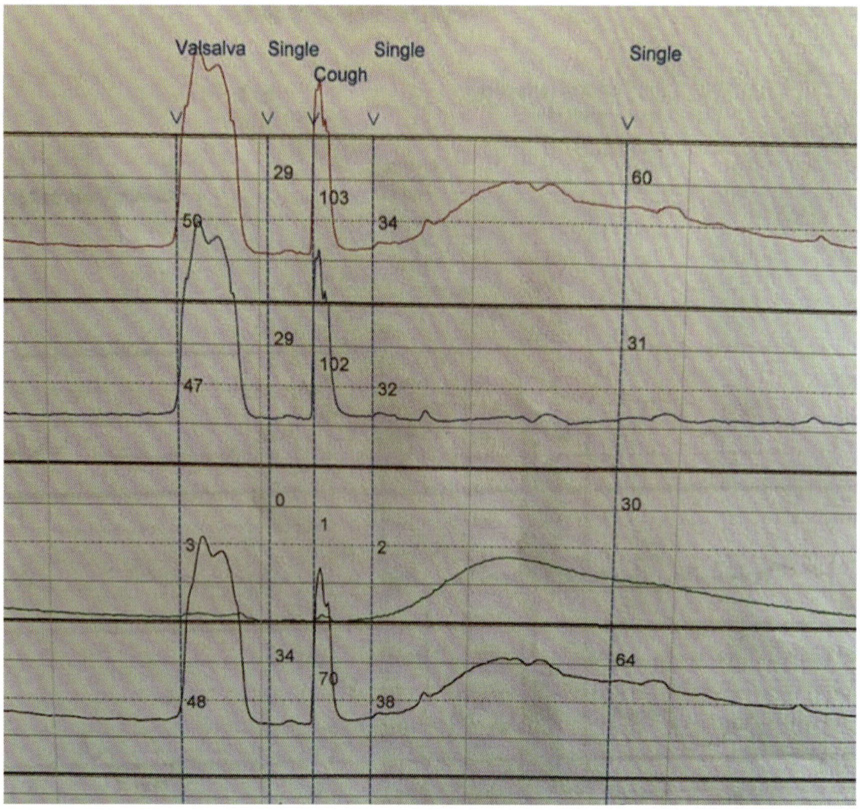

◀ 图 4-5 咳嗽相关逼尿肌过度活动：在咳嗽和 Valsalva 加压测试中"咳嗽相关活动"后立即发生逼尿肌过度活动，该女性因咳嗽后漏尿而得出压力性尿失禁的主观诊断

可能导致 Pabd 短暂下降[23]。此外，与压力性尿失禁类似，逼尿肌过度活动更可能发生在站立位，因此患者至少应处于坐位来进行尿流动力学检查[10]。

九、逼尿肌收缩力不足及无反射膀胱

女性膀胱不能完全排空、排尿困难、排尿缓慢或尿潴留的原因可能是膀胱出口梗阻或膀胱收缩力差的结果。除了尿流动力学的压力流率检测外，其他诊断方法很难区分这两种病因。使这种诊断困境更加复杂的是，在即使进行尿流动力学检测，由于患者的焦虑或不适，一些女性也会无法产生膀胱收缩或排尿，在这些情况下同样无法做出明确的诊断。这种情况被定义为"无法像往常一样排尿的情况"，如果患者表示这种排尿事件不具有代表性，则应与患者沟通如何在检测中避免发生这种情况[10]。

逼尿肌收缩无力是一种尿流动力学检查的诊断，定义为逼尿肌在排尿过程中收缩强度和（或）持续时间降低，导致膀胱排空延长和（或）未能在正常时间跨度内实现完全膀胱排空．重要的是我们要知道，许多女性自主排尿没有任何困难，虽然逼尿肌收缩非常低，或者增加腹部用力帮助排尿，这不是病态的。用于诊断女性患者逼尿肌收缩无力的标准不同，Groutz 将其定义为，在两次及以上的自由尿流率检测中，Q_{max}（最大尿流率）<12ml/s，排尿量至少 100ml 及残余尿量在 150ml 以上[33]。Abarbanel 和 Marcus 在压力流率检测中使用 $PdetQ_{max}$<30cmH$_2$O 和 Q_{max}<10ml/s 的标准[34]，Gammie 等则使用 $PdetQ_{max}$<20cmH$_2$O 和 Q_{max}<15ml/s，排尿量低于膀胱容量的 90%，临床没有任何下尿路梗阻的标准[35]。在男性中，膀胱收缩指数（BCI）<100 作为诊断被用来定义逼尿肌收缩无力（DU）[13]（图 4-6）。

膀胱收缩指数（BCI）=$PdetQ_{max}+5Q_{max}$
收缩力亢奋：BCI>150
收缩力正常：BCI 为 100～150
收缩力减弱：BCI<100
膀胱排尿效率，被称为排尿率（排尿量 %）

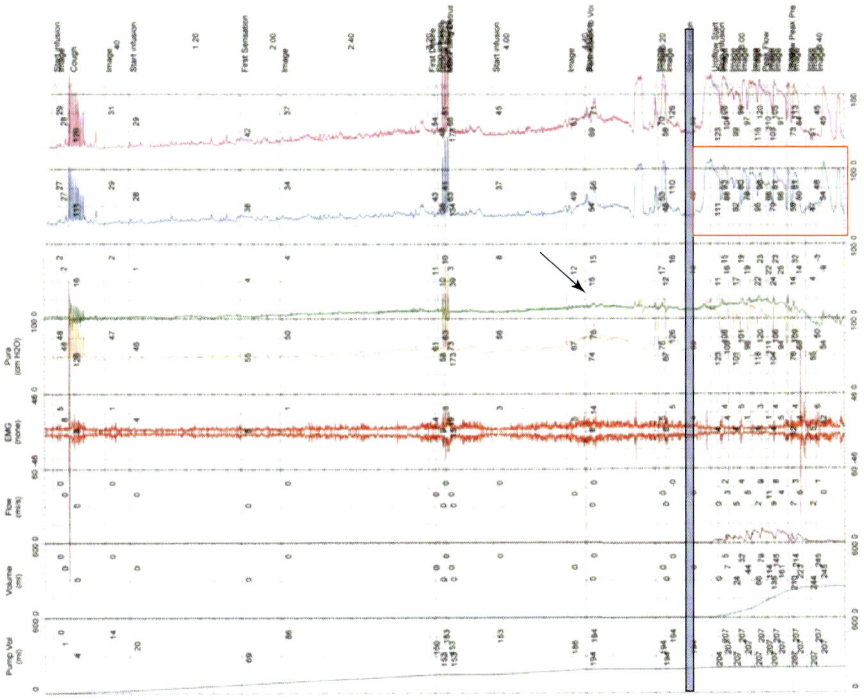

◀ **图 4-6**　逼尿肌收缩无力伴逼尿肌过度活动：**84** 岁患者，**30** 年前因宫颈癌接受放射治疗后出现尿失禁和排尿急迫。她的顺应性为 **194ml/12cmH$_2$O=16**。黑箭处有一次逼尿肌收缩但没有出现漏尿。在压力流率检测过程中，**PdetQ$_{max}$=22cmH$_2$O**，**Q$_{max}$=9ml/s**。收缩力：有（红框）**BCI=PdetQ$_{max}$ +5Q$_{max}$=22＋9×5=67**

= 总排尿量 / 总膀胱容量
= 排尿量 /（排尿量 + 残余尿量）× 100%

在 1015 例非神经源性下尿路功能障碍（LUTS）患者的大样本中，有 15% 的逼尿肌收缩无力属于 Groutz 定义，10% 属于 Ababarnel 标准，6% 属于 Gammie 标准。后两个标准都被认为在临床上作为有和无逼尿肌收缩无力 [36] 具有重要意义。收缩力被看作是膀胱压（Pves）和腹压（Pabd）的增加。这可以在体位变化或尝试排尿时观察到 [10]（图 4-6）。

十、膀胱出口梗阻

膀胱出口梗阻（BOO）也被称作膀胱流出道梗阻 [10]。由于尿流动力学检查诊断缺乏共识，女性膀胱出口梗阻的诊断比男性更困难 [37]。目前尿流动力学检查中判断膀胱出口梗阻存在几种列线图，但都将膀胱出口梗阻描述为逼尿肌压力增加和尿流率降低。

Groutz 等将尿道梗阻定义为自由尿流率持续＜12ml/s，且压力流率检测中最大尿流率时逼尿肌压力＞20cmH$_2$O [33]。Lemack 和 Zimmern 认为，排尿期逼尿肌压力＞25cmH$_2$O 或尿流率＜12ml/s 的女性被认为是尿道梗阻 [38]。Kuo 将膀胱出口梗阻定义为排尿期逼尿肌压力＞50cmH$_2$O，同时在排尿期膀胱尿道造影中尿道狭窄 [39]。Blaivas 和 Groutz 根据排尿期压力流率检测中逼尿肌最大压力的统计分析，以及多次自由尿流检测得到的最大尿流率数值 Q$_{max}$，开发了一种常用的膀胱出口梗阻列线图 PdetQ$_{max}$＞57cmH$_2$O 的患者被划分为中度或重度梗阻。PdetQ$_{max}$＜57cmH$_2$O 的患者被划分为轻度阻塞或无阻塞，该划分还需参考自由尿流率时 Q$_{max}$ 的值。在一组 600 例女性的样本统计中，6% 为轻度梗阻，2% 为中度梗阻，不到 1% 为严重梗阻 [40]。Nitti 等定性地将梗阻定义为存在持续逼尿肌收缩且具有明确的尿道狭窄的影像学证据。对于阻塞的女性 PdetQ$_{max}$ 和 Q$_{max}$ 的平均值分别为 43cmH$_2$O 和 9ml/s [41]。

Akikwala [42] 通过对 91 例女性采用上述不同诊断方法进行比较，发现其中 25 例可能有梗阻，Nitti 提出的定义具有最大的一致性 [42]。最近，Solomon 和 Greenwell [43] 创建了一个新的列线图，提出了一个女性膀胱出口梗阻系数（fBOOI），计

算方法为 $PdetQ_{max}-2.2Q_{max}$。如果 fBOOI<0，则梗阻的概率<10%，如果 fBOOI>5，则梗阻的概率为 50%。该列线图在接受手术以缓解梗阻的女性患者群体中得到验证，其中列线图准确预测了手术后的症状缓解情况[44]。图 4-2 是由于吊带引起的膀胱出口梗阻示例（解剖性）和图 4-4 由于排尿功能障碍引起的膀胱出口梗阻（功能性）。

只有少数几种可能的病因会导致女性出现膀胱出口梗阻，其中包括几种固定的解剖性梗阻，如过紧的尿道吊带、尿道狭窄、盆腔器官脱垂或恶性肿瘤。有人建议，在吊带手术后疑似梗阻的情况下不需要进行尿流动力学检查，因为新出现的排尿症状结合临床病史基本上可以诊断为梗阻，仅在具有潜在症状的情况下才需要尿流动力学检查[45]。膀胱出口梗阻的另一大类是功能性障碍，即出口不能放松。这些功能性障碍包括功能性排尿障碍，这是由于“在正常的排尿时，由于尿道周围横纹肌不自觉的间歇性收缩而引起的间歇性和（或）波动的尿流阻力”[27]，或者逼尿肌/括约肌协同失调，这是由于“逼尿肌收缩的同时尿道和（或）尿道周围横纹肌不自主收缩”。有时，尿流会被完全阻隔。区分这些疾病的最简单方法是临床病史，因为一个人只有神经系统疾病才会出现逼尿肌括约肌协调失调（DSD），无一例外。

尿流动力学测压管可能会影响尿流率速度。Groutz 观察对比了 7F 测压管在与自由尿流率时尿流率的数值，发现在插入测压管后尿流率会降低[46]。然而，其他研究并未发现同样的影响[47]。然而，谨慎的做法是，如果临床医生怀疑尿流动力学检查期间放置测压管对尿流率有影响，可以进行自由尿流率检测以确保不会由于测压管引起梗阻或患者排尿不适，影响检查结果。

十一、神经源性膀胱安全保障或顺应性差

逼尿肌漏尿点压力（DLPP）是在没有逼尿肌收缩或腹压升高的情况下发生尿液渗漏的最低逼尿肌压力值[48]。在骨髓增生异常的儿童中引入逼尿肌漏尿点压力测量作为上尿路恶化风险的指标[48]。在这些患者和其他神经源性下尿路功能障碍的患者中，逼尿肌漏尿点压力很重要，因为较高的逼尿肌漏尿点压力值与较高的上尿路病变风险相关。根据统计存在严重风险的逼尿肌漏尿点压力绝对值是 $40cmH_2O$[48]，但在成年人群中该值可能更高[32]。非神经源性患者不存在逼尿肌漏尿点压力，该术语容易在逼尿肌过度活动发生漏尿时与腹部漏尿点压力混淆。

对于神经源性下尿路功能障碍的患者进行尿流动力学检查的主要原因是他们的上尿路可能面临疾病风险，并且其中一些在尿流动力学检查中并没有发现明显的症状。在一个大型的评估系统中[32]，那些被诊断为脊柱裂和脊髓损伤的神经系统障碍的患者上尿路恶化的风险高于多发性硬化症，特别是肾积水的风险更高。膀胱顺应性差和逼尿肌漏尿点压力高都使患者处于风险之中。

膀胱顺应性的定义为膀胱容积压力测定过程中逼尿肌压力升高时膀胱容量的变化（图 4-7）。

$$顺应性 =\Delta 膀胱容量 /\Delta 逼尿肌压力$$

该计算忽略了逼尿肌过度活动所出现的逼尿肌压力变化，因为逼尿肌过度活动造成的逼尿肌压力变化会使顺应性的计算变得非常困难。此外，持续的膀胱收缩会使膀胱顺应性的计算失败，在膀胱容积压力测定过程停止膀胱灌注，也会使膀胱顺应性降低。这是确定压力上升的原因是由于逼尿肌过度活动还是膀胱顺应性降低造成的好方法。顺应性的正常值从 $<10ml/cmH_2O$ 到 $<30ml/cmH_2O$，但在大多数神经功能正常的人中，顺应性远远超过 $100ml/cmH_2O$。

逼尿肌过度活动在神经源性下尿路患者中是常见症状，发生率约为 60%[32] 并且是他们出现尿失禁的明确原因。最大逼尿肌压收缩力为 $35\sim115cmH_2O$，并且压力值 $>75cmH_2O$ 是上尿路扩张的风险因素[32]。收缩持续时间为 48～236s，

更长的时间预示肾积水的风险（236s vs. 114s），高达 44% 的神经源性下尿路功能障碍患者出现逼尿肌 / 括约肌协同失调，是上尿路扩张的另一个可预知的因素。

十二、通过影像学进行解剖诊断

在进行尿流动力学检查时，膀胱灌注溶液加入对比剂，同步进行影像检查，可获得额外的解剖信息，但会增加影像检查的操作负担以及对患者和尿流动力学检查人员的辐射显露风险。影像信息可以清楚地看到膀胱输尿管反流和膀胱颈异常。对诊断非常有帮助，特别是对于神经源性下尿路功能障碍患者[49]，影像尿流动力学检查可以帮助我们确定梗阻的来源，有助于诊断吊带造成梗阻的位置，盆腔器官脱垂造成的梗阻来源，以及功能障碍型排尿的尖陀螺膀胱尿道。其他发现可能包括尿道憩室、膀胱憩室或小梁（图 4–8 和图 4–9）。

总结

尿流动力学检查是诊断女性下尿路功能障碍的有力工具，当无创检查无法诊断时最好使用，准确的诊断对患者的治疗很重要。尿流动力学检查最好系统地进行，在检查过程中要谨慎地观察伪像，并了解患者的临床情况，以确保结果一致。如果在进行检测之前制订了一个清晰和简明的诊断问题，以确保获得最准确的结果，这样尿流动力学检查对临床也更有帮助。尿流动力学检查可以可靠地诊断压力性尿失禁、逼尿肌过度活动、逼尿肌收缩无力、膀胱出口梗阻和膀胱顺应性差，而影像学的加入可以进一步识别那些需要进行影像尿流动力学检查的特定患者的解剖异常。

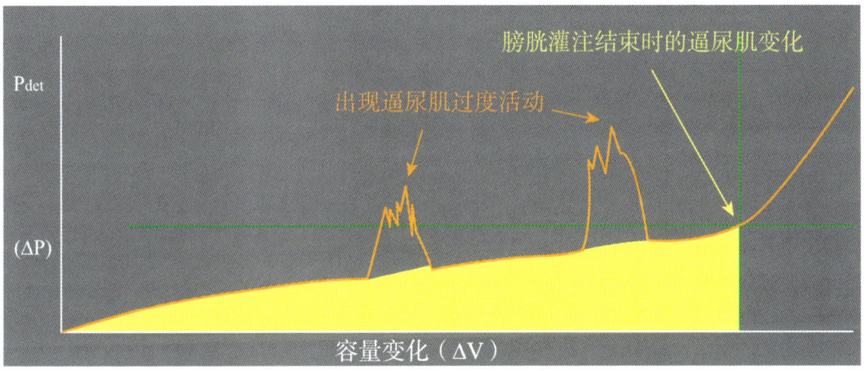

◀ 图 4–7 顺应性计算：黄色实心区域表示用于计算顺应性的最合适的体积关系。请注意，计算中仅使用初始顺应性曲线，而不是最终顺应性以及出现逼尿肌过度活动的情况

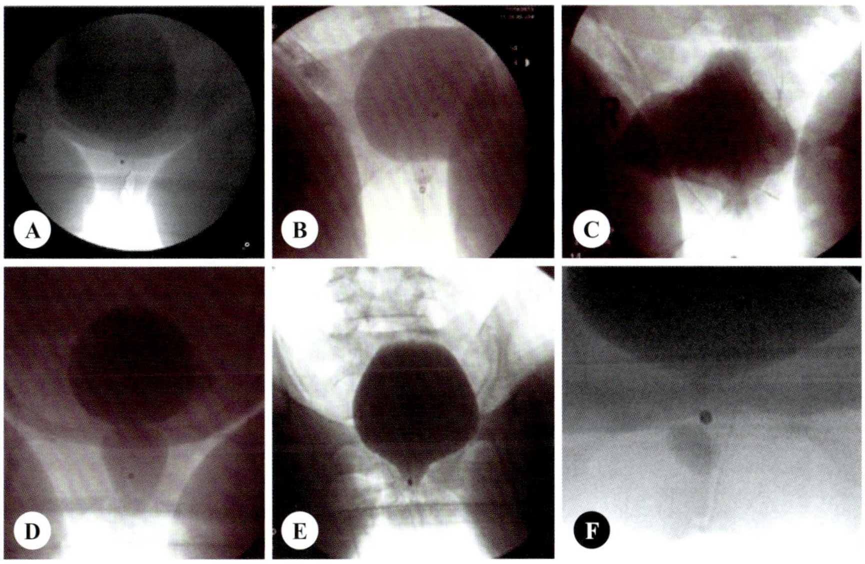

◀ 图 4–8 尿道造影检查结果：排尿时出现原发性膀胱颈梗阻（A），吊带固定的水平位置（B），多发性硬化症女性患者的逼尿肌 / 括约肌系统失调及形成膀胱小梁（C），严重的膀胱出口梗阻，并在尿道远端放置吊带，导致尿道梗阻和尿道扩张（D），排尿功能障碍伴尖陀螺膀胱尿道（E），偶然发现尿道憩室（F）

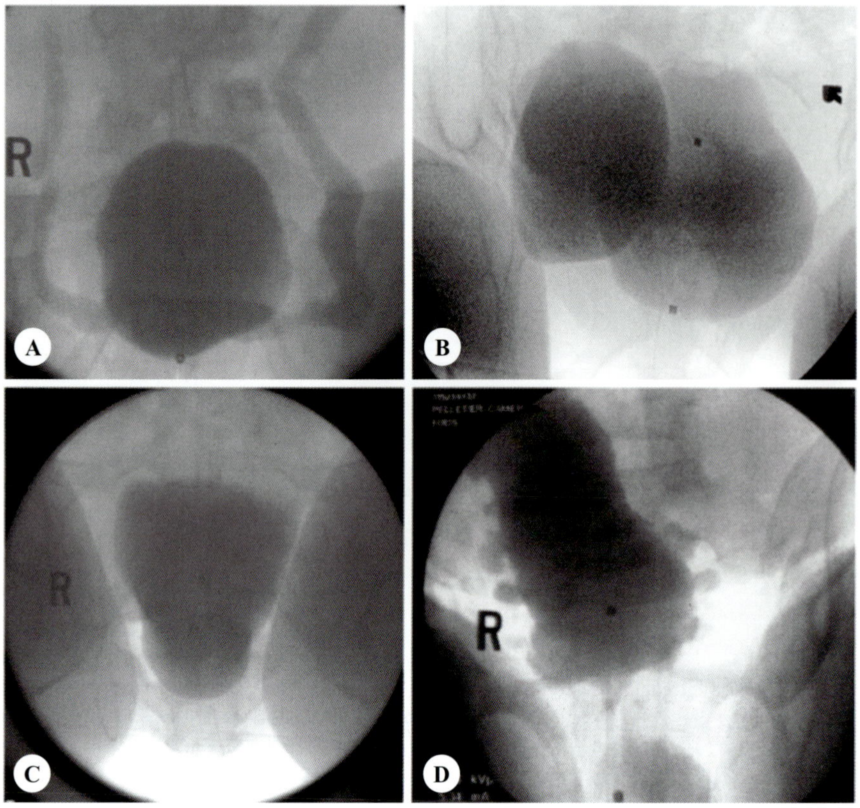

◀ 图 4-9 膀胱及输尿管造影结果：神经源性膀胱 4 级双侧反流（A），巨大膀胱憩室（B），引起排尿期膀胱出口梗阻的膀胱膨出（C），严重的膀胱小梁形成导致与膀胱顺应性差相关的圣诞树状膀胱（D）

参考文献

[1] Nager CW, FitzGerald MP, Kraus SR, Chai TC, Zyczynski H, Sirls L, et al. Urodynamic measures do not predict stress continence outcomes after surgery for stress urinary incontinence in selected women. J Urol. 2008;179(4):1470–4.

[2] Lloyd JC, Dielubanza E, Goldman HB. Trends in urodynamic testing prior to midurethral sling placement—what was the value of the VALUE trial? Neurourol Urodyn. 2018;37(3):1046–52.

[3] Chughtai B, Hauser N, Anger J, Asfaw T, Laor L, Mao J, et al. Trends in surgical management and pre-operative urodynamics in female medicare beneficiaries with mixed incontinence. Neurourol Urodyn. 2017;36(2):422–5.

[4] Suskind AM, Cox L, Clemens JQ, Oldendorf A, Stoffel JT, Malaeb B, et al. The value of urodynamics in an academic specialty referral practice. Urology. 2017;105:48–53.

[5] Nobrega RP, Solomon E, Jenks J, Greenwell T, Ockrim J. Predicting a successful outcome in sacral neuromodulation testing: are urodynamic parameters prognostic? Neurourol Urodyn. 2018;37(3):1007–10.

[6] Rachaneni S, Champaneria R, Latthe P. Does the outcome of botulinum toxin treatment differ in OAB patients with detrusor overactivity compared to those without detrusor overactivity?: a systematic review. Int Urogynecol J Pelvic Floor Dysfunct. 2015;26:S32–3.

[7] Subak LL, Brown JS, Kraus SR, Brubaker L, Lin F, Richter HE, et al. The "costs" of urinary incontinence for women. Obstet Gynecol [Internet]. 2006;107(4):908–16. Available from: http://www.pubmedcentral.nih.gov/articlerender.fcgi?artid=1557394&tool=pmcentrez&rend ertype=abstract

[8] Gormley EA, Lightner DJ, Faraday M, Vasavada SP. Diagnosis and treatment of overactive bladder (non-neurogenic) in adults: AUA/SUFU guideline amendment. J Urol [Internet]. 2015;193(5):1572–80. Available from: https://doi.org/10.1016/j.juro.2015.01.087

[9] Kobashi KC, Albo ME, Dmochowski RR, Ginsberg DA, Goldman HB, Gomelsky A, et al. Surgical treatment of female stress urinary incontinence: AUA/SUFU guideline. J Urol [Internet]. 2017;198(4):875–83. Available from: http://linkinghub.elsevier.com/retrieve/pii/ S0022534717748574

[10] Rosier PFWM, Schaefer W, Lose G, Goldman HB, Guralnick M, Eustice S, et al. International continence society good urodynamic practices and terms 2016: urodynamics, uroflowmetry, cystometry, and pressure-flow study. Neurourol Urodyn. 2017;36(5):1243–60.

[11] Peterson AC, Smith AR, Fraser MO, Yang CC, JOL DL, Gillespie BW, et al. The distribution of post-void residual volumes in people seeking care in the symptoms of lower urinary tract dysfunction network observational cohort study with comparison to asymptomatic populations. Urology. 2019;130:22–8.

[12] Al Afraa T, Mahfouz W, Campeau L, Corcos J. Normal lower urinary tract assessment in women: I. Uroflowmetry and post-void residual, pad tests, and bladder diaries. Int Urogynecol J. 2012;23(6):681–5.

[13] Abrams P. Bladder outlet obstruction index, bladder contractility index and bladder voiding efficiency: three simple indices to define bladder voiding function. BJU Int. 1999;84(1):14–5.

[14] Cameron AP, Wiseman JB, Smith AR, Merion RM, Gillespie BW, Bradley CS, et al. Are three-day voiding diaries feasible and reliable? Results from the symptoms of lower urinary tract dysfunction research network (LURN) cohort. Neurourol Urodyn. 2019;38(8):2185–93.

[15] Glass D, Lin FC, Khan AA, Van Kuiken M, Drain A, Siev M, et al. Impact of preoperative urodynamics on women undergoing pelvic organ prolapse surgery. Int Urogynecol J. 2020;31(8):1663–8.

[16] Suskind AM, Cox L, Clemens JQ, Oldendorf A, Stoffel JT, Malaeb

B, et al. The value of urodynamics in an academic specialty referral practice. Urology [Internet]. 2017;105:48–53. Available from: https://doi.org/10.1016/j.urology.2017.02.049

[17] Hooton TM, Bradley SF, Cardenas DD, Colgan R, Geerlings SE, Rice JC, et al. Diagnosis, prevention, and treatment of catheter-associated urinary tract infection in adults: 2009 international clinical practice guidelines from the Infectious Diseases Society of America. Clin Infect Dis [Internet]. 2010;50(5):625–63. Available from: http://cid.oxfordjournals.org/lookup/ doi/10.1086/650482

[18] Cameron AP, Campeau L, Brucker BM, Clemens JQ, Bales GT, Albo ME, et al. Best practice policy statement on urodynamic antibiotic prophylaxis in the non-index patient. Neurourol Urodyn. 2017;36(4):915–26.

[19] Litza JA, Brill JR. Urinary tract infections. Prim Care Clin Off Pract [Internet]. 2010;37(3):491–507. Available from: https://doi.org/10.1016/j.pop.2010.04.001

[20] Suskind AM, Clemens JQ, Kaufman SR, Stoffel JT, Oldendorf A, Malaeb BS, et al. Patient perceptions of physical and emotional discomfort related to urodynamic testing: a questionnaire-based study in men and women with and without neurologic conditions. Urology. 2015;85(3):547–51.

[21] Solomon ER, Ridgeway B. Interventions to decrease pain and anxiety in patients undergoing urodynamic testing: a randomized controlled trial. Neurourol Urodyn. 2016;35(8):975–9.

[22] Shaw C, Williams K, Assassa PR, Jackson C. Patient satisfaction with urodynamics: a qualitative study. J Adv Nurs. 2000;32(6):1356–63.

[23] Raz O, Tse V, Chan L. Urodynamic testing: physiological background, setting-up, calibration and artefacts. BJU Int. 2014;114(S1):22–8.

[24] Mahfouz W, Al Afraa T, Campeau L, Corcos J. Normal urodynamic parameters in women: part II – invasive urodynamics. Int Urogynecol J. 2012;23(3):269–77.

[25] D'Ancona CAL, Gomes MJ, Rosier PFWM. ICS teaching module: Cystometry (basic module). Neurourol Urodyn. 2017;36(7):1673–6.

[26] Drake MJ. Fundamentals of terminology in lower urinary tract function. Neurourol Urodyn. 2018;37(July):S13–9.

[27] Haylen BT, Freeman RM, Swift SE, Cosson M, Davila GW, Deprest J, et al. An international Urogynecological Association (IUGA) / International Continence Society (ICS) joint terminology and classification of the complications related directly to the insertion of prostheses (meshes, implants, tapes) & grafts in female pelvic flo. Int Urogynecol J. 2011;22(1):3–15.

[28] Seo YH, Kim SO, Yu HS, Kwon D. Leak point pressure at different bladder volumes in stress urinary incontinence in women: comparison between Valsalva and cough-induced leak point pressure. Can Urol Assoc J. 2016;10(1–2):E23–7.

[29] Maniam P, Goldman HB. Removal of transurethral catheter during urodynamics may unmask stress urinary incontinence. J Urol. 2002;167(5):2080–2.

[30] Parrillo LM, Ramchandani P, Smith AL. Can intrinsic sphincter deficiency be diagnosed by urodynamics? Urol Clin North Am [Internet]. 2014;41(3):375–81. Available from: https://doi. org/10.1016/j.ucl.2014.04.006

[31] D'Ancona C, Haylen B, Oelke M, Abranches-Monteiro L, Arnold E, Goldman H, et al. The International Continence Society (ICS) report on the terminology for adult male lower urinary tract and pelvic floor symptoms and dysfunction. Neurourol Urodyn. 2019;38(2):433–77.

[32] Musco S, Padilla-Fernández B, Del Popolo G, Bonifazi M, Blok BFM, Groen J, et al. Value of urodynamic findings in predicting upper urinary tract damage in neuro-urological patients: a systematic review. Neurourol Urodyn. 2018;37(5):1522–40.

[33] Groutz A, Blaivas JG, Chaikin DC. Bladder outlet obstruction in women: definition and characteristics. Neurourol Urodyn. 2000;19(3):213–20.

[34] Abarbanel J, Marcus EL. Impaired detrusor contractility in community-dwelling elderly presenting with lower urinary tract symptoms. Urology. 2007;69(3):436–40.

[35] Gammie A, Kaper M, Dorrepaal C, Kos T, Abrams P. Signs and symptoms of detrusor Underactivity: an analysis of clinical presentation and urodynamic tests from a large group of patients undergoing pressure flow studies. Eur Urol. 2016;69(2):361–9.

[36] Jeong SJ, Lee JK, Kim KM, Kook H, Cho SY, Oh SJ. How do we diagnose detrusor underactivity? Comparison of diagnostic criteria based on an urodynamic measure. Investig Clin Urol. 2017;58(4): 247–54.

[37] Rademakers K, Apostolidis A, Constantinou C, Fry C, Kirschner-Hermanns R, Oelke M, et al. Recommendations for future development of contractility and obstruction nomograms for women. ICI-RS 2014. Neurourol Urodyn. 2016;35(2):307–11.

[38] Defreitas GA, Zimmern PE, Lemack GE, Shariat SF. Refining diagnosis of anatomic female bladder outlet obstruction: comparison of pressure-flow study parameters in clinically obstructed women with those of normal controls. Urology. 2004;4(4):675–9.

[39] Kuo HC. Videourodynamic characteristics and lower urinary tract symptoms of female bladder outlet obstruction. Urology. 2005;66(5):1005–9.

[40] Blaivas JG, Groutz A. Bladder outlet obstruction nomogram for women with lower urinary tract symptomatology. Neurourol Urodyn. 2000;19(5):553–64.

[41] Nitti VW, Tu LM, Gitlin J. Diagnosing bladder outlet obstruction in women. J Urol. 1999;161(5):1535–40.

[42] Akikwala TV, Fleischman N, Nitti VW. Comparison of diagnostic criteria for female bladder outlet obstruction. J Urol. 2006;176(5): 2093–7.

[43] Solomon E, Yasmin H, Duffy M, Rashid T, Akinluyi E, Greenwell TJ. Developing and validating a new nomogram for diagnosing bladder outlet obstruction in women. Neurourol Urodyn. 2018;37(1):368–78.

[44] Lindsay J, Solomon E, Nadeem M, Pakzad M, Hamid R, Ockrim J, et al. Treatment validation of the Solomon-Greenwell nomogram for female bladder outlet obstruction. Neurourol Urodyn. 2020;39(5):1371–7.

[45] Aponte MM, Shah SR, Hickling D, Brucker BM, Rosenblum N, Nitti VW. Urodynamics for clinically suspected obstruction after anti-incontinence surgery in women. J Urol. 2013;190(2):598–602.

[46] Groutz A, Blaivas JG, Sassone AM. Detrusor pressure uroflowmetry studies in women: effect of a 7Fr transurethral catheter. J Urol. 2000;164(1):109–14.

[47] Harding C, Horsburgh B, Dorkin TJ, Thorpe AC. Quantifying the effect of urodynamic catheters on urine flow rate measurement. Neurourol Urodyn. 2012;31(1):139–42.

[48] McGuire EJ. Urodynamics of the neurogenic bladder. Urol Clin N Am. 2010;37(4):507–16.

[49] Winters JC, Dmochowski RR, Goldman HB, Herndon CDA, Kobashi KC, Kraus SR, et al. Urodynamic studies in adults: AUA/SUFU guideline. J Urol. 2012;188(6 SUPPL):2464–72.

第 5 章　历史上用于治疗女性压力性尿失禁和急迫性尿失禁的相关技术

Historical Treatment of SUI and UUI in Women

Justina Tam　Una J. Lee　著

女性尿失禁非常普遍，据报道影响了 5%～70% 的人口，随着年龄的增长，患病率不断增加[1]。由于其高患病率，患者渴望得到有效的治疗，同时更好的理解排尿的病理生理机制。尿失禁的原理随着时间的推移而发展。这些机制反映在当时各种手术技术中，同时也体现了当时人们对尿失禁的解剖和功能的理解。尽管许多这些历史上的外科手术不再进行，但对这些技术的机制了解对于理解女性尿失禁手术的现状很重要。此外，一些患者可能曾接受过目前开展的导致解剖或生理改变的抗失禁手术，因此了解这些手术对于既往接受过手术并现在需要治疗女性至关重要。本章的目的是回顾历史上一些治疗女性压力性尿失禁和急迫性尿失禁的方法。

关于尿失禁的第一个书面资料是公元前 2000 年的埃及手稿，其中描述了男性尿液收集装置和女性子宫托[2]。从那时起，一些非侵入性治疗就用于治疗压力性尿失禁，如女性尿道塞、电疗、手术切除部分尿道壁以缩小尿道直径，以及尿道松解术和尿道扭转等[2]。在本章中，我们描述了现代医生可能遇到的治疗尿失禁的历史上曾使用的技术。

一、原生组织扩张

由 Howard A. Kelly 于 1900 年实施的 Kelly 折叠术是第一个用于治疗女性压力性尿失禁的手术技术，该技术已成为临床常规手术。Kelly 折叠术在 19 世纪末由 Schultz 首次报道[3]，该技术涉及前阴道修补术，以及在盆腔内筋膜中的褥式缝合来折叠膀胱颈[2, 4]来缩小膀胱颈及后尿道角[5]。在手术过程中，在阴道壁上做一个垂直切口并从侧面组织间隙解剖，露出膀胱颈和阴道旁间隙[3]。将骨盆内筋膜缝合在一起，在中线形成一个组织桥，以支撑膀胱颈和近端尿道（图 5-1）。

整个 20 世纪 80 年代使用和改进了前侧阴道缝合术 –Kelly 折叠术，并有多个出版物记录了其有效性。然而，长期结果并没有那么理想，5 年目标成功率为 37%[7] 和 5 年客观压力性尿失禁率为 46.81%[8]。到 21 世纪初，Kelly 折叠术已在很大程度上被其他尿失禁手术取代[9, 10]（表 5-1）。

1947 年描述的 Ingelman-Sundberg 耻骨尾骨修复术[11]是在阴道前壁的外尿道口下方使用弓形切口，然后将膀胱韧带、耻骨尾骨肌和球海绵体肌缝合到中线以支撑尿道[12]（图 5-2）。3 年随访的结果显示，这种手术后尿失禁的治愈率为 92%[14]。在 10～20 年的随访中，患者报告的治愈率为 56.2%～84%[12, 15]。但同时直肠前突发生率及直肠前突修复后复发率较高（54.9%）。作者推测可能是由于肛提肌内侧部分或相关底层组织切除导致的结缔组织功能不全所至[12]。

二、自体组织耻骨后悬吊术

自体组织耻骨后悬吊术。这种手术最先使用的是自体的肌肉，当时的术者认为肌肉会像括约肌一样收缩[5]。这种术式由 Van Giordano 在 1907 年第一次报道，他使用股薄肌。然后 Goebell 在

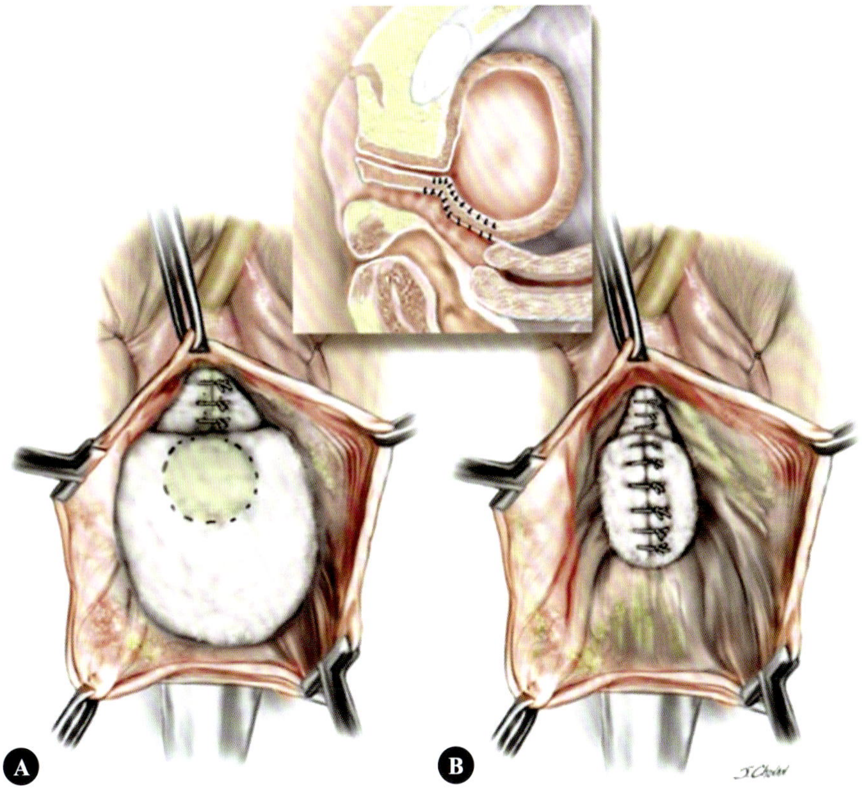

◀ 图 5-1 Kelly 折叠术中阴道前壁修补术

A. 把阴道黏膜切开，在尿道的下方缝合；B. 尿道周围的缝线最终在中线处打结缝合，用于支撑尿道近端上方的膀胱颈（图片由 Maher 和 Karram 提供[6]）

1910 年使用了锥体肌。Frangenheim 在 1914 年使用了锥体肌和直肌筋膜[2, 3, 5]。1917 年，Stoeckel 进一步将锥体肌 – 直肌筋膜吊带与膀胱颈的经阴道肌肉折叠缝合。这个术式现在被称为 Goebell-Frangenheim-Stoeckel 手术[2]。在这个术式中，把一条带有锥体肌的带蒂垂直直肌筋膜分开并旋转到尿道下，从两侧包围尿道。据报道，这个术式的成功率为 84%～88%[16, 17]，有报道 2 年后有效率会下降[16]。在平均 68 个月的随访中，有文献报道这种术式的成功率为 91.5%～96%，而在另一个文献中[17] 报道这种术式后有 73% 的患者有中等及以上的治疗效果，只有 27% 的患者治疗效果较差。该手术的术后并发症包括需要导尿缓解的暂时性尿潴留（60%）、排尿刺激症状（37.5%）和轻微尿道梗阻（12.5%）[17]。

在历史上人们还曾经使用过（包括阴道上皮在内）一条阴道组织的阴道吊带手术[18]。这条组织放置在尿道后部，组织的末端穿过前腹壁后缝合在一起，正好在耻骨联合上方[18]（图 5-3）。作者报道的 19 例患者中有 16 例治愈，2 例好转，1 例术后后腹部外伤导致吊带破裂和失禁复发[18]。

虽然利用肌肉组织和阴道上皮做吊带的手术已不再普遍使用，但使用筋膜作为吊带的改良版手术目前仍在开展，这些筋膜包括自体阔筋膜。1933 年，Price 将其改良为耻骨后方法，这种术式使用阔筋膜组织带通过尿道下方固定到直肌[19]。1942 年，Aldridge 也将这种手术进行了改良。他使用前直肌筋膜的横向组织带通过尿道下方的耻骨后入缝合在中线上[20, 21]。据报道，Aldridge 筋膜吊带术后的治愈率为 78%～86%[22-24]，在 16 年的随访中有效率可能降至 71%[25]。有关这种术式与目前仍在使用的现代手术（利用耻骨后自体直肌筋膜和阔筋膜作为吊索）的长期效果与并发症将在第 17 章描述。

三、膀胱尿道固定术

Marshall-Marchetti-Krantz 膀胱尿道固定术（MMK）于 1949 年被开创。这是一种耻骨后手术，这种术式的缝合线主要位于尿道周围组织和膀胱颈，耻骨骨膜或耻骨联合软骨上，尿道和膀

表 5-1 在医疗保险数据中反映的因压力性尿失禁接受治疗的女性患者的数量趋势 [a]

手术方式	2002 年	2003 年	2004 年	2005 年	2006 年	2007 年	总 数
耻骨阴道悬吊术	25 840（5270）	28 580（5749）	31 480（6269）	31 640（6185）	33 300（6525）	33 880（6693）	184 720
尿道膨胀术	14 100（2875）	12 100（2434）	11 300（2250）	10 160（1986）	10 980（2151）	11 320（2236）	69 960
尿道固定术	4340（885）	2480（499）	1820（362）	1360（266）	1080（212）	820（162）	11 900
包括全子宫切除的阴道尿道固定术	2900（591）	3320（668）	2740（546）	2280（446）	2440（478）	3100（612）	16 780
Raz- 形悬吊术	1100（224）	680（137）	480（96）	320（63）	220（43）	100（20）	2900
腹腔镜下修补术	680（139）	600（121）	540（108）	480（94）	500（98）	560（111）	3360
Pereyra 术式	240（49）	140（28）	100（20）	160（31）	40（8）	40（8）	720
Kelly 折叠术	140（29）	120（24）	140（28）	220（43）	140（27）	80（16）	840
总 数	**49 340**	**48 020**	**48 600**	**46 620**	**48 700**	**49 900**	**291 180**

a. 数据用具体数字展示，其中未加权的数据乘 20 计算。括号中的数是医疗系统中每 10 万女性患者以尿失禁未主要诊断接受治疗的人数

引自 Rogo-Gupta et al.[10]

胱颈部上方和前方[26]（图 5-4）。额外的缝合线也被放置到膀胱和直肌的浆膜中，以将膀胱向前拉入 Retzius 的空隙，以帮助患者在咳嗽或提举时将膀胱与膀胱颈一起抬高[26]。据报道，在一些既往接受尿失禁手术并失败的患者中，进行 MMK 后的主观尿失禁率分别为 92% 和 84.5%[27]。在文献报道中，5 年长期主观失禁率为 85.7%，15 年为 75%[28]。文献中报道的 MMK 并发症包括耻骨骨炎（发生率为 0.74%～2.5%）[27, 29]、继发于缝合的输尿管梗阻，以及膀胱 – 输尿管交界处梗阻[30]。

Burch 手术开创的灵感起源于 John C. Burch 的报道，他指出由于可视化不良和耻骨后联合骨膜在 MMK[31] 期间没有将缝合线固定到位而导致缝合线放置困难。最初，在 Burch 阴道悬吊术中，将缝合线放置在膀胱颈和近端尿道外侧的阴道旁组织中，并将这些组织用缝合线悬吊在筋膜骨盆的腱弓上。后来又进行了修改，利用了骨盆侧壁上的同侧髂耻（库珀）韧带[32]（图 5-5）。额外的缝合线也可以放置在外侧阴道穹窿水平并固定到髂耻韧带上，为外侧或阴道旁缺损提供支撑。Cochrane 分析报道称，Burch 手术后第一年尿失禁总体控制率为 85%～90%，在 5 年后为 70%[34]。该术式可以通过开放式或腹腔镜方法进行，Cochrane 分析的数据表明开放式和腹腔镜阴道悬吊术在短期内治疗尿失禁同样有效[35]。报告指出与 Burch 阴道悬吊相关的并发症包括术后血肿或出血，发生率为 2%[36]（这被认为与由于缝合时前组织暴露不足导致的阴道旁静脉损伤有关[32]），膀胱损伤（高达 9.6%，更常见于之前的盆腔手术），输尿管扭结（高达 2%），尿路感染（UTI）

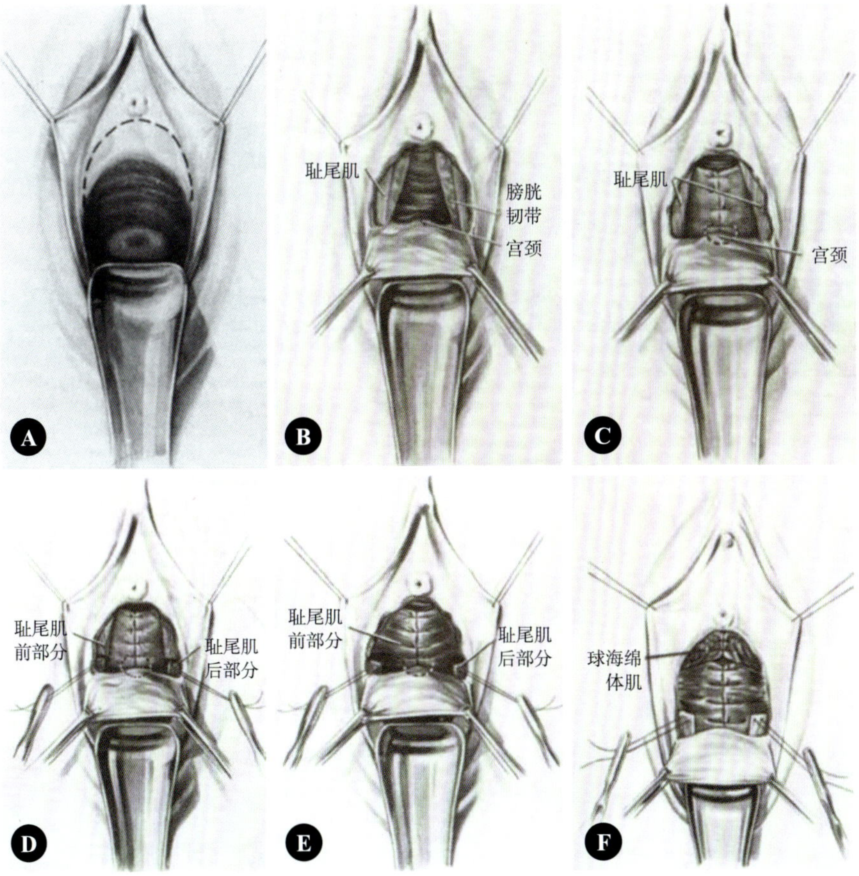

◀ **图 5-2　Ingleman-Sundberg 耻骨尾骨修补术**

A 和 B. 切开阴道前壁黏膜暴露膀胱韧带，耻骨尾骨肌，球海绵体肌；C 至 F. 将这些组织缝合至中线处来支撑尿道

图片由 Ingelman-Sundberg 提供[13]

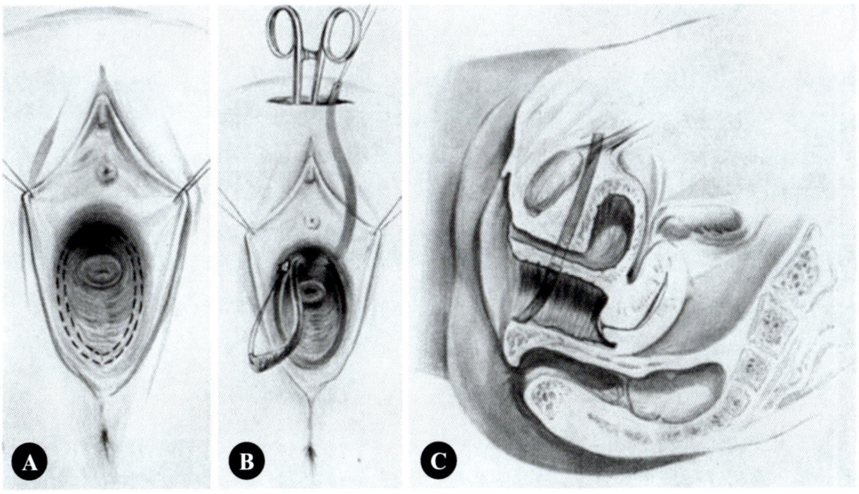

◀ **图 5-3　阴道悬吊术式由 Ingelman-Sundberg 开创**

A. 切两片大约 15mm 的包括阴道全层组织；B. 尿管放置到膀胱后，在耻骨联合上方做一个小切口，用一把手术钳通过 Retzius 空隙与阴道内尿道旁组织内的术者手指相汇合；C. 将两侧先前切下的阴道组织分别通过前腹壁到达耻骨联合上方缝合在一起

图片由 Ingelman-Sundberg 提供[18]

（高达 40%，取决于尿路感染的定义），伤口感染（高达 10.8%），尿潴留（＜3%）、逼尿肌不稳定（高达 8%）、性交困难（高达 4%）和术后小肠膨出或其他生殖器官脱垂（7.6%～26.7%）[36-40]。关于 Burch 阴道悬吊相关的生殖器脱垂，病因尚不明确。然而，这种相关的上位器官脱垂可能与盆腔器官脱垂的自然发展[32, 39]导致阴道方向的受力变化[40]有关，或者可能与手术导致的盆底肌肉神经损伤相关[41]。该术式仍在使用，详细描述见第 15 章。

四、探针悬吊术式

历史上还有许多针悬吊手术。所有这些手术都是通过用针穿过下腹部和阴道切口，在尿道旁

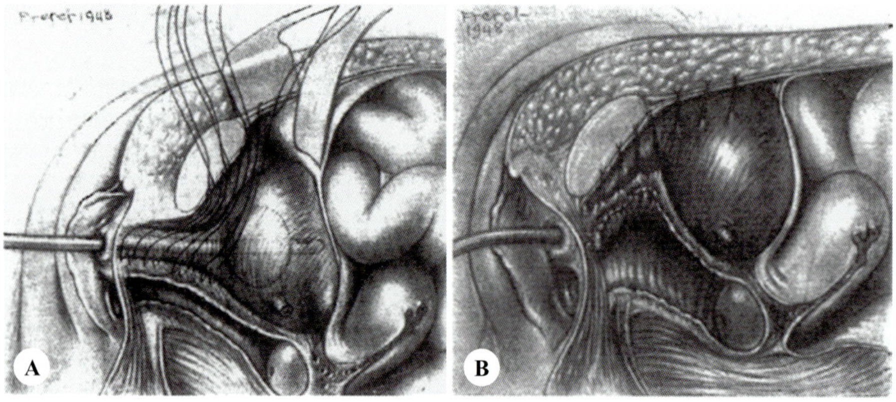

◀ 图 5-4 **Marshall-Marchetti-Krantz 膀胱尿道固定术（MMK）**

A. 矢状面展示左侧尿道旁的缝合位点；B. 缝合线向下显露尿道，膀胱颈使膀胱的位置向上向前移动

图片由 Marshall et al. 提供[26]

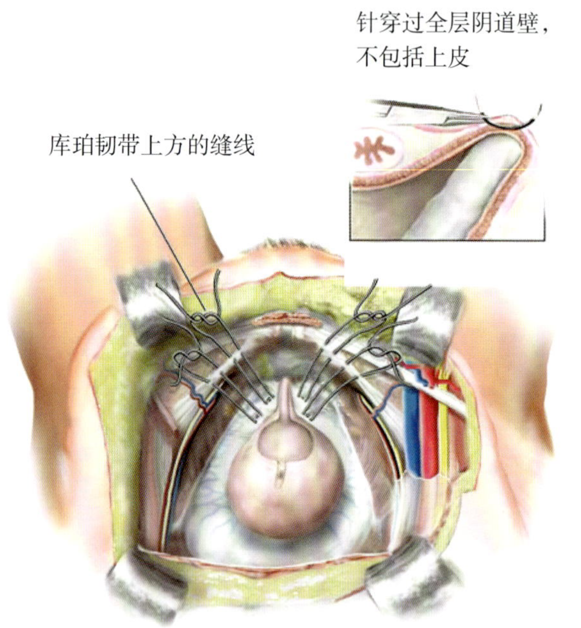

▲ 图 5-5 **Burch 阴道悬吊术，在尿道及膀胱颈的近端做 8 字缝合，并向上将尿道及膀胱颈周围组织缝合至同侧腰髂处的库珀韧带上**

图片由 Baggish 和 Karram 提供[33]，Fig.34.4

组织中放置缝合线来将尿道恢复到良好支撑的位置从而纠正压力性尿失禁。1959 年，Pereyra 开创了一种术式，用特殊针穿过耻骨上小切口[42-44]。将阴道上皮与尿道旁组织分离后，将针从耻骨后面穿过尿道外侧并引导到手指上，穿过尿道旁组织（图 5-6）。最初的术式中用钢丝来支撑组织，从而形成两圈钢丝，每条钢丝穿过腹壁、尿道旁组织，然后回到腹壁。然后将金属丝拉紧使尿道和膀胱颈适当抬高，并系在直肌筋膜水平。由于这些金属丝预计会随着时间的推移穿过阴道和尿道旁组织。当金属丝的位置改变，而由原来金属丝所在位置产生的瘢痕组织会继续支撑尿管及膀胱颈。术中沿近端侧尿道也进行了烧灼，以帮助形成瘢痕组织。由于膀胱镜检查未作为该术式的一部分进行，导致导线通过膀胱时可能损伤膀胱，因此该手术后面被进一步改良，如使用铬缝线代替钢丝。Stamey 和 Raz 修改对这个术式进行了经验改良，在术中暴露耻骨尿道韧带，然后与缝合线一起悬吊[45, 46]，详细描述见下文。报道的成功率参差不齐，据 Peyrera 和 Lebherz 报道，在 12～24 个月的随访中治愈或显著改善率为 94%[44]，在长达 36.3 个月[47]的长期随访中，数据显示在无并发症的复发性压力性尿失禁的女性中，治愈率为 81.6%。然而，其他作者的文献报道 1 年治愈率<50%，平均随访 23.2 个月的治愈率<53.6%[43, 48]。与改良 Pereyra 探针悬吊手术相关的并发症包括伤口感染（5.5%）、尿路感染（3.7%）、阴道壁血肿（3.7%）、新发急迫性尿失禁和新发逼尿肌不稳定（11.1%）、术后需自行导尿的间歇性阻塞性排尿困难（9.3%）、肠膨出（5.6%），以及复发性膀胱膨出或直肠膨出（5.6%）[47]。

1973 年，Stamey 手术开始应用，在阴道内切口，通过在尿道两侧放置 1cm 直径 5mm 的聚对苯二甲酸涤纶管作为支撑物的尼龙单丝缝合线完成对尿道和膀胱颈悬吊（图 5-7）。缝合线在同侧相系，不越过中线，张力适中[46]。Stamey 首先在这种手术中引进了膀胱镜的使用，以评估缝合线的

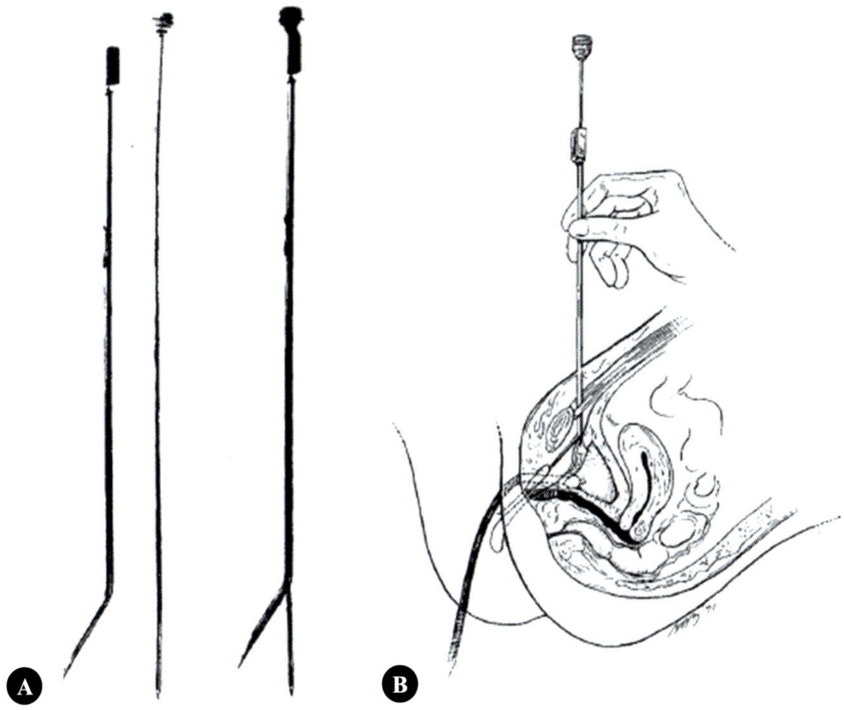

◀ 图 5-6　**Peyrera 探针装置**

A. Peyrera 导管它包括一个有倾斜尖端的针；一个中空的手柄。探针和手柄的针眼是对称的，这样探针能通过手柄来实施缝合。B. Peyrera 导管通过耻骨联合上方的切口进入一侧的尿道周围组织中，再将探针通过导管的第二个孔进入尿道周围组织，将尿道周围组织缝合至腹直肌前筋膜。同法处理对侧

图片由 Kursh et al. 提供[43]

位置和引导针的通过。长期随访评估表明，治愈率随着时间的推移而下降，成功率参差不齐。报道的 10 年治愈率为 33%～76.4%[50, 51]，15 年治愈率为 47.9%[52]。一项平均随访 66 个月的研究表明，50% 的患者在整个随访期间保持完全自主小便，11.5% 的患者最初失败，38.5% 的患者在初始完全自主小便的情况下在 6～90 个月后尿失禁复发[53]。患者还被问及他们对手术结果的满意度，35.7% 报告完全治愈，27% 有明显改善，12.7% 有轻微改善，12.7% 没有变化，11.9% 有更差的结果。这种术式并发症包括腹膜穿孔伴急腹症需要剖腹探查（1.1%）、出血 / 血肿（2.7%）、感染（31.1%）、耻骨上疼痛延长（6.5%）和尿流梗阻（8.2%）[53]。

1981 年，Raz 手术被报道，这种术式利用倒 U 形阴道切口放置耻骨上导管。穿孔盆内筋膜并通过阴道切口形成耻骨后间隙[54]，包括耻骨颈筋膜、尿道骨盆韧带的内侧切割边缘和阴道壁，不包括阴道上皮（图 5-8），以螺旋方式双侧放置不可吸收的聚丙烯缝合线。然后进行耻骨上切口并向下解剖至前直肌筋膜。将结扎针穿过耻骨上切口进入阴道，然后将阴道缝线转移到耻骨上切口以最小的张力穿过前直肌筋膜的中线[46, 54] 系在一起。膀胱镜检查作为该术式的一部分来评估膀胱或输尿管损伤。平均随访 15 个月的短期效果显示有效率为 90.3%，定义为压力性尿失禁治愈或显著改善[56]。这些结果还按失禁的严重程度进行分层，并证明 Raz 膀胱颈悬吊的成功取决于压力性尿失禁的严重程度，据报道，在轻度至中度压力性尿失禁的女性中成功率>90%，在重度压力性尿失禁的女性中成功率为 65%[56]。然而，长期研究表明成功率参差不齐，在平均 9.8 年的随访中，20% 的患者报道没有尿失禁，51% 的患者报道压力性尿失禁伴或不伴急迫性尿失禁[57]。尽管压力性尿失禁复发或持续存在，但 71% 的患者报道尿失禁显著改善，73% 的患者报道对手术结果满意[57]。短期效果较理想，主要是因为选择接受了 Raz 手术的压力性尿失禁患者伴有或不伴有轻度（1 级）膀胱膨出[56]，这表明患者的选择可能影响了手术的成功率。Raz 手术报道的并发症包括新发急迫性尿失禁（7.5%）、继发性盆腔脱垂（6%）、长期滞留（2.5%）和耻骨上疼痛（3%）[56]。

Gittes 手术在 1987 年被开创。这种术式不使用切口，用单丝缝合线通过皮肤和阴道穿孔将双侧阴道壁和尿道旁组织的深层缝合[58]。用一根

针穿过前直肌筋膜并进入阴道，将阴道壁的全层缝合，包括上皮细胞（图 5-9）。放置阴道缝线后，将缝线向上传递至前直肌筋膜。然后以最小的张力穿过中线将同侧缝合线绑在一起[46]。据报道，在 53 个月时，尿失禁完全和部分改善率为 23.1%[59]，在 5 年时为 14%[60]，在 62.5 个月为 72.6% 时[61]，在 6.4 年为 37%[51]。报道的并发症包括伤口感染（2.3%）、反复尿路感染（1.1%）、需要拆线的持续腹股沟疼痛（5.7%），以及重新出现的术后尿急和（或）急迫性尿失禁（20%）[59, 62]。

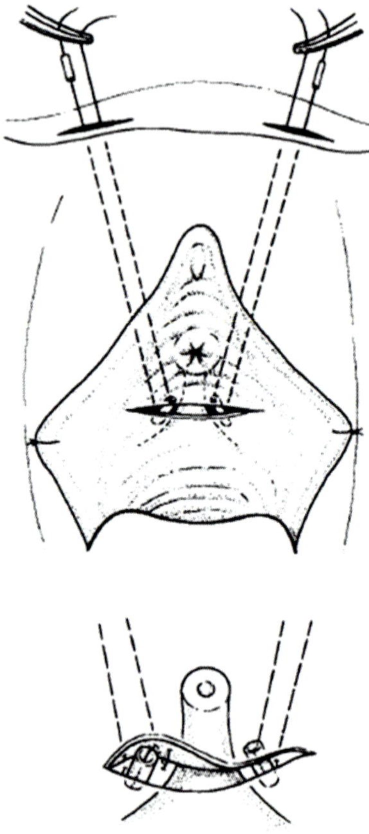

▲ 图 5-7 **Stamey 探针悬吊术式**
将尿道两侧的组织依次缝合至特定的纽扣上
图片由 Hilton 和 Mayne 提供[49]

Benderev（或 Vesica）术式开发于 1994 年[63, 64]。做 1 个切口或 2 个小切口以允许骨锚进入双侧耻骨结节，将骨锚放置在每个耻骨结节中，并使用缝线穿引器从耻骨上切口将附着的缝线穿过膀胱颈水平的阴道，将缝合线以 Z 形配置放入阴道上皮[46, 64]（图 5-10），然后通过在耻骨和缝合线结之间放置间隔装置将缝合线系在耻骨上区域。报告的完全缓解率在 6 个月时为 85%，在 12 个月时为 46%～94%[65, 66]，在 5 年时为 31%[66]。基于这些长期结果，研究人员不再提倡这种形式的膀胱颈悬吊来治疗压力性尿失禁。在复发性尿失禁患者中，70% 的症状足以再一次接受进一步的手术治疗。在随后接受 Burch 阴道悬吊术的患者中，注意到骨锚栓处的 Vesica 悬缝线磨损和断裂，这被认为是 Benderev 或 Vesica 手术失败的原因。

对于这个术式，被报道的并发症包括伤口感染（16%）、需要临时导尿的间歇性尿路梗阻（4.7%～10%）、缝合线侵蚀到膀胱（5%）、缝合线侵蚀到阴道（2.56%）、假定耻骨骨炎（1.2%～5%）和短暂的逼尿肌不稳定性（7%）[65-67]。

五、尿道膨胀术

几种经尿道注射的物质已被用于尿道扩张，目的是为了改善尿道衔接，从而改善压力性尿失

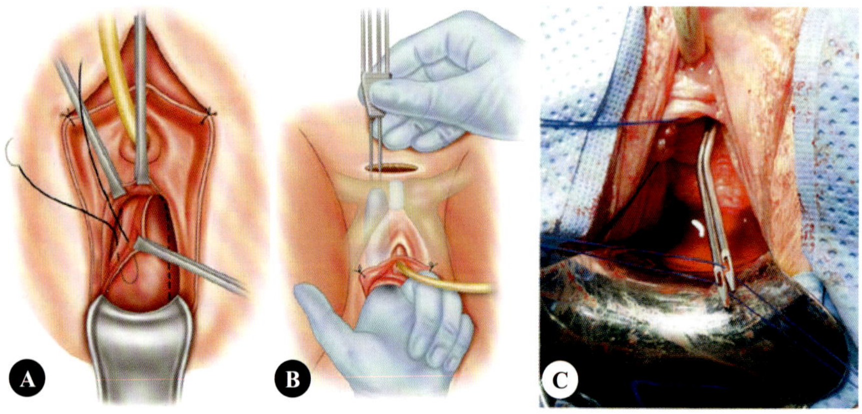

◀ 图 5-8 **Raz 探针悬吊术式**
A. 在膀胱颈旁起到悬吊作用的缝合的位点；B. 在术者手指的引导下将探针从耻骨联合上方的切口穿至阴道壁的切口，再用 Raz 探针将双层缝线从阴道内切口引导至耻骨联合上方；C. 缝线通过探针的眼通过耻骨联合上方的切口进入阴道切口最终回到耻骨联合上方
图片引自 Raz[55]，p.44，46，47，Fig.2.13，2.20，2.21

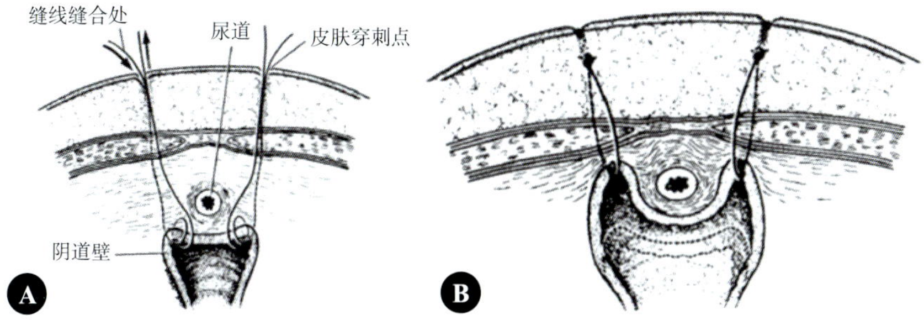

◀ 图 5-9 Gittes 探针悬吊术式

A. 没有切口，只需做皮肤到阴道的贯穿孔。探针通过腹直肌前筋膜进入阴道然后穿透阴道壁的全程包括上皮组织到达膀胱颈的水平，在阴道内缝合后缝线穿回到腹直肌前筋膜。B. 缝线最后在耻骨上方的脂肪组织中打结

图片由 Gittes 和 Loughlin 提供[58]

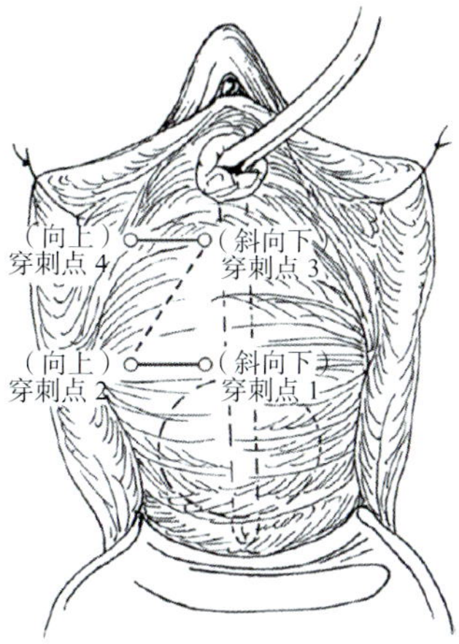

▲ 图 5-10 如图展示 Benderev（Vesica）探针悬吊术中缝合线穿过阴道壁的位点

图片由 Bodell 和 Leach 提供[46]

禁。19 世纪末，Gersuny 首先提出在尿道周围注射石蜡[2]。1938 年报道了注射鱼肝油，1 年治愈率为 60%，改善率为 25%[63]。1973 年，Politano 和 Berg[69, 70] 首次报道了 Tefon 的应用。据报道，24 个月时尿失禁的治愈率或改善率为 30%～38%[71]，但同时会导致尿道梗阻和纤维化，或者 Tefon 迁移至淋巴结，引起肉芽肿[2, 3]。1989 年，Gonzalez de Gariby 开创了自体脂肪组织注射，3 个月时尿失禁的治愈率或改善率为 22.2%，与注射盐水没有区别，但有可能导致肺脂肪栓塞[72, 73]。1989 年，Shortliffe 开创了胶原蛋白注射液，在 9～23 个月的随访中发现，其治愈率或改善率为 53%[74]。目前已经开创了一些较新的尿道填充剂（以上试剂不再使用），详细讨论见第 14 章。

六、膀胱神经组织切除术

1959 年，Ingelman-Sundberg 报道了通过单侧或双侧切除下腹下神经丛来切除膀胱神经，以治疗神经源性原因引起的急迫性尿失禁或间质性膀胱炎引起的膀胱收缩[75]（图 5-11）。在进行去神经支配之前需要进行术前测试。进行膀胱测压后，将含有肾上腺素的木卡因溶液单侧注射到前穹窿宫颈外侧 1cm，深度 3cm 处，使膀胱去神经。注射后 5min 重复膀胱测压，检查后排尿残留。如果单侧注射后膀胱测压显示无抑制收缩和膀胱容量有所改善，则进行单侧切除。如果膀胱测压没有改善，则在对侧进行相同的注射，重复膀胱测压和残余尿。如果第二次注射后膀胱测压有所改善，则进行双侧切除。如果后空隙残留量升高，则仅进行单侧切除。如果单侧麻醉后残余尿量＞150ml，则不应进行该手术。该手术是经阴道进行的，首先在外尿道口下方行横向切口。阴道前壁从尿道口一直到子宫颈，将膀胱韧带与肛提肌钝性分离，将腹下神经丛从外侧显露于直肠，内侧往下分离膀胱血管[76]，然后暴露并切除神经。在 44.1 个月的平均随访中，报告的中指出手术后的完全或部分缓解率为 67.8%（54% 完全缓解者）[76]，而 Inglman-Sundberg 报告的长期缓解率为 70%（未明确平均随访时间）[77]。

膀胱旁神经丛的经膀胱苯酚注射，通过注射苯酚损伤膀胱的节后神经纤维来治疗难治性逼尿肌不稳定性 / 逼尿肌反射亢进。这种术式的缓解率为 11%～82%[78-80]，而且手术过程中可能导致的严重并发症，如逼尿肌痉挛和瘘管形成[81, 82]。既往有盆腔放疗史的被认为是这种治疗的绝对禁忌证[83]。由于疗效差和并发症的风险大，这种治疗不被推荐并且不再使用[78]。鉴于神经消融手术的潜在长期影响和去神经组织可能比手术前处于更

病理状态[84]，其他方式神经调节技术可能会变得更受青睐。

七、逼尿肌切除术

逼尿肌切除术，也称为自动增强术，由 Cartwright 和 Snow 于 1989 年首次开创，为了避免与肠道增强术相似的并发症，其中包括电解质紊乱、肠瘘、脓肿、黏液产生和腹膜粘连[85]，在这个手术中，切除膀胱圆顶上的逼尿肌来保持膀胱上皮完整（图 5-12）。切除逼尿肌后形成一个大的、宽口的、引流良好的膀胱上皮憩室隆起。据报道，长期有效率为 60%～80%[86-88]，特发性膀胱过度活动症患者的成功率高于神经源性逼尿肌过度活动症患者（70%～79% vs. 33%～50%）[86, 87]。该术式的并发症包括需要导尿的间歇性尿路梗阻（45%）和尿路感染（31.5%）[87]。一些研究者指出，在治疗神经源性排尿功能障碍的患者时，不建议使用该术式[89]。但也有研究者推荐这种术式，因为泌尿科医师的医疗设备使这种手术变得简单且降低了并发症的发生率。即使逼尿肌切除术 / 肌切开术失败了，也可进行肠膀胱成形术进行修补[90, 91]。

总结

早在公元前 2 世纪，尿失禁的治疗就已有文献记载，范围从侵入性较小的治疗（如尿道塞）到尿道和膀胱颈的折叠，再到各种迭代的针头悬吊术、阴道悬吊术、自动增强和膀胱去神经。上文回顾了历史上用于治疗女性压力性尿失禁的手

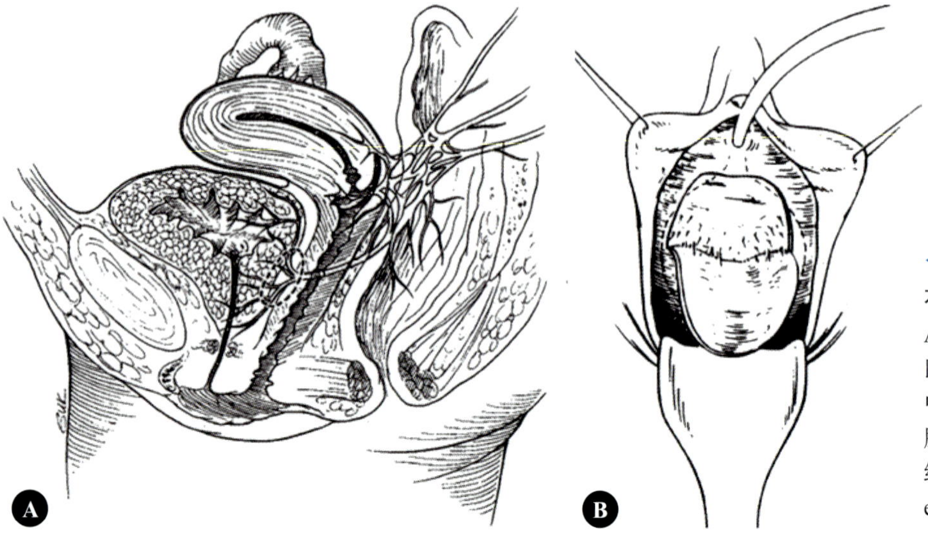

◀ 图 5-11 膀胱神经组织切除术用于治疗急迫性尿失禁

A. 盆腔的神经末梢在膀胱三角区进入膀胱分布示意图；B. 图中展示了阴道壁上皮的解剖和膀胱三角区水平的膀胱周围组织筋膜的解剖（图片由 Westney et al. 提供[76]）

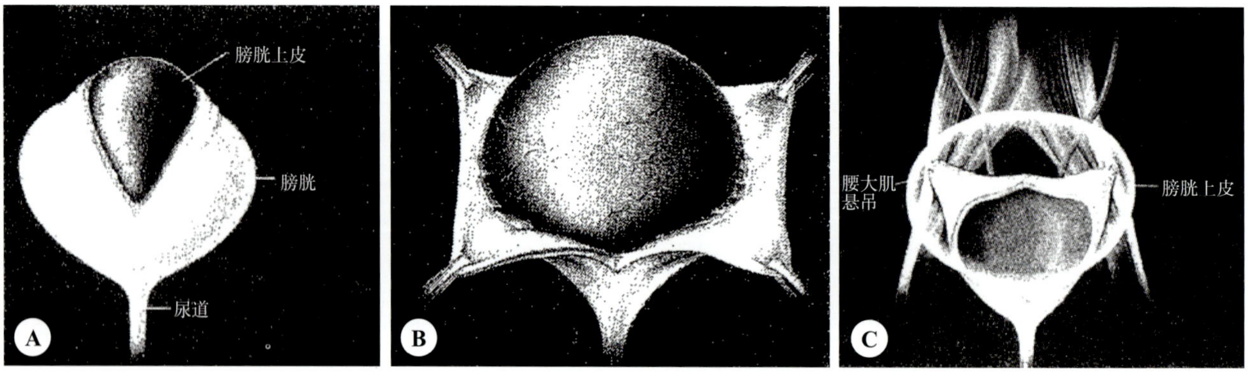

▲ 图 5-12 膀胱逼尿肌的切除也被称为膀胱自体扩充术

A. 切开膀胱上的逼尿肌，同时保留膀胱上皮组织的完整性；B. 从完整的膀胱上皮剥离的逼尿肌；C. 当膀胱充盈时可自体扩大隆起（图片引自 Cartwright and Snow[85]；discussion520–1）

术，强调了各种技术如何来支撑和稳定尿道和周围组织，但以上所记载的方法没有涵盖用于治疗压力性尿失禁的所有技术。文献中引用的成功率取决于当时对治疗成功的定义，因此有可能与当代的治疗成功定义不同。现在对治疗成功的评估，主要基于患者的感受或以患者为中心的主观和客观结果的组合。

1998年，随着尿道中段吊带的引入，这些技术的使用率已显著下降[8]。但仍有患者在经过详细的咨询后选择非网状手术治疗方案（如Burch阴道悬吊术和自体吊带）。此外，了解先前的治疗方法是为了了解当前技术原理及演变的关键。这些历史背景对于外科医生的知识也很重要，因为目前的患者在过去数十年中有可能已经接受过上述某种用于治疗尿失禁的手术了。建立在先前知识和经验的基础上，我们的理解也将进一步加深，也将推动尿失禁手术治疗的继续发展和改进。

参考文献

[1] Milsom I, Gyhagen M. The prevalence of urinary incontinence. Climacteric. 2019;22:217.
[2] Schultheiss D, Hofner K, Oelke M, et al. Historical aspects of the treatment of urinary incontinence. Eur Urol. 2000;38:352.
[3] Hinoul P, Roovers JP, Ombelet W, et al. Surgical management of urinary stress incontinence in women: a historical and clinical overview. Eur J Obstet Gynecol Reprod Biol. 2009;145:219.
[4] Kelly HA, D. W. Urinary incontinence in women without manifest injury to the bladder. Am Coll Surg. 1914;18:444.
[5] Schreiner G, Beltran R, Lockwood G, et al. A timeline of female stress urinary incontinence: how technology defined theory and advanced treatment. Neurourol Urodyn. 2020;39:1862.
[6] Maher CF, Karram M. Surgical management of pelvic organ prolapse, Chapter 8. p. 117–37.
[7] Bergman A, Elia G. Three surgical procedures for genuine stress incontinence: five-year follow- up of a prospective randomized study. Am J Obstet Gynecol. 1995;173:66.
[8] Thaweekul Y, Bunyavejchevin S, Wisawasukmongchol W, et al. Long term results of anterior colporrhaphy with Kelly plication for the treatment of stress urinary incontinence. J Med Assoc Thail. 2004;87:357.
[9] Anger JT, Weinberg AE, Albo ME, et al. Trends in surgical management of stress urinary incontinence among female Medicare beneficiaries. Urology. 2009;74:283.
[10] Rogo-Gupta L, Litwin MS, Saigal CS, et al. Trends in the surgical management of stress urinary incontinence among female Medicare beneficiaries, 2002–2007. Urology. 2013;82:38.
[11] Ingelman-Sundberg A. Extravaginal plastic repair of the pelvic floor for prolapse of the bladder neck; a new method to operate for stress incontinence. Gynaecologia. 1947;123:242.
[12] Obrink A. Pubococcygeal repair ad modum Ingelman-Sundberg. A retrospective investigation with 10–20 years time of observation. Acta Obstet Gynecol Scand. 1977;56:391.
[13] Ingelman-Sundberg A. Urinary incontinence in women, excluding fistulas. Acta Obstet Gynecol Scand. 1952;31(3):266–91.
[14] Gomes da Silveira G, Eduardo Piccoli C. Ingelman-Sundberg operation for urinary incontinence. Our experience. Acta Obstet Gynecol Scand. 1977;56:399.
[15] Debodinance P. Comparison of the Bologna and Ingelman-Sundberg procedures for stress incontinence associated with genital prolapse: ten-year follow-up of a prospective randomized study. J Gynecol Obstet Biol Reprod (Paris). 2000;29:148.
[16] Mazeman E, Wemeau L, Biserte J, et al. Bladder neck suspension for stress incontinence: long-term evaluation. Eur Urol. 1978;4:123.
[17] Chefchaouni MC, Thiounn N, Conquy S, et al. Treatment of stress urinary incontinence in women using the Goebell-Stoeckel surgical method. Study of 59 operated patients. Long-term review. J Urol (Paris). 1995;101:215.
[18] Ingelman-Sundberg A. A vaginal sling operation; for cases of stress incontinence and for women who cannot use a diaphragm due to prolapse of the anterior vaginal wall. J Obstet Gynaecol Br Emp. 1957;64:849.
[19] Price P. Plastic operations for incontinence of urine and feces. Arch Surg. 1933;26:1043.
[20] Aldridge AH. Transplantation of fascia for relief of urinary stress incontinence. Am J Obstet Gynecol. 1942;44:398.
[21] Chai TC. Edward McGuire's influence in the field of stress urinary incontinence and bladder storage symptoms. Neurourol Urodyn. 2010;29 Suppl 1:S32.
[22] Mc LH. Fascial slings for stress incontinence. J Obstet Gynaecol Br Emp. 1957;64:673.
[23] Jeffcoate TN. The results of the Aldridge sling operation for stress incontinence. J Obstet Gynaecol Br Emp. 1956;63:36.
[24] McIndoe GA, Jones RW, Grieve BW. The Aldridge sling procedure in the treatment of urinary stress incontinence. Aust N Z J Obstet Gynaecol. 1987;27:238.
[25] McLaren HC. Late results from sling operations. J Obstet Gynaecol Br Commonw. 1968;75:10.
[26] Marshall VF, Marchetti AA, Krantz KE. The correction of stress incontinence by simple vesicourethral suspension. Surg Gynecol Obstet. 1949;88:509.
[27] Mainprize TC, Drutz HP. The Marshall-Marchetti-Krantz procedure: a critical review. Obstet Gynecol Surv. 1988;43:724.
[28] McDuffie RW Jr, Litin RB, Blundon KE. Urethrovesical suspension (Marshall-Marchetti-Krantz). Experience with 204 cases. Am J Surg. 1981;141:297.
[29] Kammerer-Doak DN, Cornella JL, Magrina JF, et al. Osteitis pubis after Marshall-Marchetti-Krantz urethropexy: a pubic osteomyelitis. Am J Obstet Gynecol. 1998;179:586.
[30] Persky L, Guerriere K. Complications of Marshall-Marchetti-Krantz urethropexy. Urology. 1976;8:469.
[31] Burch JC. Urethrovaginal fixation to Cooper's ligament for correction of stress incontinence, cystocele, and prolapse. Am J Obstet Gynecol. 1961;81:281.
[32] Sohlberg EM, Elliott CS. Burch colposuspension. Urol Clin North Am. 2019;46:53.

[33] Baggish MS, Karram MM, editors. Atlas of pelvic anatomy and gynecologic surgery. 5th ed. p. 421.
[34] Lapitan MCM, Cody JD, Mashayekhi A. Open retropubic colposuspension for urinary incontinence in women. Cochrane Database Syst Rev. 2017;7:CD002912.
[35] Freites J, Stewart F, Omar MI, et al. Laparoscopic colposuspension for urinary incontinence in women. Cochrane Database Syst Rev. 2019;12:CD002239.
[36] Demirci F, Petri E. Perioperative complications of Burch colposuspension. Int Urogynecol J Pelvic Floor Dysfunct. 2000;11:170.
[37] Kenton K, Oldham L, Brubaker L. Open Burch urethropexy has a low rate of perioperative complications. Am J Obstet Gynecol. 2002;187:107.
[38] Wee HY, Low C, Han HC. Burch colposuspension: review of perioperative complications at a women's and children's hospital in Singapore. Ann Acad Med Singap. 2003;32:821.
[39] Wiskind AK, Creighton SM, Stanton SL. The incidence of genital prolapse after the Burch colposuspension. Am J Obstet Gynecol. 1992;167:399.
[40] Burch JC. Cooper's ligament urethrovesical suspension for stress incontinence. Nine years' experience-results, complications, technique. Am J Obstet Gynecol. 1968;100:764.
[41] Kjolhede P. Genital prolapse in women treated successfully and unsuccessfully by the Burch colposuspension. Acta Obstet Gynecol Scand. 1998;77:444.
[42] Pereyra AJ. A simplified surgical procedure for the correction of stress incontinence in women. West J Surg Obstet Gynecol. 1959;67:223.
[43] Kursh ED, Wainstein M, Persky L. The Pereyra procedure and urinary stress incontinence. J Urol. 1972;108:591.
[44] Pereyra AJ, Lebherz TB. Combined urethrovesical suspension and vaginourethroplasty for correction of urinary stress incontinence. Obstet Gynecol. 1967;30:537.
[45] Pereyra AJ, Lebherz TB, Growdon WA, et al. Pubourethral supports in perspective: modified pereyra procedure for urinary incontinence. Obstet Gynecol. 1982;59:643.
[46] Bodell DM, Leach GE. Needle suspension procedures for female incontinence. Urol Clin North Am. 2002;29:575.
[47] Holschneider CH, Solh S, Lebherz TB, et al. The modified Pereyra procedure in recurrent stress urinary incontinence: a 15-year review. Obstet Gynecol. 1994;83:573.
[48] Crist T, Shingleton HM, Roberson WE. Urethrovesical needle suspension: postoperative loss of vesical neck support demonstrated by chain cystography. Obstet Gynecol. 1969;34:489.
[49] Hilton P, Mayne CJ. The Stamey endoscopic bladder neck suspension: a clinical and urodynamic investigation, including actuarial follow-up over four years. Br J Obstet Gynaecol. 1991;98(11):1141–9.
[50] Mills R, Persad R, Handley Ashken M. Long-term follow-up results with the Stamey operation for stress incontinence of urine. Br J Urol. 1996;77:86.
[51] Kondo A, Kato K, Gotoh M, et al. The Stamey and Gittes procedures: long-term followup in relation to incontinence types and patient age. J Urol. 1998;160:756.
[52] Clemens JQ, Stern JA, Bushman WA, et al. Long-term results of the Stamey bladder neck suspension: direct comparison with the Marshall-Marchetti-Krantz procedure. J Urol. 1998;160:372.
[53] Conrad S, Pieper A, De la Maza SF, et al. Long-term results of the Stamey bladder neck suspension procedure: a patient questionnaire based outcome analysis. J Urol. 1997;157:1672.
[54] Raz S. Modified bladder neck suspension for female stress incontinence. Urology. 1981;17:82.
[55] Raz S. Atlas of vaginal reconstructive surgery
[56] Raz S, Sussman EM, Erickson DB, et al. The Raz bladder neck suspension: results in 206 patients. J Urol. 1992;148:845.
[57] Trockman BA, Leach GE, Hamilton J, et al. Modified Pereyra bladder neck suspension: 10-year mean followup using outcomes analysis in 125 patients. J Urol. 1995;154:1841.
[58] Gittes RF, Loughlin KR. No-incision pubovaginal suspension for stress incontinence. J Urol. 1987;138:568.
[59] Elkabir JJ, Mee AD. Long-term evaluation of the Gittes procedure for urinary stress incontinence. J Urol. 1998;159:1203.
[60] Nigam AK, Otite U, Badenoch DF. Endoscopic bladder neck suspension revisited: long-term results of Stamey and Gittes procedures. Eur Urol. 2000;38:677.
[61] Kuo HC. Long-term results of surgical treatment for female stress urinary incontinence. Urol Int. 2001;66:13.
[62] Theodorou C, Floratos D, Katsifotis C, et al. Transvaginal incisionless bladder neck suspension. A simplified technique for female genuine stress incontinence. Int Urol Nephrol. 1998;30:273.
[63] Benderev TV. A modified percutaneous outpatient bladder neck suspension system. J Urol. 1994;152:2316.
[64] Appell RA, Rackley RR, Dmochowski RR. Vesica percutaneous bladder neck stabilization. J Endourol. 1996;10:221.
[65] Rackley RR, Winters JC, Appell RA. Percutaneous bladder neck/urethra stabilization with bone-anchor suture fixation for type II genuine stress urinary incontinence. Presented at the 91st Meeting of the American Urologic Association, 1996.
[66] Reid SV, Parys BT. Long-term 5-year followup of the results of the vesica procedure. J Urol. 2005;173:1234.
[67] Matkov TG, Hejna MJ, Coogan CL. Osteomyelitis as a complication of vesica percutaneous bladder neck suspension. J Urol. 1998;160:1427.
[68] Murless BC. The injection treatment of stress incontinence. J Obstet Gynaecol Br Emp. 1938;45:67.
[69] Politano VA, Small MP, Harper JM, et al. Periurethral teflon injection for urinary incontinence. Trans Am Assoc Genitourin Surg. 1973;65:54.
[70] Berg S. Polytef augmentation urethroplasty. Correction of surgically incurable urinary incontinence by injection technique. Arch Surg. 1973;107:379.
[71] Benshushan A, Brzezinski A, Shoshani O, et al. Periurethral injection for the treatment of urinary incontinence. Obstet Gynecol Surv. 1998;53:383.
[72] Santiago Gonzalez de Garibay AM, Castro Morrondo J, Castillo Jimeno JM, et al. Endoscopic injection of autologous adipose tissue in the treatment of female incontinence. Arch Esp Urol. 1989;42:143.
[73] Lee PE, Kung RC, Drutz HP. Periurethral autologous fat injection as treatment for female stress urinary incontinence: a randomized double-blind controlled trial. J Urol. 2001;165:153.
[74] Shortliffe LM, Freiha FS, Kessler R, et al. Treatment of urinary incontinence by the periurethral implantation of glutaraldehyde cross-linked collagen. J Urol. 1989;141:538.
[75] Ingelman-Sundberg A. Partial denervation of the bladder, a new operation for the treatment of urge incontinence and similar conditions in women. Acta Obstet Gynecol Scand. 1959;38:487.
[76] Westney OL, Lee JT, McGuire EJ, et al. Long-term results of Ingelman-Sundberg denervation procedure for urge incontinence refractory to medical therapy. J Urol. 2002;168:1044.
[77] Ingelman-Sundberg A. Partial bladder denervation for detrusor dyssynergia. Clin Obstet Gynecol. 1978;21:797.
[78] Chapple CR, Hampson SJ, Turner-Warwick RT, et al. Subtrigonal phenol injection. How safe and effective is it? Br J Urol. 1991;68:483.
[79] Blackford HN, Murray K, Stephenson TP, et al. Results of transvesical infiltration of the pelvic plexuses with phenol in 116 patients. Br J Urol. 1984;56:647.
[80] Wall LL, Stanton SL. Transvesical phenol injection of pelvic nerve plexuses in females with refractory urge incontinence. Br J Urol. 1989;63:465.

[81] Harris RG, Constantinou CE, Stamey TA. Extravesical subtrigonal injection of 50 per cent ethanol for detrusor instability. J Urol. 1988;140:111.
[82] McInerney PD, Vanner TF, Matenhelia S, et al. Assessment of the long-term results of subtrigonal phenolisation. Br J Urol. 1991;67:586.
[83] Cameron-Strange A, Millard RJ. Management of refractory detrusor instability by transvesical phenol injection. Br J Urol. 1988;62:323.
[84] Petrou SP. Long-term results of Ingelman-Sundberg denervation procedures for urge incontinence refractory to medical therapy. Int Braz J Urol. 2002;28:491.
[85] Cartwright PC, Snow BW. Bladder autoaugmentation: early clinical experience. J Urol. 1989;142:505.
[86] Swami KS, Feneley RC, Hammonds JC, et al. Detrusor myectomy for detrusor overactivity: a minimum 1–year follow-up. Br J Urol. 1998;81:68.
[87] Kumar SP, Abrams PH. Detrusor myectomy: long-term results with a minimum follow-up of 2 years. BJU Int. 2005;96:341.
[88] Aslam MZ, Agarwal M. Detrusor myectomy: long-term functional outcomes. Int J Urol. 2012;19:1099.
[89] Karsenty G, Vidal F, Ruffion A, et al. Treatment of neurogenic detrusor hyperactivity: detrusor myomectomy. Prog Urol. 2007;17:580.
[90] Johnson EU, Singh G. Long-term outcomes of urinary tract reconstruction in patients with neurogenic urinary tract dysfunction. Indian J Urol. 2013;29:328.
[91] Chen LC, Kuo HC. Current management of refractory overactive bladder. Low Urin Tract Symptoms. 2020;12:109.

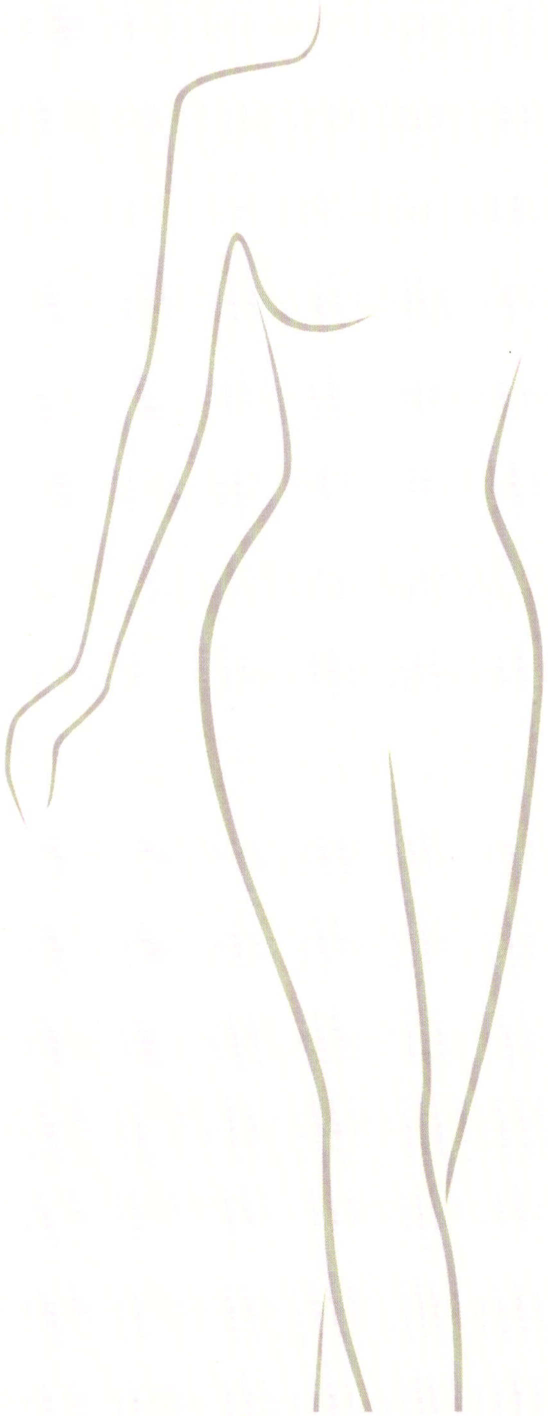

第二篇
保守疗法

Conservative Treatment

第6章　女性尿失禁的行为治疗和生活方式改变

Behavioral Therapy and Lifestyle Modifications for the Management of Urinary Incontinence in Women

Kimberly Kenne　Catherine S. Bradley　著

大多数临床实践指南推荐行为疗法作为女性尿失禁（UI）的初始治疗。这些干预措施多种多样，可能采用的方法包括液体管理、饮食变化、避免膀胱刺激物、定时排尿、膀胱训练、肠道功能管理、锻炼、减肥，以及关于吸收性物品和皮肤保护的建议。尽管支持这些干预措施的证据往往有限，因为这些干预措施很难研究，在许多情况下缺乏支持这些治疗的证据，但其风险低、费用低，因此可以将这些因素纳入早期的治疗方案。行为治疗和生活方式的改变很难标准化和监控，所以高质量的前瞻性干预研究很少。因此，围绕这一主题的许多文献本质上都是观察性的，研究结果往往被报道为行为干预的组合所致，使得结果解释起来比较困难。此外，患者的依从性也是一个挑战，因为很难评估患者对行为建议的依从性。一些证据支持将行为疗法与其他疗法结合使用。例如，在BE-DRI多中心随机试验中，在以尿急为主要症状的女性尿失禁患者的药物治疗基础上增加行为治疗（包括膀胱训练和液体管理，以及盆底肌训练），对提高患者满意度、改善感知和减少尿失禁及其他膀胱症状有益[1]。

美国泌尿外科协会（AUA）、美国泌尿妇科协会（AUGS）和美国产科医师学会（ACOG）发布的指南文件都建议妇科医生在女性尿失禁的初始治疗中使用行为疗法，通常包括盆底肌肉练习或这类训练项目[2-4]。高质量的证据确实支持使用盆底肌肉锻炼和训练来治疗压力性尿失禁和急迫性尿失禁（见第7章）。

在本章中，我们讨论了女性尿失禁的其他行为治疗，其中有许多可能被认为是生活方式的改变。在接下来的章节中，我们回顾了每一种行为干预，并总结了支持其用于治疗女性尿失禁和其他泌尿系统症状的现有证据。表6–1列出了本章讨论的干预措施、推荐使用这些措施的患者情况以及支持每种措施的证据。虽然了解与行为治疗有关的证据很重要，但是这些治疗措施通常是低风险和低成本的，并且可能对女性健康有益。因此，我们通常可以在初始侵入性或昂贵的测试之前进行评估。图6–1展示了我们在对尿失禁进行初步评估后向患者提供的宣教内容，其中包含许多与改变生活方式相关的说明和建议。

一、控制饮食

饮食和液体的控制是尿失禁行为治疗措施的一大部分。许多关于节食和膀胱功能影响的文献中把节食作为减肥的替代方法，这将在随后的章节中进一步研究。关于特定的饮食成分及其与压力性尿失禁的关系，Dallosso等[5-7]发现，摄入饱和脂肪和单不饱和脂肪可能会增加压力性尿失禁的风险，而摄入面包/淀粉和蔬菜可能会降低风险。当观察特定的营养物质时，一项大型流行病学研究发现，锌和维生素B_{12}的摄入与女性的压力不协调有关[5-7]。

由于在泌尿生殖组织（膀胱、尿道、阴道上皮、肌肉和骨盆筋膜）中发现了雌激素受体，因此就压力性尿失禁、膀胱过度活动症（OAB）和

表 6-1　推荐的女性尿失禁行为治疗

干预措施	目标人群	支持干预的证据
饮食调整	所有患者	弱：大多数观察性研究的不一致结果表明饮食和饮食成分与尿失禁之间可能存在联系
液体管理	所有患者	中度：介入性研究显示液体限制对尿失禁和膀胱过度活动症的持续益处
减少摄入咖啡因	摄入咖啡因的患者	弱：观察性研究的不一致结果支持咖啡因和尿失禁之间的联系；小型介入研究没有显示出益处
酒精减量	饮酒的患者	弱：集中于酒精和尿失禁之间联系的观察性研究的结果不一致
戒烟	吸烟的患者	弱：观察研究表明烟草使用和尿失禁之间的联系
定时 / 提示排尿	不经常排尿者	弱：介入性研究提供的益处证据不一致
膀胱训练	尿频的患者	中度：介入性研究显示膀胱训练对尿失禁的益处
肠道管理	便秘的患者	弱：观察性研究的不一致结果支持便秘和尿失禁及其他泌尿系统症状之间的联系
锻炼	所有患者	弱：有限的介入性研究提供了使用证据
失重	超重和肥胖患者	强：高质量的随机试验显示尿失禁的好处
吸收性物质	所有患者	弱：有限的介入性研究提供了使用证据
皮肤保护剂	所有患者	弱：有限的介入性研究提供了使用证据

下尿路症状（LUTS）对食用富含植物雌激素的食物之间的关系进行了研究。然而，一项评估富含大豆饮食的随机试验（假设通过植物雌激素增加循环雌激素）显示，与控制饮食相比，在总体下尿路症状或尿失禁管理方面没有改善[8]。同样，Waetjen 等[9]的报道也没有发现摄入 3 类植物雌激素（异黄酮、香豆雌酚或木脂素）的饮食与更年期女性出现任何类型的尿失禁（压力性或急迫性）之间存在关联。

关于尿急、尿频、尿失禁和膀胱过度活动症，许多关于饮食调整的建议避免涉及可能酸化尿液成分或刺激膀胱的食物，如柑橘类产品。在一项纵向队列研究中，Curto 等[6]发现，补充维生素 C 的使用量超过推荐的日摄入量与女性日间尿潴留症状的发生率较高有关，但从食物和饮料中摄入较高的基线维生素 C 与尿急症状的发生率较低有关。在一项对 2060 例女性进行的基于人群的观察性流行病学研究中也发现了类似的结果。在这项研究中，摄入高剂量维生素 C 和钙与尿失禁症状正相关，而来自食物和饮料的维生素 C 和 β- 隐黄质与排尿症状负相关[10]。总的来说，这些研究表明，维生素 C 补充剂超过中等可吸收剂量（>250mg/d）可能会刺激膀胱，应该避免摄入过量维生素 C。

Dallosso 等[6]在一项纵向研究中报道称，摄入更多维生素 D（P=0.008）、蛋白质（P=0.03）和钾（P=0.05）与新发膀胱过度活动症风险降低显著相关。这些结果没有在一项针对患有尿急和维生素 D 不足的绝经后女性的随机双盲安慰剂对照试验中得到证实。在该试验中，每周服用 50 000U 维生素 D_3 患者的尿急发作减少了 43%，但与安慰剂相比，并没有达到统计学的显著性差异（尿急发作减少了 28%），除了黑种人女性亚组（与安慰剂组的 23% 相比，其尿急发作减少了 63%）[11]。为了进一步评估维生素 D 参与调节逼尿肌收缩，Markland 等[12]在护士健康研究Ⅰ和Ⅱ中对近

帮助解决膀胱问题的方法

1. 避免膀胱刺激物。有些食物和液体可能会刺激膀胱。
   避免或减少摄入以下这些食物和饮料。
   - 酒精饮料：白酒、葡萄酒和啤酒。
   - 咖啡因：咖啡、茶、深色苏打水、深色草药茶和巧克力。
   - 非常酸的水果或果汁：橘子、柚子、柠檬、酸橙、杧果和菠萝。
   - 人造甜味剂：Equal 和 Nutrasweet。
   - 高剂量的维生素。
   - 碳酸饮料。

   最好的饮料是水。
2. 每 3～4 小时喝 4～6 盎司的液体（小杯），每天间隔均匀。将你的总液体摄入量限制在每天 48～64 盎司（6～8 盎司杯）。目标是没有强烈气味的淡黄色尿液。
3. 按时钟小便——每 2～3 小时 1 次。不要等到你觉得下腹憋胀或更方便排尿的时候。排尿时尽量放松。不要紧张或用力过猛地开始排尿或更快速地排空膀胱。
4. 减少夜间排尿的次数。
   - 晚饭后限制液体摄入，减少夜间排尿。
   - 白天休息时，穿上支撑袜或抬高双腿，避免小腿肿胀。
5. 建立规律的排便习惯。便秘影响膀胱控制。膳食纤维补充剂、粪便软化剂或泻药（如 Miralax）是帮助保持肠道正常和轻松的选择。
6. 注意你的体重。肥胖使膀胱控制更加困难。
7. 如果你吸烟，这是考虑戒烟计划的又一个理由。由于慢性咳嗽和对膀胱的刺激，吸烟会使渗漏更严重。
8. 不要刺激你的外阴区域。避免使用带颜色和香味的卫生纸和卫生巾。用温水洗外阴，穿全棉内裤，或者小尿垫。

好的膀胱习惯是可以随时养成的。旧习惯可能很难打破，尤其是当我们试图一次改变太多事情的时候。慢慢开始，一次改变一件事，直到你适应新的健康习惯。

祝你好运！

▲ 图 6-1 描述尿失禁和其他泌尿症状的行为治疗和生活方式改变的患者教育讲义

73 000 例老年和中年女性进行了分析，发现几乎没有证据表明维生素 D 摄入和尿失禁发展之间存在关系。从宏量营养素的水平来看，Dallosso 等[6]发现，蔬菜、面包和鸡肉的消费量越高，膀胱过度活动症发病的风险就越低。

大多数与特定饮食成分和尿失禁相关的研究结果都是流行病学的，并且表明可能不是因果关系的关联。因此，很难对尿失禁的治疗和（或）预防提出具体的饮食建议，最好的建议可能是建议患者饮食均衡以促进总体健康和保持良好状态。

二、液体和咖啡因的管理

也许最广泛推荐的处理尿失禁和其他泌尿症状的行为改变集中在液体和咖啡因管理上。AUA 和 AUGS/ACOG 都推荐液体管理作为一线行为矫正[2-4]。建议通常强调对液体入量的全面管理，避免刺激性液体，特别是咖啡因。尽管专家们对液体管理的重要性有这些建议和共识，但是文献表述存在差异。例如，当回顾护士健康研究队列时，Townsend 等[13]发现总液体摄入量与尿失禁事件风险之间没有关联［比较液体摄入量最高和最低的 1/5，危险比（HR）为 1.04，95%CI 0.98～1.10］。在尿失禁类型的分析中，总液体摄入量与突发压力性尿失禁、急迫性尿失禁或混合性尿失禁的风险无关。

特别是关于应激性尿失禁，Dallosso 等[6]在一项前瞻性队列研究中报道称，碳酸饮料是应激性尿失禁和膀胱过度活动症发作的重要风险因素。一项为期4周的随机、前瞻性、交叉研究旨在确定咖啡因限制和液体摄入量变化对压力性尿失禁女性泌尿系统症状的影响。在该试验中，Swithinbank等[14]确定，当将液体减少的一周与基线或液体增加的一周进行比较时，减少液体摄入可减少尿失禁和尿频次数。然而，当增加液体的一周与基线相比时，尿失禁发作没有增加。作者得出结论，减少液体可以改善泌尿症状，虽然女性必须保持足够的每日液体摄入量以避免脱水，但作为保守治疗的一部分，应建议她们少喝液体以改善症状[14]。

对膀胱过度活动症和尿急患者的研究通常显示液体摄入和症状之间存在正相关[15]。随着液体增加，女性经历的频率和尿急症状增加，而随着液体减少，尿频和尿急症状减少。具体就尿失禁而言，结果往往更为复杂，一般来说，大多数患者很难坚持液量管理协议[15]。在对十项干预性和观察性研究的系统综述中，Callan等[16]报道称，减少液体摄入有利于减轻膀胱过度活动症。这些作者还发现，在观察性研究中，增加液体摄入与膀胱过度活动症恶化相关，但在干预性研究中，症状没有差异。

咖啡因是世界上消耗最多的兴奋剂，具有利尿作用，还可能通过增加逼尿肌压力和促进逼尿肌兴奋性来影响膀胱[17]。已经发表了大量关于咖啡因摄入对泌尿症状的影响的文献，并且减少咖啡因通常被认为是尿失禁行为管理的一部分。在几项研究中，咖啡因减少与尿频、尿急和膀胱过度活动症生活质量评分减少相关[15]。虽然有一些相互矛盾的文献，Bradley等[15]的系统综述指出，“总体证据表明咖啡因和尿失禁之间存在微弱的正相关，但对于尿失禁类型存在相互矛盾的结果。”

护士健康研究前瞻性地调查了总咖啡因摄入量（通过食物频率问卷确定）和尿失禁发生率之间的关系，其中包括压力、尿急和混合性尿失禁。对65 176例女性进行了为期4年的随访，在咖啡因摄入量最高与最低的女性中（＞450mg/d与＜150mg/d）比较，虽然每周发生尿失禁的风险中度，但是风险显著增加了（RR=1.19，95%CI 1.06～1.34），随着摄入量的增加，尿失禁的风险显著增加（趋势P=0.01）。较高的每日咖啡因摄入量（大致相当于每天≥4杯咖啡或≥10杯/罐含咖啡因的茶或苏打水），而不是较低的水平，与女性尿急风险适度增加相关[18]。当纵向检查护士的健康研究时，在中度尿失禁女性中，长期摄入咖啡因与超过2年的尿失禁进展风险无关[19]。

美国国家健康和营养评估调查是一项全国代表性的横断面调查，发现咖啡因摄入量最高的患者（204mg/d）与任何尿失禁相关［患病率优势比（POR）为1.47，95%CI 1.07～2.01］，但与中度/重度尿失禁无关（POR=1.42，95%CI 0.98～2.07）。作者得出结论，适度摄入咖啡因仍然是尿失禁多组分治疗的合理组成部分[17]。类似地，Maserejian等[20]发现，与减少或保持摄入的类别相比，每天增加至少2份咖啡摄入的女性出现尿急进展的概率高出64%（P=0.003）。最近增加苏打摄入的女性，特别是含咖啡因的减肥苏打，有更高的症状评分、尿急和下尿路症状进展。这些发现支持限制含咖啡因饮料摄入的建议。在一项小型Cystometry研究中，检查前30min摄入4.5mg/kg的咖啡因会导致利尿、充盈期间感觉阈值降低、流速和排尿量增加，这表明咖啡因可以促进早期尿急和尿频[21]。咖啡因摄入量和膀胱过度活动症之间可能存在剂量依赖的正相关关系[22]。

仍然存在的一个问题是，是一般的液体限制还是咖啡因限制对患有尿失禁的女性更重要。Zimmern等[23]的研究表明一般液体管理指导（每天摄入液体50～70盎司）有助于减少服用抗胆碱能药物的女性的尿急症状，但额外的个体化指导和其他行为疗法对进一步改善结果几乎没有作用。Segal等[24]发现摄入总液体量最高的患者每日排便次数增加（P＜0.001），并且摄入含咖啡因液体量最高者尿急严重程度增加（P=0.038），两者之间显著相关。液体摄入的类型和量与尿频和尿急症状显著相关。他们得出结论：总液体摄入量的增加与尿频显著相关，摄入大量含咖啡因的液体与尿急相关。

相反，两个小型随机试验没有发现咖啡因限制对尿失禁的一般液体减少有益。一项小型随机交叉研究测试了压力和尿急女性的咖啡因限制和液体摄入变化，发现从含咖啡因饮料改为无咖啡因饮料对症状没有影响，而液体总量摄入减少导致尿频和尿失禁减少[14]。最后，Schimpf 等[25]完成了一项随机试验，旨在测试避免摄入潜在刺激性饮料（包括咖啡因、人工甜味剂、柑橘和酒精），同时保持摄入量稳定来治疗膀胱过度活动症的常见临床建议。作者报道说，与对照组相比，减少潜在刺激性饮料的摄入不会导致排尿频率降低[26]。尿急症状和烦恼评分也没有变化。总之，目前的证据表明，减少摄入潜在刺激性饮料（包括含咖啡因的饮料）可能不如减少摄入总液体量对尿失禁和膀胱过度活动症的影响大。

三、酒精和烟草

考虑到酒精的镇静作用、损害活动性的能力和利尿作用，酒精消费也被认为是治疗尿失禁的一种可改变行为[27]。2017 年发表的一项系统综述称，关于酒精和泌尿症状的研究信息有限，其结论并不相同[15]。尽管酒精可能会影响当前饮酒者的尿急和尿频，但摄入水平和症状亚型的研究结果并不一致。未发现尿失禁类型与酒精摄入之间的关联[15]。

此外，还研究了烟草使用及其对下尿路症状的影响，戒烟仍然是推荐改善泌尿系统症状的行为疗法。一些研究提供的证据表明，烟草使用与压力性尿失禁[28, 29]、急迫性尿失禁和混合性尿失禁[30]，以及任何（未指明）类型的尿失禁之间存在正相关[30-32]。六项研究没有发现这种关联，一项研究发现偶尔的尿失禁和当前吸烟之间存在负相关[15]。Hannestad 等[31]显示了当前、以前和重度吸烟患者与各种尿失禁之间的关系。

以前和现在吸烟与尿失禁有关，但仅适用于那些每天吸烟超过 20 支的人。无论吸烟多少，严重尿失禁与吸烟的关联很小。

Dallosso 等[6]发现，吸烟与膀胱过度活动症之间存在显著关联，当前吸烟者患膀胱过度活动症的可能性是非吸烟者的 1.44 倍。在膀胱过度活动症或下尿路症状的广义证据范畴内（而不是具体的失禁），结论并不一致。少量证据表明，以前和（或）现在吸烟与女性吸烟频率有关。两项研究表明，尿急与当前烟草使用呈正相关[33, 34]，而另两项研究则没有[35, 36]。Maserejian 等[37]发现，与从不吸烟者相比，女性吸烟者患下尿路症状的可能性是男性的 2 倍，尤其是尿储存期症状（OR=2.15，95%CI 1.30～3.56，P=0.003），并建议戒烟。

单一研究表明，吸烟与女性咳嗽时最大尿流率峰值[28]、咳嗽漏点压力和咳嗽时最大膀胱压之间存在正相关[38]。两项检查严重尿失禁的研究显示了正相关[15]。综合来看，研究表明烟草和泌尿系统症状之间可能存在联系。尽管不是决定性的，但考虑到戒烟对健康的额外益处，将其纳入尿失禁的行为建议是合理的。

四、定时排尿

除了液体摄入的改变之外，一种常见的控制尿失禁的行为改变是定时或敦促排尿。与膀胱训练（如下所述）不同，目的不是增加排尿间隔时间、排尿量或膀胱容量，而是鼓励定期排空膀胱，以减少在膀胱容量较高时经常发生的尿失禁[39]。大多数与这种做法相关的证据是“提示排尿”，一种经常用于认知功能障碍患者和辅助生活情况下的定时排尿，在这种情况下，护理人员或家庭成员会定期敦促患者排尿。

在对 674 例患者（大多数为女性）进行的九项试验的回顾中，比较了敦促排尿和非敦促性排尿，没有足够的证据表明这两种方法是否改善了尿失禁[40]。作者从理论上认为，敦促排尿会在短期内减少尿失禁的发生。在最近的 Cochrane 综述中，研究了固定间隔或定时排尿对认知能力下降和活动能力受损的老年女性尿失禁的治疗作用，两项包含 298 例女性的试验没有提供足够的证据支持这种治疗。然而，考虑到该人群中潜在危害的低风险和其他治疗的高风险可能性（如药物不良反应），即使提示无效仍被视为合理的治疗选择[41]。

Holroyd-Leduc 等[42] 报道称，几项检查由护理人员启动的敦促排尿的随机试验显示，其效果优于通常的尿失禁相关护理（包括定期检查和更换湿衣物和被褥）。

虽然缺乏证据，但大多数专家建议患有尿急和膀胱过度活动症的患者定时或有计划地排尿，特别是那些没有明显尿频的患者，或者其膀胱日记显示排尿间隔较长或在排尿前经常发生尿失禁的患者。

五、膀胱训练

膀胱训练是一种行为治疗策略，其鼓励患有尿急和尿频症状，以及混合性尿失禁和压力性尿失禁的患者逐渐增加排尿间隔时间，从而增加他们的膀胱容量，并可能减少漏尿和尿急感[39]。这项技术于 1966 年首次被描述，患者最初被告知每隔 1～2h 排尿 1 次。根据其症状的严重程度，排尿间隔时间以半小时为增量增加，直到达到 3.5h[43]。膀胱训练通常需要完整的认知、活动自如的患者和固定的排尿时间表，而不考虑排尿的迫切感。确切的训练技术在不同的研究中有所不同，但都涉及逐渐增加排尿间隔时间的策略。在 ESTEEM 试验的协议中，膀胱训练被描述为“多种干预措施，其中包括关于下尿路功能的患者教育、设定递增间隔排尿时间表，以及教授尿急时排尿控制技术以推迟排尿，并且遵守排尿时间表”[44]。

1996 年，Davies 等[43] 对 50 例患有长期尿频、尿急和急迫性尿失禁的患者开展了住院研究。在出院时，他们报告说 80% 的女性主观感觉治愈，改善令人满意。然而，在 12～29 个月后回复邮件调查的患者中，这一成功率下降到 32%。Visco 等[45] 得出结论，膀胱训练的实际成功率可能远远低于临床试验中的描述，因为 55% 的研究对象从未开始膀胱训练或不遵从治疗，这与保持严格的排尿计划的困难性相一致。Newman 等[44] 报道称，使用意向性治疗模型的随机试验显示，膀胱训练后，尿失禁平均降低 60%～80%。2004 年的一篇 Cochrane 综述报道说，膀胱训练可能有助于愿意使用这种方法的患者，但可能需要几个月才能取得效果[46]。作者得出初步结论，有限的证据表明膀胱训练可能有助于治疗尿失禁；这一建议有所保留，因为研究的质量不一、规模小，因此结果不太确定[46]。

一项研究检查了膀胱训练后尿流动力学参数的变化，没有发现可测量的变化。基于此，Elser 等[47] 得出结论，膀胱训练临床改善的机制仍然未知。膀胱训练有效的可能机制包括：①改善对膀胱感觉和尿道闭合的中央控制；②随着对导致膀胱漏尿原因的了解，以增加下泌尿系统“储备能力”的方式改变个体的行为[44]。患有尿失禁的患者，特别是有尿急的患者，经常频繁排尿以避免这种症状。这种行为会导致功能性膀胱容量减少，从而可能使尿急症状持续存在。

许多研究者研究了膀胱训练和其他治疗尿失禁的策略。例如，Mattiasson 等[48] 报道称，服用托特罗定并进行膀胱训练的患者减少的排尿频率百分比中位数大于单独服用托特罗定的患者（33% vs. 25%，$P<0.001$）。联合治疗组的每次排尿量增加的中位数百分比也更大（31% vs. 20%，$P<0.001$）。Wyman 等[49] 研究了膀胱训练、生物反馈骨盆肌肉锻炼或联合治疗是否更有利于治疗尿失禁，发现无论尿流动力学诊断如何，联合治疗都具有最大的即时疗效。然而，在治疗后的 3 个月，3 种干预都有相似的结果，这表明特定的治疗可能没有个体化的干预计划重要。在 Cochrane 综述中，作者报道说，没有足够的证据来确定膀胱训练作为其他疗法的补充是否有用[46]。

排尿策略（包括定时或敦促排尿和膀胱训练）的好处在于其风险最小、成本低和对所有类型尿失禁（压力性尿失禁、急迫性尿失禁和混合性尿失禁）的潜在疗效。因此，排尿策略仍然是一种理想的一线疗法，应该在更具侵入性和（或）更昂贵的诊断测试或治疗措施之前考虑采用。

六、肠道管理

治疗尿失禁和其他下尿路症状的常见行为建议是肠功能的管理 / 调节。在儿科人群中，便秘与泌尿系统症状的共存已得到很好的证实，称为功能失调综合征[50, 51]。事实上，治疗便秘有 90% 的儿童缓解了日间尿失禁，并消除了尿路感染的复发[50]。虽然这种联系在成年女性中并不确定，但文献通常支持正常肠功能有助于正常膀胱功能的理论。在对 2812 例社区女性进行的二次分析中，Cameron 等[52] 发现排便困难的女性下尿路症状发病率增加[52]。具体来说，排便困难的女性更有可能经历夜尿症（平均 1.8 ± 0.1 vs. 1.3 ± 0.0）、尿急（47.6% vs. 29.2%）、日间排尿频率增加（平均 8.2 ± 0.3 vs. 7.2 ± 0.1）、排尿困难（22.9% vs. 13.7%）和尿不尽感（55.6% vs. 28.2%）。

膀胱和肠功能之间关系的确切病理生理学仍不清楚。一种提出的机制认为延迟粪便排泄需要肛门外括约肌和耻骨直肠肌收缩，直到排便紧迫性消退。如果这种行为持续一段时间，直肠会变得过度扩张，盆底肌肉组织会过度紧张，这本身会导致泌尿症状的进展[53]。此外，完整的直肠和乙状结肠可能会对膀胱施加外部压力、降低功能容量或刺激膀胱壁的拉伸感受器，从而引发逼尿肌收缩[53, 54]。最后，脊髓或骨盆神经的共享神经通路中出现的排便功能障碍相关信号也可能导致调节膀胱功能的中枢神经系统发生变化[55]。通过在 S_3 孔放置相同的导线刺激骶神经成功使肠道和膀胱症状得到缓解，支持了认为存在影响两个器官功能（或功能障碍）共同神经通路的理论[56]。

虽然需要进一步的研究来证实治疗成年女性的肠道症状可以改善膀胱症状，但这些措施仍然是初步治疗建议的一部分，肯定是无害的。最常见的是，推荐治疗便秘的肠道疗法，如根据患者的具体情况和症状，定期使用大便软化剂、纤维补充剂或泻药。应该询问患有令人讨厌的下尿路症状的女性是否存在排便症状，并且应当考虑到它们可能的联系，这些问题应该被同时处理。

七、锻炼

通过锻炼来改善尿失禁的大多数证据涉及通过锻炼来减轻体重，从而缓解尿失禁症状。然而，研究也表明，那些认为自己比同龄的其他人（缺少锻炼的人）更有可能患压力性尿失禁，并且低身体活动水平与膀胱过度活动症发展风险的增加显著相关[6]。此外，有一个极端，参加高强度体育活动的女性，如力量举重或交叉训练，可能会出现较高的尿失禁发生率[57-59]。这些女性报道称，她们采取了预防措施来防止在锻炼过程中出现尿失禁，如在锻炼前排空膀胱、穿深色裤子，以及在锻炼过程中进行 Kegel 锻炼[59]。

锻炼盆底肌治疗尿失禁在第 7 章进行了综述。然而，一些研究已经检验了改进的普拉提或瑜伽项目的效果，这些项目增强了骨盆底的顺应性和力量，以提高完成骨盆底锻炼方案的成功率。Hein 等[60] 在一项为期 12 周的试点研究中提出，鉴于维持盆底分离患者盆底完整性的难度，进行盆底强化普拉提计划可能是有益的。

他们报道了尿失禁评分的改善和对该计划的高度依从性。同样，在一项随机试验中，Lausen 等[61] 报道了将盆底肌肉练习作为改良普拉提课程的一部分，以增加进行这些练习的动力。最后，在一项针对压力性尿失禁老年女性的小型随机试验中，与单独进行盆底肌训练相比，负重训练结合盆底肌训练能更早改善尿失禁[62]。

在一项单中心随机试点试验中，Huang 等[63] 发现，居住在社区的女性尿失禁患者通过集体课程和家庭练习成功实施了以瑜伽为基础的干预。完成 3 个月瑜伽计划的女性尿失禁频率平均降低了 76%，而完成同等时间肌肉拉伸和强化计划的女性尿失禁频率平均降低了 56%。他们得出结论，瑜伽有可能为女性提供基于社区的尿路感染管理，尽管尚不清楚这是否优于其他体育活动。尽管有这些有希望的研究，最近的Cochrane综述得出结论，瑜伽或改良的普拉提疗法在治疗尿失禁中的作用仍然不确定，因为大多数试验规模较小，存在较高的偏倚风险[64]。

八、减肥

肥胖是一个严重的公共健康问题，对女性生活的许多方面都有负面影响（包括控制排尿）。肥胖是压力性尿失禁发作的一个公认的风险因素[6]。事实上，在整个成年生活中，女性较高的体重指数（BMI）与压力和严重失禁的症状有关。从成年早期开始，超重或肥胖的女性比正常体重女性患严重尿失禁的风险超过2倍[65]。因此，重要的是鼓励女性在所有年龄保持正常体重，这既是防止尿失禁发展的一种手段，也是缓解尿失禁的一种手段。

肥胖症和尿急性尿失禁之间的联系还不清楚，但是将肥胖症和急迫性尿失禁联系起来的作用机制可能是体重指数和腹围，以及几种尿液动力学检查参数之间的正相关联系。Richter等[66]发现，在一个有急迫性尿失禁的超重和肥胖队列中，腹内压和膀胱内压随着体重指数或腹围的增加而增加。随着体重的增加，女性在可能增加膀胱压力的事件中，其膀胱压力似乎越来越接近她们的排尿阈值。Fuganti等[38]证明，与体重指数较低的女性相比，肥胖女性咳嗽时的最大膀胱内压力峰值更高。这些研究表明，体重减轻可以通过降低咳嗽和其他活动期间的膀胱内压来减少尿失禁。

通过饮食调整和加强锻炼减少尿失禁的里程碑式项目（PRIDE）试验[66]证明了体重减轻对尿失禁的影响。在PRIDE中，每周至少有10次尿失禁发作的超重和肥胖女性被随机分组参加为期6个月的减肥计划或精心组织的教育计划。在6个月时，干预组的平均体重减轻了8%（7.8kg），平均每周尿失禁发作减少了47%，而对照组的体重减轻了1.6%（1.5kg），尿失禁发作减少了28%（P=0.01）。与对照组相比，干预组压力性尿失禁发作的频率也降低更明显，但是急迫性尿失禁发作的频率降低不大。作者得出结论，减肥干预的行为疗法降低了超重和肥胖女性自我报告的尿失禁发作频率[67]。

在18个月的随访中，PRIDE研究了人群体重减轻和尿失禁改善之间的联系[67]。在12个月时，干预组报告每周压力性尿失禁发作减少的百分比更大（65% vs. 47%，P<0.001），与基线相比，减重更大比例的患者每周总压力性尿失禁发作减少至少70%。在18个月时，干预组中减重更大比例的女性在急迫性尿失禁发作方面也有超过70%的改善，但两组之间在压力性尿失禁改善和总尿失禁发作方面的差异不显著。作者得出结论，减重干预在12个月内降低了压力性尿失禁发作的频率，在18个月内改善了患者对尿失禁的满意度[68]。

虽然不属于行为矫正领域，但减肥手术的减肥结果也已被证明可以改善肥胖女性的尿失禁。几项研究表明，减肥手术后的体重减轻改善了具有临床意义的尿失禁[69–71]，并且这种改善似乎在减肥手术后1～5年保持不变[72, 73]。

AUGS系统综述小组研究了减肥干预对超重和肥胖女性下尿路症状和尿失禁的影响[74]。他们的证据高度确定，即在1～2.9年，行为干预减肥将压力性尿失禁的患病率降低15%～18%，总体尿失禁降低12%～17%。在体重减轻5%～10%后，可以察觉改善了尿失禁，进一步减轻体重的额外益处很小。有关这些干预措施的长期影响的证据的确定性较低：效果似乎随着时间的推移而减弱，这可能是体重反弹的原因。关于行为减肥对尿急和膀胱过度活动症的益处，证据的确定性为中到低。没有随机试验评估手术减肥对泌尿系统症状的影响，这方面的证据水平很低[74]。

九、吸收性物品和皮肤保护

对于治疗后仍持续出现尿失禁的女性而言，吸收性物品和皮肤保护对于维持生活质量和避免尿失禁相关皮炎非常重要。约9%的失禁治疗年度费用用于吸收性物品[75, 76]，87%的60岁及以上的社区生活女性使用护垫来控制尿失禁[77]。这些物品要求效果可靠，并且较为隐蔽[77, 78]。女性从许多渠道来获得有关这类物品的信息，但是大多数情况下，她们最终求助于试错法来选择应用何种物品。因此，医疗服务提供者应在尿失禁评估期间提供有关吸收性物品的信息[79]。

患有轻度尿失禁的女性可以从四类主要的吸收物品中进行选择：一次性插入垫、一次性月经垫、带一体式衬垫的可洗内衣和可洗衬垫[80]。Cochrane 综述发现比较这些产品的数据有限，但根据一项合格的研究得出结论，就防漏、整体可接受性和偏好而言，一次性衬垫优于月经垫，月经垫优于带一体式衬垫的可洗内衣，一体式衬垫优于可洗衬垫。就皮肤健康而言，可洗或一次性选择之间没有明显差异。大多数女性更喜欢一次性卫生巾，但这类物品通常费用更高[80]。

根据 Cochrane 对两个合格试验的综述，经历中度至重度失禁的女性可能从一次性“套穿型”产品中受益最大，尽管费用昂贵。一次性插入物是一种更便宜的选择，但可能无法提供同样多的保护。同样，没有任何特定的设计看起来对皮肤健康更好或更坏。最终，女性对吸收性产品设计有不同的选择和偏好，使用多种选择的组合可能是最合适和最具成本效益的[81]。

还应该考虑对尿失禁女性的外阴和会阴皮肤进行清洁、保湿和保护。当尿液（或粪便）与皮肤接触时，会发生与尿失禁相关的皮炎，范围从发红、肿胀、渗出、结痂和鳞屑变化到皮肤完整性丧失[39]。可能发生继发性感染，如局部念珠菌病。为了避免这种并发症，应该为尿失禁患者推荐皮肤护理方案。皮肤护理方案包括在每次尿失禁发作后使用会阴清洁剂（不是肥皂或洗手液）进行清洗，保湿（使用甘油、羊毛脂或矿物油），以及使用防潮材料（如凡士林、羊毛脂、氧化锌）来抵御刺激物和水分[39]。

有限的研究验证了用于预防成人尿失禁相关皮炎的护肤品的效果[82]。在 Pather 等[83]的综述中，作者得出结论，包括使用局部屏障产品在内的皮肤护理方案有利于预防和治疗与尿失禁相关的皮炎，但没有证据表明哪种特定产品的效果更好。一项系统性综述表明，与传统的肥皂和水相比，会阴皮肤清洁剂可有效预防失禁相关性皮炎并保持皮肤屏障功能[84]。不管有限的证据如何，对于尿失禁的女性来说，清洁、保湿，以及保护外阴和会阴皮肤是尿失禁护理方案的一个重要方面。

总结

各种各样的行为疗法和生活方式的改变被推荐作为女性尿失禁的初始治疗方法。支持这些建议的证据强度总体上是薄弱的，主要是观察性的试验研究，在这一领域，很少有随机试验。

参考文献

[1] Burgio KL. Behavioral therapy to enable women with urge incontinence to discontinue drug treatment: a randomized trial. Ann Intern Med. 2008;149:161.

[2] Lightner DJ, Gomelsky A, Souter L, Vasavada SP. Diagnosis and treatment of overactive bladder (non-neurogenic) in adults: AUA/SUFU guideline amendment 2019. J Urol. 2019;202:558–63.

[3] Kobashi KC, Albo ME, Dmochowski RR, et al. Surgical treatment of female stress urinary incontinence: AUA/SUFU guideline. J Urol. 2017;198:875–83.

[4] ACOG practice bulletin no. 155: urinary incontinence in women. Obstet Gynecol. 2015;126:e66–81.

[5] Dallosso HM, McGrother CW, Matthews RJ, Donaldson MMK, The Leicestershire MRC Incontinence Study Group. Nutrient composition of the diet and the development of overactive bladder: a longitudinal study in women. Neurourol Urodyn. 2004;23:204–10.

[6] Dallosso HM, McGrother CW, Matthews RJ, Donaldson MMK, the Leicestershire MRC Incontinence Study Group. The association of diet and other lifestyle factors with overactive bladder and stress incontinence: a longitudinal study in women. BJU Int. 2003;92:69–77.

[7] The Leicestershire MRC Incontinence Study Group, Dallosso H, Matthews R, McGrother C, Donaldson M. Diet as a risk factor for the development of stress urinary incontinence: a longitudinal study in women. Eur J Clin Nutr. 2004;58:920–6.

[8] Manonai J, Songchitsomboon S, Chanda K, Hong JH, Komindr S. The effect of a soy-rich diet on urogenital atrophy: a randomized, cross-over trial. Maturitas. 2006;54:135–40.

[9] Waetjen LE, Leung K, Crawford SL, Huang M-H, Gold EB, Greendale GA. Relationship between dietary phytoestrogens and development of urinary incontinence in midlife women. Menopause. 2013;20(4):428–36.

[10] Maserejian NN, Giovannucci EL, McVary KT, McKinlay JB. Intakes of vitamins and minerals in relation to urinary incontinence, voiding, and storage symptoms in women: a cross-sectional analysis from the Boston Area Community Health Survey. Eur Urol. 2011;59:1039–47.
[11] Markland AD, Tangpricha V, Mark Beasley T, Vaughan CP, Richter HE, Burgio KL, Goode PS. Comparing vitamin D supplementation versus placebo for urgency urinary incontinence: a pilot study. J Am Geriatr Soc. 2019;67:570–5.
[12] Markland AD, Vaughan C, Huang A, Tangpricha V, Grodstein F. Vitamin D intake and the 10-year risk of urgency urinary incontinence in women. J Steroid Biochem Mol Biol. 2020;199:105601.
[13] Townsend MK, Jura YH, Curhan GC, Resnick NM, Grodstein F. Fluid intake and risk of stress, urgency, and mixed urinary incontinence. Am J Obstet Gynecol. 2011;205:73.e1–6.
[14] Swithinbank L, Hashim H, Abrams P. The effect of fluid intake on urinary symptoms in women. J Urol. 2005;174:187–9.
[15] Bradley CS, Erickson BA, Messersmith EE, et al. Evidence of the impact of diet, fluid intake, caffeine, alcohol and tobacco on lower urinary tract symptoms: a systematic review. J Urol. 2017;198: 1010–20.
[16] Callan L, Thompson DL, Netsch D. Does increasing or decreasing the daily intake of water/ fluid by adults affect overactive bladder symptoms? J Wound Ostomy Continence Nurs. 2015;42:614–20.
[17] Gleason JL, Richter HE, Redden DT, Goode PS, Burgio KL, Markland AD. Caffeine and urinary incontinence in US women. Int Urogynecol J. 2013;24:295–302.
[18] Jura YH, Townsend MK, Curhan GC, Resnick NM, Grodstein F. Caffeine intake, and the risk of stress, urgency and mixed urinary incontinence. J Urol. 2011;185:1775–80.
[19] Townsend MK, Resnick NM, Grodstein F. Caffeine intake and risk of urinary incontinence progression among women. Obstet Gynecol. 2012;119:950–7.
[20] Maserejian NN, Wager CG, Giovannucci EL, Curto TM, McVary KT, McKinlay JB. Intake of caffeinated, carbonated, or citrus beverage types and development of lower urinary tract symptoms in men and women. Am J Epidemiol. 2013;177:1399–410.
[21] Lohsiriwat S, Hirunsai M, Chaiyaprasithi B. Effect of caffeine on bladder function in patients with overactive bladder symptoms. Urol Ann. 2011;3:14.
[22] Selo-Ojeme D, Pathak S, Aziz A, Odumosu M. Fluid and caffeine intake and urinary symptoms in the UK. Int J Gynecol Obstet. 2013;122:159–60.
[23] Zimmern P, Litman HJ, Mueller E, Norton P, Goode P. Effect of fluid management on fluid intake and urge incontinence in a trial for overactive bladder in women. BJU Int. 2009;105:1680–5.
[24] Segal S, Saks EK, Arya LA. Self-assessment of fluid intake behavior in women with urinary incontinence. J Women's Health. 2011;20: 1917–21.
[25] Schimpf MO, Smith AR, Miller JM. Fluids affecting bladder urgency and lower urinary symptoms (FABULUS): methods and protocol for a randomized controlled trial. Int Urogynecol J. 2020;31:1033–40.
[26] Schimpf MO, Smith AR, Hawthorne K, Garcia C, Miller JM. Fluids affecting bladder urgency and lower urinary symptoms (FABULUS): results from a randomized controlled trial. Female Pelvic Med Reconstr Surg. 2020;26((105)Supplement 1):S5.
[27] Karram MM, Walters MD, Elsevier (Amsterdam). Urogynecology and reconstructive pelvic surgery. Philadelphia: Elsevier/Saunders; 2015.
[28] Bump RC, McClish DK. Cigarette smoking and urinary incontinence in women. Am J Obstet Gynecol. 1992;167:1213–8.
[29] Richter HE, Burgio KL, Brubaker L, et al. Factors associated with incontinence frequency in a surgical cohort of stress incontinent women. Am J Obstet Gynecol. 2005;193:2088–93.
[30] Tampakoudis P, Tantanassis T, Grimbizis G, Papaletsos M, Mantalenakis S. Cigarette smoking and urinary incontinence in women—a new calculative method of estimating the exposure to smoke. Eur J Obstet Gynecol Reprod Biol. 1995;63:27–30.
[31] Hannestad YS, Rortveit G, Daltveit AK, Hunskaar S. Are smoking and other lifestyle factors associated with female urinary incontinence? The Norwegian EPINCONT Study. BJOG Int J Obstet Gynaecol. 2003;110:247–54.
[32] Danforth KN, Townsend MK, Lifford K, Curhan GC, Resnick NM, Grodstein F. Risk factors for urinary incontinence among middle-aged women. Am J Obstet Gynecol. 2006;194:339–45.
[33] Tähtinen RM, Auvinen A, Cartwright R, Johnson TM, Tammela TLJ, Tikkinen KAO. Smoking and bladder symptoms in women. Obstet Gynecol. 2011;118:643–8.
[34] Nuotio M, Jylhä M, Koivisto A-M, TLJ T. Association of smoking with urgency in older people. Eur Urol. 2001;40:206–12.
[35] Aydin Y, Hassa H, Oge T, Yalcin OT, Mutlu FŞ. Frequency and determinants of urogenital symptoms in postmenopausal Islamic women. Menopause. 2014;21:182–7.
[36] de Boer TA, Slieker-ten Hove MCP, Burger CW, Vierhout ME. The prevalence and risk factors of overactive bladder symptoms and its relation to pelvic organ prolapse symptoms in a general female population. Int Urogynecol J. 2011;22:569–75.
[37] Maserejian NN, Kupelian V, Miyasato G, McVary KT, McKinlay JB. Are physical activity, smoking and alcohol consumption associated with lower urinary tract symptoms in men or women? Results from a population based observational study. J Urol. 2012;188:490–5.
[38] Fuganti PE, Gowdy JM, Santiago NC. Obesity and smoking: are they modulators of cough intravesical peak pressure in stress urinary incontinence? Int Braz J Urol. 2011;37:528–33.
[39] Cameron AP, Jimbo M, Heidelbaugh JJ. Diagnosis and office-based treatment of urinary incontinence in adults. Part two: treatment. Ther Adv Urol. 2013;5:189–200.
[40] Eustice S, Roe B, Paterson J. Prompted voiding for the management of urinary incontinence in adults. Cochrane Database Syst Rev. 2000; https://doi.org/10.1002/14651858.CD002113.
[41] Ostaszkiewicz J, Johnston L, Roe B. Timed voiding for the management of urinary incontinence in adults. In: The Cochrane Collaboration, editor. Cochrane Database Syst. Rev. Chichester: Wiley; 2000. p. CD002802.
[42] Holroyd-Leduc JM, Straus SE. Management of urinary incontinence in women: scientific review. JAMA. 2004;291:986.
[43] Davies JA, Hosker G, Lord J, Smith ARB. An evaluation of the efficacy of in-patient bladder retraining. Int Urogynecol J. 2000;11:271–6.
[44] Newman DK, Borello-France D, Sung VW. Structured behavioral treatment research protocol for women with mixed urinary incontinence and overactive bladder symptoms. Neurourol Urodyn. 2018;37:14–26.
[45] Visco AG, Weidner AC, Cundiff GW, Bump RC. Observed patient compliance with a structured outpatient bladder retraining program. Am J Obstet Gynecol. 1999;181:1392–4.
[46] Wallace SA, Roe B, Williams K, Palmer M. Bladder training for urinary incontinence in adults. Cochrane Database Syst Rev. 2004; https://doi.org/10.1002/14651858.CD001308.pub2
[47] Elser DM, Wyman JF, McClish DK, Robinson D, Fantl JA, Bump RC. The effect of bladder training, pelvic floor muscle training, or combination training on urodynamic parameters in women with urinary incontinence. Continence Program for Women Research Group. Neurourol Urodyn. 1999;18:427–36.
[48] Mattiasson A, Blaakaer J, Høye K, Wein AJ, The Tolterodine Scandinavian Study Group. Simplified bladder training augments the effectiveness of tolterodine in patients with an overactive bladder. BJU Int. 2003;91:54–60.
[49] Wyman JF, Fantl JA, McClish DK, Bump RC. Comparative efficacy

of behavioral interventions in the management of female urinary incontinence. Continence Program for Women Research Group. Am J Obstet Gynecol. 1998;179:999–1007.
[50] Loening-Baucke V. Urinary incontinence and urinary tract infection and their resolution with treatment of chronic constipation of childhood. Pediatrics. 1997;100:228–32.
[51] Feng WC, Churchill BM. Dysfunctional elimination syndrome in children without obvious spinal cord diseases. Pediatr Clin N Am. 2001;48:1489–504.
[52] Cameron A, Fenner DE, DeLancey JOL, Morgan DM. Self-report of difficult defecation is associated with overactive bladder symptoms: difficult defecation in OAB. Neurourol Urodyn. 2010;29:1290–4.
[53] Franco I. Overactive bladder in children. Part 2: management. J Urol. 2007;178:769–74; discussion 774.
[54] Fernandes E, Vernier R, Gonzalez R. The unstable bladder in children. J Pediatr. 1991;118:831–7.
[55] Warne SA, Godley ML, Wilcox DT. Surgical reconstruction of cloacal malformation can alter bladder function: a comparative study with anorectal anomalies. J Urol. 2004;172:2377–81; discussion 2381.
[56] Jarrett MED. Neuromodulation for constipation and fecal incontinence. Urol Clin North Am. 2005;32:79–87.
[57] Hagovska M, Švihra J, Buková A, Dračková D, Horbacz A. The impact of different intensities of exercise on body weight reduction and overactive bladder symptoms- randomised trial. Eur J Obstet Gynecol Reprod Biol. 2019;242:144–9.
[58] Wikander L, Cross D, Gahreman DE. Prevalence of urinary incontinence in women powerlifters: a pilot study. Int Urogynecol J. 2019;30:2031–9.
[59] Yang J, Cheng JW, Wagner H, Lohman E, Yang SH, Krishingner GA, Trofimova A, Alsyouf M, Staack A. The effect of high impact crossfit exercises on stress urinary incontinence in physically active women. Neurourol Urodyn. 2019;38:749–56.
[60] Hein JT, Rieck TM, Dunfee HA, Johnson DP, Ferguson JA, Rhodes DJ. Effect of a 12–week pilates pelvic floor-strengthening program on short-term measures of stress urinary incontinence in women: a pilot study. J Altern Complement Med. 2020;26:158–61.
[61] Lausen A, Marsland L, Head S, Jackson J, Lausen B. Modified Pilates as an adjunct to standard physiotherapy care for urinary incontinence: a mixed methods pilot for a randomised controlled trial. BMC Womens Health. 2018;18:16.
[62] Virtuoso JF, Menezes EC, Mazo GZ. Effect of weight training with pelvic floor muscle training in elderly women with urinary incontinence. Res Q Exerc Sport. 2019;90:141–50.
[63] Huang AJ, Chesney M, Lisha N, Vittinghoff E, Schembri M, Pawlowsky S, Hsu A, Subak L. A group-based yoga program for urinary incontinence in ambulatory women: feasibility, tolerability, and change in incontinence frequency over 3 months in a single-center randomized trial. Am J Obstet Gynecol. 2019;220:87.e1–87.e13.
[64] Wieland LS, Shrestha N, Lassi ZS, Panda S, Chiaramonte D, Skoetz N. Yoga for treating urinary incontinence in women. Cochrane Database Syst Rev. 2019; https://doi.org/10.1002/14651858. CD012668.pub2
[65] Mishra GD, Hardy R, Cardozo L, Kuh D. Body weight through adult life and risk of urinary incontinence in middle-aged women: results from a British prospective cohort. Int J Obes. 2008;32:1415–22.
[66] Richter HE, Creasman JM, Myers DL, Wheeler TL, Burgio KL, Subak LL, for the Program to Reduce Incontinence by Diet and Exercise (PRIDE) Research Group. Urodynamic characterization of obese women with urinary incontinence undergoing a weight loss program: the Program to Reduce Incontinence by Diet and Exercise (PRIDE) trial. Int Urogynecol J. 2008;19:1653–8.
[67] Subak LL, Wing R, West DS, et al. Weight loss to treat urinary incontinence in overweight and obese women. N Engl J Med. 2009;360:481–90.
[68] Wing RR, West DS, Grady D, et al. Effect of weight loss on urinary incontinence in overweight and obese women: results at 12 and 18 months. J Urol. 2010;184:1005–10.
[69] Ait Said K, Leroux Y, Menahem B, Doerfler A, Alves A, Tillou X. Effect of bariatric surgery on urinary and fecal incontinence: prospective analysis with 1–year follow-up. Surg Obes Relat Dis. 2017;13:305–12.
[70] O'Boyle CJ, O'Sullivan OE, Shabana H, Boyce M, O'Reilly BA. The effect of bariatric surgery on urinary incontinence in women. Obes Surg. 2016;26:1471–8.
[71] Whitcomb EL, Horgan S, Donohue MC, Lukacz ES. Impact of surgically induced weight loss on pelvic floor disorders. Int Urogynecol J. 2012;23:1111–6.
[72] Anglim B, O'Boyle CJ, O'Sullivan OE, O'Reilly BA. The long-term effects of bariatric surgery on female urinary incontinence. Eur J Obstet Gynecol Reprod Biol. 2018;231:15–8.
[73] Gabriel I, Tavakkoli A, Minassian VA. Pelvic organ prolapse and urinary incontinence in women after bariatric surgery: 5–year follow-up. Female Pelvic Med Reconstr Surg. 2018;24:120–5.
[74] Yazdany T, Jakus-Waldman S, Jeppson PC, et al. American Urogynecologic Society systematic review: the impact of weight loss intervention on lower urinary tract symptoms and urinary incontinence in overweight and obese women. Female Pelvic Med Reconstr Surg. 2020;26:16–29.
[75] Hu T-W, Wagner TH, Bentkover JD, Leblanc K, Zhou SZ, Hunt T. Costs of urinary incontinence and overactive bladder in the United States: a comparative study. Urology. 2004;63:461–5.
[76] Wilson L. Annual direct cost of urinary incontinence. Obstet Gynecol. 2001;98:398–406.
[77] Fader M, Bliss D, Cottenden A, Moore K, Norton C. Continence products: research priorities to improve the lives of people with urinary and/or fecal leakage. Neurourol Urodyn. 2010;29:640–4.
[78] Teunissen TAM, Lagro-Janssen ALM. Sex differences in the use of absorbent (incontinence) pads in independently living elderly people: do men receive less care? Int J Clin Pract. 2009;63:869–73.
[79] Smith N, Hunter KF, Rajabali S, Milsom I, Wagg A. Where do women with urinary incontinence find information about absorbent products and how useful do they find it? J Wound Ostomy Continence Nurs. 2019;46:44–50.
[80] Fader M, Cottenden AM, Getliffe K. Absorbent products for light urinary incontinence in women. Cochrane Database Syst Rev. 2007; https://doi.org/10.1002/14651858. CD001406.pub2
[81] Fader M, Cottenden AM, Getliffe K. Absorbent products for moderate-heavy urinary and/ or faecal incontinence in women and men. Cochrane Database Syst Rev. 2008; https://doi. org/10.1002/14651858. CD007408
[82] Beeckman D, Van Damme N, Schoonhoven L, et al. Interventions for preventing and treating incontinence-associated dermatitis in adults. Cochrane Database Syst Rev. 2016; https://doi. org/10.1002/14651858. CD011627.pub2
[83] Pather P, Hines S, Kynoch K, Coyer F. Effectiveness of topical skin products in the treatment and prevention of incontinence-associated dermatitis: a systematic review. JBI Database Syst Rev Implement Rep. 2017;15:1473–96.
[84] Lachance CC, Argaez C. Perineal skin cleansers for adults with urine incontinence in long-term care or hospital settings: a review of the clinical effectiveness and guidelines. Ottawa: Canadian Agency for Drugs and Technologies in Health; 2019.

第7章 物理治疗和止尿装置

Physical Therapy and Continence Inserts

Paige De Rosa　Ilana Bergelson　Elizabeth Takacs　著

女性尿失禁的发病率为25%～45%[1]，并随年龄增长、妊娠和产后次数增加而增加，严重影响生活质量。盆底肌训练（PFMT）和其他保守治疗（如子宫托）经常因未被充分利用而被认为无效。盆底肌训练最早于1936年由英国学者Margaret Morris提出，但直到1948年Arthur Kegel运用该技术成功治疗了64例患者后，才得到更加广泛地应用[2]。Kegel训练本质上是盆底肌训练的一种形式，最初是通过会阴压力计测量并指导肌肉正确的放松和收缩，但是，随着时间的推移，Kegel训练发展为一个家庭治疗方案，但因缺乏正确的指导和监督，常常导致不正确的肌肉收缩锻炼，因此曾被认为无效[3]。和其他疾病的治疗一样，尿失禁的预防和保守治疗需要患者和医疗服务提供者积极配合，而且服务提供者必须对患者进行个体化指导并确保盆底肌肉锻炼（PFME）的正确性。进行盆底肌肉治疗监督的物理治疗师需要经过盆底康复专门培训和资格认证，当然，这可能是一个挑战，尤其在农村地区。此外，患者必须愿意接受治疗效果不是立竿见影的，并且需要坚持才能维持治疗效果。除了应用方面存在的问题外，不论是在预防还是治疗方面，尚没有研究证实尿失禁保守治疗的有效性和效果如何。鉴于文献数量少，且存在试验设计和干预的异质性，目前的Meta分析和系统性回顾研究还不能对尿失禁的保守治疗提供建议。

一、尿失禁的一级预防

大多数关于尿失禁的研究都集中在治疗，通常是手术或过程干预。目前尿失禁的研究目标逐渐转变为关注尿失禁的预防和改善控尿能力[4]，研究关注重点之一是不同社会阶层人群的风险因素和保护因素[5]。根据个体化差异和基于教育程度、身份识别、干扰因素、嵌入式变量，以及观察指标等因素的流行病学调查，已初步建立了尿失禁多层次预防模型[4]。第六届国际尿失禁咨询委员会（ICI）对尿失禁一级预防的结论是：迄今为止，除了老年女性、妊娠期女性和分娩后女性外，以预防为主要干预措施的数据有限[4]。

二、老年女性尿失禁的预防

众所周知，随着人口年龄的增长，尿失禁患病率增加。已有一系列研究致力于55岁以上女性尿失禁的预防干预措施，其中包括尿失禁在内的盆底疾病的一般教育[6]、开发风险人群的识别工具[7]，以及个人和群体行为训练等[8, 9]。基于这些和其他的一些研究，ICI得出的结论是：有Ⅰ级证据支持应为老年女性提供教育方案（A级推荐）[4]。

三、妊娠期和分娩后女性尿失禁的预防

妊娠期尿失禁的发病率为18.6%～75%，并随着胎龄的增加而增长[10]。识别风险因素对于了解谁有发生尿失禁的风险至关重要，干预措施可以针对高危人群或增加风险的事件。妊娠期尿失禁和分娩后尿失禁的可干预因素可分为母体因素、分娩前和分娩时因素、胎儿因素和分娩方式。通常确定的危险因素包括母亲年龄、体重指数增加、妊娠前吸烟和尿失禁[10, 11]、妊娠期体重增加[10]和妊娠期糖尿病[10]。第六届ICI建议应停止吸烟、

达到正常的分娩后体重并避免妊娠期便秘（B级推荐）[4]。目前无准确的数据证明会阴撕裂伤/会阴切开术、第二产程延长、新生儿出生体重大是否增加尿失禁发生率[11]。分娩方式，特别是阴道分娩和选择性剖宫产的影响，仍然是一个有争议的话题，因此不在本章的讨论范围。

此外，盆底肌力、既往压力性尿失禁病史、新生儿体重和妊娠期间新发压力性尿失禁已被确定为分娩后尿失禁的危险因素[12]。既往的压力性尿失禁和新发压力性尿失禁与盆底肌肌力直接相关，可能是预防尿失禁发生的干预目标。盆底肌肉锻炼的整体目标是最小风险的增加盆底肌肉强度，从而改善对膀胱、膀胱颈和尿道[10, 12]的支撑。2020年科克伦数据库系统审查和第六届ICI得出如下结论：有足够的证据支持女性妊娠早期使用结构化盆底肌训练可以预防妊娠后期和分娩后尿失禁[4, 13]，盆底肌肉锻炼应该提供给所有孕妇[4]。

四、阴道和尿道装置

压力性尿失禁的保守治疗包括使用阴道内装置，如子宫托。虽然子宫托经常被用于盆腔器官脱垂（POP），但有几种类型的子宫托可以用于压力性尿失禁。子宫托是一种具有中央开口的支撑装置，根据作用方式可分为支撑型和填充型。支撑型子宫托，如MILEX子宫托、尿失禁盘（图7-1）、带或不带把手的环形子宫托均可有效治疗压力性尿失禁。用于治疗压力性尿失禁的子宫托装置通过抬高膀胱颈，以及在耻骨后支撑尿道并尽量减少尿道活动过度来稳定尿道[14, 15]。Valsalva动作下的磁共振成像（MRI）证实子宫托使尿道长度增加，而尿道-膀胱后角变小[16]。尿流动力学研究（UDS）表明：带有子宫托的压力性尿失禁患者逼尿肌压力增加且最大尿流率降低，提示子宫托增加了尿道阻力[15]。

子宫托非一次性使用，使用后症状改善、满意度和持续使用情况依赖于子宫托是否成功放置[15]。对子宫托放置采取个性化的方法是很重要的，佩戴后不适、出血和反复脱出是停用的常见原因[17]。子宫托是一种低成本、低风险、非手术的治疗方法，几乎可以提供给几乎所有患者。子宫托的禁忌证包括活动性盆腔或阴道感染、严重溃疡、硅胶或橡胶过敏，以及可能无法进行适当随访的患者[15]。建议绝经后的女性使用阴道雌激素。已经证明，使用阴道雌激素乳膏的女性更有可能继续使用子宫托并且阴道分泌物较少，但它不能避免阴道上皮被侵蚀[18]。子宫托使用的轻微并发症包括阴道分泌物增加和异味、自发性脱出、排尿困难和阴道上皮侵蚀[14, 15]。严重的并发症包括出血、严重的阴道排液、便秘、疼痛、嵌顿、磨损和侵蚀邻近器官，这通常与使用时间长（6～10年）、用于盆腔器官脱垂的子宫托，以及遗忘或忽视子宫托有关。结果显示，超过50%的压力性尿失禁女性使用子宫托能得到满意的症状改善[17, 19, 20]。与行为治疗（包括监督性盆底肌训练）对比，在治疗3个月和12个月时，子宫托治疗组和行为治疗组之间没有差异[19, 20]。较高的子宫托失败率与患者之前进行过尿失禁手术相关[17]。

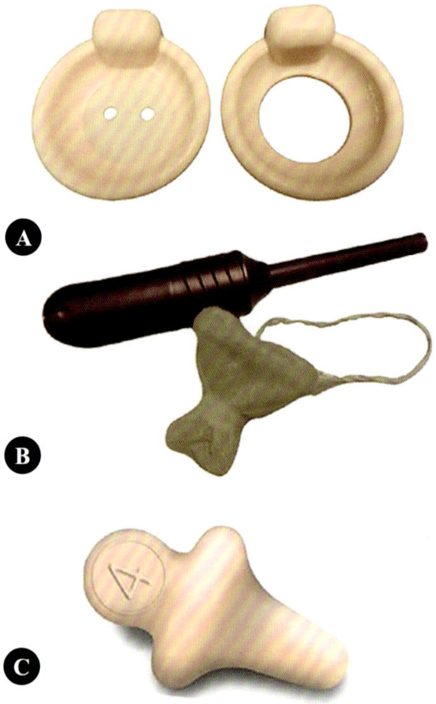

▲ 图7-1 **A. MILEX尿失禁盘（有或无支架）；B. Poise® Impressa® 膀胱支架；C. Uresta® 膀胱支架**

子宫托使用的局限性主要是缺乏关于子宫托佩戴的知识、患者能否正确定位和放置子宫托。Uresta 是一种医用级橡胶钟形子宫托，专门用于压力性尿失禁，插入阴道内，在膀胱颈处提供尿道支持[21]。通过抓住手柄，并将锥形部分（必要时使用润滑剂）插入阴道（图 7-1）。患者通过购买启动装来确定适当的尺寸，并尝试逐步增大尺寸。正确的大小不会引起不适，可以减轻或缓解压力性尿失禁的症状，并且没有排尿或排便困难（https://www.uresta.com/pages/support）。停止治疗的原因与其他子宫托类似，其中包括无法改善症状和子宫托脱出，这可能是由于子宫托佩戴不当所致[21]。研究没有记录其他不良事件或明显不适[21, 22]（https://myuresta.com/wp-content/uploads/2019/08/023099-Uresta-IFU-NA-2018-PRF.pdf）。结果研究仅限于单一的前瞻性研究和使用尿垫试验的单一前期评估。在第一个研究中，66% 的患者（压力性尿失禁或以压力性尿失禁为主的混合性尿失禁）成功地进行了前瞻性随访，所有类型的尿失禁症状均显著改善，76% 的患者在 1 年时继续使用该设备[21]。第二项研究是使用 Uresta 或阴道硅胶环安慰剂进行的尿垫试验，与安慰剂相比，放置 Uresta 后尿垫重量减少 50% 或更多[22]。目前还没有长期研究或更大患者群体的研究。

Impressa 是另一种治疗尿失禁的装置。该装置是一个类似卫生棉条的尼龙网覆盖的树脂芯（图 7-1）。将 Impressa 放置在阴道内，展开后以无张力的方式提供尿道下段支持，有绳子连接在远端便于抓住以取出[23]。像 Uresta 一样，使用 Impressa 的患者应购买适当的尺寸在减少或解决漏尿的同时增加舒适性。使用 Impressa 的并发症包括阴道腐蚀、阴道疼痛、阴道和尿路感染，以及可能的中毒性休克综合征。建议每天放置的时间不超过 12h（https://www.poise.com/-/media/poise/fles/poise-impressa-instructions-for-use.pdf）。在文献中，我们注意到是否使用 Impressa 的尿流率和残余尿量没有显著差异。最常见的不良反应是不适、疼痛和腐蚀[23]。在一项维持 28 天的短期研究中发现使用 Impressa 的女性减少了 70% 以上的漏尿量，仅 8% 的女性在佩戴过程中感到不适[23]。此外，平均生活质量评分和其他问卷评分有显著提高[24]。

值得注意的是，尿道置入物 FemSoft 也曾被用于治疗女性压力性尿失禁。这个装置包括一根顶端带有球囊的管子插入尿道，用矿物油充盈顶端球囊固定。虽然研究发现尿垫重量和尿失禁发作次数在统计学上显著减少，但并发症包括尿路感染、插入造成的损伤，甚至需要膀胱镜检查才能解决装置移位。因此 FemSoft 已被停产[25]。

五、盆底肌训练

盆底肌训练的目标是增加盆底肌肉的力量，目前已经成为治疗压力性尿失禁、急迫性尿失禁和混合性尿失禁的重要方法，禁忌证主要为患者盆腔肌肉功能障碍、盆底肌高张力或盆腔疼痛。2010 年，第四届国际尿失禁咨询委员会提出了以下建议：尿失禁的初始治疗应包括生活方式的建议、物理治疗、定期排尿方案、行为治疗和药物治疗。盆底肌训练建议用于尿失禁及膀胱过度活动症女性（A 级推荐）。

盆底肌训练最大的挑战之一是患者接受教育和评估的频率和形式，因为包括培训技巧、培训工具和设备，以及培训方法在内，都存在显著的差异。42%～73% 非妊娠患者接受过盆底肌训练指导，指导方式常见于口头或书面，体检指导率为 7%～28%[26, 27]。妊娠期或分娩后女性能意识到盆底肌肉锻炼的重要性。然而，大多数教育指导是通过口头或书面，很少接受体检指导[28, 29]。女性进行正确盆底肌肉收缩的能力是有差异的，一项触诊评估显示，66% 的分娩前女性无法正确收缩盆底肌肉达到测试基线[30]，在 55 岁及以上的女性中，23%～60% 能够达到 3 级以上的肌力，8%～16% 无法完成盆底肌肉收缩，9%～44% 使用辅助肌肉收缩，而 6%～12% 进行 Valsalva 动作[26, 27]。因此，为了确保患者能够正确地识别盆底肌肉，并进行正确的盆底肌训练，治疗师通过阴道触诊指导是非常重要的[31]。

六、盆底肌收缩评估

阴道触诊是评估盆底肌肌力的常用方法。阴道触诊价格低、无创、不需要特殊设备、患者耐受性好，且可以和常规盆腔检查同时进行。目前常用的盆底功能评估方法有 3 种：改良牛津肌力分级（MOS）[32]、Brink 量表[33] 和 PERFECT 量表[34]（表 7-1）。改良牛津肌力分级是通过阴道指诊下收缩阴道完成的，按照收缩强度从弱到强分为 0～5 级。有作者报道，改良牛津肌力分级的评估者间信度仅轻到中等[31, 35, 36]。Brink 量表包括 3 个方面的评分：收缩力、持续时间和垂直平面的移动度，评估后计算总分[33]。采用 Brink 量表的评估者用双指触诊，示指靠着中指水平置于阴道内[34]。Brink 量表的各项评价指标都表现出良好的评估者间信度，与收缩持续时间的相关性最低[33, 37, 38]，且有较好的重复检测间信度[33]。Brink 总分和收缩力评分与会阴压力计检测到的最大收缩力中度相关（0.67～0.71）[37]。与改良牛津肌力分级和 Brink 量表相比，PERFECT 量表可以评估盆底肌肉的快肌和慢肌纤维。在这个评估模式中，通过阴道（女性）或直肠（男性）的单指触诊对盆底肌肉的力量（或压力）、耐力、重复次数和快速收缩进行评估[34]。

会阴压力计和超声是用于评估盆腔肌力的辅助工具。会阴压力计是一种阴道压力测量计，可以测量阴道收缩压力、静息压力和耐力[30]。已证明压力测量有较高的评价者间信度和评分者内部的可靠性[36, 37]，并且常用于研究目的而非临床实践。经腹超声成像目前主要用于研究设计；然而，随着可用性的增加，它成为临床实践中的一项新兴技术。超声可以通过显示患者的膀胱后壁抬高[39] 来评估阴道收缩和提升情况，但是不能用于评估盆底肌肌力。

表 7-1　常用盆底肌肉收缩评估量表比较

改良牛津肌力分级[a]	Brink 量表[b]	PERFECT 量表[c]
压力 • 0 级：无反应 • 1 级：肌肉颤动 • 2 级：不完全收缩 • 3 级：完全收缩，无对抗 • 4 级：完全收缩，轻微对抗 • 5 级：完全收缩，持续对抗	**收缩力** • 1 分：无反应，无法感知挤压 • 2 分：弱收缩力 / 指尖感到微弱的挤压 • 3 分：中度收缩力 / 指尖感到明显挤压 • 4 分：强烈收缩力 / 指尖感到强烈挤压 **位移** • 1 分：无 • 2 分：指尖向前移动 • 3 分：整个指节向前移动 • 4 分：整个手指向前移动 **持续时间** • 无 • ≥1s 且≤3s • ＞3s	**压力（P）** • 0 级：无反应 • 1 级：肌肉颤动 • 2 级：不完全收缩 • 3 级：完全收缩，无对抗 • 4 级：完全收缩，轻微对抗 • 5 级：完全收缩，持续对抗 **耐力（E）** • 肌肉保持最大自主收缩的时间（最高 10s） **重复性（R）** • 患者在 1 次检测中可以进行多少次最大程度自主收缩（最大 10 次） **快速收缩（F）** • 患者可以连续进行的 1s 快速有力收缩的次数（最多 10 次） **ECT** • 每次收缩时间

a. Schüssler et al.[32]；b. Brady et al.[5]；c. Laycock and Jerwood[34]

七、指导盆底肌收缩

成功执行盆底肌肉锻炼和盆底肌训练的第二个关键因素是，通过书面和口头交流指导女性正确地进行盆底肌肉锻炼，包括或不包括触诊、中断排尿或使用生物反馈的工具和设备。在过去，宣教是通过授课、视频和纸质材料向患者提供的。TULIP 项目证明，在尿急和尿失禁方面，通过 2h 授课和 20min 视频进行宣教的效果是没有差异的[40]。随着信息技术和互联网的进步，人们对基于网络或移动应用程序进行盆底肌肉锻炼的宣教越来越感兴趣。研究人员进行了一系列的研究来评估教育材料的影响，这些材料包括关于压力性尿失禁的信息、盆底肌训练、Knack 操作教程、图形练习，以及对自我报告有压力性尿失禁的女性进行每日 3 次的锻炼计划。基于互联网的教育材料与纸质邮寄材料一样有效，两组都报道了症状、状况和具体生活质量问题得到显著改善，并维持了 2 年时间[41.42]；并且不仅对诊断为压力性尿失禁的女性，被提供宣教材料的所有女性都有改善[43]。来自上述研究的在线教育材料现在是一款名为“Tät（®）”的移动应用程序，其不仅设置了提醒功能，还通过对 App 影响的评估，有效地改善了参与者的 QOL 评分和症状严重程度，并提高了依从性[44]。接受基于网络的盆底治疗方案也得到了第二项独立研究的支持[45]。研究证实，报告有改善的女性有较高的治疗期望值、体重控制和自我评估肌力的改善[46]。

指导正确的收缩对所有类型的尿失禁都至关重要。不正确的收缩包括那些不能产生任何收缩、使用辅助肌群或 Valsalva 动作。正确的收缩包括收紧阴道口周围，然后向内向头顶方向抬起[30]，检查时阴道肌肉应该向上和向内牵拉，而不使用包括腹部和臀部肌肉在内的辅助肌肉[27]。由一组物理治疗师和一名专业护士进行的定性研究发现，在盆底治疗中需设置特定的训练提示和语言提示，需要一定的沟通技巧使患者理解治疗方案及其安全性。大多数参与者一致认为，需要建立一个提示和言语提示的“信息库”，并且对女性和男性使用不同的语言[47]。一项研究发现，患者对提示“收紧你用来憋尿的阴道肌肉”最容易做出正确收缩动作；而对“向上向内抬起你的阴道肌肉”则很少引出正确的收缩[27]。表 7-2 列出了有助于引出患者正确收缩的语言提示。

排尿中断技术已被用于帮助女性验证她们是否启用了正确的盆底肌，并正确的进行了盆底肌肉锻炼[26]。在这项技术中，女性被指示在排尿时停止尿流。最近的一项研究表明，中断排尿的连续性会导致残余尿量（PVR）增加（36.7ml vs. 8.2ml）和最大尿流率降低（17.8ml/min vs. 26.9ml/min），由此作者得出结论排尿中断不应用于盆底肌训练[48]。中断尿流可能会中断正常的排尿周期，并有可能导致排尿功能障碍，由于这一假设性担心导致该技术使用频率较低。建议女性在进行盆底肌肉锻炼时不要常规中断排尿[48.49]。

虽然阴道触诊是用来评估和指导正确收缩的经典方法，但目前生物反馈已经成为一种辅助和（或）替代方法。在广义上，生物反馈可以使认知可视化，普遍认为生物反馈是使用各种工具、计算机分析以及物理视觉图像来帮助识别和正确执行所需要的练习。生物反馈的使用，特别是所使用的技术，取决于物理治疗师。尽管少数个体研究显示生物反馈在盆底肌肌力和尿失禁治疗效果上的优势[50.51]，但 2019 年对使用生物反馈进行盆底肌训练的随机对照试验的 Meta 分析得出结论：生物反馈并不能提供全面治疗益处[52]。

八、结果

有很多方法可以让患者进行盆底肌肉锻炼和盆底肌训练，其中包括有监督或无监督的环境、小组治疗与个人治疗，以及使用电刺激和生物反馈等辅助手段。关于非监督方案成功与否，现有数据结论并不一致。早期研究表明，非监督治疗方案在尿垫试验、排尿日记、问卷调查和主观报告的改善情况劣于监督方案，而非治疗组对改善结果的满意度较低[53-56]。最近的一些文献证实，在开始治疗前确认正确进行盆底肌锻炼能改善实施家庭治疗方案的患者的预后指标[57.58]。这强调了非监督治疗方案的患者能够正确进行盆底肌肉锻炼的重要性。为了维持症状的改善，患者需要继续进行盆底肌训练，即使对完成了全部盆底肌训练监督方案的患者也是如此[59]。

盆底肌训练的个体治疗（IT）和小组治疗（GT）在减轻症状严重程度方面同样有效[60-62]，而且可能有更高的成本效益[61]。在已报道的文献中，对于客观指标的评估存在差异。Figueiredo 等报道，与只接受小组治疗的患者相比，接受至少部分个体治疗的患者盆底功能有更好的改善[62]。相反，de Oliveira 等证明接受个体治疗与小组治疗的患者在盆底肌肌力或尿垫试验方面没有差异[60]。

在探讨盆底肌训练的效果时，即使患者的盆底肌肌力没有明显改善，她们的生活质量仍有可能得到改善[57]。表 7–3 列出了国际尿失禁咨询委员会的具体建议。

九、反向支撑和尿意抑制

反向支撑或“the Knack 方法”是指在估计要漏尿时收缩盆底肌。最初由 Burgio 等在 1986 年提出，这一方法需要在压力动作发生前或发生时

表 7–2　有助于引出患者正确收缩的语言提示[a]

通用提示	女性特定提示
口头提示 “收缩和抬起。” • “收缩和抬起你的盆底肌肉。” • “想象关闭和提升，把你的尾骨拉向耻骨上。” • 想象提示 • “像电梯上升一样，往上抬升。” • “想象一下，你提示自己阻止尿流，我认为这可以帮助大多数人。” • “想象一下，你在一个拥挤的电梯里，有一些风，你试图抓住它，因为你不想让任何人听到或闻到你要放手的东西。” • “想象海洋，或者想象看到海浪进来，然后感觉它消失，释放出来，离开。” • “想象钟表盘，12 在顶部，6 在尾部，3 和 9 在两旁，想象你坐在一个一定大小的时钟上，把所有这些数字画出来，把这些数字抓在一起，然后放下来，放松，让这些数字漂移到时钟的位置上。” • “把一根吸管拉进去，把所有的东西都拉进去。” • “如果你想更向前移动，像飞机一样起飞。”	**口头提示** • “收缩和抬起。” • “向上向内抬起你的阴道肌肉。” • “你坐在上面，在你的肛门和阴道之间，想象你的马鞍在里面拉着。” • “向前摆动尾骨，停止排尿，关闭阴道。” • “如果坐着，尝试从椅子上起来，收缩并离开椅子，然后慢慢放松，再次坐回去。” • “吸吮吸管，体会这是一个更长更慢的收缩。” • “收缩你用来抑制排气的阴道肌肉。” • “收缩你用来抑制排尿的阴道肌肉。” **智能提示** • “你能感觉到我的手指吗？想象那里有一条卫生棉条。” • “你能感觉到我的手指吗？你能尝试推动或拉动手指吗？” • “好的，收缩这里”，在阴道内触诊时 • “收缩我手指周围的阴道肌肉。” **想象提示** • “想象你的内裤里有个棉球，你想让它往上提升，然后让它缓慢下降、慢慢地、柔和的下降，至远离内裤。” • “想想你尝试将阴道远离内裤。” • “想象一下电梯上升，电梯下来。” • “想象一下，你正在拉动一颗豌豆，从阴道向你的头部。” • “想象一下你正在将卫生棉条往阴道里边塞。” • “想象一下，有人试图拉出卫生棉条绳，而你却试图抵制它。” • “想象一下有东西在阴道里，你试图把它挤出来。”

a. Slade et al.[47]

有目的地收缩盆底肌肉[63.64]。已证实在咳嗽时收缩盆底肌会移动膀胱颈和降低其活动度[65]。该方法可减少 71%～98.2% 的漏尿量，并使 18.8% 的漏尿症状消失[64, 66, 67]。行为矫正和膀胱训练是急迫性尿失禁保守治疗的主要手段。在膀胱训练中，需指导患者进行下尿路功能训练，其中包括设定递增的排尿计划、指导尿意抑制技巧或“收紧并维持”的动作等（附图 7–1）。盆底肌训练在膀胱训练中非常重要，以促进尿意抑制和最大限度减少漏尿[68]。已经证实，盆底肌的收缩增加了尿道内压力，并抑制了排尿反射[69]。根据目前已经发表的研究，有证据表明，盆底肌训练可以减少膀胱过度活动症症状和急迫性尿失禁；然而，由于研究的异质性，清楚地确定其效果是不太可能的[70]。

十、制订个性化方案

参与盆底肌训练培训计划的患者是有不同的基础知识、技能和期望的。认识到这些差异并理解患者的意愿对于制订诊断患者的个性化培训计划至关重要，因此，通用治疗方案的作用是有限的[47]。有效的教育可以通过传统授课、书面材料、视频、基于网络的程序以及移动应用程序来实现。训练可以在个人或小组环境中进行，但评估患者能够和正确的收缩盆底肌肉必不可少。辅助性监督、生物反馈和其他设备可能是帮助患者正确进行锻炼所必需的。文献提供的锻炼方案更为复杂，但由于研究中缺乏标准化锻炼方案，很难得出什么方案是最有效的结论[34]；我们在附图 7–2 中提供了一个常规强化方案。在评估和确认正确地盆底肌收缩后，提供者可以使用常规强化方案为患者设定初始参数和目标。然而，如果患者在办公室训练时不能进行正确收缩，在放弃盆底肌训练前应该考虑转诊给物理治疗师。物理治疗师对接受监督性盆底肌训练的患者，应该根据反复的重新评估进行个性化家庭治疗方案的指导。

总结

尿失禁给医疗系统和患者带来了巨大的经济负担，随着人口老龄化，其经济影响将会持续增加。2007 年，仅膀胱过度活动症造成的总负担（包括工作能力的丧失）就达 659 亿美元，2020 年估计为 826 亿美元[5]。随着尿失禁医疗费用和经济负担的增加，考虑非手术干预非常重要。成本分析研究表明，对于支付意愿高的患者，手术干预最具成本效益，但对于支付意愿低的患者，子宫托最具成本效益[71]。在非手术干预手段中，盆底肌训练似乎具有最大的经济效益[72]，手术失败的患者也应考虑保守治疗[73]。尿失禁保守治疗或非手术治疗的成功与否取决于患者的选择。研究发现，绝经、受教育程度高、尿失禁前无手术史、漏尿发生率低是压力性尿失禁非手术干预成功的相关因素[74]，老年患者和规律进行盆底肌训练的患者远期成功率更高[75]。在向患者提供非手术治疗干预手段时，可能需要考虑这些因素。

凯格尔训练

重要提醒：有盆腔疼痛的女性不应进行凯格尔训练，如果您在进行训练时感到疼痛，请立即停止。

什么是凯格尔运动?

- 凯格尔运动是一种加强盆底肌肉的锻炼。
- 加强盆底肌肉可以预防尿液或粪便的泄漏，如果已经存在，也可以帮助减少泄漏。

你的盆底肌有什么作用?

这些肌肉支撑着子宫（如果未切除）、膀胱、阴道、直肠和小肠。

盆底肌为什么会变弱?

妊娠、分娩、手术，年龄增长，过度用力（便秘），长期咳嗽以及超重等原因。

哪些人应该做凯格尔运动?

任何人都可以从凯格尔运动中受益，尤其是发生以下情况。

- 在打喷嚏、笑或咳嗽时会漏出几滴尿液（强调性尿失禁）。
- 在大量排尿之前会突然强烈地想要排尿（紧迫性尿失禁）。
- 漏粪（肛门失禁）。

如何进行盆底肌肉锻炼?

找到正确的肌肉。

- 刚开始时，可以放松身体，如躺着或坐着练习。
- 挤压或缩紧肌肉时呼气，松弛时吸气。
- 你应该能够感受到肌肉的升起。
  - 缩紧肌肉就像尽可能地避免放屁或假装停止尿液流动。不要开始和停止你的尿流。
  - 假装阴道夹着卫生棉条收缩肌肉。
  - 试图将阴道向上提到肚脐或头部。
  - 插入一个手指到你的阴道里并收缩。您应该感觉到阴道紧缩以及骨盆底部向上移动。
- 确保在紧缩后完全放松。

最佳的方法或理想的做法

- 你应该感到骨盆区域后面（靠近直肠）的收缩较为明显，而不是前面。
- 不要用力挤压腹部肌肉（肚子）、臀部肌肉或者内侧大腿肌肉。将手放在腹部、臀部下方或者内侧大腿上。如果你在挤压时感到这些肌肉有运动，那么你错用了肌肉。
- 在进行挤压时，你的身体不应该抬起。

增加收缩次数和时间。就像任何新的运动一样，需要慢慢开始，逐渐增加强度。

- 先进行慢速肌肉收缩训练。
  - 挤压并保持3～5s，然后休息3～5s，这是1个凯格尔运动。
  - 看看你能连续做多少个，但不要挤压超过10次。如果你无法进行10次有质量的挤压，逐渐训练到超过10次挤压松弛周期。
  - 1组为10个挤压，每个挤压保持3～5s，然后休息3～5s。
  - 目标是每天进行2～3组，每组进行10次收缩，总共进行30～40次锻炼。
  - 如果你感到疼痛，请停止锻炼，及时咨询医生。
- 在你正确完成慢速收缩练习之后，增加快收缩肌肉训练练习。短时间内完成收缩，快速进行2～3s的收缩和释放。
  - 简短收缩。快速进行2～3s的收缩和放松。
- 完整的锻炼方案包括以下内容。
  - 3组，每组10次挤压并保持5s放松5s。
  - 3组，每组10次快速挤压并松开。
  - 质量比数量更重要。

我可以什么时候做凯格尔运动?

- 可以分散到一整天进行。
- 随时随地可以进行：电梯、红绿灯、排队等待、刷牙、进餐，甚至在开会中。但不要在小便时进行。

如果我不能做凯格尔运动或觉得我没有做对怎么办?

请与您的医生或其他医护人员进行沟通。

可能需要与物理治疗师合作，使用生物反馈传感器或负重锥。

- 物理治疗师－盆底治疗师接受了专门的培训。请向您的医护人员咨询以寻求推荐。
- 生物反馈传感器－将压力传感器放置在阴道或直肠中，当您放松和收缩盆底肌肉时，显示屏上就会显示出来。
- 负重锥－插入阴道中的阴道负重器。在日常活动中收缩盆底肌肉以保持其位置稳定。

需要多长时间才能看到效果?

通过定期进行锻炼，可能需要几个星期到几个月才能注意到改善。

一开始改善可能很小。

- 每次上厕所的时间间隔更长。
- 出现的意外事故更少。
- 能够更长时间地收缩或进行更多次数的重复。
- 内裤更干燥或使用更少或更小的护垫。
- 为了持续获得益处和改善，你需要将这些纳入你的日常生活中。

▲ 附图 7-1　凯格尔训练

表 7-3　第五届国际尿失禁咨询委员会的推荐[a]

分　类		推荐等级	推　荐
盆底肌训练	初产妇 – 预防尿失禁	A	产前应该提供一个有监督的、高强度的强化训练，以防止分娩后尿失禁
	产后 3 个月治疗尿失禁	A	一线保守治疗方法
		B	强化盆腔肌力训练可能会增加治疗效果
	育龄女性的预防与治疗	B	考虑由卫生专业人员基于成本 / 效益或人群，提供分娩前或分娩后盆底肌训练
	一般人群的尿失禁治疗	A	作为压力性尿失禁、急迫性尿失禁或混合性尿失禁的一线保守治疗。尽可能提供最大强度的盆底肌训练方案
		A	由训练有素的卫生专业人员进行监督和教学，比自我指导训练效果更好
生物反馈辅助盆底肌训练	临床生物反馈	A	没有明确推荐
		B	没有明确推荐
阴道哑铃	压力性尿失禁	B	对于能够和准备使用阴道哑铃的女性，由训练有素的卫生专业人员进行监督培训是一线方案
膀胱锻炼	一般人群的尿失禁	A	可能是一种合适的一线治疗方法
	急迫性尿失禁或混合性尿失禁	B	有效的一线保守治疗
	压力性尿失禁	B	盆底肌训练优于膀胱训练
	逼尿肌过度活动或急迫性尿失禁	B	膀胱训练或抗胆碱能药物可能有效

a. Dumoulin et al.[76]

膀胱再训练

催尿波[a]
膀胱向大脑传递信息

随着膀胱的充盈，膀胱会向大脑发出如厕的需求信号。我们会感受到排尿的冲动。随着膀胱的持续充盈，冲动会变得越来越强烈，直到达到顶峰。在顶峰时会出现漏尿的情况，我们会赶快去洗手间，或者这种感觉会逐渐消失。

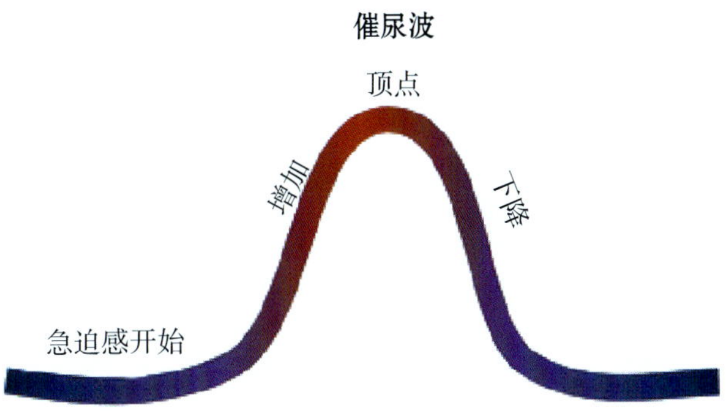

▲ 附图 7-2　膀胱再训练

a. Urge wave image from Newman DK, Burgio KL, Markland AD, Goode PS. Urinary Incontinence: Nonsurgical Treatments. In: Griebling TL, editor. Geriatric Urology. New York, NY: Springer New York; 2014. p. 141–68. Original: Urge suppression strategy: patient handout. Burgio KL, Pearce KL, Lucco AJ. Staying Dry: A Practical Guide to Bladder Control. Baltimore, MD: Johns Hopkins Press, 1989; 67–100

膀胱再训练 [b]

膀胱再训练是一种旨在帮助您掌握膀胱控制，并在无紧迫感时进行排尿的方法

急迫地冲往洗手间
这可能会使这种感觉更糟糕
增加对膀胱充盈的意识
可能会让膀胱收缩并排空（尿湿你的裤子或垫子）

目标：每 3～4 小时排尿 1 次，避免严重的紧迫感。

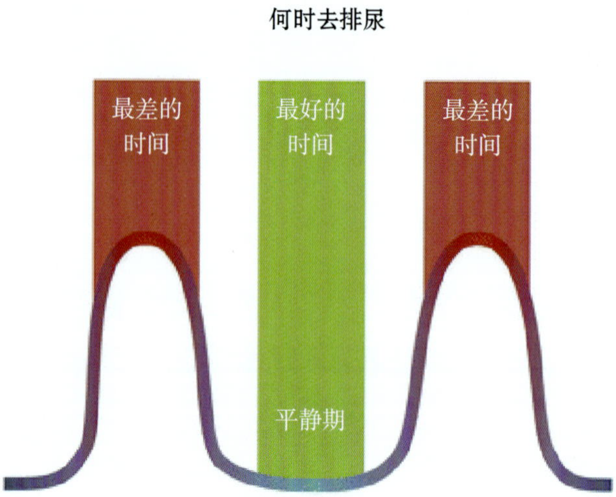

当紧迫感来袭时：冲动抑制技术 [c]

1. 如有可能，请停下来坐下。
2. 快速收缩盆底肌（凯格尔运动）3～5 次，不要在收缩之间放松。
3. 深呼吸，尝试放松自己，并分散注意力。让尿意自然消失。
   - 分散注意力的方法。
     i. 以每七个数字为一递减的方式倒数。
     ii. 吟唱自己喜欢的歌曲。
     iii. 专注于其他身体感觉，如深呼吸。
     iv. 看手机、其他设备或玩游戏。
4. 在尿意消失后以正常步伐走到厕所。
5. 如果冲动再次出现，请停止并重复步骤 1～4。
6. 在步骤 1～5 成功后，尝试将排尿延迟 5min，逐渐延长延迟的时间。
7. 继续拖延，直到两次上厕所之间有 3～4h。

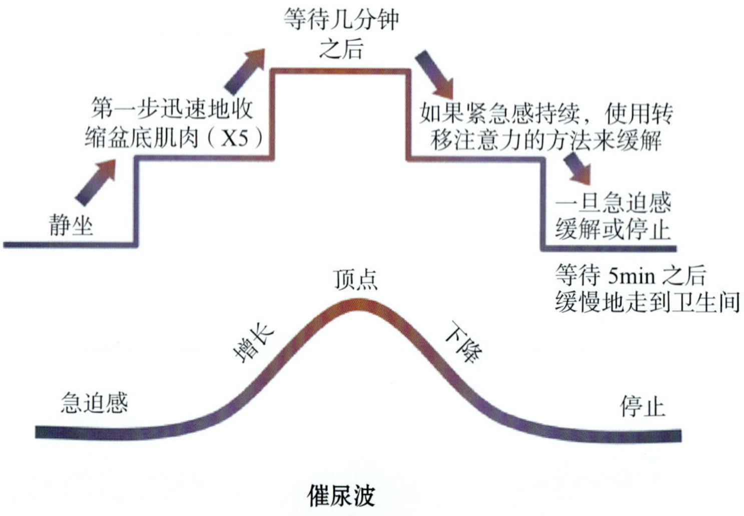

▲ 附图 7-2（续） 膀胱再训练

b. When to Void image from Newman DK, Burgio KL, Markland AD, Goode PS. Urinary Incontinence: Nonsurgical Treatments. In: Griebling TL, editor. Geriatric Urology. New York, NY: Springer New York; 2014. p. 141-68. Original: Urge suppression strategy: patient handout. Burgio KL, Pearce KL, Lucco AJ. Staying Dry: A Practical Guide to Bladder Control. Baltimore, MD: Johns Hopkins Press, 1989; 67–100

c. Urge Wave image from Skokan A, Newman DK. Behavioral Intervention for Lower Urinary Tract Symptoms in Older Adults. In: Guzzo TJ, Drach GW, Wein AJ, editors. Primer of Geriatric Urology. New York, NY: Springer New York; 2016. p. 149-

参考文献

[1] Altman D, Cartwright R, Lapitan MC, Milsom I, Nelson R, Sjöström S, Tikkinen KAO. Epidemiology of urinary incontinence (UI) and other lower urinary tract symptoms (LUTS), pelvic organ prolapse (POP) and anal incontinence (AI). In: Abrams P, Cardozo L, Wagg A, Wein A, editors. Incontinence: 6th international consultation on incontinence, Tokyo, September 2016. Bristol: International Continence Society; 2017. p. 1–141.

[2] Price N, Dawood R, Jackson SR. Pelvic floor exercise for urinary incontinence: a systematic literature review. Maturitas. 2010;67(4): 309–15.

[3] Lamin E, Parrillo LM, Newman DK, Smith AL. Pelvic floor muscle training: underutilization in the USA. Curr Urol Rep. 2016;17(2):10.

[4] Palmer MH, Cockerell R, Griebling TL, Rantell A, van Houten P, Newman DK. Review of the 6th international consultation on incontinence: primary prevention of urinary incontinence. Neurourol Urodyn. 2020;39(1):66–72.

[5] Brady SS, Bavendam TG, Berry A, Fok CS, Gahagan S, Goode PS, et al. The Prevention of Lower Urinary Tract Symptoms (PLUS) in girls and women: developing a conceptual framework for a prevention research agenda. Neurourol Urodyn. 2018;37(8):2951–64.

[6] Geoffrion R, Robert M, Ross S, van Heerden D, Neustaedter G, Tang S, et al. Evaluating patient learning after an educational program for women with incontinence and pelvic organ prolapse. Int Urogynecol J Pelvic Floor Dysfunct. 2009;20(10):1243–52.

[7] Diokno AC, Ogunyemi T, Siadat MR, Arslanturk S, Killinger KA. Continence Index: a new screening questionnaire to predict the probability of future incontinence in older women in the community. Int Urol Nephrol. 2015;47(7):1091–7.

[8] Diokno AC, Newman DK, Low LK, Griebling TL, Maddens ME, Goode PS, et al. Effect of group-administered behavioral treatment on urinary incontinence in older women: a randomized clinical trial. JAMA Intern Med. 2018;178(10):1333–41.

[9] Tannenbaum C, Agnew R, Benedetti A, Thomas D, van den Heuvel E. Effectiveness of continence promotion for older women via community organisations: a cluster randomised trial. BMJ Open. 2013;3(12):e004135.

[10] Sangsawang B. Risk factors for the development of stress urinary incontinence during pregnancy in primigravidae: a review of the literature. Eur J Obstet Gynecol Reprod Biol. 2014;178:27–34.

[11] Kissler K, Yount SM, Rendeiro M, Zeidenstein L. Primary prevention of urinary incontinence: a case study of prenatal and intrapartum interventions. J Midwifery Womens Health. 2016;61(4):507–11.

[12] Baracho SM, Barbosa da Silva L, Baracho E, Lopes da Silva Filho A, Sampaio RF, Mello de Figueiredo E. Pelvic floor muscle strength predicts stress urinary incontinence in primiparous women after vaginal delivery. Int Urogynecol J. 2012;23(7):899–906.

[13] Woodley SJ, Lawrenson P, Boyle R, Cody JD, Mørkved S, Kernohan A, et al. Pelvic floor muscle training for preventing and treating urinary and faecal incontinence in antenatal and postnatal women. Cochrane Database Syst Rev. 2020;5(5):CD007471.

[14] Jones KA, Harmanli O. Pessary use in pelvic organ prolapse and urinary incontinence. Rev Obstet Gynecol. 2010;3(1):3–9.

[15] Al-Shaikh G, Syed S, Osman S, Bogis A, Al-Badr A. Pessary use in stress urinary incontinence: a review of advantages, complications, patient satisfaction, and quality of life. Int J Women's Health. 2018;10:195–201.

[16] Komesu YM, Ketai LH, Rogers RG, Eberhardt SC, Pohl J. Restoration of continence by pessaries: magnetic resonance imaging assessment of mechanism of action. Am J Obstet Gynecol. 2008;198(5):563 e1–6.

[17] Farrell SA, Singh B, Aldakhil L. Continence pessaries in the management of urinary incontinence in women. J Obstet Gynaecol Can. 2004;26(2):113–7.

[18] Dessie SG, Armstrong K, Modest AM, Hacker MR, Hota LS. Effect of vaginal estrogen on pessary use. Int Urogynecol J. 2016;27(9):1423–9.

[19] Richter HE, Burgio KL, Brubaker L, Nygaard IE, Ye W, Weidner A, et al. Continence pessary compared with behavioral therapy or combined therapy for stress incontinence: a randomized controlled trial. Obstet Gynecol. 2010;115(3):609–17.

[20] Kenton K, Barber M, Wang L, Hsu Y, Rahn D, Whitcomb E, et al. Pelvic floor symptoms improve similarly after pessary and behavioral treatment for stress incontinence. Female Pelvic Med Reconstr Surg. 2012;18(2):118–21.

[21] Farrell SA, Baydock S, Amir B, Fanning C. Effectiveness of a new self-positioning pessary for the management of urinary incontinence in women. Am J Obstet Gynecol. 2007;196(5):474 e1–8.

[22] Lovatsis D, Best C, Diamond P. Short-term Uresta efficacy (SURE) study: a randomized controlled trial of the Uresta continence device. Int Urogynecol J. 2017;28(1):147–50.

[23] Ziv E, Stanton SL, Abarbanel J. Efficacy and safety of a novel disposable intravaginal device for treating stress urinary incontinence. Am J Obstet Gynecol. 2008;198(5): 594 e1–7.

[24] Ziv E, Stanton SL, Abarbanel J. Significant improvement in the quality of life in women treated with a novel disposable intravaginal device for stress urinary incontinence. Int Urogynecol J Pelvic Floor Dysfunct. 2009;20(6):651–8.

[25] Sirls LT, Foote JE, Kaufman JM, Lightner DJ, Miller JL, Moseley WG, et al. Long-term results of the FemSoft urethral insert for the management of female stress urinary incontinence. Int Urogynecol J Pelvic Floor Dysfunct. 2002;13(2):88–95; discussion

[26] Moen MD, Noone MB, Vassallo BJ, Elser DM, Urogynecology N. Pelvic floor muscle function in women presenting with pelvic floor disorders. Int Urogynecol J Pelvic Floor Dysfunct. 2009;20(7):843–6.

[27] Kandadai P, O'Dell K, Saini J. Correct performance of pelvic muscle exercises in women reporting prior knowledge. Female Pelvic Med Reconstr Surg. 2015;21(3):135–40.

[28] Ismail SI. An audit of NICE guidelines on antenatal pelvic floor exercises. Int Urogynecol J Pelvic Floor Dysfunct. 2009;20(12): 1417–22.

[29] Fine P, Burgio K, Borello-France D, Richter H, Whitehead W, Weber A, et al. Teaching and practicing of pelvic floor muscle exercises in primiparous women during pregnancy and the postpartum period. Am J Obstet Gynecol. 2007;197(1):107 e1–5.

[30] Ahlund S, Nordgren B, Wilander EL, Wiklund I, Friden C. Is home-based pelvic floor muscle training effective in treatment of urinary incontinence after birth in primiparous women? A randomized controlled trial. Acta Obstet Gynecol Scand. 2013;92(8):909–15.

[31] Bo K, Finckenhagen HB. Vaginal palpation of pelvic floor muscle strength: inter-test reproducibility and comparison between palpation and vaginal squeeze pressure. Acta Obstet Gynecol Scand. 2001;80(10):883–7.

[32] Schüssler B, Laycock J, Hesse U, Hilton P, Kölbl H, Debus-Thiede G, et al. Evaluation of the pelvic floor. In: Schüssler B, Laycock J, Norton PA, Stanton SL, editors. Pelvic floor re-education. London: Springer; 1994.

[33] Brink CA, Wells TJ, Sampselle CM, Taillie ER, Mayer R. A digital test for pelvic muscle strength in women with urinary incontinence. Nurs Res. 1994;43(6):352–6.

[34] Laycock J, Jerwood D. Pelvic floor muscle assessment: the PERFECT

scheme. Physiotherapy. 2001;87(12):631–42.
[35] Ferreira CH, Barbosa PB, de Oliveira SF, Antonio FI, Franco MM, Bo K. Inter-rater reliability study of the modified Oxford Grading Scale and the Peritron manometer. Physiotherapy. 2011;97(2):132–8.
[36] Navarro Brazalez B, Torres Lacomba M, de la Villa P, Sanchez Sanchez B, Prieto Gomez V, Asunsolo Del Barco A, et al. The evaluation of pelvic floor muscle strength in women with pelvic floor dysfunction: a reliability and correlation study. Neurourol Urodyn. 2018;37(1):269–77.
[37] Hundley AF, Wu JM, Visco AG. A comparison of perineometer to brink score for assessment of pelvic floor muscle strength. Am J Obstet Gynecol. 2005;192(5):1583–91.
[38] Boyles SH, Edwards SR, Gregory WT, Denman MA, Clark AL. Validating a clinical measure of levator hiatus size. Am J Obstet Gynecol. 2007;196(2):174 e1–4.
[39] Sherburn M, Murphy CA, Carroll S, Allen TJ, Galea MP. Investigation of transabdominal real-time ultrasound to visualise the muscles of the pelvic floor. Aust J Physiother. 2005;51(3):167–70.
[40] Sampselle CM, Newman DK, Miller JM, Kirk K, DiCamillo MA, Wagner TH, et al. A randomized controlled trial to compare 2 scalable interventions for lower urinary tract symptom prevention: main outcomes of the TULIP study. J Urol. 2017;197(6):1480–6.
[41] Sjostrom M, Umefjord G, Stenlund H, Carlbring P, Andersson G, Samuelsson E. Internet-based treatment of stress urinary incontinence: a randomised controlled study with focus on pelvic floor muscle training. BJU Int. 2013;112(3):362–72.
[42] Sjostrom M, Umefjord G, Stenlund H, Carlbring P, Andersson G, Samuelsson E. Internet-based treatment of stress urinary incontinence: 1– and 2–year results of a randomized controlled trial with a focus on pelvic floor muscle training. BJU Int. 2015;116(6):955–64.
[43] Bokne K, Sjostrom M, Samuelsson E. Self-management of stress urinary incontinence: effectiveness of two treatment programmes focused on pelvic floor muscle training, one booklet and one internet-based. Scand J Prim Health Care. 2019;37(3):380–7.
[44] Asklund I, Nystrom E, Sjostrom M, Umefjord G, Stenlund H, Samuelsson E. Mobile app for treatment of stress urinary incontinence: a randomized controlled trial. Neurourol Urodyn. 2017;36(5):1369–76.
[45] Barbato KA, Wiebe JW, Cline TW, Hellier SD. Web-based treatment for women with stress urinary incontinence. Urol Nurs. 2014;34(5):252–7.
[46] Nystrom E, Asklund I, Sjostrom M, Stenlund H, Samuelsson E. Treatment of stress urinary incontinence with a mobile app: factors associated with success. Int Urogynecol J. 2018;29(9):1325–33.
[47] Slade SC, Hay-Smith J, Mastwyk S, Morris ME, Frawley H. Strategies to assist uptake of pelvic floor muscle training for people with urinary incontinence: a clinician viewpoint. Neurourol Urodyn. 2018;37(8):2658–68.
[48] Chesnel C, Charlanes A, Tan E, Turmel N, Breton FL, Ismael SS, et al. Influence of the urine stream interruption exercise on micturition. Int J Urol. 2019;26(11):1059–63.
[49] Lukacz ES, Santiago-Lastra Y, Albo ME, Brubaker L. Urinary incontinence in women: a review. JAMA. 2017;318(16):1592–604.
[50] Bertotto A, Schvartzman R, Uchoa S, Wender MCO. Effect of electromyographic biofeedback as an add-on to pelvic floor muscle exercises on neuromuscular outcomes and quality of life in postmenopausal women with stress urinary incontinence: a randomized controlled trial. Neurourol Urodyn. 2017;36(8):2142–7.
[51] Aksac B, Aki S, Karan A, Yalcin O, Isikoglu M, Eskiyurt N. Biofeedback and pelvic floor exercises for the rehabilitation of urinary stress incontinence. Gynecol Obstet Investig. 2003;56(1):23–7.
[52] Nunes EFC, Sampaio LMM, Biasotto-Gonzalez DA, Nagano R, Lucareli PRG, Politti F. Biofeedback for pelvic floor muscle training in women with stress urinary incontinence: a systematic review with meta-analysis. Physiotherapy. 2019;105(1):10–23.
[53] Felicissimo MF, Carneiro MM, Saleme CS, Pinto RZ, da Fonseca AM, da Silva-Filho AL. Intensive supervised versus unsupervised pelvic floor muscle training for the treatment of stress urinary incontinence: a randomized comparative trial. Int Urogynecol J. 2010;21(7):835–40.
[54] Wong KS, Fung BKY, Fung LCW, Ma S. Pelvic floor exercises in the treatment of stress urinary incontinence in Hong Kong Chinese women. September 1997; Yokohama Japan. In: Proceedings of the 27 Annual Meeting of the International Continence Society; 1997. p. 23–6.
[55] Sugaya K, Owan T, Hatano T, Nishijima S, Miyazato M, Mukouyama H, et al. Device to promote pelvic floor muscle training for stress incontinence. Int J Urol. 2003;10(8):416–22.
[56] Zanetti MR, Castro Rde A, Rotta AL, Santos PD, Sartori M, Girao MJ. Impact of supervised physiotherapeutic pelvic floor exercises for treating female stress urinary incontinence. Sao Paulo Med J. 2007;125(5):265–9.
[57] Al Belushi ZI, Al Kiyumi MH, Al-Mazrui AA, Jaju S, Alrawahi AH, Al Mahrezi AM. Effects of home-based pelvic floor muscle training on decreasing symptoms of stress urinary incontinence and improving the quality of life of urban adult Omani women: a randomized controlled single-blind study. Neurourol Urodyn. 2020;39(5):1557–66.
[58] Cavkaytar S, Kokanali MK, Topcu HO, Aksakal OS, Doganay M. Effect of home-based Kegel exercises on quality of life in women with stress and mixed urinary incontinence. J Obstet Gynaecol. 2015;35(4):407–10.
[59] Kruger AP, Luz SC, Virtuoso JF. Home exercises for pelvic floor in continent women one year after physical therapy treatment for urinary incontinence: an observational study. Rev Bras Fisioter. 2011;15(5):351–6.
[60] de Oliveira CF, Rodrigues AM, Arruda RM, Ferreira Sartori MG, Girao MJ, Castro RA. Pelvic floor muscle training in female stress urinary incontinence: comparison between group training and individual treatment using PERFECT assessment scheme. Int Urogynecol J Pelvic Floor Dysfunct. 2009;20(12):1455–62.
[61] Lamb SE, Pepper J, Lall R, Jorstad-Stein EC, Clark MD, Hill L, et al. Group treatments for sensitive health care problems: a randomised controlled trial of group versus individual physiotherapy sessions for female urinary incontinence. BMC Womens Health. 2009;9:26.
[62] Figueiredo VB, Nascimento SL, Martinez RFL, Lima CTS, Ferreira CHJ, Driusso P. Effects of individual pelvic floor muscle training vs individual training progressing to group training vs group training alone in women with stress urinary incontinence: a randomized clinical trial. Neurourol Urodyn. 2020;39(5):1447–55.
[63] Burgio KL, Robinson JC, Engel BT. The role of biofeedback in Kegel exercise training for stress urinary incontinence. Am J Obstet Gynecol. 1986;154(1):58–64.
[64] Miller JM, Ashton-Miller JA, DeLancey JO. A pelvic muscle precontraction can reduce cough-related urine loss in selected women with mild SUI. J Am Geriatr Soc. 1998;46(7):870–4.
[65] Miller JM, Perucchini D, Carchidi LT, DeLancey JO, Ashton-Miller J. Pelvic floor muscle contraction during a cough and decreased vesical neck mobility. Obstet Gynecol. 2001;97(2):255–60.
[66] Miller JM, Sampselle C, Ashton-Miller J, Hong GR, DeLancey JO. Clarification and confirmation of the Knack maneuver: the effect of volitional pelvic floor muscle contraction to preempt expected stress incontinence. Int Urogynecol J Pelvic Floor Dysfunct. 2008;19(6):773–82.
[67] Miller JM, Hawthorne KM, Park L, Tolbert M, Bies K, Garcia C, et al. Self-perceived improvement in bladder health after viewing a novel tutorial on knack use: a randomized controlled trial pilot study. J Womens Health (Larchmt). 2020;29(10):1319–27.
[68] Burgio KL. Update on behavioral and physical therapies for

incontinence and overactive bladder: the role of pelvic floor muscle training. Curr Urol Rep. 2013;14(5):457–64.
[69] Shafik A, Shafik IA. Overactive bladder inhibition in response to pelvic floor muscle exercises. World J Urol. 2003;20(6):374–7.
[70] Bo K, Fernandes A, Duarte TB, Brito LGO, Ferreira CHJ. Is pelvic floor muscle training effective for symptoms of overactive bladder in women? A systematic review. Physiotherapy. 2020;106:65–76.
[71] Von Bargen E, Patterson D. Cost utility of the treatment of stress urinary incontinence. Female Pelvic Med Reconstr Surg. 2015;21(3):150–3.
[72] Simpson AN, Garbens A, Dossa F, Coyte PC, Baxter NN, McDermott CD. A cost-utility analysis of nonsurgical treatments for stress urinary incontinence in women. Female Pelvic Med Reconstr Surg. 2019;25(1):49–55.
[73] Kavanagh A, Sanaee M, Carlson KV, Bailly GG. Management of patients with stress urinary incontinence after failed midurethral sling. Can Urol Assoc J. 2017;11(6Suppl2):S143–S6.
[74] Schaffer J, Nager CW, Xiang F, Borello-France D, Bradley CS, Wu JM, et al. Predictors of success and satisfaction of nonsurgical therapy for stress urinary incontinence. Obstet Gynecol. 2012;120(1):91–7.
[75] Lindh A, Sjostrom M, Stenlund H, Samuelsson E. Non-face-to-face treatment of stress urinary incontinence: predictors of success after 1 year. Int Urogynecol J. 2016;27(12):1857–65.
[76] Dumoulin C, Hunter KF, Moore K, Bradley CS, Burgio KL, Hagen S, Imamura M, Thakar R, Williams K, Chambers T. Conservative management for female urinary incontinence and pelvic organ prolapse review 2013: Summary of the fifth International Consultation on Incontinence. Neurourol Urodyn. 2016;35(1):15–20. https://doi.org/10.1002/nau.22677. Epub 2014 Nov 15. PMID: 25400065.

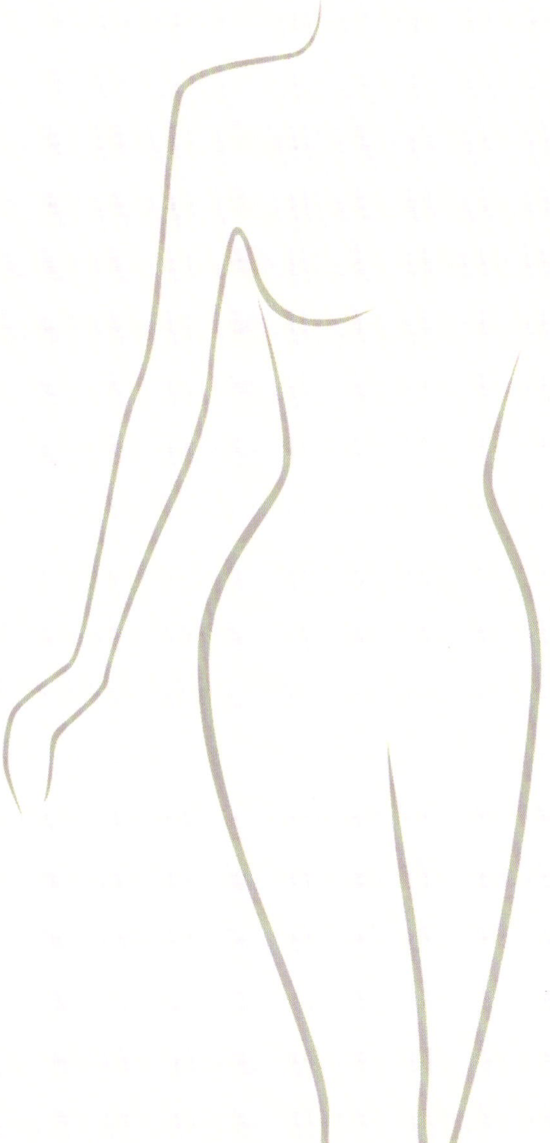

第三篇
急迫性尿失禁的药物和手术治疗

Medical and Surgical Treatment of UUI

第 8 章　药物治疗：抗胆碱类药和 β_3 受体激动药
Medical Therapy with Antimuscarinics and β_3-Agonists

Sophia Delpe Goodridge　Leslie M. Rickey　著

膀胱过度活动症（OAB）是一种良性下尿路疾病，影响 10%～17% 的人群，其患病率随着受试者年龄的增长而增加[1, 2]。仅在北美，膀胱过度活动症影响了 3400 万人，并带来了巨大的经济负担。据估计，在美国每年有 120 亿美元用于管理膀胱过度活动的人群[3]。非致命性的下尿路功能障碍可使人精神衰弱，对生活质量产生相应的影响，包括行动障碍、家庭和工作效率下降、社交孤立、睡眠障碍、抑郁和性功能受损等[4-6]。虽然男性和女性的总体患病率相似，但女性报告的症状更严重，急迫性尿失禁（UUI）的发生率更高[4]。

联合国国际学会将膀胱过度活动症定义为尿急及存在或不存在急迫性尿失禁时突然需要排尿，包括日间尿频和夜尿频繁[7]。关于膀胱过度活动的潜在病理有几种理论（包括神经源性和肌源性）[8]。年龄、传染病和炎症可影响逼尿肌通透性和神经元功能，个别微生物群也可导致膀胱过度活动症[9-11]。这些理论可能与膀胱过度活动症多层次和异质性的病因相互关联。

在 AUA/SUFU 指南中，有一些行为矫正和盆腔肌肉干预的方法，口服药物治疗是治疗膀胱过度活动症的二线药物[12]。已确定有两类药物可用于治疗膀胱过度活动症：抗毒蕈碱类药和 β_3 受体激动药。本章的目的是回顾药物的药理学用于膀胱过度活动症的不良反应和疗效。

一、药物药理学

膀胱功能受副交感神经和交感神经系统的调节。正常情况下，交感神经系统促进膀胱壁舒张、储存尿液，副交感神经系统介导膀胱壁收缩及尿液排空[8]。

抗毒蕈碱类药通过胆碱能阻断逼尿肌毒蕈碱受体抑制副交感神经通路，从而减轻或消除逼尿肌收缩的严重程度。已知毒蕈碱受体亚型有 5 种（M1～M5）[13]，而逼尿肌平滑肌主要含有 M2 和 M3 受体。M3 受体介导胆碱能诱导的膀胱收缩，而 M2 受体的作用尚不明确，但认为其与 M3 协同作用[14-16]。M2 和 M3 受体在整个尿路上皮和神经纤维中都有发现，它们可能对 A-delta 和 C-fiber 神经纤维的传入通路也有影响[17]。目前抗毒蕈碱药物治疗方法与其他受体亚型相比对 M3 有不同程度的亲和力，这导致了不同的不良反应[18]。毒蕈碱受体在口腔、眼睛和肠道中也大量存在，是造成口干、便秘和视觉障碍这些常见不良反应的原因。此外，毒蕈碱受体还存在于中枢神经系统，其中 M1 和 M2 对高级认知过程很重要[19]。

肾上腺素受体是介导儿茶酚胺作用的一类组织受体（包括去甲肾上腺素和肾上腺素），刺激 β_3 受体致逼尿肌松弛。这里描述了 3 个 β 肾上腺素受体：β_1、β_2 和 β_3。β_3 受体主要存在于逼尿肌和尿路上皮，并能被肾上腺素刺激激活。逼尿肌黏膜层和肌层表达的 β 肾上腺素受体有 97% 为 β_3 受体[20]。

二、抗胆碱类药的功效

AUA/SUFU 指南认可 6 种口服抗胆碱类药可用于膀胱过度活动症的受试者（表 8-1）[12]。这些药物包括奥昔布宁、托特罗定、达非那新、索利那新、弗斯特罗定和曲司氯胺。奥昔布宁速释

表 8-1　抗胆碱类药用于治疗膀胱过度活动症

用于膀胱过度活动症的口服抗胆碱类药	剂　量	给药方式	不良反应	特殊人群用药
达非那新	• 7.5mg，每日 1 次 • 根据反应和耐受性可增加至 15mg，每日最多 1 次	缓释剂	• 7.5mg – 口干 20.5% – 便秘 14.8% – 尿路感染 4.7% • 15mg – 口干 35.3% – 便秘 21.3% – 消化不良 8.4% – 尿路感染 4.5%	• 中度肝损害受试者（Child-Pugh B 级）或服用强效 CYP3A4 抑制药的受试者不建议超过 7.5mg • 严重肝损害受试者（Child-Pugh C 级）不建议使用 • 肾损害受试者调整剂量
弗斯特罗定	• 4mg，每日 1 次 • 根据反应和耐受性可增加到 8mg，每日最多 1 次	缓释剂	• 4mg – 口干 18.8% – 便秘 4% • 8mg – 口干 19% – 便秘 6%	• 严重肾损害（CrCl<30ml/min）或服用强效 CYP3A4 抑制药的受试者不建议超过 4mg • 肝硬化严重者不推荐使用（Child-Pugh C 级） • 中度肝损伤受试者不建议调整剂量（Child-Pugh B 级）
奥昔布宁	• 成人：5～15mg，每日 1 次，每天不超过 30mg • 儿童（6 岁及以上）：5mg，每日 1 次，每天不超过 20mg	缓释剂	• 口干 71.4% • 便秘 15.1% • 头痛 7.5% • 嗜睡 14.0% • 头晕 16.6%	• 不适用于有肾或肝损害的患者 • 不建议不能咀嚼或不能吞咽的儿童使用 • 服用 CYP3A4 抑制药时应小心 • 同时服用酮康唑时，奥昔布宁的剂量约为最高剂量的 2 倍
索利那新	• 5mg，每日 1 次 • 根据反应和耐受性可增加到 10mg，每日 1 次	薄膜衣剂	• 5mg – 口干 10.9% – 便秘 5.4% • 10mg – 口干 27.6% – 便秘 13.4% – 尿路感染 4.8%	对于严重肾功能损害（CrCl<30ml/min）、中度肝损害（Child-Pugh B 级）或服用强力 CYP3A4 抑制药的受试者，不要超过 5mg
托特罗定	• 速释剂：1～2mg，每日 2 次 • 缓释剂：2～4mg，每日 1 次	速释剂和缓释剂	• 口干 30% • 便秘 7% • 头痛 7% • 眩晕 / 头晕 5% • 腹痛 5%	• 速释剂 – 严重肾损害受试者减少剂量至 1mg，每日 2 次（CrCl 10～30ml/min） – 严重肝损害受试者减少剂量至 1mg，每日 2 次 • 缓释剂 – 严重肾损害受试者减少剂量至 2mg，每日 1 次（CrCl 10～30ml/min），CrCl<10ml/min 不推荐

（续表）

用于膀胱过度活动症的口服抗胆碱类药	剂　量	给药方式	不良反应	特殊人群用药
托特罗定				- 对于轻度至中度肝损伤（Child-Pugh A 级或 Child-Pugh B 级）受试者，减少剂量至 2mg，每日 1 次，Child-Pugh C 级不推荐 - 参见与 CYP3A4 抑制药共同给药的剂量
曲司氯铵	• 速释剂：20mg，每日 2 次 • 缓释剂：60mg，每日早晨 1 次	速释剂和缓释剂	• 口干 5.8% • 便秘 4.6%	• 速释剂 - 对于严重肾功能损害受试者（CrCl＜30ml/min），减少剂量至每日 20mg，有肝损害者不推荐使用 - 根据耐受性，75 岁以上的老年受试者可滴注每日 20mg • 缓释剂 - 不推荐严重肾功能损害受试者使用（CrCl＜30ml/min） - 不推荐肝功能损伤的受试者使用

注：包括所有在患病率≥4% 时测量的不良反应
引自参考文献 [21–28]

（IR）是目前使用的最古老的药物配方。已进行大量实验将其与安慰剂进行对比，以评估药物的疗效和不良反应。在膀胱过度活动症的改善方面，研究表明通过药物可治疗的急迫性尿失禁的比例为 49%（四分位差，35.6%～58%）[29]。无尿失禁受试者的急迫性、频率和夜尿症状改善程度较低（15%～35%）[30, 31]。

最近的一项 Meta 分析随机比较了 128 项合格的研究结果。总体而言，与安慰剂相比，积极治疗的受试者更有可能报告漏尿次数和排尿次数有所改善（OR 为 1.42～2.20），而积极治疗的受试者之间差异性不显著[32]。另一项针对女性抗胆碱类药试验的系统综述和 Meta 分析中发现，服用了抗胆碱类药可每天减少 2 次尿失禁和 1.73 次尿失禁，这说明药物在疗效优越性这方面并没有差异[33]。值得注意的是，82% 符合纳入分析标准的研究是由行业赞助的。记录了增加膀胱细胞容量（平均 54ml，43～66ml）和膀胱首次收缩体积（平均 52ml，38～67ml）与安慰剂相比排尿后残余尿量的平均增加没有临床意义（0.1～6.8ml）[18]。

通过尿失禁影响问卷、King 的健康问卷和膀胱过度活动症问卷（OAB-q）的评分评估受试者症状对生活的干扰和影响的变化，结果显示与安慰剂相比，下尿路症状（LUTS）相关的生活质量都有所改善，抗胆碱类药之间无差异[34]。

所有抗胆碱类药最常见的不良反应是口干（与安慰剂相比，OR 为 3～5），其中奥昔布宁（OR=9.5）的发生率最高[32]。其次最常见的不良反应是便秘和视力变化。不良事件的报告在各个临床试验中是不同的，但一项系统综述报告显示在试验参与者中口干的发生率为 6.3%～13.6%，便秘的发生率为 2.2%～5.1%，视物模糊的发生率为

0.8%～6.2%[35]。

还应该注意的是，尽管药物对膀胱过度活动症有效，但受试者对药物依从性的差异很大。在临床试验中，停药率为 4%～31%，而医疗索赔研究显示更高的停药率为 43%～83%。大多数受试者在 30 天内停止用药，随着时间的推移，停药率逐渐增加，其主要原因是缺乏疗效和药物的不良反应[36, 37]。

从受试者的角度出发，主观结果反映了受试者的整体改善情况和满意度，这在衡量治疗效果的方面是很重要的[38]。评估受试者生活质量的改善情况和整体结局指标可能同时需要考虑到受试者症状的改善和带来的不良反应，这与单独记录膀胱数据相比，可能是记录成功治疗受试者和受试者对药物依从性的优越指标。

相对有效性

对上述 6 种抗胆碱类药进行了一些随机对照试验，其大多数实验是由制药公司赞助的。Hsu 等最近更新了 2012 年的 Cochrane Review，在总结比较数据后，证实虽然抗胆碱药在不良反应方面存在差异，但疗效是相似的[35]。

在评估托特罗定与奥昔布宁疗效的研究中，受试者每天尿失禁发作、排尿频率或生活质量没有统计学差异。托特罗定的不良事件较少，导致停药率降低（RR=0.52，95%CI 0.40～0.66），报告中口干舌燥的事件较少（RR=0.65，95%CI 0.60～0.71）[39]。一项试验发现，服用奥昔布宁 10mg 缓释剂的受试者相比于服用托特罗定 4mg 缓释剂的受试者更有可能发生尿失禁（23% vs. 17%，P=0.03）[40]。

曲司氯铵和奥昔布宁的速释剂对症状的改善率相似；然而服用曲司氯铵的受试者不太可能出现口干的症状（RR=0.64，95%CI 0.52～0.77），这可能是因为停药率较低。其中一项比较索利那新和奥昔布宁速释剂的试验也显示，服用索利那新的受试者口干和停药率较低。

在一项比较达非那新 7.5mg 和曲司氯胺 60mg 速释剂的药物作用小型试验，发现在所有膀胱过度活动症状评分亚量表（OABSS）（尿急、尿频、夜尿和急迫性尿失禁）和便秘增加率方面都有所提高。

在比较索利那新 5mg 和托特罗定 4mg 的试验中，索利那新组受试者的生活质量有比较好的改善，漏尿事件发生较少，24h 排尿情况没有差异。两项试验的汇总结果显示索利那新改善症状和治愈疾病的效果更好（RR=1.25，95%CI 1.13～1.39）。由于不良反应和不良事件在停药的受试者中没有差异。与托特罗定速释剂相比，索利那新的口干率较低，但与托特罗定缓释剂相比，索利那新的口干率较高。一项新的试验比较了 4mg 非索罗定和 5mg 索利那新的疗效，报道的 OABSS 有类似的改善。虽然非索罗定组有较高的便秘率（5.1% vs. 1.7%）和口干率（13.6% vs. 5.0%）但没有统计学意义，相对于索利那新组在非索罗定组有更多的受试者退出（10.2% vs. 0%）[35]。

当比较弗斯特罗定 8mg 和托特罗定 4mg 缓释剂时，弗斯特罗定组的受试者报道在生活质量（QOL）、漏尿事件、频率和紧迫性增加的方面有所改善。虽然弗斯特罗定的改善率 / 治愈率较高（RR=1.11，95%CI 1.06～1.16），但由于口干舌燥不良反应发生率较高，所以其停药率也较高[39]。

Reynolds 等对托特罗定速释剂 / 缓释剂、曲司氯铵、达非那新、索非那新和弗斯特罗定对女性的疗效进行了系统评价。发现所有药物对改善一种或多种膀胱过度活动症有一定的疗效。总体而言，缓释剂具有绝对优势。最终，没有一种药物优于另一种，这与其他系统评价和 Meta 分析一致[40]。

三、经皮抗胆碱类药的使用

奥昔布宁是美国市场上最广泛使用的抗胆碱类药，在过去 40 年里从口服剂型发展到透皮贴剂和凝胶。这在很大程度上受到了口服速释形式奥昔布宁的不良反应影响[41]。奥昔布宁速释剂首先通肝脏代谢，产生一种活性的初级代谢物，对腮腺 M3 受体的亲和力高于逼尿肌抗毒蕈碱受体[42]。

为了改善药代动力学和降低不良事件的发生率，经皮抗毒蕈碱药物治疗应运而生。

经皮奥昔布宁（OXY-TDS）通过真皮小毛细血管进入体循环，保持稳定96h，避免了其首先通过肝脏代谢，减少了主要代谢物，减少口干舌燥（7.0%）和便秘（2.1%）的发生[43]。皮肤部位反应是最常见的不良反应，其中包括红斑（8.3%）和瘙痒（14.0%）。应用部位的轮换减少了皮肤相关的不良事件，并在很大程度上可自行缓解。经皮奥昔布宁和长效托特罗定的随机对照研究显示，二者在减少尿失禁发作和尿频方面疗效相同，且均优于安慰剂[44]。

奥昔布宁氯化物外用凝胶（OTG）每日1次，其利用乙醇作为皮肤渗透促进剂。应用后1周内可达到稳态血浆水平。药动力学特征不会受到沐浴或防晒霜的影响。总的来说，使用奥昔布宁氯化物外用凝胶后尿频和急迫性尿失禁发作频率明显减少，据报告的口干率为6.9%、应用部位反应较少（5.4%）[45-47]。奥昔布宁氯化物外用凝胶与安慰剂或抗毒蕈碱类药物比较的数据有限。到目前为止，在美国还没有与奥昔布宁氯化物外用凝胶治疗效果的报告。

四、β_3受体激动药有效性

（一）米拉贝隆

β_3受体激动药作为抗毒蕈碱类药物治疗膀胱过度活动症的替代治疗方案（表8-2）。美国食品药品管理局（FDA）批准了两种β_3受体激动药（第一种就是2012年批准的米拉贝隆）。

与安慰剂相比，米拉贝隆50mg和100mg可改善急迫性尿失禁发作［-1.13（-1.35，-0.91），-1.47（-1.69，-1.25），-1.63（-1.86，-1.40）］ 和24h空白组［-1.05（-1.31，-0.79），-1.66（-1.92，-1.40）和-1.75（-2.01，-1.48）］（$P<0.05$）。12个月时，米拉贝隆50mg组和米拉贝隆100mg组的尿失禁平均发作数较基线下降≥50%的有效率分别为63.7%和66.3%。与安慰剂对照相比，使用OAB-q和受试者膀胱状况感知表（PPBC）的治疗满意度和受试者报告的改善也有显著改善[50]。

在接受50mg和100mg的受试者中，报道便秘和口干的不良反应少于2%，无尿潴留。50mg组和100mg组分别有2.7%和3.7%的受试者报道尿路感染（无培养记录），而安慰剂组尿路感染为1.8%。总体而言，米拉贝隆与安慰剂发生口干舌燥、便秘和视物模糊的风险相似[51]。

β_3受体存在于心血管系统，激活可能对心房组织产生正性肌力作用，心室组织产生负性肌力作用[20]。一项评估米拉贝隆对心血管系统影响的Meta分析发现，在治疗12周时，25%的25mg组参与者、8.7%的50mg组参与者和8.5%的安慰剂组参与者出现高血压，收缩压和舒张压平均增加1mmHg。停药后发现血压升高是可逆的[52]。在100mg组中，观察到心率呈剂量依赖性增加，每分钟增加<3次。显然在某些情况下，很难将药物作用与疾病的自然进程区分开来。当观察高血压状态之间的变化时，检测出从正常血压到高血压的比例为2.6%的安慰剂组、2.6%的25mg米拉贝隆组和6.4%的50mg米拉贝隆组。在那些首次诊断为安慰剂的受试者中，出现高血压恶化的人18.3%为安慰剂组，16.3%的人服用25mg的米拉贝隆，21%的人服用50mg的米拉贝隆[53]。

在一项基于人群的队列研究中，新使用米拉贝隆和抗毒蕈碱类药的受试者心律失常或心动过速的发生率相似（3.6% vs. 3.8%）。米拉贝隆组没有发现心肌梗死（MI）或卒中风险增加（HR=1.06，95%CI 0.89～1.27）[54]。在一项≥65岁受试者的二次分析中，5例（1.1%）安慰剂受试者和9例（2.0%）米拉贝隆受试者报道了心脏疾病[55]。米拉贝隆组和安慰剂组受试者的主要不良心脏事件相似（0.4%），有3例受试者报告非致命性中风（安慰剂组2例，米拉贝隆50mg组1例），米拉贝隆50mg组1例非致命性心肌梗死[53]。需要更多的研究来阐明还存在更高风险的受试者群体，这将影响是否使用β_3受体激动药治疗膀胱过度活动症。

表 8-2　$β_3$ 受体激动药用于治疗膀胱过度活动症

用于膀胱过度活动症的口服 $β_3$ 受体激动药	剂　量	剂　型	不良反应	特殊人群用药
米拉贝隆	每日 25～50mg	缓释剂	• 25mg – 高血压 11.3% – 尿路感染 4.2% • 50mg – 高血压 7.5%	• 避免高血压控制不良的患者（收缩压≥180mmHg 或舒张压≥110mmHg，或者两者都有） • 严重肾功能损害［CrCl 15～29ml/min 或 GFR 15～29ml/(min・1.73m^2)］的患者不超过 25mg • 轻度或中度肾功能损害［CrCl 30～89ml/min 或 eGFR 30～89ml/(min・1.73m^2)］的患者无须调整剂量 • 中度肝损害的患者不超过 25mg（Child-Pugh B 级） • 通过 CYP2D6 酶监测药物代谢 • 轻度、中度或严重肾功能损害［15ml/(min・1.73m^2)≤eGFR＜90ml/(min・1.73m^2)］的患者无须调整 GEMTESA（维贝格龙）剂量 • 轻度至中度肝损害的患者无须调整 GEMTESA 的剂量（Child-Pugh A 级和 Child-Pugh B 级）
维贝格龙	每日 75mg	缓释剂	头痛 4%	

注：包括所有在患病率≥4% 时测量的不良反应
引自参考文献 [48, 49]

（二）维贝格龙

维贝格龙是一种新型 $β_3$ 受体激动药，于 2020 年 12 月获得美国食品药品管理局（FDA）批准治疗膀胱过度活动症（剂量 75mg 每日 1 次）。值得注意的是，该药物对肝同工酶无影响，可以降低 CYP2D6 代谢药物与药物相互作用的风险 [56]。在Ⅲ期 EMPOWUR 研究中，将 75mg 的维贝格龙与安慰剂、托特罗定 4mg 缓释剂作为有效对照，在 12 周时，维贝格龙组在排尿频率和尿失禁发作方面有更好的改善（分别为 –1.8 vs. –1.3，P＜0.001 和 –2.0 vs. –1.4，P＜0.0001）[57]。在尿失禁的受试者中，52% 服用维贝格龙的受试者每日急迫性尿失禁降低≥75%，而安慰剂组为 37%（P＜0.0001），在一项扩展研究中，改善保持在 52 周 [58]。与安慰剂相比，维贝格龙治疗的不良事件发生率较高的是头痛、鼻咽炎、腹泻和恶心。两组的高血压发生率相似（1.7%），血压升高也相似（维贝格龙组为 0.7%，安慰剂组为 0.9%）。最后，维贝格龙组的停药率为 1.7%，安慰剂组为 1.1%，托特罗定组为 3.3%。

五、$β_3$ 受体激动药与抗毒蕈碱类药单药治疗的比较

Kelleher 等进行了一项 Meta 分析，将抗毒蕈碱类药与 50mg 米拉贝隆进行了比较，包括 64 项研究。关于排尿频率，除了发现索利那新 10mg 更有效外，米拉贝隆 50mg 和抗毒蕈碱类药单药治疗之间没有显著差异。与米拉贝隆相比，弗斯特罗 8mg 能降低急迫性尿失禁的发生率，其余的药剂同样有效。所有的药都可以实现减少 50% 尿失禁的发生率，而曲司氯铵 60mg（OR=1.62）、索利那新 10mg（OR=1.28）和弗斯特罗 8mg（OR=1.27）口干的发生率都比米拉贝隆 50mg 高 [59]。

本 Meta 分析中研究的不良反应包括口干、便秘、视物模糊、高血压和尿潴留。与其他有效的治疗相比，除了奥昔布宁 5mg 速释剂（OR=2.99；

0.68，13.75）外。米拉贝隆显著降低了口干的发生频率。与大多数抗毒蕈碱类药物相比，米拉贝隆组的便秘和尿潴留风险也显著降低。两类药物在视物模糊和高血压发生率上无显著差异[59]。

总而言之，这项Meta分析表明，米拉贝隆治疗膀胱过度活动症的疗效与抗毒蕈碱类药相似，在某些情况下耐受性增加。英国临床实践的一项大型数据库研究表明，与抗毒蕈碱类药相比，米拉贝隆的停留时间更长（169天 vs. 30～78天）和12个月的持久性更强（38% vs. 8.3%～25%，$P<0.0001$）[60]。美国的一项数据库分析显示，在12个月里，米拉贝隆（44%）和抗毒蕈碱类药（31%）的受试者的依从率都很低[61]。

在药物转换方面，报道显示30%的受试者此前坚持使用抗毒蕈碱类药治疗（至少3个月）的患者在改用米拉贝隆后，有中度至显著改善，25%报道有轻微改善，31%报道无变化，10%报道结果恶化[62]。最后，在之前至少使用一种抗毒蕈碱类药治疗失败的女性中，将米拉贝隆50mg作为二线药治疗后，37%的患者是有效的，未接受治疗组为75%（$P<0.00001$）[63]。

关于一、二、三线治疗各种膀胱过度活动症结果的预测因素数据有限。下尿路功能障碍症状研究网络（LURN）正在膀胱过度活动症症状谱中开发更多受试者的离散亚型，这可能有助于改善针对特殊受试者的治疗建议。此外，应在风险分层的模型中考虑到体弱、年龄、生物学、合并症和生活方式等因素的影响[64]。

六、联合治疗

膀胱过度活动症指南于2019年修订，其中包括考虑对单药治疗症状改善不理想的受试者使用抗毒蕈碱类药治疗和β受体激动药进行联合治疗。已经试验了索利那新和米拉贝隆联合疗法的各种组合，总的来说，与安慰剂和单一药物疗法相比，联合疗法可以更好地改善排尿频率和尿失禁发作等。总体口干发生率更高（46%～52% vs. 38%～46%）[65, 66]。

在BESIDE试验中，服用索利那新5mg时持续尿失禁的受试者被随机分为索利那新5mg、索利那新10mg或索利那新5mg+米拉贝隆25mg联合治疗等治疗组。与索利那新10mg单药治疗相比，联合组急迫性尿失禁发作率较低（–1.82 vs. –1.63，$P=0.014$），且更多受试者在3天记录中显示"零尿失禁"［46% vs. 40%，OR=1.28（1.02～1.61，$P=0.033$）］[66]。一项随机对照试验评估了米拉贝隆50mg、索利那新10mg、米拉贝隆50mg、索利那新10mg联合用药与安慰剂的疗效。通过尿流动力学评估，以及治疗前后的膀胱过度活动症问卷来衡量治疗的反应。两个单药治疗组的疗效相似，联合治疗组在尿失禁、频率和急迫性尿失禁方面有更大的改善，且不良反应没有增加[67]。在联合组中，29%的受试者报道有不良反应，米拉贝隆组为33%，索利那新组为21%，安慰剂组为24%。SYNERGY研究进一步支持了这一数据，表明联合治疗不仅改善了客观结果，也改善了主观的、与患者相关的结果[68]。

七、膀胱过度活动症的治疗与认知障碍

最新研究表明，服用抗胆碱能药的人有患认知障碍的风险[69]。如前所述，中枢神经系统中存在毒蕈碱受体，治疗膀胱过度活动症的药有可能穿过血脑屏障。用于治疗膀胱过度活动症的抗毒蕈碱类药包括叔胺和季胺。叔胺较小，亲脂性，中性，因此能够穿过血脑屏障。已知的叔胺有达非那新、弗斯特罗、奥昔布宁、索非那新和托特罗定。季胺类，如曲司氯铵，具有净正电荷，亲水，亲脂性较低，因此不太可能穿过血脑屏障[70]。研究还表明，作为渗透性糖蛋白（P-gp）系统一部分的药物可以穿过血脑屏障。达非那新、弗斯特罗和曲司氯铵是渗透性糖蛋白系统底物，在动物研究中显示其穿透血脑屏障的能力较差[71]。创伤、帕金森病、阿尔茨海默病、糖尿病、多发性硬化症、高血压、癫痫、偏头痛、压力和年龄等多种因素都会增加血脑屏障的通透性[72]。

2019年，发表在《美国医学会杂志》（*JAMA*）

上的一项大型病例对照研究表示，在 11 年的研究期间，使用抗胆碱能药物是 55 岁以上受试者诊断为痴呆症的一个危险因素。膀胱过度活动症抗毒蕈碱类药对痴呆症的 OR 调整为 1.20～1.65，这一发现似乎与早期研究一致，该研究显示治疗膀胱过度活动症抗胆碱药使用者在痴呆诊断前 4～20 年的 OR=1.2[69, 73]。虽然抗胆碱能药物的使用和认知障碍（CI）的风险相关的证据已经联系起来，但其个体风险和因果关系还不太清楚。膀胱过度活动症受试者有更多的系统性神经、心理、心肺和肌肉骨骼疾病，并且更可能有中枢神经系统和心血管系统的合并症，从而增加其认知障碍的风险[74, 75]。然而，基于人群的队列研究显示，与新的 β_3 受体激动药使用者相比，尽管其总体风险较低[76]。新的膀胱过度活动症抗毒蕈碱类药使用者患痴呆症的风险更高（HR=1.23，95%CI 1.12～1.35），有趣的是，性别似乎起了一定的作用，因为增加的风险主要见于男性，而在亚组分析中，女性没有显著差异。

在对服用抗毒蕈碱类药物治疗膀胱过度活动症的临床人群进行的短期研究中，对认知测量有不同的影响。在一项针对老年人的随机研究中，与安慰剂相比，随机接受弗斯特罗的受试者的 PPBC 有显著改善，满意度较高。在 12 周时，两组的简易精神状态测试（MMSE）均保持稳定，但弗斯特罗组有 2 例受试者报告了主观记忆受损，1 例受试者因轻度混淆而退出[77]。在一项≥75 岁的轻度认知障碍受试者的小型研究中，他们被随机分配到索利那新、奥昔布宁或安慰剂组，只有奥昔布宁与注意力指标下降有关[55]。当对年龄≥60 岁的随机接受达非那新、奥昔布宁缓释剂或安慰剂的受试者进行认知测试时，只有奥昔布宁在使用 3 周后[78]与记忆障碍相关。一项评估≥55 岁膀胱过度活动症女性的前瞻性研究表明，根据霍普金斯 V 语言学习测试（修订版）（Hopkins Verbal Learning Test-Revised），使用曲司氯铵缓释剂后，人的认知功能开始出现衰退。认知功能在治疗第 4 周恢复到基础水平，并保持稳定，直到第 12 周研究结束[79]。有作者进行了一项随机对照随访研究，在 4 周的时间内，曲司氯铵组和安慰剂组在认知功能上没有发现任何差异[80]。

中枢神经系统中几乎没有 β_3 受体，β_3 受体激动药是有认知障碍风险患者潜在的治疗选择。米拉贝隆也是渗透性糖蛋白体系的已知底物。最近一项评估米拉贝隆安全性和耐受性的研究发现，认知功能损伤在治疗组和安慰剂组之间结果相似，蒙特利尔认知评估与基线相比没有显著调整[81]。

许多处方药和非处方药，都有抗胆碱能受体的作用。老年人群多种药物联用风险增加，抗胆碱能负荷可增加老年受试者认知障碍的风险[80]。尽管存在有多种抗胆碱能负荷量表[82]，但临床应用中并没有理想的量表，并且现有的量表对抗胆碱能药物活性和负荷的分级存在差异[83]。最佳实践指南比尔斯标准对老年受试者建议，应避免在老年人中使用抗毒蕈碱类药，或者在必要时尽量少使用，老年病学协会建议在痴呆受试者中停止使用抗毒蕈碱类药[83]。但是重要的是权衡药物治疗的潜在风险与不治疗膀胱过度活动症的风险，包括焦虑和抑郁、摔倒和骨折的增加，以及身体功能的恶化[84]。有报告显示接受膀胱过度活动症治疗的老年患者相关生活质量更好，活动障碍更少；因此，接受治疗至关重要[85]。美国妇科泌尿学会建议考虑替代药物（目前考虑 β_3 受体激动药），70 岁以上的女性避免使用抗毒蕈碱类药，考虑到抗毒蕈碱类药通过血脑屏障的可能性较低，并讨论使用肉毒杆菌毒素 A 或神经调节的三线治疗[86]。AUA/SUFU 指南同样建议在体弱的老年受试者使用这两类药物时要谨慎[87]。

总结

随着年龄的增长，膀胱过度活动症越来越普遍，并严重影响生活质量、身体功能和心理健康。膀胱过度活动症既有个人负担也有社会成本，应该在所有报道烦恼的受试者中得到解决。但是，必须仔细考虑抗毒蕈碱类药的不良反应。尤其应该考虑老年受试者神经认知功能改变的可能，因为在这类人群中，即使是认知功能的轻微下降也可能导致其独立性的丧失[88]。

对于一线膀胱过度活动症干预后症状改善不完全的受试者，药物治疗可减轻症状并对其生活质量有重要影响[89]。在美国，治疗膀胱过度活动症的药物主要包括抗毒蕈碱类药和越来越多 β_3 受体激动药，目前 FDA 批准了两种配方可供患者使用。在某些受试者中，联合治疗可能比单药治疗有更好的疗效，而且没有复合的不良反应。评估不良反应风险（包括认知障碍）和共同决策对于优化风险平衡收益非常重要[90]。更多受试者特异性结果的进一步研究和预测工具的开发是必要的，用以帮助提供者更好地为他们的受试者提供咨询，并最终降低与膀胱过度活动症相关的负担。

参考文献

[1] Irwin DE, Kopp ZS, Agatep B, Milsom I, Abrams P. Worldwide prevalence estimates of lower urinary tract symptoms, overactive bladder, urinary incontinence and bladder outlet obstruction. BJU Int. 2011;108(7):1132–8.

[2] Stewart WF, Van Rooyen JB, Cundiff GW. Prevalence and burden of overactive bladder in the United States. World J Urol. 2003;20(6):327–36. https://doi.org/10.1007/s00345-002- 0301-4.

[3] Hu TW, Wagner TH, Bentkover JD. Costs of urinary incontinence and overactive bladder in the United States: a comparative study. Urology. 2004;63(3):461–5.

[4] Milsom I, Kaplan SA, Coyne KS. Effect of bothersome overactive bladder symptoms on health-related quality of life, anxiety, depression, and treatment seeking in the United States: results from EpiLUTS. Urology. 2012;80(1):90–6. https://doi.org/10.1016/j.urology.2012.04.004.

[5] Kinsey D, Pretorius S, Glover L. The psychological impact of overactive bladder: a systematic review. J Health Psychol. 2014; https://doi.org/10.1177/1359105314522084.

[6] Stuart Reynolds W, et al. The burden of overactive bladder on US public health. Curr Bladder Dysfunct. 2016;11:8–13. https://doi.org/10.1007/s11884-016- 0344-9.

[7] Abrams P, Cardozo L, Fall M, et al. The standardization of terminology in lower urinary tract function: report from the standardization sub-committee of the international continence society. Urology. 2003;61: 37–49.

[8] Abrams P, Anderson KE. Muscarinic receptor antagonists for overactive bladder. BJUI. 2007;100(5):987–1006. https://doi.org/10.1111/j.1464-410X. 2007.07205.x.

[9] Pratt TS, Suskind AM. Management of overactive bladder in older women. Curr Urol Rep. 2018;19:92. https://doi.org/10.1007/s11934-018- 0845-5.

[10] Fok CS, Gao X, Lin H. Urinary symptoms are associated with certain urinary microbes in urogynecologic surgical patients. Int Urogynecol J. 2018;29:1765–71. https://doi.org/10.1007/ s00192-018- 3732- 1

[11] Curtiss N, Balachandran A, Krska L. A case-controlled study examining the bladder microbiome in women with Overactive Bladder (OAB) and healthy controls. Eur J Obstet Gynecol Reprod Biol. 2017;214:31–5. https://doi.org/10.1016/j.ejogrb.2017.04.040.

[12] Gormley EA, Lightner DJ, Burgio KL, Chai TC, American Urological Association; Society of Urodynamics, Female Pelvic Medicine & Urogenital Reconstruction, et al. Diagnosis and treatment of overactive bladder (non-neurogenic) in adults: AUA/SUFU guideline. 2012; amended 2014. http://www.auanet.org/guidelines/overactive-bladder-(oab)-(aua/ sufu-guideline- 2012- amended- 2014).

[13] Andersson KE, Cardozo L, Cruz F, et al. Pharmacological treatment of urinary incontinence. In: Abrams P, Cardozo L, Wagg A, editors. Incontinence. 6th ed; 2017. p. 805–97.

[14] Fetscher C, Fleichman M, Schmidt M. M(3) muscarinic receptors mediate contraction of human urinary bladder. Br J Pharmacol. 2002;136:641–3.

[15] Igawa Y, Zhang X, Nishizawa O. Cystometric findings in mice lacking muscarinic M2 or M3 receptors. J Urol. 2004;172:2460–4.

[16] Andersson KE. Antimuscarinics for treatment of overactive bladder. Lancet Neurol. 2004;3:46–53.

[17] Mukerji G, Yiangou Y, Grogono J. Localization of M2 and M3 muscarinic receptors in human bladder disorders and their clinical correlations. J Urol. 2006;176:367–73.

[18] Herbison P, Hay-Smith J, Moor K. Effectiveness of anticholinergic drugs compared with placebo in the treatment of overactive bladder: a systematic review. BMJ. 2003;326:841–4.

[19] Kay GG, Granville LJ. Antimuscarinic agents: implications and concerns in the management of overactive bladder in the elderly. Clin Ther. 2005;27(1):127–38.

[20] Goodridge SD, Dmochowski RR. B3-agonist for overactive bladder. In: Cox L, Rovner E, editors. Contemporary pharmacotherapy of overactive bladder. Cham: Springer; 2019. p. 115–31.

[21] Darifenacin [prescribing information]. India: Jubilant Cadista Pharmaceuticals Inc; September 2017.

[22] TOVIAZ (fesoterodine fumarate) [prescribing information]. Ireland: Pfizer Inc; October 2020.

[23] Oxybutynin chloride [prescribing information]. Philadelphia: Lannett Company Inc; October 2019.

[24] Solifenacin succinate [prescribing information]. Israel: Teva Pharmaceuticals USA, Inc; June 2020.

[25] DETROL LA (tolterodine tartrate extended release) [prescribing information]. New York: Pharmacia and Upjohn Company LLC; 2020.

[26] Tolterodine tartrate [prescribing information]. Peapack: Greenstone LLC; 2017.

[27] Trospium chloride extended release [prescribing information]. Chantily: BluePoint Laboratories; 2020.

[28] Trospium chloride [prescribing information]. Warren: Cipla USA Inc; 2020.

[29] Riemsma R, Hagen S, Kirschner-Hermanns R. Can incontinence be cured? A systematic review of cure rates. BMC Med. 2017;15:63. https://doi.org/10.1186/s12916-017- 0828-2.

[30] Lukacz ES, Santiago-Lastra Y, Albo ME. Urinary incontinence in women: a review. JAMA. 2017;318(16):1592–604. https://doi.org/10.1001/jama.2017.12137.

[31] Abrams P, Swift S. Solifenacin is effective for the treatment of OAB dry patients: a pooled analysis. Eur Urol. 2005;48(3):483–7. https://

doi.org/10.1016/j.eururo.2005.06.007.

[32] Herbison P, McKenzie JE. Which anticholinergic is best for people with overactive bladders? A network meta-analysis. Neurourol Urodyn. 2019;38(2):525–34. https://doi.org/10.1002/ nau.23893.

[33] Reynolds WS, McPheeters M, Blume J. Comparative effectiveness of anticholinergic therapy for overactive bladder in women. Obstet Gynecol. 2015;125(6):1423–32. https://doi. org/10.1097/ AOG.0000000000000851.

[34] Khullar V, Chapple C, Gabriel Z. The effects of antimuscarinics on health-related quality of life in overactive bladder: a systematic review and meta-analysis. Urology. 2006;68(2):38–48. https://doi.org/10.1016/ j.urology.2006.05.043.

[35] Hsu FC, Weeks CE, Selph SS. Updating the evidence on drugs to treat overactive bladder: a systematic review. Int Urogynecol J. 2019;30:1603–17. https://doi.org/10.1007/ s00192–019– 04022–8.

[36] Sexton CC, Notte SM, Maroulis C. Persistence and adherence in the treatment of overactive bladder syndrome with anticholinergic therapy: a systematic review of the literature. Int J Clin Pract. 2011;65(5):567–85. https://doi.org/10.1111/j.1742–1241.2010.02626. x.

[37] Benner JS. Patient-reported reasons for discontinuing overactive bladder medication. BJUI. 2010;105(9):1283–90.

[38] Akino H, Namiki M, Suzuki K. Factors influencing patient satisfaction with antimuscarinic treatment of overactive bladder syndrome: results of a real-life clinical study. Int J Urol. 2014;21(4):389–94. https://doi. org/10.1111/iju.12298.

[39] Madhuvrata P, Cody JD, Ellis G. Which anticholinergic drug for overactive bladder symptoms in adults. Cochrane Database Syst Rev. 2012; https://doi.org/10.1002/145618.CD005429.pub2.

[40] Diokno AC, Appell RA, Sand PK. Prospective, randomized, double-blind study of the efficacy and tolerability of the extended-release formulations of oxybutynin and tolterodine for overactive bladder: results of the OPERA trial. Mayo Clin Proc. 2003;78(6):687–95.

[41] Thuroff JW, Chartier-Kastler E, Corcus J. Medical treatment and medical side effects in urinary incontinence in the elderly. World J Urol. 1998;16(suppl 1):S248–61.

[42] Waldeck K, Larsson B, Andersson KE. Comparison of oxybutynin and its active metabolite N-desethyloxybutynin in the human detrusor and parotid gland. J Urol. 1997;157(3):1093–7.

[43] Dmochowski RR, Davila GW, Zinner NR. Efficacy and safety of transdermal oxybutynin in patients with urge and mixed incontinence. J Urol. 2002;168:580–6.

[44] Dmochowski RR, Sand PK, Zinner NR. Comparative efficacy and safety of transdermal oxybutynin and oral tolterodine versus placebo in previously treated patients with urge and mixed urinary incontinence. Urology. 2003;62:237–42.

[45] Staskin DR, Dmochowksi RR, Sand PK. Efficacy and safety of oxybutynin chloride topical gel for overactive bladder: a randomized, double-blind, placebo controlled, multicenter study. Adult Urol. 2009;181(4):1764–72.

[46] Caramelli KE, Staskin DR, Volinn W. Steady-state pharmacokinetics of an investigational oxybutynin gel in comparison with oxybutynin transdermal system. Poster presented at: Annual Meeting of the American Urological Association; May 17–22, 2008.

[47] Caramelli KE, Stanworth S, Volinn W, Hoel G. Pharmacokinetics of oxybutynin topical gel: effects of showering, sunscreen application, and person-to-person transference. Poster presented at: Annual Meeting of the American College of Clinical Pharmacy; October 19–22, 2008; Louisville.

[48] Mybetriq (Mirabegron extended-release tablets) [prescribing information]. Northbrook. Astella Pharma; 2012.

[49] Gemtesa (Vibegron) [prescribing information]. Irvine. Urovant Sciences, Inc.; 2020.

[50] Chapple CR, Kaplan SA, Mitcheson D. Randomized double-blind, active-controlled Phase 3 study to assess 12–month safety and efficacy of Mirabegron, a β3–adrenoceptor agonist, in overactive bladder. Eur Urol. 2013;63(2):296–305. https://doi.org/10.1016/ j.eururo.2012.10.048.

[51] Nitti VW, Auerbach S, Martin N. Results of a randomized phase III trial of mirabegron in patients with overactive bladder. J Urol. 2013;189(4):1388–95.

[52] Chapple CR, Dvorak V, Radziszewski P, Dragon Investigator Group. A phase II doseranging study of mirabegron in patients with overactive bladder. Int Urogynecol J. 2013;24(9):1447–58.

[53] Herschorn S, Staskin D, Schermer CR. Safety and tolerability results from the PILLAR study: a Phase IV, double-blind, randomized, placebo-controlled study of mirabegron in patients ≥65 years with overactive bladder-wet. Drugs Aging. 2020;37:665–76. https://doi. org/10.1007/ s40266–020– 00783– w.

[54] Tadrous M, Matta R, Greaves S. Association of mirabegron with the risk of arrhythmia in adult patients 66 years or older- a population-based cohort study. JAMA Int Med. 2019;179(10):1436–9.

[55] Wagg A, Staskin D, Engel E. Efficacy, safety, and tolerability of mirabegron in patients aged ≥65yr with overactive bladder wet: a phase IV, double-blind, randomized, placebo-controlled study (PILLAR). Eur Urol. 2020;77(2):211–20. https://doi.org/10.1016/ j.eururo.2019.10.002.

[56] Rutman MP, King JR, Bennet N. Once-daily vibegron, a novel oralB3 agonist does not inhibit CYP2D6, a common pathway for drug metabolism in patients on OAB medications. J Urol. 2019;201:4S.

[57] Staskin D, Frankel J, Varano S. International phase III, randomized, double-blind, placebo and active controlled study to evaluate the safety and efficacy of vibegron in patients with symptoms of overactive bladder: EMPOWUR. J Urol. 2020;204(2):316–24.

[58] Staskin D, Frankel J, Varano S. Once-daily vibegron 75 mg for overactive bladder: double-blind 52–week results from an extension study of the international phase 3 trial (EMPOWUR). J Urol. 2021;205(5):1421–9.

[59] Kelleher C, Hakimi Z, Zur R, et al. Efficacy and tolerability of Mirabegron compared with antimuscarinic monotherapy or combination therapies for overactive bladder: a systematic review and network meta-analysis. Eur Urol. 2018;74:334–5.

[60] Chapple CR, Nazir J, Hakimi Z. Persistence and adherence with mirabegron versus antimuscarinic agents in patients with overactive bladder: a retrospective observational study in UK clinical practice. Eur Urol. 2017;72(3):389–99. https://doi.org/10.1016/ j.eururo.2017.01.037.

[61] Sussman D, Yehoshua A, Kowalksi J. Adherence and persistence of mirabegron and anticholinergic therapies in patients with overactive bladder: a real-world claims data analysis. Int J Clin Pract. 2017;71:3–4.

[62] Liao CH, Kuo HC. High satisfaction with direct switching from antimuscarinics to mirabegron in patients receiving stable antimuscarinic treatment. Medicine. 2016;95(45):e4962. https:// doi. org/10.1097/MD.0000000000004962.

[63] Serati M, Leone Roberti Maggiore U, Sorice P, et al. Is mirabegron equally as effective when used as first- or second-line therapy in women with overactive bladder? Int Urogynecol J. 2017;28:1033–9. https://doi.org/10.1007/s00192–016– 3219– x.

[64] Adreev VP, Liu G, Yang C. Symptoms based clustering of women in the LURN observational cohort study. J Urol. 2018;200(6):1323–31.

[65] Herschorn S, Chapple CR, Abrams P. Efficacy and safety of combinations of mirabegron and solifenacin compared with monotherapy and placebo in patients with overactive bladder. (SYNERGY study). BJU. 2017;120(4):562–75.

[66] Drake JM, Chapple C, Esen AA. Efficacy and safety of mirabegron add-on therapy to solifenacin in incontinent overactive bladder patients with an inadequate response to initial 4–week solifenacin

monotherapy: a randomized double-blind multicenter phase 3B study (BEDSIDE). Eur Urol. 2016;70(1):136–45. https://doi.org/10.1016/j.eururo.2016.02.030.
[67] Kosilov K, Loparev S, Ivanovskaya M, Kosilova L. A randomized, controlled trial of effectiveness and safety of management of OAB symptoms in elderly men and women with standard-dosed combination of solifenacin and mirabegron. Arch Gerontol Geriatr. 2015;61(2):212–6.
[68] Robinson D, Kelleher C, Staskin D, Mueller ER, Falconer C, Wang J, et al. Patient-reported outcomes from SYNERGY, a randomized, double-blind, multicenter study evaluating combinations of mirabegron and solifenacin compared with monotherapy and placebo in OAB patients. Neurourol Urodyn. 2018;27(1):394–406.
[69] Coupland CAC, Hill T, Dening T. Anticholinergic drug exposure and the risk of dementia: a nested case-control study. JAMA Intern Med. 2019;179(8):1084–93. https://doi.org/10.1001/ jamainternmed.2019.0677.
[70] Rosenberg GA. Neurological diseases in relation to the blood-brain barrier. J Cereb Blood Flow Metab. 2012;32(7):1139–1151. https://doi.org/10.1038/jcbfm.2011.197.
[71] Griebling TL, Campbell NL, Mangel J, et al. Effect of mirabegron on cognitive function in elderly patients with overactive bladder: moCA results from a phase 4 randomized, placebo-controlled study (PILLAR). BMC Geriatr. 2020;20(1):1. https://doi.org/10.1186/s12877–020– 1474–7.
[72] Chancellor, M.B., Staskin, D.R., Kay, G.G. et al. Blood-Brain Barrier Permeation and Efflux Exclusion of Anticholinergics Used in the Treatment of Overactive Bladder. Drugs Aging 2012;29:259–273.
[73] Richardson K, Fox C, Maidment I. Anticholinergic drugs and risk of dementia: case-control study. BMJ. 2018;25(361):K1315.
[74] Lai HH, Vetter J, Jain S. Systemic nonurological symptoms in patients with overactive bladder. J Urol. 2016;196(2):467–72.
[75] Asche CV, Kim J, Kulkarni AS. Presence of central nervous system, cardiovascular and overall co-morbidity burden in patients with overactive bladder disorder in a real-world setting. BJUI. 2012;109(4):572–80.
[76] Welk B, McArthur E. Increased risk of dementia among patients with overactive bladder treated with an anticholinergic medication compared to a beta-3 agonist: a population-based cohort study. BJUI. 2020;126(1):183–90.
[77] Dubeau CD, Kraus SR, Griebling TL. Effect of fesoterodine in vulnerable elderly subjects with urgency incontinence: a double-blind, placebo controlled trial. J Urol. 2014;191(2):395–404. https://doi.org/10.1016/j.juro.2013.08.027.
[78] Kay G, Crook T, Rekeda L. Differential effects of the antimuscarinic agents darifenacin and oxybutynin ER on memory in older subjects. Eur Urol. 2006;20(2):317–26.
[79] Arklalitis G, Robminson D, Cardozo L. Cognitive effects of anticholinergic load in women with overactive bladder. Clin Interv Aging. 2020;15:1493–503.
[80] Geller EJ, Crane AK, Wells EC. Effect of anticholinergic use for the treatment of overactive bladder on cognitive function in postmenopausal women. Clin Drug Investig. 2012;32(10):697–705.
[81] Geller EJ, Dumond JB, Bowling JM, et al. Effect of trospium chloride on cognitive function in women aged 50 and older: a randomized trial. Female Pelvic Med Reconstr Surg. 2017;23(2):118–23.
[82] Villalba-Moreno AM, Alfaro-Lara ER, Perez-Guerrero MC. Systematic review on the use of anticholinergic scales in poly pathological patients. Arch Gerontrol Geriatr. 2016;62:1–8. https://doi.org/10.1016/j.archger.2015.10.002.
[83] Welsh TJ, van der Wardt V, Ojo G, et al. Anticholinergic drug burden tools/scales and adverse outcomes in different clinical settings: a systematic review of reviews. Drugs Aging. 2018;35:523–38.
[84] Challegari E, Malotra B, Bungay PJ. A comprehensive non-clinical evaluation of the CNS penetration potential of antimuscarinic agents for the treatment of overactive bladder. Br J Clin Pharmacol. 2011;72(2):235–46.
[85] Fick, D. M., T. P. Semla, and J. Beizer. “American Geriatrics Society 2015 Beers Criteria Update Expert Panel. American Geriatrics Society 2015 updated beers criteria for potentially inappropriate medication use in older adults.” J Am Geriatr Soc 63.11 (2015):2227–46.
[86] Chiarelli PE, Mackenzie LA, Osmotherly PG. Urinary incontinence is associated with an increase in falls: a systematic review. Aust J Pysiother. 2009;55(2):89–5. https://doi. org/10.1016/s0004–9514(09)70038–8.
[87] Lee LK, Goren A, Zou KH. Potential benefits of diagnosis and treatment on health outcomes among elderly people with symptoms of overactive bladder. Int J Clin Pract. 2016;70(1):66–81.
[88] Thomas TN, Walters MD. Clinical consensus statement: association of anticholinergic medication use and cognition in women with overactive bladder. Female Pelvic Med Reconstr Surg. 2021;27(2):69–71.
[89] Lightner DJ, Gomelsky A, Souter L. Diagnosis and treatment of overactive bladder (non-neurogenic) in adults: AUA/SUFU guideline amendment 2019. J Urol. 2019;202:558–63.
[90] Gray SL, Anderson ML, Dublin S, et al. Cumulative use of strong anticholinergics and incident dementia: a prospective cohort study. JAMA Intern Med. 2015;175(3):401–7.

第 9 章 胫后神经刺激对于女性急迫性尿失禁治疗的应用

Posterior Tibial Nerve Stimulation for Female Urge Urinary Incontinence

Giulia Lane 著

在传统针灸技术中，覆盖在腓总神经和胫后神经上的皮肤与盆底疾病的治疗相关[1, 2]。1983 年，Ed McGuire 博士及其同事论证了对胫后神经进行电刺激［他称之为胫后神经刺激（PTNS）］可以抑制逼尿肌收缩，并治疗因逼尿肌不稳定引起的急迫性尿失禁[1-3]。随后，Marshall Stoller 博士开发了早期动物模型和商业化设备[1-3]。从那时起，已有强有力的证据评估胫后神经刺激术对患有急迫性尿失禁的女性的疗效。2016 年，一项包括胫后神经刺激在内的对于膀胱过度活动症（OAB）的非置入式电刺激进行的系统评价和Meta 分析发现，与未接受治疗的患者相比，接受治疗患者的症状改善或治愈率增加了约 2 倍[4]。2019 年美国泌尿外科学会（AUA）关于膀胱过度活动症的指南认为胫后神经刺激是治疗膀胱过度活动症的三线疗法，该疗法已获得 FDA 批准[5]。本章将回顾胫后神经刺激治疗女性膀胱过度活动症和急迫性尿失禁的作用机制、技术、证据和不良反应。

一、作用机制

胫神经是坐骨神经最大的远端分支，起源于 L_4、L_5、S_1、S_2 和 S_3 神经根，并携带运动和感觉纤维[6]（图 9–1）。胫神经位于内踝后方的部分称为胫后神经，因此，胫后神经不是胫神经的分支[6]。胫神经延伸至足部，然后产生分支，并最终形成内足底神经、外足底神经和跟骨神经[6]。胫神经的分支为足底提供感觉[6]。胫骨末端神经分支的运动纤维支配控制趾骨和足底的肌肉[6]（图 9–2）。

神经调节改善膀胱过度活动和急迫性尿失禁症状的机制尚不清楚。在 1983 年最初版本的出版物中，McGuire 描述了动物充盈时逼尿肌反射的反应可以通过对胫后神经[1]进行针灸来延迟。最近有几个研究假设被提出，其中包括刺激 Onuf 核的运动刺激，通过传入神经的中枢抑制或感觉神经的激活[7]。与此相一致的是，动物研究发现了从膀胱组织水平（蛋白质表达和细胞募集）到中央皮质重组都发生了变化[8]。

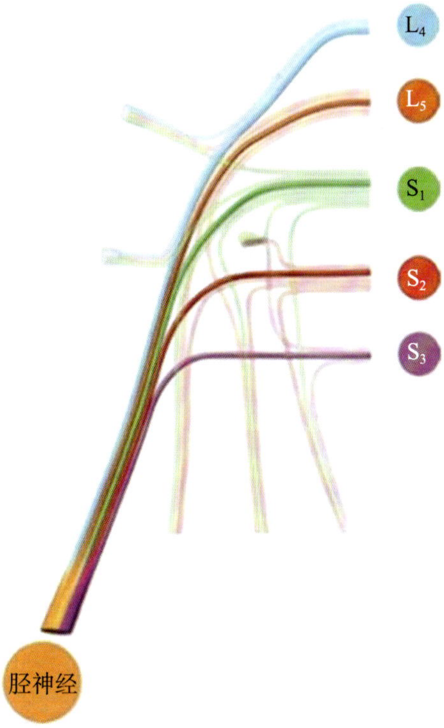

▲ 图 9–1 胫神经的起点

胫神经是坐骨神经的一个分支，两条神经都起源于 L_4、L_5、S_1、S_2 和 S_3 神经根（改编自 Rigoard[33]）

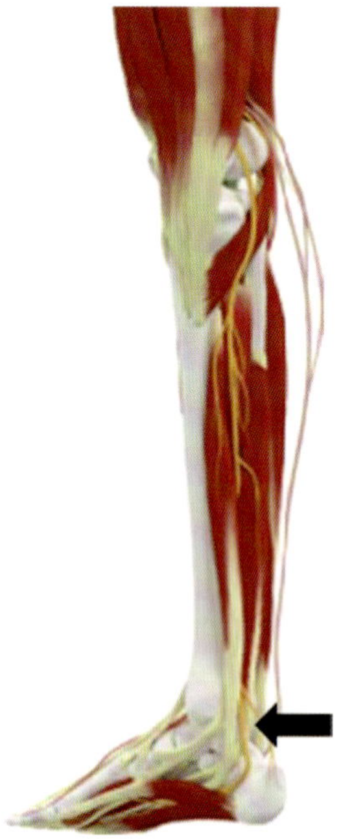

▲ 图 9-2 胫神经的走行

胫神经是坐骨神经最大的远端分支，走行于腘窝并终止于内足底神经、外足底神经和跟骨神经。箭头指示了胫神经在内踝后方的部分（改编自 Rigoard[33]。https://doi-org.proxy.lib.umich.edu/10.1007/978-3-319-43089-8_16）

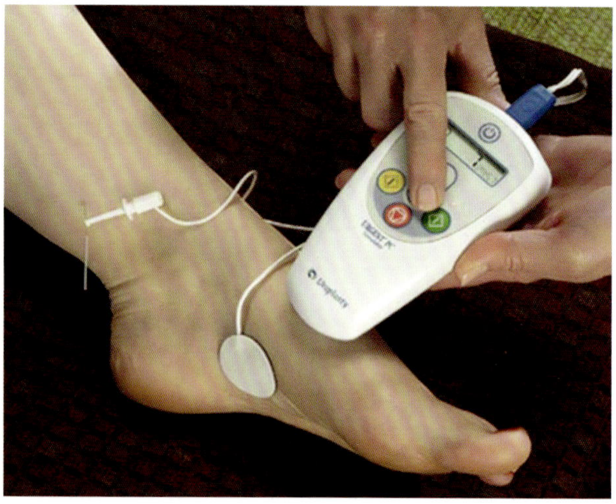

▲ 图 9-3 经皮穿刺胫后神经器放置

将一根 34 号实心针以 60° 角在距内踝头侧约 5cm 处插入胫骨稍后方。将来自刺激仪的电极连接到针上。随附的表面电极放置在同侧跟骨上（图片由 Dr. Priyanka Gupta 和 Dr. Kenneth Peters 提供）

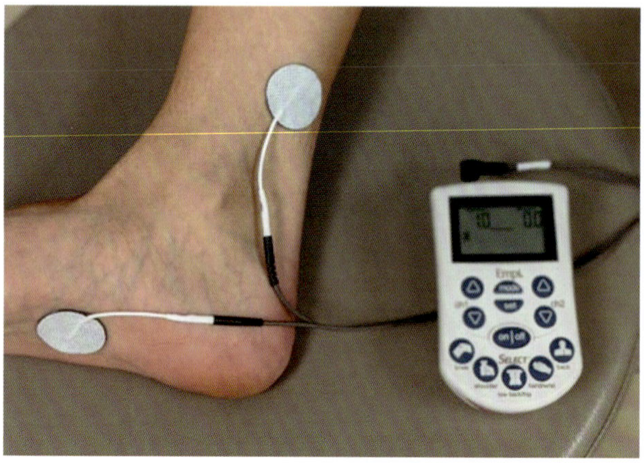

▲ 图 9-4 经皮电极胫后神经刺激

经皮电极胫后神经刺激使用施加在胫后神经和足底面的表面电极进行，并连接到经皮神经电刺激仪（图片由 Dr. Giulia Lane 提供）

二、技术

胫后神经刺激术可通过经皮穿刺或经皮电极途径进行。胫后神经刺激最常见的方式是单侧治疗，也有双侧胫后神经刺激治疗的研究[4, 9]。

在经皮穿刺方式中，会将一根 34 号实心针以 60° 的角度在距内踝头侧约 5cm[10, 11] 处插入胫骨稍后方。来自刺激仪的电极将连接到针上。随附的表面电极放置在同侧跟骨上[10, 11]（图 9-3）。

经皮电极胫后神经刺激（T-PTNS）使用表面电极而不是针头传递，施加在同一区域的胫后神经上，并连接到经皮神经电刺激仪（TENS）上[12]（图 9-4）。

在经皮穿刺和经皮电极方法中，刺激是通过低压神经刺激器进行传导的。经皮穿刺胫后神经刺激的电流强度为 0.5～0mA，经皮电极胫后神经刺激为 10～50mA；两者都以 20Hz 的方波传输，持续时间为 200μs[4, 8, 10, 11, 13, 14]。可以增加电压以确认适当的感觉和运动反应。与准确的针屈曲一致的运动反应包括大脚趾的屈曲或足趾的扇形展开，而感觉反应包括脚底的感觉。一旦达到适当的反应，刺激就会逐渐增加到患者可以忍受的强度水平[2, 11, 15]。

胫后神经刺激的治疗通常每周 1 次，每次 30min，连续进行 12 周[8, 10, 11]。然而，也有关于治疗频率和持续时间的替代方案[4, 16, 17]。症状有所改善的患者可以通过维持疗程继续治疗。维持性的 PTNS 治疗通常每月进行 1 次；然而，文献中描述的维护疗程的频率和持续时间是可变的[18, 19]。在美国，有两种用于经皮穿刺胫后神经刺激的商业经皮神经电刺激仪：Urgent PC（Cogenix, Minneapolis, MN）和 Nuvo（Medtronic, Minneapolis, MN）。许多市售的经皮神经电刺激仪可用于经皮胫后神经刺激，但并未经过 FDA 批准。

三、有效性证据

（一）经皮穿刺胫后神经刺激

2016 年，一项关于外部电刺激治疗膀胱过度活动症的系统回顾和 Meta 分析发现，有中等质量的证据表明，经皮穿刺胫后神经刺激在改善膀胱过度活动症方面比假治疗或安慰剂更有效（RR=3.19，95%CI 2.22～4.58）[4]。同一篇综述发现，与对照组相比，接受胫后神经刺激治疗的女性，她们的急迫性尿失禁（UUI）症状的改善是对照组的两倍多（RR=2.23，95%CI 1.46～3.40）[4]。为经皮穿刺胫后神经刺激的有效性提供大量证据的随机对照试验总结如下。

2010 年，Peters 及其同事发表了一项多中心、随机对照试验的结果，该试验为期 12 周，每次 30min，进行经皮穿刺胫后神经刺激或假治疗，被称为 SUmmiT 试验[11]。该试验包括患有急迫性尿失禁 3 个月以上，并且有严重症状的门诊成年男性和女性，通过 OAB-q 简表（SF）得分 4 分或以上，来衡量尿急和平均每天排尿 10 次或更多的排尿频率。患者保守治疗失败，治疗前有 2 周的抗毒蕈碱治疗洗脱期。这项研究排除了神经源性膀胱患者、使用第三线治疗膀胱过度活动症、当前泌尿系或阴道感染的患者，以及使用起搏器或置入式除颤器的患者。主要结果是胫后神经刺激与假治疗相比的疗效，在完成连续 12 次每周干预治疗（每次持续 30min）后，在第 13 周通过七级整体反应评估（GRA）的测量。在整体反应评估中报道膀胱症状为中度或显著改善的患者被视为反应者。

共有 220 例成人被随机分组（每组 110 例），在 13 周时使用意向治疗分析，胫后神经刺激组 55% 的患者整体反应评估报道中度或显著改善，而对照组为 21%（$P<0.001$）[11]。该研究评估了排尿日记的结果，整体反应评估子集症状成分、OAB-q 简表和 SF-36 问卷作为次要结果。这些是根据符合方案集结果进行分析的，胫后神经刺激组分析了 103 例患者，对照组分析了 106 例患者。研究发现，在对照组和干预组之间，膀胱的胫后神经刺激亚组症状组成中，尿急、尿频和急迫性尿失禁的症状有显著改善。胫后神经刺激组 OAB-q 简表严重程度评分平均下降（改善）36.7（SD=21.5）分，而对照组为 29.2（SD=20.7）分（$P=0.01$）。既往研究发现，OAB-q 简表的最小重要差异为 11 分，表明该差异不仅具有统计学意义，还具有临床意义[20]。与对照组相比，胫后神经刺激组的 OAB-q 简表中健康相关生活质量评分基线与 13 周之间的平均差异也有统计学意义上的改善。然而，在接受胫后神经刺激治疗与假治疗的患者之间，13 周的 SF-36 身体和心理领域量表上基线之间的平均差异没有差别。排尿日记结果显示，胫后神经刺激组每天平均排尿减少 2.4（SD=2.5）次，而对照组每天减少 1.5（SD=2.4）次（$P=0.01$）[11]。

Peters 及其同事的经皮胫神经刺激（STEP）持续疗效研究招募了 50 例随机参与者接受胫后神经刺激的治疗，并在 SUmmiT 试验中达到了疗效的主要结果[18]。STEP 研究中的患者接受了以下 5 次胫后神经刺激治疗的方案：28 天里每 14 天治疗 1 次（2 次治疗），42 天里每 21 天治疗 1 次（2 次治疗），以及 28 天后接受 1 次治疗。基于膀胱过度活动症随着治疗间隔的症状变化情况，患者继续接受常规胫后神经刺激治疗，以维持治疗效果。每 3 个月收集 1 次整体反应评估数据，共 36 个月。主要结果是 36 个月时整体反应评估显示中度或显著改善。

在上述方案之后，研究参与者每月接受 1 次平均值的治疗（IQR 为 1.0～1.6），这取决于他们保持治疗效果的时间间隔[18]。在总共 36 个月，每

6个月时随访时间点发现，排尿日记的参数均有所改善，在36个月时，排尿平均值从每天12次减少到8.7次。在36个月时，29例患者仍在研究中，其中28例（97%）达到了治疗反应的主要终点。尽管该研究有大量流失，但作者指出，50例患者中只有2例由于难以参加治疗退出了研究[18]。

2010年，Finazzi-Agrò及其同事发表了一项比较经皮穿刺胫后神经刺激与安慰剂治疗的随机对照试验结果。该研究包括那些患有急迫性尿失禁和尿流动力学诊断为逼尿肌过度活动性尿失禁的成年女性，保守治疗和抗胆碱药物对这些女性无效。该试验排除了那些使用起搏器或除颤器、患有活动性或复发性尿路感染、糖尿病、神经源性膀胱、膀胱容量＜100ml的患者，以及有其他泌尿科诊断的女性。胫后神经刺激组的女性每周接受3次30min的治疗，共12个疗程，而对照组的女性接受相同频率和持续时间的治疗，但将胫后神经刺激针置于腓肠肌头部。

主要结果测量是指在基线和随访（4周）之间，在3天排尿日记中，女性急迫性尿失禁发作至少减少50%的比例。该研究随机分配了35例女性，并发现胫后神经刺激组中71%的女性符合反应标准，而对照组中没有女性符合（P=0.001）；胫后神经刺激组3天平均尿失禁发作次数从4.1次降至1.8次，而对照组为4.2次降至3.8次。胫后神经刺激组每天排尿的平均值从13.6减少到9.5，而对照组从14.7减少到13.9。通过尿失禁生活质量量表（I-QOL）衡量，胫后神经刺激组的生活质量显著提高。

（二）经皮电极胫后神经刺激

至少有3项经皮电极胫后神经刺激治疗急迫性尿失禁的随机对照试验。每篇文章的作者都得出结论，随机分配至经皮电极胫后神经刺激治疗的患者，他们的泌尿系统症状在统计学上有显著改善。

2010年，Lucas Schreiner及其同事将51例60岁以上患有急迫性尿失禁的女性随机分配到每周1次的经皮电极胫后神经刺激（12min）+ Kegels膀胱训练与单独使用Kegels膀胱训练组中（30min）[14]。两组白天排尿次数、夜尿次数和3天急迫性尿失禁发作次数的排尿日记均有所改善；与对照组相比，经皮电极胫后神经刺激组在3个方面都有更显著的改善（排尿次数：平均差 −1.4 vs. −0.2，P=0.013；夜尿次数：平均差 −1.6 vs. 0.4，P＜0.001；急迫性尿失禁发作次数：平均差 −6.3 vs. −1.3，P＜0.001）[14]。研究人员发现，两组在国际尿失禁咨询问卷 – 尿失禁简表（ICIQ-UI-SF）上都有显著改善；然而，经皮电极胫后神经刺激组的改善大于对照组（7.2 vs. 2.6，P＜0.001）[14]。先前的研究人员发现，该问卷的最小重要差异是在12个月时降低了5分[21]。研究人员报告说，接受经皮电极胫后神经刺激治疗的患者在King健康问卷（King’s Health Questionnaire）中对尿失禁、日常活动限制、身体限制、情绪、睡眠 / 供给和严重程度测量的影响方面在统计学上有更大的改善[14]。

Booth及其同事将30例65岁以上患有膀胱或肠道功能障碍并在养老院中生活的老人随机分为经皮电极胫后神经刺激组和对照组，每周两次接受经皮电极胫后神经刺激与假治疗30min，持续6周（共12次）[22]。他们在6周时测量结果发现，美国泌尿外科协会症状指数（AUA-SI）总分在经皮电极胫后神经刺激组中平均下降了7分，而在对照组中增加了1分（P＜0.001）。根据AUA-S的发现，经皮电极胫后神经刺激组的15例患者中有13例报道症状有所改善，而对照组只有4例。研究人员没有发现两组患者从基线检查到干预后ICIQ-UI-SF评分的变化存在差异。通过超声测量，经皮电极胫后神经刺激组患者的排尿后残余尿量平均减少60ml，而对照组仅为4.8ml（P=0.048）[22]。

2019年，Baoretto及其同事将65例女性随机分配接受经皮电极胫神经刺激（n=22）、会阴锻炼（n=22）或每天10mg奥昔布宁（n=13）治疗。3天排尿日记中的排尿次数（前后对比：7.8 vs. 7.1，

P=0.015）和急迫性尿失禁发作次数（1.7 vs. 0.05，*P*=0.015）在经皮电极胫后神经刺激组中都有显著减少。作者发现这三组的 OAB-q 简表评分都有显著改善，但三组之间的改善没有显著差异[23]。

最近，Inés Ramírez-García 及其同事将 68 例男性和女性随机分配到经皮电极胫后神经刺激组和胫后神经刺激组中，每周 30min 的疗程，持续 12 周。他们进行了非劣效性分析，发现经皮电极胫后神经刺激并不比胫后神经刺激劣势[12]。

这些研究提供了一致的 I 级证据，表明与假干预相比，胫后神经刺激显著改善了膀胱过度活动症，患者报告的结果测量和排尿日记的定量分析证明了这一点。

四、不良反应 / 并发症

胫后神经刺激的优点之一是它可以在门诊环境中进行，并且健康风险很小，几乎没有排除的标准。然而，胫后神经刺激禁用于使用起搏器或置入式除颤器的患者、妊娠患者或在治疗期间打算备孕的患者。易发生过度出血的患者也禁用经皮穿刺胫后神经刺激治疗。

经皮穿刺胫后神经刺激的不良事件很少见，如果存在，也是轻微和暂时的。大多数不良事件与进针部位的疼痛或不适有关。在 Peters 等的胫后神经刺激与假治疗的研究中（2010 年），有 6 例胫后神经刺激受试者（共 110 例）报道了 9 项轻度或中度与治疗相关的不良事件。这些不良事件包括脚踝瘀伤（*n*=1，0.9%）、针头部位不适（*n*=2，1.8%）、针头部位出血（*n*=3，2.7%）和腿部刺痛（*n*=1，0.9%）[11]。Finazzi Agro 的假治疗 - 对照试验发现，没有患者出现严重并发症，但报告了针插入部位的短暂疼痛[16]。一项研究报告了 4 周的自限性神经病变，对应于胫神经足底内侧支的分布，没有相关的传导延迟或神经损伤的超声检查证据[19]。经皮电极胫后神经刺激的不良事件可能更少；然而，在两种疗法正面交锋的比较中，两组均未报告严重的不良事件[12]。

获得治疗和治疗依从性可能是接受胫后神经刺激治疗的重大障碍。鉴于需要医疗提供者放置针头，患者必须能够每周预约前往。研究人员已经评估了养老院中的胫后神经刺激治疗，这可能会减轻患者的前往治疗负担。更新的技术已经应用到可以减轻这种负担的可置入设备。然而，在开始治疗的患者中，治疗的总体依从性很高，并且在经皮穿刺或经皮电极方法之间没有显示出不同[12]。

五、胫后神经刺激病理生理学及治疗失败

在最初的随机试验中，只有 5%～6% 的患者在 12 周的胫后神经刺激治疗结束前退出[11, 24]。在随机对照试验之外，据报道，在完成初始治疗之前的损耗率高达 22%[25]。在完成初始胫后神经刺激治疗的患者中，48%～76% 的患者会持续每月进行 1 次维持治疗疗程，在大型回顾性研究中发现，平均维持时间约为 1 年[18, 19, 25, 26]。一项对 400 例在荷兰单一中心接受胫后神经刺激的患者回顾性研究发现，所有患者的平均治疗时间约为 4 个月[26]。这与约 50% 的患者在完成最初 3 个月的治疗后，停止治疗的事实是一致的。然而，在接受胫后神经刺激且治疗反应良好，并未因其他原因退出的患者中，平均治疗持续时间要长得多，约为 4 年[26]。在模型中，作者发现，在随访的 6 年里，由于前往治疗原因（前往预约的途中出现问题）或身体原因（踝关节部位疼痛）而放弃胫后神经刺激治疗的风险超过 40%[26]。

关于膀胱过度活动症患者经皮胫后神经刺激成功结果的预测因素的文献很少。Brandon 及其同事进行了一项前瞻性、开放性研究，以评估胫后神经刺激维持进展是否与总体感知改善［通过患者整体改善印象（PGII）衡量］相关，而不是与 OAB-q 简表衡量的症状特异性改善相关[25]。在 90 例开始胫后神经刺激治疗的男性和女性中，其中 70 例（78%）完成了治疗，38 例（54%）继续每月进行 1 次维护疗程，其中不到 50%（*n*=17，45%）完成了 12 个月的每月维护疗程，占开始治

疗的初始患者的 19%[25]。作者发现，完成治疗和未完成治疗的患者在人口统计学、到门诊的距离、健康状况和泌尿症状评分方面没有差异。他们确实发现，完成并选择每月维持治疗的患者在第 12 周时 BMI（24 vs. 28，$P<0.01$）和 PGII 评分较低（3.0 vs. 4.0，$P<0.01$），但与那些没有进行每月维持治疗的人相比，基线或 12 周 OAB-q 简表没有评分[25]。

两项研究阐明了停止每月经皮胫后神经刺激治疗的原因[25, 26]。其中，近 50% 的患者对治疗不满意（21 例患者中有 10 例，48%），而很大一部分没有列出他们停止胫后神经刺激的原因（21 例患者中有 8 例，38%）[25]。同样，一项针对经皮胫后神经刺激患者的大型回顾性研究发现，9% 的患者无缘无故停止治疗，而 40% 的患者因交通原因或踝关节疼痛而停止治疗[26]。

对于初次经皮胫后神经刺激治疗没有明显疗效的患者，可以提供一线、二线或第三线替代疗法[5]。然而，文献表明，这些患者往往不寻求进一步治疗。例如，在一项对 402 例开始胫后神经刺激治疗的荷兰患者展开的研究中，有 228 例患者没有进行维持性的胫后神经刺激治疗，其中大多数人选择不进一步治疗（57%），其次是药物治疗（27%）[26]。类似的，Brandon 等发现选择反对每月维持胫后神经刺激治疗的人群中，最多的一组接受了药物治疗（19%，n=13），其次是失访或选择不治疗的人，约 15%[25]。只有 11%（n=7）的患者选择接受其他三线治疗，如骶神经调节（4%，n=3）或肉毒杆菌毒素 A（7%，n=5）[25]。患有急迫性尿失禁的女性如果停止经皮胫后神经刺激治疗或不每月进行胫后神经刺激治疗，可能会面临停止对其急迫性尿失禁症状进行进一步干预的高风险，并可能受益于更密切的随访。

六、胫后神经刺激的新技术

置入式胫后神经刺激装置是女性急迫性尿失禁神经调节的最前沿技术。在仅使用局部麻醉的门诊手术中，这些装置将被放置在胫后神经上。有 3 种可用的技术：完全置入设备、无线接收器设备，以及由外部刺激仪供电的置入式有线设备[27, 28]。

由外部脉冲发射器供电的置入导线，如 Stimrouter® 外周神经刺激系统（Bioness, United States），已用于慢性疼痛患者的神经调节[28]。然而，现在有正在进行的试验来评估这种技术对急迫性尿失禁患者的疗效（NCT02873312）[29]。无线设备，如 BlueWind RENOVA™（BlueWind Medical, Herzliya, Israel），涉及置入一个接收器“天线”，然后由放置在脚踝周围的袖带供电[27, 30]。完全置入的设备（eCoin™, Valencia Technologies, California）则不需要外部能源[27, 31]。

除了置入式装置外，目前正在开发移动式经皮胫神经刺激装置（geko™, Firstkind Ltd., California）[28, 32]。患者在家时，可将这些装置固定在胫后神经上方的皮肤上。该设备以 1Hz 的频率提供 27mA 的电流，并具有 7 个设置，对应 70～560μs 的脉冲宽度[32]。

总结

胫后神经刺激是治疗女性急迫性尿失禁的一种可行方法，可以通过经皮电极或经皮穿刺进行。然而，经皮穿刺方法具有更可靠的结果数据。这些方法造成不良事件的风险最小。更新颖的技术正在出现，以提高女性在家中治疗的便利性。

参考文献

[1] Mcguire EJ, Shi-chun Z, Horwinski ER, Lytton B. Treatment of motor and sensory detrusor instability by electrical stimulation. J Urol. 1983;129:78–9.

[2] Heesakkers J, Blok B. Electrical stimulation and neuromodulation in storage and emptying failure. In: Partin AW, Dmochowski RR, Kavoussi LR, Peters CA, editors. Campbell Walsh Wein urology. Elsevier; 2021. p. 2739–2755.e3.

[3] Stoller ML, Copeland S, Millard RJ, Murnaghan GF. The efficacy of acupuncture in reversing the unstable bladder in pig-tailed monkeys. J Urol. 1987;137(6):104A.

[4] Stewart F, Gameiro OLF, El Dib R, Gameiro MO, Kapoor A, Amaro JL. Electrical stimulation with non-implanted electrodes for overactive bladder in adults. Cochrane Database Syst Rev. 2016;4:CD010098. https://doi.org/10.1002/14651858.cd010098.pub3.
[5] Lightner DJ, Gomelsky A, Souter L, Vasavada SP. Diagnosis and treatment of overactive bladder (non-neurogenic) in adults: AUA/SUFU guideline amendment 2019. J Urol. 2019;202:558–63.
[6] Granger CJ, Cohen-Levy WB. Anatomy, bony pelvis and lower limb, posterior tibial nerve. StatPearls;2020.
[7] van der Pal F, Heesakkers JPFA, Bemelmans BLH. Current opinion on the working mechanisms of neuromodulation in the treatment of lower urinary tract dysfunction. Curr Opin Urol. 2006;16:261–7.
[8] Gaziev G, Topazio L, Iacovelli V, Asimakopoulos A, Di Santo A, De Nunzio C, Finazzi-Agrò E. Percutaneous Tibial Nerve Stimulation (PTNS) efficacy in the treatment of lower urinary tract dysfunctions: a systematic review. BMC Urol. 2013;13:61.
[9] Takano S. Bilateral transcutaneous posterior tibial nerve stimulation for functional anorectal pain. 2014 IEEE 19th International Functional Electrical Stimulation Society Annual Conference (IFESS). 2014. https://doi.org/10.1109/ifess.2014.7036731
[10] MacDiarmid SA, Peters KM, Shobeiri SA, Wooldridge LS, Rovner ES, Leong FC, Siegel SW, Tate SB, Feagins BA. Long-term durability of percutaneous tibial nerve stimulation for the treatment of overactive bladder. J Urol. 2010;183:234–40.
[11] Peters KM, Carrico DJ, Perez-Marrero RA, Khan AU, Wooldridge LS, Davis GL, Macdiarmid SA. Randomized trial of percutaneous tibial nerve stimulation versus Sham efficacy in the treatment of overactive bladder syndrome: results from the SUmmiT trial. J Urol. 2010;183:1438–43.
[12] Ramírez-García I, Blanco-Ratto L, Kauffmann S, Carralero-Martínez A, Sánchez E. Efficacy of transcutaneous stimulation of the posterior tibial nerve compared to percutaneous stimulation in idiopathic overactive bladder syndrome: randomized control trial. Neurourol Urodyn. 2019;38:261–8.
[13] Nuhoğlu B, Fidan V, Ayyildiz A, Ersoy E, Germiyanoğlu C. Stoller afferent nerve stimulation in women with therapy resistant overactive bladder; a 1-year follow up. Int Urogynecol J Pelvic Floor Dysfunct. 2006;17:204–7.
[14] Schreiner L, dos Santos TG, Knorst MR, da Silva Filho IG. Randomized trial of transcutaneous tibial nerve stimulation to treat urinary incontinence in older women. Int Urogynecol J. 2010;21:1065–70.
[15] van Balken MR, Vandoninck V, Gisolf KW, Vergunst H, Kiemeney LA, Debruyne FM, Bemelmans BL. Posterior tibial nerve stimulation as neuromodulative treatment of lower urinary tract dysfunction. J Urol. 2001;166:914–8.
[16] Finazzi Agrò E, Campagna A, Sciabica F, Petta F, Germani S, Zuccalà A, Miano R. Posterior tibial nerve stimulation: is the once-a-week protocol the best option? Minerva Urol Nefrol. 2005;57:119–23.
[17] Yoong W, Ridout AE, Damodaram M, Dadswell R. Neuromodulative treatment with percutaneous tibial nerve stimulation for intractable detrusor instability: outcomes following a shortened 6-week protocol. BJU Int. 2010;106:1673–6.
[18] Peters KM, Carrico DJ, Wooldridge LS, Miller CJ, MacDiarmid SA. Percutaneous tibial nerve stimulation for the long-term treatment of overactive bladder: 3-year results of the STEP study. J Urol. 2013;189:2194–201.
[19] Yoong W, Shah P, Dadswell R, Green L. Sustained effectiveness of percutaneous tibial nerve stimulation for overactive bladder syndrome: 2-year follow-up of positive responders. Int Urogynecol J. 2013;24:795–9.
[20] Blanker MH, Alma HJ, Devji TS, Roelofs M, Steffens MG, van der Worp H. Determining the minimal important differences in the International Prostate Symptom Score and Overactive Bladder Questionnaire: results from an observational cohort study in Dutch primary care. BMJ Open. 2019;9:e032795.
[21] Sirls LT, Tennstedt S, Brubaker L, Kim H-Y, Nygaard I, Rahn DD, Shepherd J, Richter HE. The minimum important difference for the International Consultation on Incontinence Questionnaire-Urinary Incontinence Short Form in women with stress urinary incontinence. Neurourol Urodyn. 2015;34:183–7.
[22] Booth J, Hagen S, McClurg D, Norton C, MacInnes C, Collins B, Donaldson C, Tolson D. A feasibility study of transcutaneous posterior tibial nerve stimulation for bladder and bowel dysfunction in elderly adults in residential care. J Am Med Dir Assoc. 2013;14:270–4.
[23] Boaretto JA, Mesquita CQ, Lima AC, Prearo LC, Girão MJBC, Sartori MGF. Comparison of oxybutynin, electrostimulation of the posterior tibial nerve and peroneal exercises in the treatment of overactive bladder syndrome. Fisioter Pesqui. 2019;26:127–36.
[24] Finazzi-Agrò E, Petta F, Sciabica F, Pasqualetti P, Musco S, Bove P. Percutaneous tibial nerve stimulation effects on detrusor overactivity incontinence are not due to a placebo effect: a randomized, double-blind, placebo controlled trial. J Urol. 2010;184:2001–6.
[25] Brandon C, Oh C, Brucker BM, Rosenblum N, Ferrante KL, Smilen SW, Nitti VW, Pape DM. Persistence in percutaneous tibial nerve stimulation treatment for overactive bladder syndrome is best predicted by patient global impression of improvement rather than symptom-specific improvement. Urology. 2021;148:93–9. https://doi.org/10.1016/j. urology.2020.12.009.
[26] Te Dorsthorst MJ, Heesakkers JPFA, van Balken MR. Long-term real-life adherence of percutaneous tibial nerve stimulation in over 400 patients. Neurourol Urodyn. 2020;39:702–6.
[27] Yamashiro J, de Riese W, de Riese C. New implantable tibial nerve stimulation devices: review of published clinical results in comparison to established neuromodulation devices. Res Rep Urol. 2019;11:351–7.
[28] Te Dorsthorst M, van Balken M, Heesakkers J. Tibial nerve stimulation in the treatment of overactive bladder syndrome: technical features of latest applications. Curr Opin Urol. 2020;30:513–8.
[29] Overactive bladder treatment using StimRouter neuromodulation system: a prospective randomized trial. https://clinicaltrials.gov/ct2/show/NCT02873312?term=stimrouter&cond=oab &draw=2&rank=1. Accessed 28 Jan 2021.
[30] Heesakkers JPFA, Digesu GA, van Breda J, Van Kerrebroeck P, Elneil S. A novel leadless, miniature implantable Tibial Nerve Neuromodulation System for the management of overactive bladder complaints. Neurourol Urodyn. 2018;37:1060–7.
[31] MacDiarmid S, Staskin DR, Lucente V, et al. Feasibility of a fully implanted, nickel sized and shaped tibial nerve stimulator for the treatment of overactive bladder syndrome with urgency urinary incontinence. J Urol. 2019;201:967–72.
[32] Seth JH, Gonzales G, Haslam C, Pakzad M, Vashisht A, Sahai A, Knowles C, Tucker A, Panicker J. Feasibility of using a novel non-invasive ambulatory tibial nerve stimulation device for the home-based treatment of overactive bladder symptoms. Transl Androl Urol. 2018;7:912–9.
[33] Rigoard P. The tibial nerve. In: Rigoard P, editor. Atlas of anatomy of the peripheral nerves. Cham: Springer; 2017.

第10章 骶神经和阴部神经调节
Sacral and Pudendal Neuromodulation (SNM)

Priyanka Gupta 著

神经调节是对神经的电或化学调节，用于影响由该神经支配的终末器官的生理行为[1]。在排尿功能障碍方面，神经调节是一种微创的第三线治疗，可用于治疗难治性膀胱过度活动症（OAB）、大便失禁和非梗阻性尿潴留。在本章中，我们将重点关注难治性膀胱过度活动症。

一、骶神经和阴部神经调节的作用机制

20世纪70年代，Tanagho和Schmidt率先对使用电刺激治疗膀胱功能障碍进行了初步研究[2]。1988年，他们在犬类模型上进行了背根切断术和选择性腹侧神经切断术的研究被广泛引用。然后，他们进行了骶神经刺激，从而使膀胱排空恢复了正常[3]。他们的研究最终促成了用于治疗急迫性尿失禁的置入式神经假体的发展。第一个出现的装置是Pisces Quad神经孔电极，该电极通过棘突旁的切口放置到S_3神经孔中，并切开腰背筋膜和棘突旁的肌肉组织。电极必须缝合到骶骨后部骨膜上，并通过管道贯穿连接到置入腹壁的发生器。这最终让FDA于1997年批准其作为治疗急迫性尿失禁的设备[4]。手术技术和设备随后都进行了改进，出现了更细致的微创放置技术和具有更长电池寿命的新型电流发生器。

神经调节的作用机制尚未完全清楚。有多种神经通路会影响膀胱、胃肠道和盆底的反应。腰神经、骨盆神经和阴部神经由传入轴突和传出轴突组成。在充盈阶段，交感神经系统是活跃的，会允许膀胱放松以储存尿液和收缩尿道括约肌以防止尿失禁。正常排尿时，膀胱充盈的感觉通过传入轴突传递到骶脊髓，到达脑桥排尿中心。然后通过副交感神经系统（通过$S_{2\sim4}$神经根传递）发送传出信号，从而使膀胱收缩和尿道放松，以允许排尿。在排尿阶段，阴部神经被激活，以放松外括约肌[5]。

骶神经调节（SNM）被认为参与了抑制膀胱反射通路的神经元间的传递。两种被广泛提出的骶神经调节作用机制是：①选择性激活传入纤维，抑制脊髓内和脊髓上的排尿信号；②直接激活横纹肌尿道括约肌的传出纤维，抑制逼尿肌的收缩[5, 6]。

阴部神经调节（PNM）经研究表明是通过周围神经刺激用作解决排尿功能障碍的另一种方法。阴部神经由$S_{1\sim3}$的纤维组成，支配尿道外括约肌、肛门括约肌和盆底肌，因此在膀胱充盈和排空、排便功能和盆底感觉中不可或缺[7]。类似地，阴部神经模拟被认为会影响脊髓和皮质中心的存储和控制。具体而言，在动物研究中发现阴部神经调节可抑制伤害感受和非伤害感受的膀胱信号[8, 9]。由于阴部神经的组成，它被认为具有更广泛的骶神经根刺激，并被作为骶神经调节治疗失败患者的潜在靶点来研究。

二、骶神经和阴部神经调节的手术方法

（一）骶神经调节

该过程分为两个阶段进行。第一阶段可以在门诊进行操作，称为经皮神经评估（PNE），也可以在手术室中进行第一阶段电极放置（FSLP）。这两种方法都允许患者在植入完整的设备和电池之

前有一段试验期来测试治疗的临床有效性。PNE 和 FSLP 的操作步骤详述如下。

1. 经皮神经评估[10]

(1) 让患者俯卧。

(2) 如果无法进行荧光检查法，可使用解剖标志来确定 S_3 神经孔，方法是沿脊柱中线从尾骨开始测量 10cm，然后从侧面测 2cm，再从该点上方测 3cm ❶。

(3) 在针头插入点注射局部麻醉剂。

(4) 以 30°～60° 角插入针头。

(5) 通过让患者报告刺激感觉的位置来确认电极的放置。应在阴道、阴囊或直肠区域感觉到刺激。患者可能表现出大踇趾的屈曲。

(6) 一个临时电极通过针头并贴在皮肤上。

(7) 将电极与外部临时脉冲发生器连接 3～7 天，同时完成排尿日记和症状评分。

2. 第一阶段电极放置（FSLP）[10]

(1) 让患者俯卧。

(2) 给予静脉注射镇静。

(3) 在荧光检查法的帮助下，使用定位导丝定位中线并由用垂直线来标记。然后确定骶髂关节和棘突的交点并用横线标记。这定义了 S_3 神经孔的区域（图 10–1）。

(4) 如果前 / 后视图中 S_3 神经孔在荧光检查法下清晰可见，则标记神经孔的上内侧（图 10–2）。

(5) 如果由于肠道内容物覆盖而无法识别 S_3 神经孔，则从两条线交叉点外侧约 2cm 和上方约 3cm（取决于体型）开始（见步骤 3）。在左右两侧标记（图 10–2）。

(6) 将针以 60° 角穿过入口点，进入神经孔，并将其推进至骶骨下板边缘（图 10–3）。

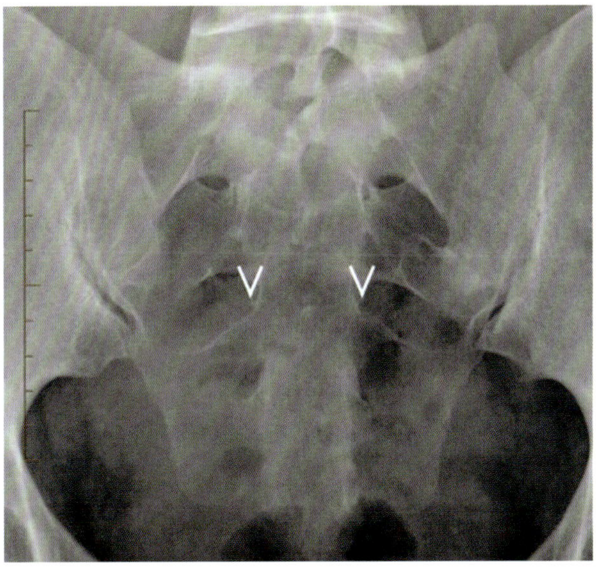

▲ 图 10–2　确定 S_3 神经孔的内侧
图片来自 Medtronic

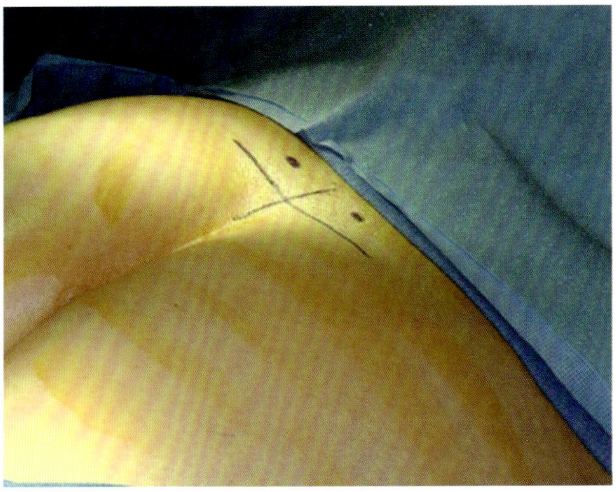

▲ 图 10–1　确定 FSLP 标志
图片来自 Kenneth Peters MD

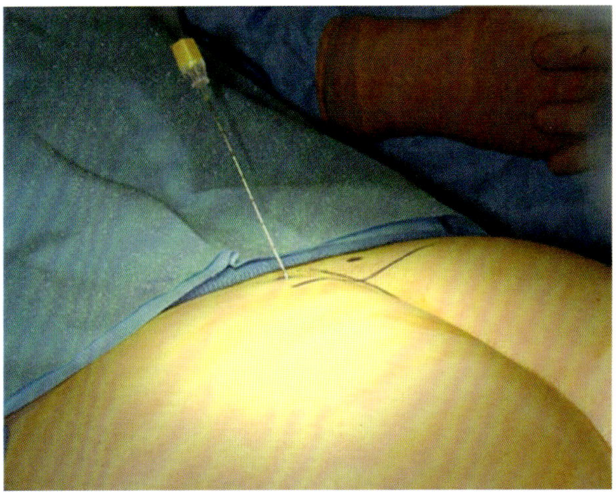

▲ 图 10–3　针刺的位置
图片来自 Kenneth Peters MD

❶ 如果外科医生不喜欢使用荧光检查法帮助，这种方法可以用于下面的第一阶段电极放置，并且测量 3cm 的高度取决于体型，组织较厚需要更多距离。

(7) 进行电刺激。理想的反应是在<2V 的刺激下盆底肌发生的波纹管状收缩，然后是大脚趾发生屈曲。S_2 刺激将通过整个足部的弯曲和脚后跟旋转来体现，S_4 刺激将单独导致波纹管状收缩。

(8) 带有运动反应的荧光检查法可帮助确认适当的神经孔。在图 10-4 中，成像首先显示皮肤位置过高，然后太低，然后刚刚好。在侧视图上，目标区域应该在 S_3 小丘上方约 1cm 处。如侧位 X 线片所示，小丘是从骶骨前表面向前突出的骨，位于 S_3 水平（图 10-4）。

(9) 然后将定位导丝穿过套管，并使用引导鞘扩张尿道。引导鞘不应超过下骨板。

(10) 然后在荧光检查法引导下，展开带有弯曲探针的倒刺电极并将其放置于下方和侧面。它有 4 个编号为 0～3 的圆柱形电极。电极 2 和电极 3 应该横跨骨缘。然后分别刺激每个电极。评估运动反应的目标应该是在低电压（理想情况下<2V）下实现所有 4 个电极的响应。

(11) 通过荧光检查法在侧位和前后位确定电极位置（图 10-5 和图 10-6）。

(12) 在同侧臀部确定置入式脉冲发生器（IPG）的潜在位置，做一个 2cm 的切口并创建一个皮下囊袋。如果测试阶段成功，置入式脉冲发生器将被放置在这里。

(13) 经皮延伸导线连接到倒刺电极，倒刺电极从对侧臀部引出，连接到外部神经调节系统（ENS），并设置编程参数。

(14) 闭合切口，电极的外部使用 4×4 无菌敷料和绷带固定。

(15) 使用外部神经调节系统，患者在 14 天的测试期间试验各种刺激参数，并保持排尿日记和症状评分，以评估改善情况。

3. 永久置入式脉冲发生器的第二阶段放置 [10]

(1) 症状改善超过 50% 且对反应满意的患者被视为反应者，应接受Ⅱ期置入。

(2) 先前的囊袋部位重新打开，且切口扩大。然后将电极连接到永久置入式脉冲发生器。这可以是不可充电或可充电的置入式脉冲发生器。

(3) 设备连接在手术室进行测试和确认。囊袋切口用可吸收缝线缝合。

(4) 测试特定的刺激程序，然后在术后将其编程到设备中，以实现最佳设备设置。

（二）阴部神经调节

阴部神经调节也分 2 个阶段进行。由于放置技术和所需的电极长度，这必须使用第一阶段电极放置完成。该技术需要增加肌电图监测，如下所述，阴部神经的最佳刺激点在坐骨棘水平。Ⅱ阶段的放置与骶神经调节相似，但必须将电极从臀部下方的切口部位通过管道贯穿到背部下方的置入式脉冲发生器位置 [10]。

1. 第一阶段电极放置

(1) 让患者采用俯卧位，确保所有受压点适当

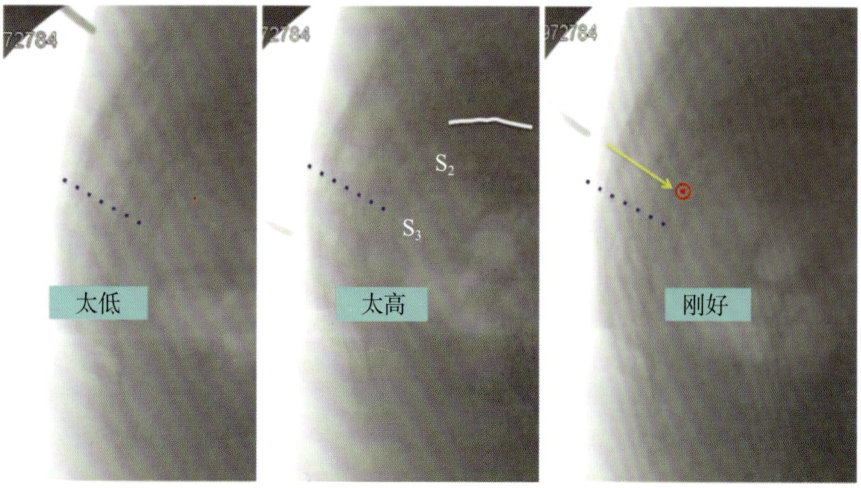

◀ 图 10-4　理想的横向放置
图片由 Medtronic 提供（will need to obtain permission）

地垫好了。

(2) 使用静脉注射镇静，采用无菌技术准备并使用手术洞巾覆盖患者，建议在穿刺部位的注射局部麻醉剂。

(3) 将电极针放置在肛门括约肌的 3 点钟和 9 点钟位置。这些将用于术中肌电图（EMG）监测。

(4) 通过坐骨直肠窝使用经皮穿刺进入阴部神经，将一根神经孔针从坐骨结节的内侧沿内侧到外侧方向穿过坐骨棘（图 10–7）。当针通过时，以 5Hz 的频率和 5V 的电压进行刺激，以识别神经。可以通过在肌电图上看到复合肌肉动作电位（CMAP）和在检查中看到肛门收缩来识别神经。

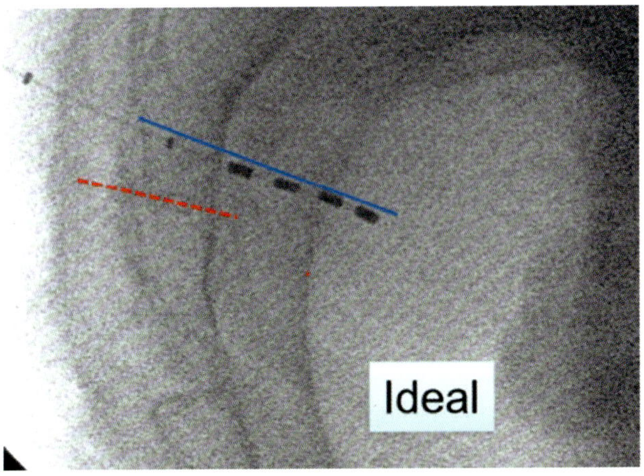

▲ 图 10–5　X 线片显示理想的横向位
图片由 Medtronic 提供

(5) 沿着神经推进针头，同时刺激，以确认它是平行于神经而不是垂直于神经。这将允许永久电极上的多个电极刺激神经。

(6) 在荧光检查法下检验针头的位置（图 10–8）。然后放置定向导丝和电极引导鞘，类似于骶神经调节程序。

(7) 在荧光检查法下将倒刺电极推进到位。由于从电极到神经刺激器部位的轨迹较长，因此将使用较长的 41cm 导线。刺激每个电极并记录获得运动和肌电响应所需的电压；理想情况下，在复合肌肉动作电位和肛门收缩的情况下，所有 4 个电极上的刺激电压都低于 2V。当每个电极都获得满意的响应时，部署倒刺电极。

(8) 电极位置应在荧光检查法下，对前后（图 10–9）和横向（图 10–10）位置进行确认。

(9) 在同侧臀部上识别神经刺激器的潜在位置，并切开一个 1cm 的切口，然后创建一个皮下囊袋。如果测试阶段成功，神经刺激器将被放置在这里。

(10) 将电极穿过管道贯穿至神经刺激器部位，并将经皮延伸导线连接到管道并从对侧臀部引出，用于临时外部刺激。

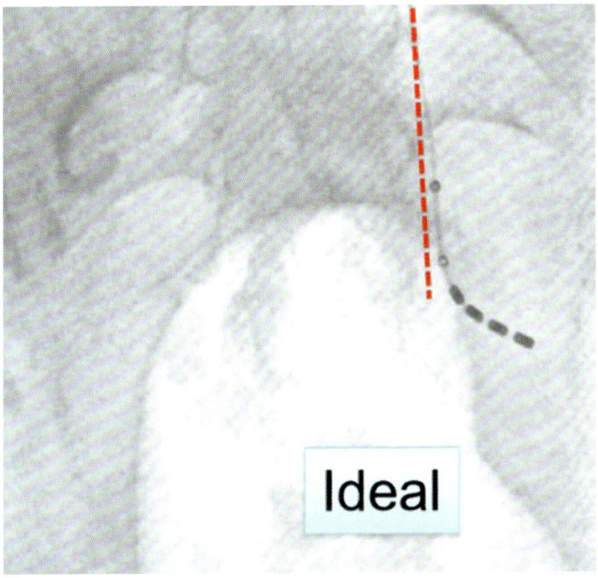

▲ 图 10–6　X 线片显示理想的前后位
图片由 Medtronic 提供

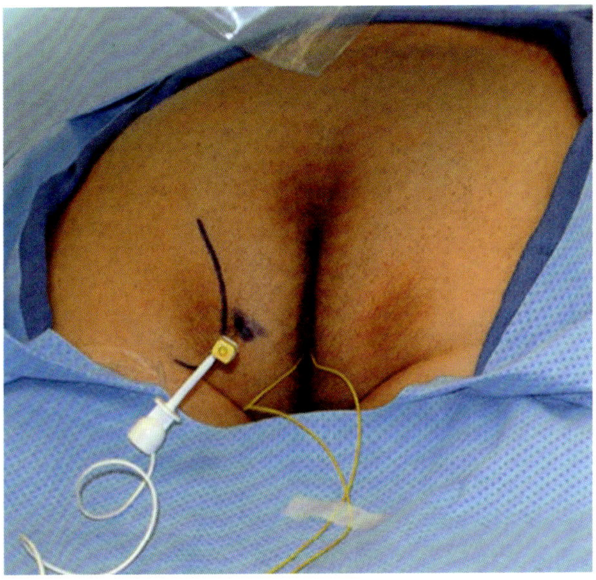

▲ 图 10–7　阴部针插入
图片由 Kenneth Peters MD 提供

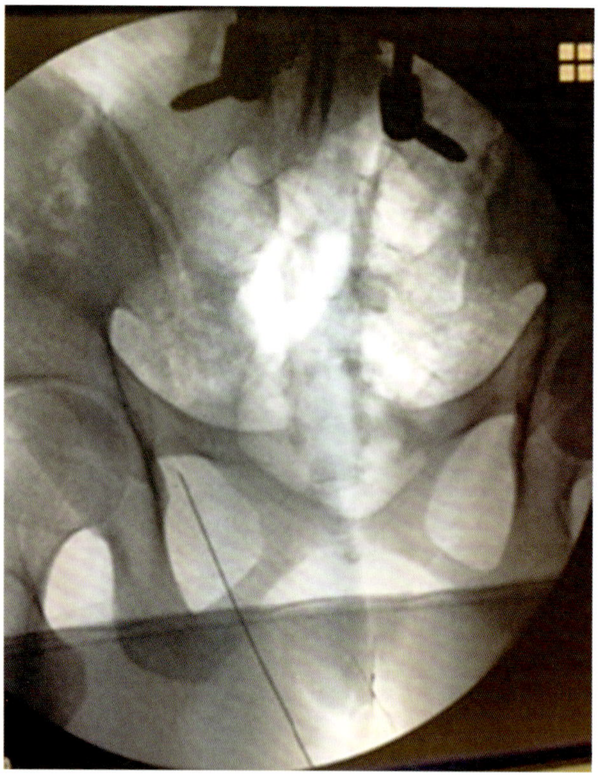

▲ 图 10-8　荧光检查法下的针头位置
图片由 Kenneth Peters MD 提供

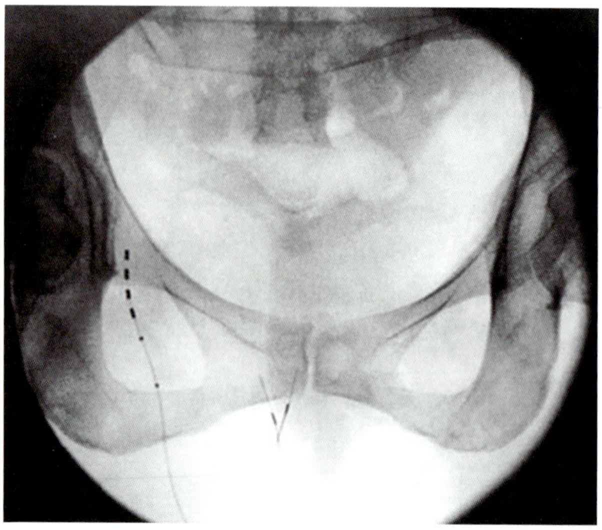

▲ 图 10-9　前后电极位置
图片由 Kenneth Peters MD 提供

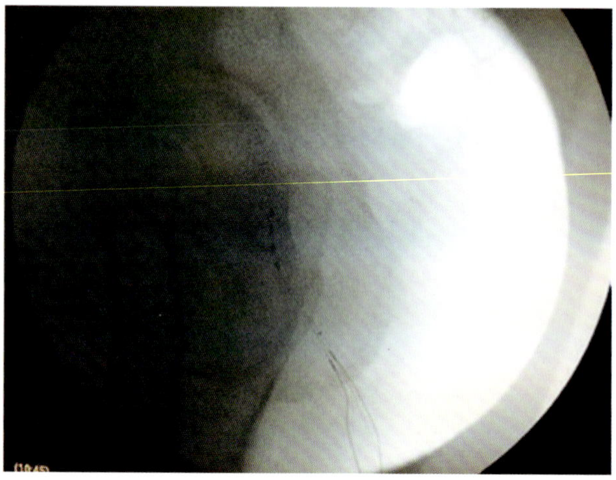

▲ 图 10-10　横向电极位置
图片由 Kenneth Peters MD 提供

(11) 闭合切口，外部连线部分使用敷料和绷带固定。

三、最近的技术进步

目前，2 种骶神经调节设备已获得 FDA 批准在美国和欧洲上市（Interstim® Medtronic 设备和 Axonics® 骶神经调节系统）。2 种系统都使用经皮四极倒刺电极。他们最近对该技术进行了升级，因为两者都兼容磁共振成像，并提供了可充电电池选项。不可充电置入式脉冲发生器的寿命通常为 3～5 年，新型可充电置入式脉冲发生器的寿命为 10～15 年，但需要定期充电。

磁共振成像兼容性将扩大该设备用于可能需要磁共振检查的患者接受其他疾病治疗的能力。据估计，至少有 50% 置入神经刺激器或起搏器装置的患者终其一生可能都需要进行磁共振检查[11]。此外，由于需要磁共振检查，约 23% 的骶神经调节解释被执行[12]。骶神经调节作为神经系统疾病患者（如多发性硬化症和不完全脊髓损伤患者以及腰痛患者）的治疗选择，以前由于需要定期进行磁共振检查而受到限制[12]。这种技术的进步将使这些患者能够尝试治疗他们的泌尿系统症状。未来的研究将需要评估这些特殊人群的疗效和功效。

骶神经调节的第二个改进是可充电的置入式脉冲发生器。可充电电池的优点是允许使用更小体积的置入式脉冲发生器，可以使患者更舒适，和有更长的电池使用寿命，这可能减少再次手术的必要。目前可用的系统包括：不可充电 Interstim Ⅱ 系统（容量 12.5cm³）、可充电 Interstim Micro

系统（容量 2.8cm^3）和可充电 Axonics 系统（容量 5.5cm^3）。容量较小的置入式脉冲发生器可能适用于体重指数较低、对器械外观和舒适度更有意识的患者。然而，对于大多数体重指数值处于平均值或高于平均值的患者来说，一旦置入皮肤下，尺寸上的差异就可能不太明显了。此外，为了给设备充电，充电线和充电器必须靠近置入式脉冲发生器，对于肥胖患者来说是否能够准确地做到这一点，可能是更具挑战性的。在老年患者中，这也可能是一个问题，因为灵巧度和记忆问题可能会降低患者对器械准确充电的能力。最后，对技术的信心可能也是一个需要考虑的重要因素，因为一些患者可能对执行充电的过程感到不舒服。

置入式脉冲发生器的使用寿命是另一个需要考虑的因素，因为理论上的优势可能是减少电池更换所需的操作次数。但是，这可能不适用于所有情况。在一项对 325 例使用骶神经调节治疗大便失禁患者进行的纵向研究报道（平均随访时间为 7.1 年），21.7% 的患者因治疗无效、设备问题或感染等而移除了设备[13]。因此，再次手术率可能受到与器械功能相关的其他因素的影响，而不仅仅是电池寿命。此时，尚不清楚电池是否会随时间衰减。已知一些设备会经历电池老化，寿命可能短于 10～15 年。

为了在不可充电置入式脉冲发生器或可充电置入式脉冲发生器之间做出决定，临床医生必须与患者共同参与决策过程，以确保考虑这些因素并帮助选择能够为患者带来最佳结果的治疗方法。在一项对 352 例使用脊髓刺激器的患者进行的多中心研究中，他们发现使用可充电设备的患者会比那些使用不可充电设备的患者提前结束治疗[14]。对脊髓刺激器和脑深部电刺激器空间的研究表明，充电系统的治疗管理负担更大，可能导致患者提前中止治疗[12]。在未来的数年里，这仍有待于在骶神经调节领域进行研究。

四、骶神经调节的结果

已经发表的几项研究确定了，骶神经调节对难治性湿性 – 膀胱过度活动症和干性 – 膀胱过度活动症患者的疗效。InSite 试验是一项前瞻性的多中心试验，在 6 个月时将骶神经调节与标准药物治疗进行比较。然后随访患者以评估 5 年时的骶神经调节结果。共有 340 例患者接受了刺激测试，其中 272 例患者进行了置入。在湿性 – 膀胱过度活动症患者中，他们的基线（尿失禁）为（3.1 ± 2.7）次 / 天。进行骶神经调节治疗的患者，平均每天减少（2.2 ± 2.7）次尿失禁。在干性 – 膀胱过度活动症患者中，他们的基线（排尿）为（12.6 ± 4.5）次 / 天。进行骶神经调节治疗的患者，平均每天减少（5.1 ± 4.1）次排尿，这具有统计学意义。80% 的受试者报道称其在 12 个月时的泌尿系统症状有所改善[15]。在同一患者队列的 5 年随访中，使用改良完成者分析的治疗成功率为 67%，使用完成者分析的治疗成功率为 82%。患者的所有生活质量指标均有所改善[16]。在一项全球性多中心的骶神经调节试验中，接受刺激组中的干性 – 膀胱过度活动症患者的排尿次数显著改善，从基线时的 16.9 ± 9.7 到接受刺激后 6 个月时的 9.3 ± 5.1（$P<0.0001$）。在这项研究中，88% 刺激组的患者的排尿紧迫程度有所改善。有趣的是，在这项研究中，有患者在治疗 6 个月后关闭了设备，然而他们的症状恶化且回到了基线。该组的所有患者在试验结束时均重新开始治疗[17]。因此，骶神经调节的主动刺激在改善难治性膀胱过度活动症方面具有治疗作用，但不能永久治愈它们。

文献也强烈支持骶神经调节在改善湿性 – 膀胱过度活动症患者的尿失禁和尿垫使用方面的有效性。在 Schmidt 等的一项随机试验的 34 例患者中，75% 的患者在临床上取得成功，其中 16 例（47%）是完全干性 – 膀胱过度活动症患者，其中 10 例（29%）的尿失禁发作减少了 50% 以上。57% 的患者不再需要尿布或尿垫[18]。在 Sutherland 等的回顾性研究中，他们观察到平均每日失禁次数从 5.0 下降到 1.0，平均每日尿垫使用次数从 2.3 下降到 0.3（$P<0.05$）[19]。在 Weil 等进行的一项随

机试验中，他们注意到主要尿失禁事件每天减少 3.8 次（P=0.0039），每日尿垫使用平均减少 4.4 次（P=0.0011）[20]。

尽管目前膀胱过度活动症不是 FDA 批准的治疗适应证，但骶神经调节也被证明对间质性膀胱炎和盆腔疼痛患者有效。2020 年，在骶神经调节治疗骨盆疼痛综合征的 Meta 分析中，对 6 项前瞻性队列研究和 4 项回顾性病例系列进行了研究。研究发现平均 69% 的患者进行了置入（52%～91%）。此外，被纳入的所有研究均报道了骶神经调节可降低疼痛评分[21]。在 Peters 对 26 例难治性间质性膀胱炎（IC）患者进行的一项研究中，71% 的患者盆腔疼痛有所改善，68% 的患者尿急症状有所改善，72% 的患者尿频症状有所改善。96% 的患者表示他们将再次接受置入手术，并将向朋友推荐该疗法[22]。在 Marinkovic 的一项回顾性研究中，他们注意到骶神经调节治疗间质性膀胱炎取得了类似的成功，根据 VAS 量表显示，评分从 6.5 分降低到 2.4 分（P<0.01），平均随访时间为 89 个月[23]。

五、阴部神经调节的结果

阴部神经调节目前尚未获得 FDA 批准用于治疗排尿障碍，因此这是一种用于治疗膀胱过度活动症、尿潴留和盆腔疼痛的指征外治疗。2005 年，在一项骶神经调节与阴部神经调节的前瞻性随机对照试验中，更多的患者选择了骶神经调节治疗。在试验阶段，骶骨和阴部都置入了电极。每根电极都试验 7 天，患者并不知道刺激的是哪根电极。收集每条电极对于有关症状改善的数据。然后，患者可以选择将置入式脉冲发生器连接到哪条电极。在 24 例患者中，19 例选择了阴部神经调节，5 例选择了骶神经调节。阴部神经调节在整体症状改善（P=0.02）、尿急（P=0.005）、尿频（P= 0.007）和肠功能（P=0.049）方面都更具有优势[24]。在另一项针对难治性间质性膀胱炎患者的骶神经调节与阴部神经调节的对比试验中，对骶骨和阴部电极放置进行了与上述类似的设计。在这项对 22 例患者的研究中，77% 接受了永久性电极置入，59% 选择了阴部电极，18% 选择了骶骨电极。阴部神经调节治疗和骶神经调节治疗的总体症状减轻率分别为 59% 和 44%[25]。在另一项对 19 例接受阴部神经调节治疗的阴部神经痛患者进行的研究中，36% 的患者完全或几乎完全缓解，52% 的疼痛明显缓解，15% 的患者报告疼痛轻度缓解，所有患者均接受了置入式脉冲发生器[26]。在这些关于阴部神经调节的小型研究中，似乎对治疗排尿功能障碍和盆腔疼痛有效。

六、骶神经调节治疗失败

一些研究估计，有 10%～25% 的患者会经历骶神经调节治疗失败[15, 27]。而阴部神经调节治疗，对于骶神经调节治疗失败的患者特别有效，因为对于这一类具有挑战性的人群来说，几乎没有其他治疗选择。在一项对骶神经调节治疗难治性的膀胱过度活动症和间质性膀胱炎 / 梨状腹综合征（PBS）患者的研究中，93%（44 例患者中有 41 例）的患者对阴部神经调节治疗有反应。在 1 年的随访中，83% 的患者仍在使用他们的设备，74% 的患者表示他们将再次接受该手术[28]。Carmel 报道了 3 例因慢性盆腔 – 会阴疼痛的患者在骶神经调节治疗失败后，重新接受了阴部神经调节治疗，他们报告在 2 年的随访后症状显著改善[29]。阴部神经调节对骶神经调节治疗困难的患者是一种有效的治疗方法，应考虑用于治疗排尿功能障碍和盆腔疼痛。

七、不良事件 / 并发症

骶神经调节和阴部神经调节的不良事件可能与设备相关的不良事件（AE）有关。我们将重点关注与当前设备相关的事件，该设备是一种带有弯曲探针的经皮四极倒刺电极。然而，一些早期的研究可能会讨论其他置入技术。InSite 试验报告的不良事件率为 30.5%[30]。最常见的不良事件是疼痛，无论是来自设备的刺激，还是与置入式脉冲发生器或电极相关的部位的疼痛。大多数不良事件通过保守治疗可以得到解决。13% 需要手术干预；这包括手术部位的疼痛（4%）、缺乏 / 丧失疗效（4%）和感染（3%）[31]。在来自法国的一项多中心研究中，他们还注意到 33% 的不良事件发生率，大多数可以通过重新编程解决。最常见的不良事件包括置入部位疼痛（5%；301 例患者中有 16 例）和置入部位感染（4%；301 例患者中有 13 例）[32]。

置入式脉冲发生器位置发生并发症往往是最常见的，并且可能由于置入式脉冲发生器位置的创伤或手术期间的次优放置而发生。重要的是要考虑患者的因素包括身体习惯、骨骼标志的位置，以及患者裤子的典型位置。如果放置在骨骼标志上方位置或过于浅表，这可能会引起疼痛。此外，如果患者体重发生变化，这也会影响置入式脉冲发生器的位置，这可能需要重新进行置入。

电极发生位移是另一个潜在的并发症。自从置入倒刺电极后，这种情况的发生率大大降低。在 Peters 等的一项研究中，他们指出，电极位移率从使用开放式放置技术的 42% 下降到使用经皮倒刺电极放置的 15%，这具有统计学意义 [33]。更常见的情况是，如果患者跌倒或受伤，可能会导致电极被破坏。使用倒刺电极的手术技术的进步大大减少了这种情况的发生。

考虑到设备置入时通常给予抗生素预防治疗，因此设备感染不太常见。在文献中估计，感染率低于 10% [33, 34]，且大多数感染在置入后早期出现。在 InSite 试验中，10 例患者中有 5 例感染出现在置入后的前 3 个月 [34]。与任何设备感染一样，建议移除置入的设备。在充分治疗和解决感染后，可以考虑重新置入。

阴部神经调节也有类似的设备相关并发症，其中包括电极或置入式脉冲发生器位置的疼痛和感染风险。阴部神经调节更容易受到电极位移的影响，因为电极穿过软组织而不是通过神经孔固定。这使得电极更容易因跌落或臀部区域的创伤而发生移位。Peters 等报道，84 例患者中有 3 例发生了电极位移，并且在 84 例患者中有 1 例发生了感染 [28]。

总结

骶神经调节和阴部神经调节是治疗难治性膀胱过度活动症的有效疗法。随着磁共振成像兼容性和可充电设备的引入，这种疗法的应用将在未来数年得到推广，并且可能会改善对其他疾病的治疗（包括神经源性膀胱疼痛和盆腔疼痛）。这种疗法与不良事件的低风险相关，并且随着时间的推移，症状得以持续改善。

参考文献

[1] Peters KM. Alternative approaches to sacral nerve stimulation. Int Urogynecol J. 2010;21(12):1559–63.
[2] Tanagho EA, Schmidt RA, Orvis BR. Neural stimulation for control of voiding dysfunction: a preliminary report in 22 patients with serious neuropathic voiding disorders. J Urol. 1989;142(2 Pt 1):340–5.
[3] Tanagho EA. Neural stimulation for bladder control. Semin Neurol. 1988;8(2):170–3.
[4] Dijkema HE, Weil EH, Mijs PT, Janknegt RA. Neuromodulation of sacral nerves for incontinence and voiding dysfunctions. Clinical results and complications. Eur Urol. 1993;24(1):72–6.
[5] Leng WW, Chancellor MB. How sacral nerve stimulation neuromodulation works. Urol Clin North Am. 2005;32(1):11–8.
[6] Barboglio Romo PG, Gupta P. Peripheral and sacral neuromodulation in the treatment of neurogenic lower urinary tract dysfunction. Urol Clin North Am. 2017;44(3):453–61.
[7] Gracely A, Gupta P. Pudendal neuromodulation for pelvic pain. Curr Bladder Dysfunct Rep. 2020;15:113–20.
[8] Gonzalez EJ, Grill WM. Sensory pudendal nerve stimulation increases bladder capacity through sympathetic mechanisms in cyclophosphamide-induced cystitis rats. Neurourol Urodyn. 2019;38(1):135–43.
[9] Ness TJ, DeWitte C, McNaught J, Clodfelder-Miller B, Su X. Spinal mechanisms of pudendal nerve stimulation-induced inhibition of bladder hypersensitivity in rats. Neurosci Lett. 2018;686:181–5.
[10] Bartley J, Gilleran J, Peters K. Neuromodulation for overactive bladder. Nat Rev Urol. 2013;10(9):513–21.
[11] Kalin R, Stanton MS. Current clinical issues for MRI scanning of pacemaker and defibrillator patients. Pacing Clin Electrophysiol. 2005;28(4):326–8.
[12] De Wachter S, Knowles CH, Elterman DS, Kennelly MJ, Lehur PA, Matzel KE, et al. New technologies and applications in sacral neuromodulation: an update. Adv Ther. 2020;37(2):637–43.
[13] Janssen PT, Kuiper SZ, Stassen LP, Bouvy ND, Breukink SO, Melenhorst J. Fecal incontinence treated by sacral neuromodulation: long-term follow-up of 325 patients. Surgery. 2017;161(4):1040–8.
[14] Pope JE, Deer TR, Falowski S, Provenzano D, Hanes M, Hayek SM, et al. Multicenter retrospective study of neurostimulation with exit of

therapy by explant. Neuromodulation. 2017;20(6):543–52.
[15] Noblett K, Siegel S, Mangel J, Griebling TL, Sutherland SE, Bird ET, et al. Results of a prospective, multicenter study evaluating quality of life, safety, and efficacy of sacral neuromodulation at twelve months in subjects with symptoms of overactive bladder. Neurourol Urodyn. 2016;35(2):246–51.
[16] Siegel S, Noblett K, Mangel J, Bennett J, Griebling TL, Sutherland SE, et al. Five-year followup results of a prospective, multicenter study of patients with overactive bladder treated with sacral neuromodulation. J Urol. 2018;199(1):229–36.
[17] Hassouna MM, Siegel SW, Nyeholt AA, Elhilali MM, van Kerrebroeck PE, Das AK, et al. Sacral neuromodulation in the treatment of urgency-frequency symptoms: a multicenter study on efficacy and safety. J Urol. 2000;163(6):1849–54.
[18] Schmidt RA, Jonas U, Oleson KA, Janknegt RA, Hassouna MM, Siegel SW, et al. Sacral nerve stimulation for treatment of refractory urinary urge incontinence. Sacral Nerve Stimulation Study Group. J Urol. 1999;162(2):352–7.
[19] Sutherland SE, Lavers A, Carlson A, Holtz C, Kesha J, Siegel SW. Sacral nerve stimulation for voiding dysfunction: one institution's 11–year experience. Neurourol Urodyn. 2007;26(1):19–28; discussion 36.
[20] Weil EH, Ruiz-Cerda JL, Eerdmans PH, Janknegt RA, Bemelmans BL, van Kerrebroeck PE. Sacral root neuromodulation in the treatment of refractory urinary urge incontinence: a prospective randomized clinical trial. Eur Urol. 2000;37(2):161–71.
[21] Cottrell AM, Schneider MP, Goonewardene S, Yuan Y, Baranowski AP, Engeler DS, et al. Benefits and harms of electrical neuromodulation for chronic pelvic pain: a systematic review. Eur Urol Focus. 2020;6(3):559–71.
[22] Peters KM, Carey JM, Konstandt DB. Sacral neuromodulation for the treatment of refractory interstitial cystitis: outcomes based on technique. Int Urogynecol J Pelvic Floor Dysfunct. 2003;14(4):223–8; discussion 8.
[23] Marinkovic SP, Gillen LM, Marinkovic CM. Minimum 6–year outcomes for interstitial cystitis treated with sacral neuromodulation. Int Urogynecol J. 2011;22(4):407–12.
[24] Peters KM, Feber KM, Bennett RC. Sacral versus pudendal nerve stimulation for voiding dysfunction: a prospective, single-blinded, randomized, crossover trial. Neurourol Urodyn. 2005;24(7):643–7.
[25] Peters KM, Feber KM, Bennett RC. A prospective, single-blind, randomized crossover trial of sacral vs pudendal nerve stimulation for interstitial cystitis. BJU Int. 2007;100(4):835–9.
[26] Peters KM, Killinger KA, Jaeger C, Chen C. Pilot study exploring chronic pudendal neuromodulation as a treatment option for pain associated with pudendal neuralgia. Low Urin Tract Symptoms. 2015;7(3):138–42.
[27] Peters KM, Killinger KA, Ibrahim IA, Villalba PS. The relationship between subjective and objective assessments of sacral neuromodulation effectiveness in patients with urgency-frequency. Neurourol Urodyn. 2008;27(8):775–8.
[28] Peters KM, Killinger KA, Boguslawski BM, Boura JA. Chronic pudendal neuromodulation: expanding available treatment options for refractory urologic symptoms. Neurourol Urodyn. 2010;29(7): 1267–71.
[29] Carmel M, Lebel M, Tu LM. Pudendal nerve neuromodulation with neurophysiology guidance: a potential treatment option for refractory chronic pelvi-perineal pain. Int Urogynecol J. 2010;21(5):613–6.
[30] Siegel S, Noblett K, Mangel J, Griebling TL, Sutherland SE, Bird ET, et al. Results of a prospective, randomized, multicenter study evaluating sacral neuromodulation with InterStim therapy compared to standard medical therapy at 6–months in subjects with mild symptoms of overactive bladder. Neurourol Urodyn. 2015;34(3):224–30.
[31] Noblett K, Benson K, Kreder K. Detailed analysis of adverse events and surgical interventions in a large prospective trial of sacral neuromodulation therapy for overactive bladder patients. Neurourol Urodyn. 2017;36(4):1136–9.
[32] Chartier-Kastler E, Le Normand L, Ruffion A, Dargent F, Braguet R, Saussine C, et al. Sacral neuromodulation with the InterStim system for intractable lower urinary tract dysfunctions (SOUNDS): results of clinical effectiveness, quality of life, patient-reported outcomes and safety in a French Multicenter Observational Study. Eur Urol Focus. 2020; https://doi. org/10.1016/j.euf.2020.06.026.
[33] Peeters K, Sahai A, De Ridder D, Van Der Aa F. Long-term follow-up of sacral neuromodulation for lower urinary tract dysfunction. BJU Int. 2014;113(5):789–94.
[34] Siegel S, Noblett K, Mangel J, Griebling TL, Sutherland SE, Bird ET, et al. Three-year follow- up results of a prospective, multicenter study in overactive bladder subjects treated with sacral neuromodulation. Urology. 2016;94:57–63.

第 11 章　肉毒杆菌毒素治疗膀胱过度活动症

Botulinum Toxin for Overactive Bladder

Sophia Janes　Sara M. Lenherr　Anne P. Cameron　著

缩略语

ACh	Acetylcholine	乙酰胆碱
ASB	Asymptomatic bacteriuria	无症状菌尿
BTXA	Onabotulinum toxin A	肉毒杆菌毒素 A
DMSO	Dimethyl sulfoxide	二甲基亚砜
GRA	global Response Assessment	全球响应评估
ICS	International Continence Society	国际尿控协会
NLUTD	neurogenic lower urinary tract dysfunction	神经源性下尿路功能障碍
OAB	overactive bladder	膀胱过度活动症
PVR	post void residual	残余尿量
SNM	sacral neuromodulation	骶神经调节
U	Units	国际单位
UTI	urinary tract infection	尿路感染
UUI	urgency urinary incontinence	急迫性尿失禁

膀胱过度活动症在本书的第 3 章和第 8 章进行了详细讨论，主要介绍了其高危因素、诊断和保守治疗的方法。简单地说，国际尿控协会（ICS）将膀胱过度活动症（OAB）定义为一种以尿急为特征的临床症候群，常伴有尿频和夜尿增多症状，伴或不伴有急迫性尿失禁，无尿路感染及其他明确的病理改变[1]。2011 年，美国食品药品管理局（FDA）批准肉毒杆菌毒素 A（BTXA）用于神经源性下尿路功能障碍（NLUTD），并于 2013 年 1 月批准用于治疗膀胱过度活动症。肉毒杆菌毒素 A 是膀胱过度活动症的三线治疗，通常在保守和药物治疗失败后使用[2]，并且肉毒杆菌毒素 A 常常联合胫后神经刺激和骶神经调节（SNM）来治疗膀胱过度活动症。因为大多数的文献都是关于肉毒杆菌毒素 A 的，所以本手稿将主要介绍肉毒杆菌毒素 A，除非另有专门说明。此外，虽然本综述主要讲的是女性特发性肉毒杆菌毒素 A，但一些研究证据仅在其他患者群体中使用而被证实。

一、肉毒杆菌毒素的作用机制

肉毒杆菌毒素是由肉毒杆菌产生的。冻干的肉毒杆菌毒素溶于无菌生理盐水中，在膀胱镜直视下注射到逼尿肌中。肉毒杆菌毒素的主要目的是阻断副交感神经传出神经中乙酰胆碱的突触前释放。然而，越来越多的证据表明，传入神经输入也受到肉毒杆菌毒素 A 的影响[3]。

当注射到组织中时，肉毒杆菌毒素 A 通过与突触囊泡蛋白 SV2 结合进入神经细胞膜，然后在神经细胞膜中被切割成重链（100kDa）和轻链（50kDa），其中轻链与 SNAP25 蛋白结合后可抑制突触囊泡前末端乙酰胆碱（ACh）的释放，从而阻止乙酰胆碱介导的肌肉收缩。此外，肉毒杆菌毒素 A 还能阻止囊泡释放其他神经肽，如 ATP、NO、降钙素相关肽和 P 物质[4]。乙酰胆碱、NO、CRP 和 P 物质会引起憋胀感、膀胱的炎症和逼尿肌的收缩。乙酰胆碱作用于毒蕈碱受体，使逼尿肌收缩。副交感神经细胞也会释放 ATP 并激活逼尿肌中的 P2X 受体以诱导收缩。

二、神经毒素在世界范围内的应用

目前，肉毒杆菌毒素 A（BTXA, Allergan, Irvine, CA）是美国唯一经 FDA 批准用于治疗膀胱过度活动症的毒素。其他具有相同作用机制且具有类似的效果的毒素也被大量使用，但是目前还没有随机对照试验来证明同等的治疗益处[5]。此外，关于膀胱过度活动症的文献对这些毒素的描述有限。下面将介绍些不同的化合物。

三、肉毒杆菌毒素 A: Dysport（Ipsen Biopharm Ltd., Slough, UK）

肉毒杆菌毒素 A 是一种在美国广泛使用的毒素，通常用于儿科神经性下尿路功能障碍。Dysport 和 Botox 的区别主要在于纯化过程。Dysport 通过柱分离方法纯化，而肉毒杆菌毒素则经过反复沉淀和溶解[5]。对于神经源性下尿路功能障碍来说，两种配方之间没有临床差异，特别是 Botox 300U 和 Dysport 750U[6]。一项单中心观察性研究比较了 Botox 与 Dysport 的治疗效果。研究发现，尿频、夜尿、尿失禁的改善和疗效持续时间相似。但 Dysport 组患者需要间歇性自我导尿的症状性尿潴留率是对照组的两倍[7]。另一项使用 Dysport 的 9 年前瞻性研究显示，与标准的肉毒杆菌毒素 A 治疗结果相似。两组中，膀胱过度活动症的严重程度改善率相似，残余尿量升高后的自导尿率相似（约 18%）。OABSS 和生活质量得分分别提高了 35% 和 41%（$P<0.001$）。26% 的参与者解除了急迫性尿失禁，44% 的参与者尿失禁严重程度降低。平均治疗间隔为 21.3 个月[8]。一个单中心队列跟踪了 33 例特发性逼尿肌过度活动的女性，她们接受了 Dysport 500U 膀胱内重复注射[9]。他们采用了保留三角肌的方法，并注意到肉毒杆菌毒素 A 的再注射间隔比我们通常预期的要长。

一项研究检查了患有神经性下尿路功能障碍的患者，他们在尿路内注射肉毒杆菌毒素 A 失败后改用 Dysport[10]。尿失禁的发生率显著降低，所有患者最大逼尿肌压力降低，56.14% 的患者认为治疗成功。虽然在膀胱过度活动症中还没有这一策略的数据，但仍有待观察的是，当其他策略（如剂量递增）对其[11]无效后，神经毒素开关是否可能是一种解决毒素耐药性的方法。

四、肉毒杆菌毒素 A: Xeomin（Merz Pharmaceutics, Frankfurt Germany）

一种不太常用的毒素——Xeomin。一组患有神经源性逼尿肌过度活动的老年男性服用 Xeomin 后，在每日尿垫使用、每日失禁发作、每日尿频、自我导尿间隔时间等方面均有显著改善[12]。最近，美国的一些供应商已经开始使用该产品，因为 Xeomin 更具成本效益（每 100U 节省约 150 美元），但其疗效尚未在特发性膀胱过度活动症的大型随机临床试验中得到证实。

其他毒素还没有被用于膀胱过度活动症或没有临床可用，如中国肉毒杆菌毒素 A：Lantox（Lanzhou Biological Products Institute, China），以及 Myobloc（NeuroBlock, RimabotulinumtoxinB, Solstice Neurosciences Inc.）和 Neuronox（BONTA, Medy-Tox Inc.）。

五、肉毒杆菌毒素注射技术

冻干的肉毒杆菌毒素 A 应用可注射的、不含防腐剂的生理盐水进行重组。为防止蛋白质变性，不得在液体中起泡或搅拌。冻干的肉毒杆菌毒素 A 可在室温下保存 5 天，但应在恢复后 5h 内使用。供应商应该仔细注意稀释、准备和储存，以防止一次和二次治疗失败。

一般在注射前 10～30min，无菌技术在膀胱内灌注 2% 利多卡因，并允许留置，进行局部麻醉。最近的一项随机对照试验研究了在注射前向标准的 20ml 2% 利多卡因中加入 10ml 8.4% 碳酸氢钠以减轻疼痛，并发现这种碱化方案在术后立即显著降低了疼痛等级。疼痛评分（0～10 分）为 2.37 ± 0.31，而溶液未碱化时为 4.44 ± 0.36（$P<0.01$）[13]。治疗后 1h 无明显差异。这是一种非常具有成本效益和简单的方法，以减少疼痛而不影响并发症或疗效，值得进一步关注。

根据制造商和对膀胱过度活动症患者的临床试验，溶解肉毒杆菌毒素 A（100U）应该用 10ml 无菌生理盐水。该针应插入逼尿肌约 2mm，在 20 个部位进行注射，每个部位注射 0.5ml，间隔约 1cm，保留三角区。

大多数供应商在临床试验中都使用的是这 20 个位点模板注射模式，但也有一些基本的修改。许多供应商已经调整了稀释度，以减少注射部位的数量，使手术更容易耐受，特别是对于那些尿路上皮脆弱的患者，应减少注射部位，以降低出血风险。

有限的证据支持注射模式的改变。一项单盲随机对照研究评价了膀胱内注射不同次数的肉毒杆菌毒素 A 治疗膀胱过度活动症患者的有效性和安全性[14]。将 67 例患者随机分为 3 组，均将 100U 肉毒杆菌毒素 A 进行 10ml 稀释后膀胱内注射 10 次（n=24）、20 次（n=22）、40 次（n=21）。全球反应评估（GRA≥1）的治疗成功率约为 80%，在治疗后 1 个月、3 个月和 6 个月组间具有可比性，不良事件无显著差异。

另一项近期的初步研究显示，在一组膀胱过度活动症患者中，沿膀胱后壁水平注射 3 个注射点（每个注射点注射 2ml）的临床疗效与之前的注射模式相似，也没有增加不良事件[15]。

在临床试验中，都会选择避开三角区的注射模式，但考虑到该区域的神经组织密度，许多供应商选择为某些患者注射三角区。最近，在 2019 年的国际尿控协会年会上，由 Allergan 资助的名为 LO-BOT 的方案展示了一种替代注射模式（Clinicaltrials.gov，NCT03052764）。在本研究方案中，100U 进行 10ml 稀释，给予 8 次三角区周注射和 2 次三角区内注射。与之前合并的 3 期和 4 期研究相比，需要间歇导尿的留置发生率较低（6.2% vs. 2.6%）。他们假设尿潴留的减少可能是由于注射更多的是针对传入的三角区神经而不是逼尿肌。

注射的另一个变量是注射的深度。调节注射深度的许多参数都是由正在使用的针头决定的。与刚性的针相比，更小的弹性针穿透逼尿肌的深度更小。虽然临床试验提供的注射深度为标准的逼尿肌 2mm，但随着膀胱充盈，尿路上皮和逼尿肌是动态变化的。一些严重小梁化的膀胱主要是Ⅲ型胶原，识别神经肌肉连接的位置是一个挑战。为了利用肉毒杆菌毒素 A 可能的传出和传入效应，一些提供者故意进行表面注射以引起更多的尿路上皮泡。这种观点认为，传入信号可能在患有膀胱过度活动症的感觉急症患者中被阻断，而不是严重的逼尿肌收缩所导致的症状。这项技术也有望用于降低尿潴留的风险，但还需要进一步的研究。

六、其他探索中的注射技术

虽然逼尿管内注射是有效的且普遍使用的，但其他的侵入性较小的给药方法仍然值得进一步的研究，将神经毒素输送到膀胱内，又能够减少疼痛、感染和出血的方法。直接膀胱内应用 BTX 是无效的，因为肉毒杆菌毒素 A 的高分子量（150kDa），使其难以通过尿路上皮屏障到达黏膜下神经。通过导尿管将药物作用于膀胱，必须采用其他方法能够使药物穿透尿路上皮并将毒素转移到神经肌肉接头处[16]。

尿路上皮屏障不能被大的肉毒杆菌毒素A分子单独穿透，而脂质体配方允许其通过尿路上皮屏障的被动扩散。在膀胱过度活动症患者中，采用双盲RCT评价脂质体肉毒杆菌毒素A灌注与生理盐水[17]的有效性。实验组给予含80mg脂质体、200U肉毒杆菌毒素A的脂毒素膀胱灌注。1个月后发现实验组患者尿频发生率明显降低（P=0.0008），尿急发作明显减少（P=0.012）。而尿失禁无明显变化（P=0.797）。与膀胱内注射相比，这种治疗对膀胱过度活动症的益处不大。

一些其他的技术已经进行了试验，其中包括膀胱内热敏聚合物水凝胶作为载体延长药物的作用时间[18]，与磷脂酰乙醇胺（HA-PE）连接的透明质酸作为大蛋白的载体，如通过尿路上皮的肉毒杆菌毒素A[19]，用1%的硫酸鱼精蛋白或二甲亚砜（DMSO）破坏尿路上皮屏障[20]，甚至电动式药物给药（EDMA）[21]或低能量冲击波[22]，并取得不同的成功。

作为膀胱内注射的替代方法，其他研究小组正在探索经阴道注射[23]的可行性。在此可行性研究中，8具女性尸体骨盆经阴道超声引导下注射墨水进入三角区和后壁。经组织学分析，墨水存在于逼尿肌层内，提示经阴道注射的可行性和准确性。虽然这种方法还没有在临床实践中被复制，但对一些女性来说，这种给药方法可能有吸引力，尽管注射区域局限于膀胱三角区和膀胱后壁。

七、疗效

早期关于膀胱过度活动症中肉毒杆菌毒素A疗效的小型安慰剂随机对照试验的报道表明，不同剂量的毒素均具有临床和尿流动力学效应[24, 25]。症状缓解主要表现为尿急、尿频和急症尿失禁发生显著变化，最早可在注射后3天或4天发生，夜尿症通常在第一周后改善[25, 26]。

早期的研究使用了较高的剂量（200U），这是神经性下尿路功能障碍的典型剂量，有很高的膀胱排空不全率[27]，但确实有很好的疗效，72%的患者尿失禁改善75%，中位反应持续时间为373天。

当代大型随机对照试验已进行Ⅱ期剂量范围研究。Dmochowski等[28]招募了313例膀胱过动症患者（288例女性），每周至少发生8次急迫性尿失禁，并给予安慰剂、50U、100U、150U、200U或300U的肉毒杆菌毒素A。12周后的结果显示，所有100U或更大剂量的药物在减少每周急迫性尿失禁发作的疗效上都比安慰剂有改善。这些效应在扩展研究中被证明持续了4年以上[29]。对各种剂量的剂量–反应曲线的进一步分析得出结论，当剂量＞150U时，没有提供可证明的额外改善。作者指出，空后残余尿量的增加和间歇导尿的使用都是剂量依赖的，因此，建议将100U作为膀胱过度活动症的剂量，以最佳地平衡收益和安全性。该研究的尿流动力学结果表明，所有肉毒杆菌毒素A的剂量均显著增加膀胱容量，然而，剂量＞150U导致排空后残余尿量＞200ml[30]。

Chapple等在2013年报道了一项大型Ⅲ期多中心随机安慰剂对照双盲试验的结果，该试验是注射100U肉毒杆菌毒素A与安慰剂治疗膀胱过度活动症。共有277例患者接受了100U肉毒杆菌毒素A治疗，报道急迫性尿失禁发生率减少了2.95次，而271例接受安慰剂治疗的患者减少了1.03次（P=0.001）。“显著改善”或“改善”治疗效益量表的阳性反应结果也非常显著，接受肉毒杆菌毒素A治疗的患者中有62.8%报道了阳性反应，而接受安慰剂治疗的患者中有26.8%报道了阳性反应（P=0.001）。Nitti等在一项类似的Ⅲ期多中心研究中，对557例膀胱过度活动症[32]患者注射100U肉毒杆菌毒素A与安慰剂进行了比较。第12周时，注射肉毒杆菌毒素A的患者每天尿失禁的次数减少了2.65次，而安慰剂组为0.87次（P＜0.001）。肉毒杆菌毒素A治疗受益量表反应为60.8%，安慰剂为29.2%（P＜0.001）。

已经将肉毒杆菌毒素A与其他治疗女性膀胱过度活动症的标准疗法进行了比较。ABC双盲随机试验比较了一组 241 例女性（n=241）接受口服索利那新（5mg，如果需要剂量增加 10mg）膀胱注射生理盐水或膀胱注射 100U 肉毒杆菌毒素 A，以及每日口服安慰剂患者的急迫性尿失禁减少情况。这些女性平均每天有 5.0 次急迫性尿失禁发作，两组的发作分别减少了 3.4 和 3.3，（P=0.81），但抗胆碱能组口干更多，这也导致更多的尿路感染和尿潴留[33]。

另一项大型随机试验在 9 个医疗中心比较了 200U 肉毒杆菌毒素 A 和骶神经调节，其中包括 364 例急迫性尿失禁[34]患者。6 个月时的早期结果显示，与骶神经调节相比，肉毒杆菌毒素 A 组每日急迫性尿失禁发生率的下降幅度略大（–3.9 vs. –3.3，P=0.01）。2 年的随访显示，两组急迫性尿失禁降低相似（–3.88 次 / 天 vs. –3.50 次 / 天，95%CI –0.14～0.89，P=0.15），急迫性尿失禁分辨率无差异，但肉毒杆菌毒素 A 组患者的满意度较高，尽管 24% 的复发性尿路感染发生率较高，而骶神经调节组为 10%（P<0.01），6% 的患者在第二次注射后需要间歇性导尿。骶神经调节翻修和切除分别发生在 3% 和 9% 的患者中[35]。

肉毒杆菌毒素 A 也被证明对那些骶神经调节失败的人有效。假设这些是更复杂的急迫性尿失禁病例，因为他们已经对三线治疗失败了。在 76 例患者中，超过 50% 的患者在随访期停止了注射，但 43% 的患者在第一次注射后报道了疗效，这使得在这种情况下肉毒杆菌毒素 A 是一个可行的选择[36]。

八、注射并发症和其他考虑事项

由肉毒杆菌毒素 A 注射引起的直接并发症可分为直接注射和延迟注射。直接的风险包括注射时的疼痛、焦虑和出血。这些直接的危险因素可以通过注射的设置来改变，在诊所或手术室或其他可以给予更多镇静的设置。在手术室中，如有必要，也有更多的电灼途径进行止血。然而，许多出血病例可以直接手动按压尖端的出血区域。肉毒杆菌毒素 A 注射的直接并发症可分为立即并发症和延迟并发症。当前的风险包括注射时的疼痛、焦虑和出血。这些直接的危险因素可以通过改变注射的设置，在诊所或手术室，以及其他可以给予更多镇静的地方进行。在手术室，如果必要的话，也可以用电灼来止血。然而，许多的出血可以用手直接按压出血末端来处理。

根据肉毒杆菌毒素 A 的包装说明，在肉毒杆菌毒素 A 注射期间禁止同时进行抗凝治疗。然而，使用更小的针头和修改一些注射参数（如注射部位的数量和注射量）通常会将出血的风险降低到最小。此外，让患者停止抗凝治疗一定要考虑到停止这种治疗的风险，这确实有助于患者的长期抗凝计划。许多供应商在考虑到患者出血风险略有增加的情况下进行注射，同时继续进行抗凝治疗[37]。

迟发性并发症包括最常见的症状性尿路感染、持续疼痛、尿失禁恶化、便秘和尿潴留。在特发性膀胱过度活动症患者注射肉毒杆菌毒素 A 之前，无症状菌尿（ASB）的管理是相当有争议的。根据肉毒杆菌毒素 A 的临床试验设计，大多数提供者可能通过评估症状和在注射时进行尿液分析来证实患者没有尿路感染。然而，全国各地的许多提供者会在不考虑尿液分析的情况下进行注射，并提供单剂量抗生素或经验性疗程，同时进行培养。在一项研究中，该策略被证明是安全的，该研究比较了一组接受注射的患者术后尿路感染的发生率，这些患者要么是尿检阴性（无血、白细胞酯酶或亚硝酸盐），要么是术前尿检阳性。值得注意的是，这些患者都没有尿路感染的症状。两组术后尿路感染发生率无明显差异[38]，即使在存在无症状菌尿时，住院率和败血症也没有差异，在一项 457 次注射的回顾性研究中疗效也没有差异。无症状菌尿患者术后发生尿路感染的风险增加[39]。

九、免疫原性：其他肉毒杆菌毒素 A 注射的时机

目前，FDA 批准的肉毒杆菌毒素 A 注射适用证主要有 4 类。除了泌尿系统疾病外，患者也可

以因运动障碍（如痉挛和颈部肌张力障碍）和皮肤病（如腋窝多汗症），以及美容应用而接受肉毒杆菌毒素A的治疗。此外，有许多适应证包括肉毒杆菌毒素A治疗盆腔张力肌痛等。虽然肉毒杆菌毒素A的效用应该被赞赏，但许多患者往往在不被告知其他提供者的情况下接受不同厂家的产品，这导致异步注射。

关于“非同步”注射的担忧是增加了免疫原性的风险。免疫原性的发生是因为机体在使用时中和或阻断肉毒杆菌毒素A，导致二次治疗失败。肉毒杆菌毒素A被宿主认为是外来的，潜在的免疫反应可以针对抗原。这种免疫原性的风险随着在“助推器”时间轴上重复给药而增加，通常间隔2～3周。究竟是实际的150kDa肉毒杆菌毒素A蛋白还是复合物蛋白刺激了免疫反应目前还不清楚[40]。一种理论认为肉毒杆菌毒素A因抗体产生而失败是因为膀胱（及其尿路上皮）是一种免疫反应器官，其被设计用于对其他抗原敏感，如尿路感染[41]。

为了降低免疫原性的风险，泌尿科医生应该询问患者最近是否接受过其他肉毒杆菌毒素A治疗。应考虑到肉毒杆菌毒素A治疗的慢性、长期性和需要反复注射的非永久性神经肌肉连接阻滞，这一点尤为重要。作者的临床实践是保持异步注射间隔在1周内或延迟至3个月。由于这种临床模式，大多数保险计划不会支付超过3个月的重复注射。如果担心中和抗体导致治疗失败，可以在颞部肌肉注射功能评价试验，寻找肌肉反应（单侧前额注射）或检测肉毒杆菌毒素[40]的中和抗体。然而，不管是否存在中和抗体，治疗失败的管理是相同的，尽管昂贵的额外测试 – 过渡到替代疗法。

十、远距离扩散

注射肉毒杆菌毒素A的一个可怕并发症是毒素会远距离传播到非靶部位。2009年，FDA发布了一个黑框警告，讨论脑瘫患者逼尿肌注射肉毒杆菌毒素治疗颈椎肌张力障碍后出现肉毒杆菌毒素中毒的症状[42]。虽然没有发现致命的不良反应，但逼尿肌注射的多种不良反应已被记录。最常见的不良反应是逼尿肌注射后的肌无力。在这些病例报道中，一份报道了2例脊髓损伤患者出现肌肉无力，导致运动障碍[43]；另一份报道了4例神经源性逼尿肌过度活动患者出现短暂的全身无力[44]。此外，1例多发性硬化症患者在注射肉毒杆菌毒素A后双侧腿部无力，后来被确定为多发性硬化症[45]。值得注意的是，所有的病例报道都是在神经功能障碍的患者中，而不是特发性膀胱过度活动症的患者。注射肉毒杆菌毒素的远处扩散是一种罕见但严重的并发症，需要进行更多的研究。

十一、禁忌证

肉毒杆菌毒素A禁用于既往对肉毒杆菌或肉毒杆菌化妆品有过敏反应的患者，且禁用于在注射部位有感染或存在尿路感染的患者。目前尚不清楚肉毒杆菌毒素A在孕妇和哺乳期女性中的作用。然而，动物研究表明，妊娠期动物肌肉注射肉毒杆菌毒素A可降低胎儿体重、增加胎儿骨骼骨钙流失、导致流产、早产和孕产妇死亡（根据Allergan肉毒杆菌毒素A产品标签）。由于抗胆碱能作用，肉毒杆菌毒素A也不建议用于肌萎缩侧索硬化症、重症肌无力或兰伯特 – 伊顿综合征患者。然而，这些情况目前还没有被标记为禁忌证。

总结

肉毒杆菌毒素是治疗膀胱过度活动症的一种非常有效的三线治疗方法，但仍有许多改进措施有助于改善结局。提供者应该了解肉毒杆菌毒素A的其他用途和患者的使用模式。患者不应每3个月注射1次，应尽量减少不同时期的注射，而采取集中注射，从而避免免疫原性的发生。肉毒杆菌毒素A的应用方法改进可能在不久的将来提高患者的安全和舒适感。

参考文献

[1] Haylen BT, Freeman RM, Swift SE, Cosson M, Davila GW, Deprest J, et al. An International Urogynecological Association (IUGA) / International Continence Society (ICS) joint terminology and classification of the complications related directly to the insertion of prostheses (meshes, implants, tapes) & grafts in female pelvic flo. Int Urogynecol J. 2011;22(1):3–15.

[2] Gormley EA, Lightner DJ, Faraday M, Vasavada SP. Diagnosis and treatment of overactive bladder (non-neurogenic) in adults: AUA/SUFU guideline amendment. J Urol [Internet]. 2015;193(5):1572–80. Available from: https://doi.org/10.1016/j.juro.2015.01.087

[3] Coelho A, Cruz F, Cruz CD, Avelino A. Spread of onabotulinumtoxinA after bladder injection. Experimental study using the distribution of cleaved SNAP-25 as the marker of the toxin action. Eur Urol. 2012;61(6):1178–84.

[4] Chen JL, Kuo HC. Clinical application of intravesical botulinum toxin type a for overactive bladder and interstitial cystitis. Investig Clin Urol. 2020;61:S33–42.

[5] Walker TJ, Dayan SH. Comparison and overview of currently available neurotoxins. J Clin Aesthet Dermatol. 2014;7(2):31–9.

[6] Stoehrer M, Wolff A, Kramer G, Steiner R, Löchner-Ernst D, Leuth D, et al. Treatment of neurogenic detrusor overactivity with botulinum toxin A: the first seven years. Urol Int. 2009;83(4):379–85.

[7] Ravindra P, Jackson BL, Parkinson RJ. Botulinum toxin type A for the treatment of non-neurogenic overactive bladder: does using onabotulinumtoxinA (Botox®) or abobotulinumtoxinA (Dysport®) make a difference? BJU Int. 2013;112(1):94–9.

[8] Craciun M, Irwin PP. Outcomes for intravesical abobotulinumtoxin A (Dysport) treatment in the active management of overactive bladder symptoms—a prospective study. Urology [Internet]. 2019;130:54–8. Available from: https://doi.org/10.1016/j.urology.2019.04.018

[9] Abeywickrama L, Arunkalaivanan A, Quinlan M. Repeated botulinum toxin type A (Dysport®) injections for women with intractable detrusor overactivity: a prospective outcome study. Int Urogynecol J Pelvic Floor Dysfunct. 2014;25(5):601–5.

[10] Bottet F, Peyronnet B, Boissier R, Reiss B, Previnaire JG, Manunta A, et al. Switch to abobotulinum toxin A may be useful in the treatment of neurogenic detrusor overactivity when intradetrusor injections of onabotulinum toxin A failed. Neurourol Urodyn. 2018;37(1):291–7.

[11] Apostolidis A, Cameron AP. Neurourological management after failed Intradetrusor onabotulinumtoxinA injections. Eur Urol Focus [Internet]. 2020;6(5):814–6. Available from: https:// doi.org/10.1016/j.euf.2019.10.003

[12] Asafu-Adjei D, Small A, McWilliams G, Galea G, Chung D, Pak J. The intravesical injection of highly purified botulinum toxin for the treatment of neurogenic detrusor overactivity. Can Urol Assoc J. 2019;14(10):520–6.

[13] Pereira e Silva R, Ponte C, Lopes F, Palma dos Reis J. Alkalinized lidocaine solution as a first-line local anesthesia protocol for intradetrusor injection of onabotulinum toxin A: results from a double-blinded randomized controlled trial. Neurourol Urodyn. 2020;39(8):2471–9.

[14] Liao C-H, Chen S-F, Kuo H-C. Different number of intravesical onabotulinumtoxinA injections for patients with refractory detrusor overactivity do not affect treatment outcome: a prospective randomized comparative study. Neurourol Urodyn. 2016;35:717–33.

[15] Martínez-Cuenca E, Bonillo MA, Morán E, Broseta E, Arlandis S. Onabotulinumtoxina reinjection for refractory detrusor overactivity using 3–4 injection sites: results of a pilot study. Urology. 2020;137:50–4.

[16] Chen P-Y, Lee W-C, Wang H-J, Chuang YC. Therapeutic efficacy of onabotulinumtoxinA delivered using various approaches in sensory bladder disorder. Toxins (Basel). 2020;12(75):1–11.

[17] Kuo HC, Liu HT, Chuang YC, Birder LA, Chancellor MB. Pilot study of liposome-encapsulated onabotulinumtoxinA for patients with overactive bladder: a single-center study. Eur Urol [Internet]. 2014;65(6):1117–24. Available from: https://doi.org/10.1016/j.eururo.2014.01.036

[18] Tyagi P, Li Z, Chancellor M, De Groat WC, Yoshimura N. Sustained intravesical drug delivery using thermosensitive hydrogel. Pharm Res. 2004;21(5):832–7.

[19] El Shatoury MG, DeYoung L, Turley E, Yazdani A, Dave S. Early experimental results of using a novel delivery carrier, hyaluronan-phosphatidylethanolamine (HA-PE), which may allow simple bladder instillation of botulinum toxin A as effectively as direct detrusor muscle injection. J Pediatr Urol [Internet]. 2018;14(2):172.e1–6. Available from: https://doi.org/10.1016/j. jpurol.2017.11.016

[20] Petrou SP, Parker AS, Crook JE, Rogers A, Metz-Kudashick D, Thiel DD. Botulinum A toxin/ dimethyl sulfoxide bladder instillations for women with refractory idiopathic detrusor overactivity: a phase 1/2 study. Mayo Clin Proc [Internet]. 2009;84(8):702–6. Available from: https:// doi.org/10.4065/84.8.702

[21] Ladi-Seyedian SS, Sharifi-Rad L, Kajbafzadeh AM. Intravesical electromotive botulinum toxin type "A" administration for management of urinary incontinence secondary to neuropathic detrusor overactivity in children: long-term follow-up. Urology [Internet]. 2018;114:167–74. Available from: https://doi.org/10.1016/j.urology.2017.11.039

[22] Nageib M, Zahran MH, El-Hefnawy AS, Barakat N, Awadalla A, Aamer HG, et al. Low energy shock wave-delivered intravesical botulinum neurotoxin-A potentiates antioxidant genes and inhibits proinflammatory cytokines in rat model of overactive bladder. Neurourol Urodyn. 2020;39(8):2447–54.

[23] Syan R, Briggs MA, Olivas JC, Srivastava S, Comiter CV, Dobberfuhl AD. Transvaginal ultrasound guided trigone and bladder injection: a cadaveric feasibility study for a novel route of intradetrusor chemodenervation. Investig Clin Urol. 2019;60(1):40–5.

[24] Flynn MK, Amundsen CL, Perevich MA, Liu F, Webster GD. Outcome of a randomized, double-blind, placebo controlled trial of botulinum a toxin for refractory overactive bladder. J Urol [Internet]. 2009;181(6):2608–15. Available from: https://doi.org/10.1016/j.juro.2009.01.117

[25] Sahai A, Khan MS, Dasgupta P. Efficacy of botulinum toxin-A for treating idiopathic detrusor overactivity: results from a single center, randomized, double-blind, placebo controlled trial. J Urol. 2007;177(6):2231–6.

[26] Kalsi V, Apostolidis A, Gonzales G, Elneil S, Dasgupta P, Fowler CJ. Early effect on the overactive bladder symptoms following botulinum neurotoxin type a injections for detrusor overactivity. Eur Urol. 2008;54(1):181–7.

[27] Brubaker L, Richter HE, Visco A, Mahajan S, Nygaard I, Braun TM, et al. Refractory idiopathic urge urinary incontinence and botulinum a injection. J Urol. 2008;180(1):217–22.

[28] Dmochowski R, Chapple C, Nitti VW, Chancellor M, Everaert K, Thompson C, et al. Efficacy and safety of onabotulinumtoxina for idiopathic overactive bladder: a double-blind, placebo controlled, randomized, dose ranging trial. J Urol [Internet]. 2010;184(6):2416–22. Available from: https://doi.org/10.1016/j.juro.2010.08.021

[29] Kennelly M, Dmochowski R, Schulte-Baukloh H, Ethans K, Del

Popolo G, Moore C, et al. Efficacy and safety of onabotulinumtoxinA therapy are sustained over 4 years of treatment in patients with neurogenic detrusor overactivity: final results of a long-term extension study. Neurourol Urodyn. 2017;36(2):368–75.

[30] Rovner E, Kennelly M, Shulte-Baukloh H, Zhou J, Haag-Molkenteller C, Dasgupta P. Urodynamic results and clinical outcomes with intradetrusor injections of onabotulinumtoxinA in a randomized, placebo-controlled dose-finding study in idiopathic overactive bladder. Neurourol Urodyn. 2011;30:556–62.

[31] Chapple C, Sievert KD, Macdiarmid S, Khullar V, Radziszewski P, Nardo C, et al. OnabotulinumtoxinA 100 U significantly improves all idiopathic overactive bladder symptoms and quality of life in patients with overactive bladder and urinary incontinence: a randomised, double-blind, placebo-controlled trial. Eur Urol [Internet]. 2013;64(2):249–56. Available from: https://doi.org/10.1016/j.eururo.2013.04.001

[32] Nitti VW, Dmochowski R, Herschorn S, Sand P, Thompson C, Nardo C, et al. OnabotulinumtoxinA for the treatment of patients with overactive bladder and urinary incontinence: results of a phase 3, randomized, placebo controlled trial. J Urol [Internet]. 2013;189(6):2186–93. Available from: https://doi.org/10.1016/j.juro.2012.12.022

[33] Visco AG, Brubaker L, Richter HE, Nygaard I, Paraiso MFR, Menefee SA, et al. Anticholinergic therapy vs. onabotulinumtoxinA for urgency urinary incontinence. N Engl J Med. 2012;367(19):1803–13.

[34] Amundsen CL, Richter HE, Menefee SA, Komesu YM, Arya LA, Gregory WT, et al. Onabotulinumtoxin a vs sacral neuromodulation on refractory urgency urinary incontinence in women: a randomized clinical trial. JAMA. 2016;316(13):1366–74.

[35] Amundsen CL, Komesu YM, Chermansky C, Gregory WT, Myers DL, Honeycutt EF, et al. Two-year outcomes of sacral neuromodulation versus onabotulinumtoxinA for refractory urgency urinary incontinence: a randomized trial [figure presented]. Eur Urol [Internet]. 2018;74(1):66–73. Available from: https://doi.org/10.1016/j.eururo.2018.02.011

[36] Baron M, Perrouin-Verbe MA, Lacombe S, Paret F, Le Normand L, Cornu JN. Efficacy and tolerance of botulinum toxin injections after sacral nerve stimulation failure for idiopathic overactive bladder. Neurourol Urodyn. 2020;39(3):1012–9.

[37] Wells H, Luton O, Simpkin A, Bullock N, KandaSwamy G, Younis A. Intravesical injection of botulinum toxin a for treatment of overactive bladder in anticoagulated patients: is it safe? Turk J Urol. 2020;46(6):481–7.

[38] Derisavifard S, Giusto LL, Zahner P, Rueb JJ, Goldman HB. Safety of intradetrusor onabotulinumtoxinA (BTX-A) injection in the asymptomatic patient with a positive urine dip. Urology. 2020;135:38–43.

[39] Aharony S, Przydacz M, Van Ba OL, Corcos J. Does asymptomatic bacteriuria increase the risk of adverse events or modify the efficacy of intradetrusor onabotulinumtoxinA injections? Neurourol Urodyn. 2020;39(1):203–10.

[40] Dressler D. Clinical presentation and management of antibody-induced failure of botulinum toxin therapy. Mov Disord. 2004;19(Suppl. 8):92–100.

[41] Schulte-Baukloh H, Bigalke H, Miller K, Heine G, Pape D, Lehmann J, et al. Botulinum neurotoxin type A in urology: antibodies as a cause of therapy failure. Int J Urol. 2008;15(5):407–15.

[42] Linsenmeyer TA. Use of botulinum toxin in individuals with neurogenic detrusor overactivity: state of the art review. J Spinal Cord Med [Internet]. 2013;36(5):402–19. Available from: http://www.ncbi.nlm.nih.gov/pubmed/23941788

[43] Wyndaele JJ, Van Dromme SA. Muscular weakness as side effect of botulinum toxin injection for neurogenic detrusor overactivity. Spinal Cord. 2002;40(11):599–600.

[44] Grosse J, Kramer G, Stöhrer M. Success of repeat detrusor injections of botulinum A toxin in patients with severe neurogenic detrusor overactivity and incontinence. Eur Urol. 2005;47(5):653–9.

[45] Kalsi V, Gonzales G, Popat R, Apostolidis A, Elneil S, Dasgupta P, et al. Botulinum injections for the treatment of bladder symptoms of multiple sclerosis. Ann Neurol. 2007;62(5):452–7.

第 12 章 非神经源性膀胱扩大成形术
Augmentation Cystoplasty in the Non-neurogenic Bladder Patient

Aisha L. Siebert　Elizabeth Rourke　Stephanie J. Kielb　著

由肠管替代的膀胱扩大成形术适用于治疗因潜在神经源性疾病而导致的低容量、顺应性差或难治性逼尿肌过度活动的膀胱。这种手术方法可以而且应该被考虑用于治疗药物和保守手术干预无效的各种非神经源性疾病导致的膀胱功能障碍。本章讨论膀胱过度活动症（OAB）、间质性膀胱炎（IC）或膀胱疼痛综合征（BPS）、良性膀胱病变或瘘管修补的膀胱部分切除，以及导致膀胱顺应性下降的特殊情况（结核病、终末期肾病和氯胺酮膀胱炎）。

一、膀胱过度活动症

美国泌尿外科协会（AUA）和泌尿动力学学会、女性盆腔医学和泌尿生殖系统重建（SUFU）指南建议仅对严重、难治、复杂的膀胱过度活动症患者进行膀胱扩大成形术。小数据病例系列报道 66%～94% 的患者术后膀胱过度活动症得到缓解，患者的满意度高于连续注射肉毒杆菌毒素，但需要注意的是，进行膀胱扩大成形术的患者术前症状往往很严重[2-5]。因患者术后排尿能力不同，高达 75% 的患者需要间歇性清洁自我导尿（CIC），术前需严格筛选患者，并告知患者这种风险[6]。少数患者诊治中记录了使用猪真皮移植，在 1 年的随访中显示干燥率为 25%，总体改善率为 83%，而且没有明显的并发症[7]，但缺乏长期随访结果。膀胱扩大成形术是一种侵入性腹部手术，需要肠切除和重新吻合，由于手术风险、长期需要间歇性清洁自我导尿，以及发生恶性肿瘤的风险，仅仅被用作难治性膀胱过度活动症的四线治疗方案。在选定的患者群中，膀胱扩大成形术可以缓解症状，患者满意度优于逼尿肌内注射肉毒杆菌毒素。

二、间质性膀胱炎 / 膀胱疼痛综合征

间质性膀胱炎或膀胱疼痛综合征是一种排他性诊断。包括膀胱次全切除术和替代性膀胱成形术的大手术在内，被认为是间质性膀胱炎或膀胱疼痛综合征患者药物和内镜治疗失败的六线治疗方案[8]。保留三角区的手术理论上可以降低尿潴留的风险，术后大多数患者能够自行排尿，很少需要间歇性清洁自我导尿。然而，采用这种方法后，33% 的女性报道继发于组织学证实的三角区受累的持续刺激症状，因此建议术前进行膀胱活检并标测，但并未被广泛采用[9]。能够预测持续刺激症状的患者因素包括以尿道疼痛为主要症状、没有 Hunner 损害，以及膀胱镜评估时膀胱容量较大[8]。一些报道显示，在不切除膀胱的情况下进行膀胱扩大成形术可以增加膀胱容量，尿频和夜尿症等贮存症状得到改善，但对膀胱疼痛几乎没有改善[10]。间质性膀胱炎 / 膀胱疼痛综合征膀胱扩大成形术包括 12% 的 Clavien Ⅲ级并发症和 29% 的持续性疼痛[11]。对于膀胱镜检查或尿流动力学显示膀胱容量下降的患者，膀胱扩大可能有作用，但证据有限。单纯的膀胱扩大成形术并不能解决膀胱疼痛，而膀胱次全切除术和替代性膀胱成形术可以不同程度的解决膀胱疼痛。

三、部分膀胱切除术后

对有症状的良性膀胱病变进行部分膀胱切除术可能导致膀胱顺应性降低和膀胱功能受损。膀胱切除术与膀胱扩大成形术相结合，以保持膀胱顺应性并降低对生活质量的影响。瘘管切除和创伤为指征的膀胱部分切除已描述[12, 13]。如果膀胱受损，无论膀胱组织丢失与否，伴或不伴顺应性改变，都可能需要膀胱扩大成形术。病例报道描述了这种手术在以前的放射治疗中的应用，术后保留了长达7个月的排尿功能[14]。虽然难治性放射性膀胱炎被认为是膀胱扩大术的禁忌证，但却是膀胱切除术或膀胱次全切除术和替代性膀胱成形术的适应证。当计划在辐射区域进行手术时，外科医生应考虑组织质量，以及辐射对伤口愈合的不良影响。

四、膀胱容量减少

膀胱顺应性差导致的终末期肾病（ESRD）可能由结核病、放射并发症、先天性畸形（包括膀胱输尿管反流和后尿道畸形）和间质性膀胱炎以及许多神经源性原因引起。当造影作为移植前常规评估的一部分时，多达2.5%的患者出现排尿性膀胱尿道造影异常，不足1%的患者需要干预，很少需要膀胱扩大成形术[15]。在移植前进行尿流动力学评估寻找病因的患者中，超过70%的患者表现出导致肾功能不全的泌尿系统病变（包括梗阻、反流或膀胱功能障碍）[16]，并且需要在移植前进行干预。在肾移植前、后或同时行膀胱扩大成形术虽然很少见，但仍有报道。输尿管移植可以与扩大的膀胱或原输尿管吻合[17]。移植物存活率很高，1年为96%～100%，2年为92%，5年为77%～100%[18-20]。虽然一些中心报道与不进行膀胱扩大术的移植患者相比，移植肾功能有下降趋势[21]，术后4年内肾功能稳定[22, 23]，移植肾功能衰竭的发生率几乎没有增加[24]，不增加尿毒症的风险，但严重尿路感染（UTI）的风险增加。

泌尿生殖系统是肺外结核最常见的侵犯部位，常导致膀胱储存功能障碍。由炎症导致的脓肿形成、输尿管和尿道狭窄，以及膀胱挛缩并发症通常需要手术治疗，严重情况下最终会出现肾功能不全。膀胱扩大成形术可提高膀胱容量和顺应性，可以保留膀胱感觉功能[25]。手术后膀胱容量>250ml，昼夜排尿频率可提高到2h以上，但是膀胱不自主收缩可能会持续存在，需要额外的药物治疗[26]。

长期使用氯胺酮是膀胱纤维化的罕见原因，会导致膀胱变小、挛缩。小数据病例系列报道称，这种情况下膀胱扩大术后膀胱容量显著增加，疼痛、尿频、尿急减轻，镇痛药使用减少[27]。

五、外科手术方法

因内科和微创介入治疗失败而接受手术的患者应由专门研究这些适应证的中心管理。选择合适的患者，以及术前、术后咨询对于患者期望值的设定和提高术后生活质量的目标至关重要。术前评估应包括尿道评估和控尿能力评估，结合膀胱镜评估、尿流率或尿流动力学检查，以及自我导尿能力评估来完成。肾功能可能受到潜在疾病进展和膀胱功能障碍的不良影响，因此建议手术前再次进行肾功能评估和术后监测。机器人膀胱扩大成形术已被许多中心描述为一种可行的选择，尽管相对于开放手术的临床获益还不确定（表12-1）。手术入路的选择应由外科医生的技能和经验决定。

回肠是膀胱扩大成形术最常用的肠管，回盲部、乙状结肠和胃也可使用。当使用回肠时，在回盲部近端15～20cm处切取20～25cm的肠管，由相应的血管弓决定切取肠管的具体位置和长度，以便保障微量营养的再分配。

若有盆腔放射病史或同时进行结肠手术（如结肠造口术）时，结肠膀胱扩大成形术可以避免肠吻合。在这种情况下，应仔细考虑手术时机及可能影响伤口愈合的其他因素，并与患者进行讨论。如果术中认为小肠置入不适合，在置入结肠前应进行结肠镜检查。

胃是较少用于膀胱扩大的组织来源。沿胃大弯楔形切除10～20cm胃窦或胃体可用于膀胱扩大

表 12-1　机器人方法在膀胱扩大成形术中的应用

作者，文献	期　刊	结　果	并发症	*N*
K. E. Al-Othman, H. A. Al-Hellow, H. M. Al-Zahrani, R. M. Seyam. Robotic augmentation enterocystoplasty	*Journal of Endourology*. 22(4): 597–600 (2008)	术后麻醉需求低	手术时间长	1
J. J. Gould, J. T. Stoffel. Robotic enterocystoplasty: technique and early outcomes	*Journal of Endourology*. 25(1): 91–95 (2011)	尿道节制，正常上尿路显像	罕见肠梗阻	5
Robotic approaches to augmentation cystoplasty: ready for prime time?Prithvi Murthy, Joshua A. Cohn, Mohan S. Gundeti	*Current Bladder Dysfunction Reports*. 9:310–317 (2014)	更快的恢复时间，减少术后麻醉剂的使用和粘连形成	费用	13
Andrew S. Flum, Lee C. Zhao, Stephanie J. Kielb, Erik B. Wilson, Tung Shu, John C. Hairston. Completely intracorporeal robotic-assisted laparoscopic augmentation enterocystoplasty with continent catheterizable channel	*Journal of Urology*. 84(6):1314–1318 (2014)	恢复时间更快，降低伤口 / 肠道并发症（如小肠梗阻和肠梗阻）	静脉血栓栓塞	22
A. C. Wiestma, C. R. Estrada Jr., P. S. Cho, M. V. Hollis, R. N. Yu. Robotic-assisted laparoscopic bladder augmentation in the pediatric patient	*Journal of Pediatric Urology*. 12(5):313. e1–e2 (2016)	增加膀胱容量	手术时间长	1

术。血管蒂由胃网膜左或右动脉供应，然后穿过横结肠和小肠系膜。与易引起慢性菌尿的肠管膀胱扩大术相比，胃膀胱扩大术分泌的黏液少，不易发生代谢性酸中毒和感染，但尿痛 – 血尿综合征使得胃膀胱扩大术不再受欢迎。

在进行膀胱扩大成形术时，选定的肠段沿肠系膜对侧缘切开，根据长度折叠肠管成 U 形、S 形或 W 形，并与原膀胱顶中的矢状切口吻合[28]。怀疑有多种疾病的患者需要进行输尿管评估。回肠替代输尿管、颊黏膜移植替代尿道成形术和回肠膀胱扩大成形术可单独或联合使用以解决多部位病变[29]。

膀胱扩大成形术技术

1. 有 / 无导管通道开放的膀胱扩大成形术

(1) 患者取仰卧位（女性呈蛙腿状，以便在手术过程中轻松进入尿道），伴或不伴肾脏松弛状。将导尿管放置在无菌区域上，选择腹中线脐下切口，可根据需要将其延伸至脐上方以便充分显露。进入腹腔后评估肠管，这一步是必需的，切开耻骨后的 Retzius 间隙并移动膀胱，用电切法打开膀胱，从膀胱颈向前延伸约 2cm，从膀胱三角向后延伸约 2cm（图 12–1A）。这可防止由于肠 / 膀胱缝合线收缩而出现沙漏结构。

(2) 确定用于扩大的肠段（回肠、升结肠或乙状结肠）。对于回肠成形术，使用距回盲瓣 15～20cm 长约 25cm 的回肠段（结肠为 15～20cm）。用缝合线标记该肠段的近端和远端，用 GIA 吻合器取肠，在所取肠管上方进行肠吻合，确保所有吻合钉都从扩大段中移除（图 12–1B）。用电凝法将肠段去管化，并使肠壁似 S 形（注：U 形、S 形和 W 形的直补片或杯形补片是膀胱扩大术的可选技术），黏膜边缘（在期望的结构中）可以用 2–0 Vicryl 缝合线或 3–0 聚二烷酮（PDS）缝合线进行缝合（图 12–1E 和 F）。为了便于冲洗和术后管理，在完成后部吻合后，将一根 16～20 号导尿管穿过逼尿肌放入原膀胱置于耻骨上（也可以使用 Malecot 导管）（图 12–1H），前部吻合完成后，冲洗膀胱 / 检测膀胱沿缝合线的渗漏情况，并根据需要进行支撑。

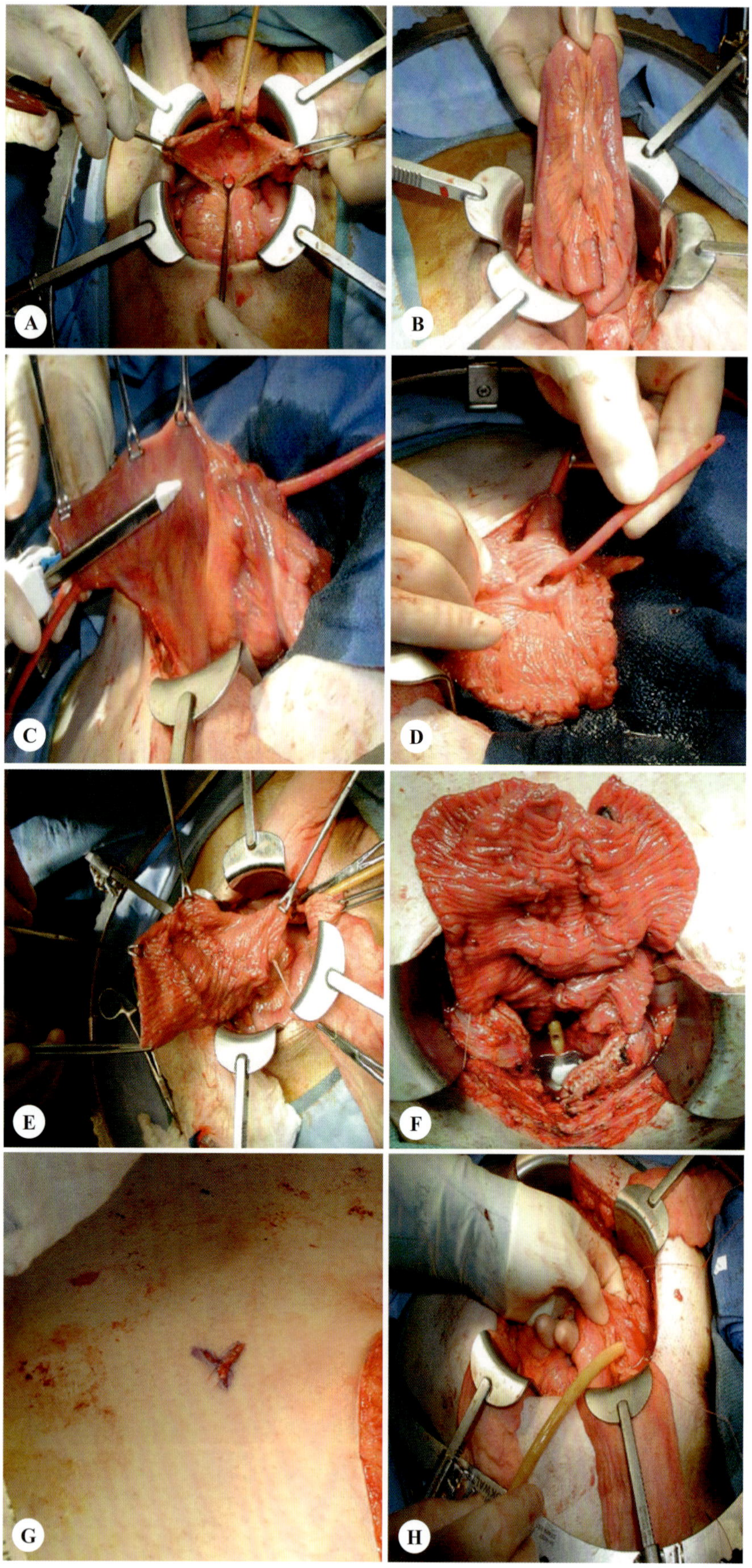

◀ 图 12-1 有导管的回肠膀胱成形术

A. 双瓣膀胱，后向三角区，前向膀胱颈；B. 回肠段长度约 45cm；C. 在盲肠系带上用 12～14 号红色橡胶导尿管塑造导管通道（Mitrofanoff）；D. 检测导管通道的松紧度；E. 回肠段去管；F. 回肠段与双瓣膀胱吻合；G. 造口 Y-V 成形；H. 耻骨上导管扩大膀胱

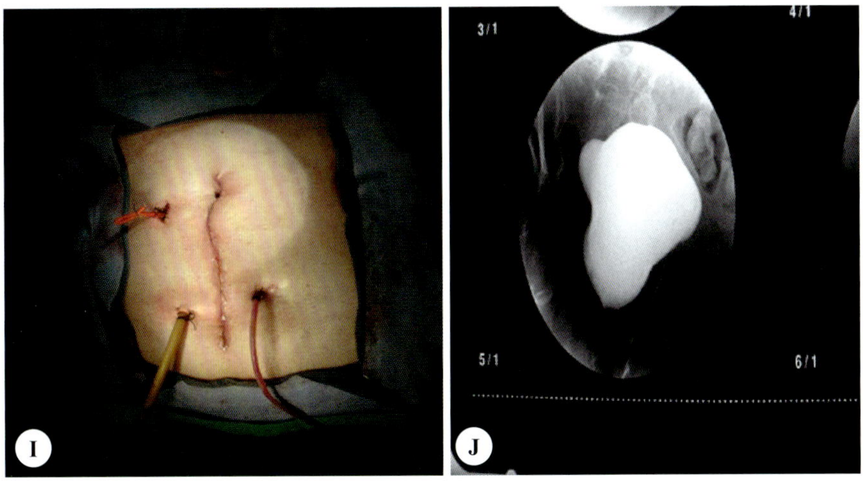

◀ **图 12-1（续） 有导管的回肠膀胱成形术**

I. 造口 12 号红色橡胶导尿管，耻骨上扩大膀胱的导管和腹腔引流管；J. 术后膀胱造影（图片由 Melissa Kaufman MD MPH 提供）

(3) 如果需要可插入导管的通道，最常见的方法是使用阑尾（如果长度足够）或带有部分回肠的阑尾。通过将阑尾与盲肠分离，同时将阑尾动脉保留在阑尾的肠系膜内并与盲肠分开，创建阑尾膀胱造口术 /Mitrofanoff。如果长度达不到需要，可以用阑尾连接部分盲肠并管状化。在通道中加入盲肠系带可以降低皮肤水平的造口狭窄风险。阑尾通道长度也可以通过阑尾连同一段盲肠一起切除来增加，并用 GIA 吻合器在导管上逐渐缩窄（图 12-1C），然后通过黏膜下隧道将阑尾置入膀胱。建议在原膀胱后外侧位置将通道与其吻合，而不在扩大的补片上吻合。阑尾也可以固定在膀胱外壁上，以防止造口回缩。造口位置可能因通道长度和患者解剖结构而异，可放置在下腹壁或脐部（首选），通道应能容纳 12～14 号红色橡胶导尿管（图 1-1D）。如果阑尾不可用，可以使用 Yang Monti（YM）技术，用长 2cm 回肠段来创建通道。将选定的肠管节段沿肠系膜方向横向切开，并分成两层（黏膜和浆膜）沿其长轴使用 3-0/4-0 可吸收缝合线进行缝合，重新管状化形成长通道（通常是截取肠管节段长度的两倍）。建议在 12～14 号导尿管引导下形成通道，如果需要更长的通道，双 YM 或螺旋 YM 是可行的选择。通过这种方法形成的管段再首尾吻合，可产生双 YM。

(4) 造口可选择 Y-V 形、V 形或 U 形切口，位于脐部或下腹部象限（图 12-1G）。最终最重要的是造口的位置便于导管插入。在造口过程中，必须对通道进行反复测试。在 Y-V 成形术中，将 V 的顶点固定在通道上（皮肤真皮层至通道黏膜）用 3-0 Vicryl 缝合线进行缝合，然后间断缝合造口。术后，在造口中保留 16 号导尿管 3 周。必须将通道固定到腹膜后 / 腹壁上，以确保正确地直接对准膀胱，从而避免导管插入困难。

(5) 如果不担心腹腔内漏尿，可以在出院前拔除膀胱周围 / 腹腔内引流管（图 12-1I）。

(6) 术后，可将导尿管留在原处，在患者出院前取出。术后 3 周内每天冲洗耻骨上导管，以防止黏液积聚，并在取出前进行膀胱造影（图 12-1J）。如果膀胱造影没有显示尿液外渗，则堵住耻骨上导管，患者将开始通过通道导尿（如果存在）。如果导尿没有问题，则拔除耻骨上导管[30, 31]。

2. 腹腔镜 / 机器人技术的膀胱扩大成形术

机器人辅助腹腔镜技术经过多年的发展，最近已经用于包括膀胱扩大成形术在内的复杂泌尿系统的微创治疗。Gundeti 等于 2008 年首次在小儿神经源性膀胱治疗中描述了机器人回肠膀胱成形术[32]。传统上膀胱扩大成形术采用开腹手术，详细说明机器人辅助腹腔镜体内膀胱扩大成形术的安全性、可行性和手术技术的出版物有限，因此，迄今为止尚未得到很好的证实。但是，为了降低膀胱扩大成形术的并发症和危险性，下面详细介绍了几种建议的技术，除了外科医生在机器人方面的必要时的经验外，在进行机器人治疗之前，必须考虑患者的选择。

(1) 将患者置于陡峭的头低足高仰卧背侧截石位。根据外科医生的喜好，使用 Veress 或 Hassan 技术将 12mm 相机端口放置在脐上方 2～5cm 处。端口放置类似于机器人辅助根治性膀胱切除术和前列腺切除术，在腹直肌左、右外侧边有两个 8mm 机器人端口，在右侧髂前上棘（ASIS）上方 2cm 处有一个额外的 8mm 机器人端口，以及左侧髂前上棘上方 2cm 处的 12mm 辅助端口。每个端口应相距约 8cm。可以根据需要放置一个 5mm 的辅助端口（图 12–2）。

(2) 首先在脐内侧韧带之间沿腹膜纵向切开，通过钝性和电切相结合的方式进入腹膜外间隙，显露膀胱顶部，膨胀膀胱以便于膀胱切开术，与开腹手术类似，在矢状面中线对膀胱进行双瓣切开。

(3) 回肠补片是通过截取距回盲部 15cm，长 15～20cm 的远端回肠形成的。该段肠管的远端用缝合线固定于腹壁，以便于收集回肠段补片[33]。使用内镜吻合器分离回肠段，并使用单、双极组合分割肠系膜，再次使用内镜吻合器将回肠段两

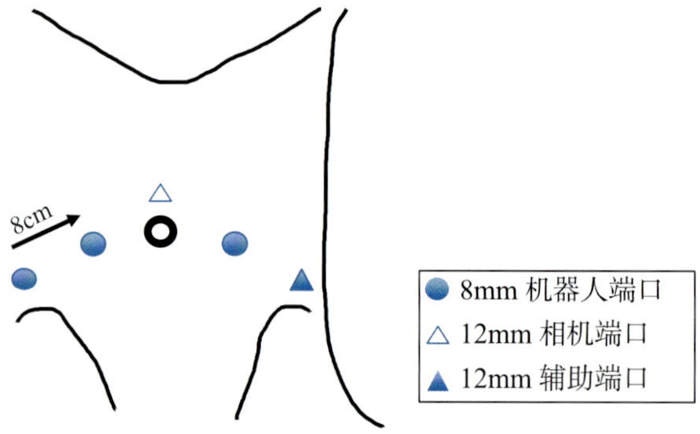

▲ 图 12–2 机器人辅助腹腔镜回肠成形术的端口放置

在气腹针或 Hassan 技术的帮助下，将 12mm 相机端口放置在脐上方 2～5cm 处。2 个 8mm 机器人端口沿腹直肌左右侧外侧边放置，还有 1 个 8mm 机器人端口放置在右侧髂前上棘上方 2cm 处，以及 1 个 12mm 辅助端口在左侧髂前上棘上方 2cm 处，端口应相距约 8cm。可根据需要放置一个 5mm 的辅助端口（图片由 Melissa Kaufman MD MPH 提供）

个断端吻合。用 3–0 Vicryl 缝合线使肠系膜窗贴近关闭，缝合针从回肠扩大段的末端移除并去管（可借助抽吸装置引导切口方向），并用 3–0 Vicryl 缝合线缝合成 U 形（或优选构形）。（注：这部分可以通过延长脐孔切口在体外进行）。

(4) 回肠 – 膀胱吻合的方式与开腹手术相似。首先进行后壁吻合，再向前缝合至膀胱颈，U 型肌的顶端应位于膀胱颈的前方，这可以用 2–0 Vicryl 缝合线单层全层封闭完成，必要时进行灌水和加固试验。

(5) 除耻骨上导尿管和尿道导尿管外，还保留有腹腔引流管。在患者出院前拔除腹腔引流管和尿道导尿管，3 周后行膀胱造影术，如果未发现并发症 / 漏尿，则拔除耻骨上导尿管[34, 35]。

扩大的膀胱自发穿孔是一种严重的风险，其发生率高达 13%，被认为是继发于慢性或急性过度膨胀，以及随后的肠壁缺血坏死[36-41]。临床患者常见于长期让膀胱过度膨胀，或者在酒精影响下膀胱过度充盈并自发破裂。

对疑似穿孔的评估应包括计算机断层扫描（CT）和采用导尿管导尿的保守治疗、静脉注射抗生素或手术探查及修复的治疗。Lee 等已经提出了一种管理算法，但由于存在败血症的风险，建议降低手术探查指征[42]，应就这种风险向患者提出建议，并鼓励患者维持常规的导尿计划。

六、跟进

因非神经源性适应证而接受膀胱扩大成形术的患者需要对肠或膀胱吻合口破裂、瘘管和功能延迟恢复进行类似的短期监测，以及对肾功能的长期监测和对恶性肿瘤的常规筛查。这包括定期电解质、全血细胞计数、尿液分析、B12 和定期超声成像。电解质紊乱和结石疾病的随访不在本章讨论范围内，但需要进行常规监测。肠置入患者，以及进行间歇性清洁自我导尿的患者被认为患恶性肿瘤的风险增加，应在该患者群体中评估有无血尿，如果没有，则不应将其视为感染迹象。

七、膀胱扩大术后妊娠

多个病例报道描述了膀胱扩大术后的无并发症妊娠[43]。肾盂肾炎的风险约为 15%，而无症状菌尿且下尿路正常孕妇的发病率为 20%～40%[44]。目前的实践模式要求在妊娠期治疗渐进性菌尿，并可放宽预防性抗生素用于可能有慢性定植的肠管膀胱吻合。与回肠导管（23%）相比，由于妊娠子宫的外部压迫导致排尿障碍相对少见（4%），通常是由于左侧输尿管压迫至骶骨所致[45]。剖宫产率为 27%，与一般人群相似，通常有产科适应证。膀胱扩大成形术的患者不会增加尿失禁的风险。值得注意的例外包括那些进行膀胱颈重建或人工尿道括约肌的患者，在这种情况下需要剖宫产。剖宫产的手术方法必须考虑覆盖子宫的肠系膜的位置，通常横向移位，并且可能粘连。尽管已有在膀胱扩大后进行子宫下段剖宫产无并发症的描述[46]，但为了避免损伤血管供应，首选高位子宫切口。

总结

膀胱扩大成形术可用于影响膀胱容量和顺应性的非神经源性疾病，尽管通常是在其他风险较低的选择已经用尽之后。回肠是最常用的肠段，手术方法类似于神经源性疾病。由于代谢异常、结石形成和膀胱穿孔的风险，需要长期随访。

参考文献

[1] Lightner DJ, Gomelsky A, Souter L, et al. Diagnosis and treatment of overactive bladder (non-neurogenic) in adults: AUA/SUFU guideline amendment 2019. J Urol. 2019;202:5.
[2] Kayigil Ö, Atahan Ö, Metin A. Experiences with clam ileocystoplasty. Int Urol Nephrol. 1998;30(1):45–8.
[3] Andersen AV, Granlund P, Schultz A, Talseth T, Hedlund H, Frich L. Long-term experience with surgical treatment of selected patients with bladder pain syndrome/interstitial cystitis. Scand J Urol Nephrol. 2012;46(4):284–9.
[4] El-Azab AS, Moeen AM. The satisfaction of patients with refractory idiopathic overactive bladder with onabotulinumtoxinA and augmentation cystoplasty. Arab J Urol. 2013;11(4):344–9.
[5] Mishra NN. Clinical presentation and treatment of bladder pain syndrome/interstitial cystitis (BPS/IC) in India. Transl Androl Urol. 2015;4(5):512–23. https://doi.org/10.3978/j. issn.2223-4683.2015.10.05.
[6] Sood A, Eilender B, Wong P, Atiemo H. Outcomes in patients with idiopathic overactive bladder undergoing augmentation cystoplasty in the era of onabotulinumtoxin-A and interstim. Neurourol Urodyn. 2019;38:S238–9.
[7] Barrington JW, Dyer R, Bano F. Bladder augmentation using Pelvicol implant for intractable overactive bladder syndrome. Int Urogynecol J Pelvic Floor Dysfunct. 2006;17(1):50–3.
[8] Hanno PM, Erickson D, Moldwin R, et al. Diagnosis and treatment of interstitial cystitis/bladder pain syndrome: AUA guideline amendment. J Urol. 2015;193:1545.
[9] Nurse DE, Parry JRW, Mundy AR. Problems in the surgical treatment of interstitial cystitis. Br J Urol. 1991;68(2):153–4.
[10] Zhang GK, Sidi AA, Reddy PK. Treatment of interstitial cystitis with augmentation cystoplasty. Neurourol Urodyn. 1990;9(2):222–3.
[11] Downey AP, Osman NI, Park JJ, et al. Contemporary outcomes of surgery for bladder pain syndrome/interstitial cystitis. Neurourol Urodyn. 2018;37:S357.
[12] Tabakov ID, Slavchev BN. Large post-hysterectomy and post-radiation vesicovaginal fistulas: repair by ileocystoplasty. J Urol. 2004;171:272–4.
[13] Hsu TH, Rackley RR, Abdelmalak JB, Madjar S, Vasavada SP. Novel technique for combined repair of postirradiation vesicovaginal fistula and augmentation ileocystoplasty. Urology. 2002;59:597–9.
[14] Miyamoto S, Takushima A, Harii K, Shimoi H, Nutahara K. Ileal patch graft used to repair a bladder injured during repair of an abdominal wall hernia. J Plast Surg Hand Surg. 2010;44(1):66–8.
[15] Glazier DB, Whang MIS, Geffner SR, et al. Evaluation of voiding cystourethrography prior to renal transplantation. Transplantation. 1996;62(12):1762–5.
[16] Theodorou C, Katsifotis C, Bocos J, Moutzouris G, Stournaras P, Kostakis A. Urodynamics prior to renal transplantation-its impact on treatment decision and final results. Scand J Urol Nephrol. 2003;37(4):335–8.
[17] Power RE, O'Malley KJ, Khan MS, Murphy DM, Hickey DP. Renal transplantation in patients with an augmentation cystoplasty. BJU Int. 2000;86(1):28–31.
[18] Martín MG, Castro SN, Castelo LA, Abal VC, Rodríguez JS, Novo JD. Enterocystoplasty and renal transplantation. J Urol. 2001;165(2): 393–6.
[19] Van Ophoven A, Oberpenning F, Hertle L. Long-term results of trigone-preserving orthotopic substitution enterocystoplasty for interstitial cystitis. J Urol. 2002;167(2 I):603–7.
[20] Slagt IK, Ijzermans JN, Alamyar M, et al. Long-term outcome of kidney transplantation in patients with a urinary conduit: a case-control study. Int Urol Nephrol. 2013;45(2):405–11.
[21] Pazik J, Wazna E, Lewandowski Z, et al. Factors predisposing to urinary tract infections in adult kidney allograft recipients with lower urinary tract reconstruction. Transplant Proc. 2009;41(8):3039–42.
[22] Barnett MG, Bruskewitz RC, Belzer FO, Sollinger HW, Uehling DT. Ileocecocystoplasty bladder augmentation and renal transplantation. J Urol. 1987;138(4):855–8.
[23] Milutinovic D, Topuzovic C, Hadzi-Djokic J. Clam ileoplasty bladder augmentation and renal transplantation. Acta Chir Iugosl. 2007;54(4):79–81.
[24] Garat JM, Caffaratti J, Angerri O, Bujons A, Villavicencio H. Kidney transplants in patients with bladder augmentation: correlation and evolution. Int Urol Nephrol. 2009;41(1):1–5.
[25] Singh V, Sinha RJ, Sankhwar SN, Sinha SM. Reconstructive surgery for tuberculous contracted bladder: experience of a center in northern India. Int Urol Nephrol. 2011;43(2):423–30.
[26] de Figueiredo AA, Lucon AM, Srougi M. Bladder augmentation for

the treatment of chronic tuberculous cystitis. Clinical and urodynamic evaluation of 25 patients after long term follow- up. Neurourol Urodyn. 2006;25(5):433–40.
[27] Yee CH, Chiu PKF, Chan YS, et al. Robotic augmentation cystoplasty for contracted bladder secondary to cystitis: a 1-year outcome assessment. J Urol. 2020;203:e1017–8.
[28] Morrison CD, Kielb SJ. Use of bowel in reconstructive urology: what a colorectal surgeon should know. Clin Colon Rectal Surg. 2017;30(3):207–14.
[29] Singh O, Gupta SS, Arvind NK. A case of extensive genitourinary tuberculosis: combined augmentation ileo-cystoplasty, ureteric ileal replacement and buccal mucosal graft urethroplasty. Updat Surg. 2013;65(3):245–8.
[30] Partin AW, Dmochowski RR, Kavoussi LR, Peters C, editors. Campbell-Walsh-Wein urology/ editor-in-chief, Alan W. Partin; editors, Roger R. Dmochowski, Louis R. Kavoussi, Craig A. Peters. 12th ed. Philadelphia: Elsevier; 2020.
[31] Montague DK, Gill I, Ross J, Angermeier KW, editors. Textbook of reconstructive urologic surgery. 1st ed. CRC Press; 2008.
[32] Gundeti MS, Eng MK, Reynolds WS, Zagaja GP. Pediatric robotic-assisted laparoscopic augmentation ileocystoplasty and mitrofanoff appendicovesicostomy: complete intracorporeal— initial case report. Urology. 2008;72(5):1144–7.
[33] Passerotti CC, Nguyen HT, Lais A, Dunning P, Harrell B, Estrada C, et al. Robot-assisted laparoscopic ileal bladder augmentation: defining techniques and potential pitfalls. J Endourol. 2008;22(2):355–60.
[34] Dogra P, Regmi S, Singh P, Bora G, Saini A, Aggarwal S. Robot-assisted laparoscopic augmentation ileocystoplasty in a tubercular bladder. Urol Ann. 2014;6(2):152–5.
[35] Grilo N, Chartier-Kastler E, Grande P, Crettenand F, Parra J, Phé V. Robot-assisted supratrigonal cystectomy and augmentation cystoplasty with totally intracorporeal reconstruction in neurourological patients: technique description and preliminary results. Eur Urol. 2021;79(6):858–65.
[36] Metcalfe PD, Casale AJ, Kaefer MA, Misseri R, Dussinger AM, Meldrum KK, et al. Spontaneous bladder perforations: a report of 500 augmentations in children and analysis of risk. J Urol. 2006;175:1466–70; discussion 1470–1.
[37] DeFoor W, Tackett L, Minevich E, Wacksman J, Sheldon C. Risk factors for spontaneous bladder perforation after augmentation cystoplasty. Urology. 2003;62:737–41.
[38] Bertschy C, Bawab F, Liard A, Valioulis I, Mitrofanoff P. Enterocystoplasty complications in children. A study of 30 cases. Eur J Pediatr Surg. 2000;10:30–4.
[39] Shekarriz B, Upadhyay J, Demirbilek S, Barthold JS, González R. Surgical complications of bladder augmentation: comparison between various enterocystoplasties in 133 patients. Urology. 2000;55:123–8.
[40] Krishna A, Gough DC, Fishwick J, Bruce J. Ileocystoplasty in children: assessing safety and success. Eur Urol. 1995;27:62–6.
[41] Rushton HG, Woodard JR, Parrott TS, Jeffs RD, Gearhart JP. Delayed bladder rupture after augmentation enterocystoplasty. J Urol. 1988;140:344–6.
[42] Lee T, Kozminski DJ, Bloom DA, Wan J, Park JM. Bladder perforation after augmentation cystoplasty: determining the best management option. J Pediatr Urol. 2017;13(3):274.e1–7.
[43] Norris JP, Wheeler JS, Norris DM, Rubenstein MA. Augmentation cystoplasty and ileal conduits in pregnancy. Int Urogynecol J. 1995;6(1):37–40.
[44] Krieger JN. Complications and treatment of urinary tract infections during pregnancy. Urol Clin North Am. 1986;13(4):685–93.
[45] Hill DE, Chantigian PM, Kramer SA. Pregnancy after augmentation cystoplasty. Surg Gynecol Obstet. 1990;170(6):485–7.
[46] Shaikh A, Ahsan S, Zaidi Z. Pregnancy after augmentation cystoplasty. J Pak Med Assoc. 2006;56(10):465–7.

第 13 章　难治急迫性尿失禁的最新治疗方法

Advanced Options for Treatment of Refractory Urgency Urinary Incontinence

Elizabeth Rourke　Alice Wang　Melissa Kaufman　著

一、耻骨上造瘘：适应证和方法

耻骨上造瘘被认为是处理膀胱异常充盈或压力性尿失禁患者的紧急替代方法[3]。然而，在急迫性尿失禁（UUI）三线治疗失败后，也可以考虑放置耻骨上造瘘管。通常经内镜或外科手术于脐下放置耻骨上造瘘管不仅可以避免留置导尿管造成的炎症，且更易护理，舒适性更佳。尽管耻骨上造瘘管的放置可以充分排空膀胱并改善尿失禁，但膀胱过度活动仍可能存在。耻骨上造瘘管最常与药物治疗和（或）肉毒杆菌毒素结合使用，如果女性有严重的压力性尿失禁，则尿道未闭，可能不会导致尿失禁。

（一）经皮耻骨上造瘘管置入

对于尿道梗阻需膀胱引流者，首选经皮局麻耻骨上造瘘管置入术。术前须对患者既往手术史评估，以防止既往腹腔手术所致腹膜破裂后肠道移位至耻骨后间隙。可以用床旁超声来观察术中导尿管及肠襻位置关系。如果超声无法清楚显示上述位置关系，则应终止操作，考虑其他替代方式。CT 引导下放置引流管目前也是临床手术中一种常用的选择。围术期需用抗生素来预防皮肤及泌尿生殖系统的细菌感染。沿腹中线耻骨联合上方约 2 指宽部位行皮肤深、浅局部麻醉。用 20 号的腰穿针沿此点穿过皮肤进入膀胱。为避免肠管干扰，膀胱应充分充盈，穿刺针应水平成 75°，向下穿刺直到抽到尿液。然后在先前标记的腹中线水平耻骨联合上方 2 指宽穿刺点处做 1cm 横切口。固定穿刺针方向及深度，沿套管针方向，使用扩张鞘依次扩张。然后取出穿刺管针，将扩张鞘固定在原位。选择合适的导管穿过扩张鞘套管，用无菌水注射气囊固定，最后将扩张鞘外套从导尿管剥离[4]。

（二）内镜耻骨上造瘘管置入

对于内镜逆行膀胱切开耻骨上造瘘管置入术，常用 Lowsley 拉钩[5]。如果患者尿道通畅，且没有下腹部手术史，这种手术方式更可取。由于女性尿道较短，这种技术在女性中通常更简单。获得患者知情同意后，在术前适当给予抗生素。虽然这种手术是内镜下进行的，但通常使用全身麻醉。无论男性还是女性，首选截石位，以便拉钩。Lowsley 拉钩经尿道进入膀胱，指向耻骨联合上方约 2cm 处的前腹壁。可借助膀胱镜来精准定位穿刺针。拉钩需固定牢固，防止尿道外伤。在耻骨上定位点处沿皮肤、皮下组织和腹直肌筋膜电切一小切口，直到内镜可见。然后将合适型号造瘘管通过不可吸收缝合线（通常是尼龙线或丝线）与 Lowsley 拉钩固定。然后将拉钩从膀胱内经尿道拉出。后拆除缝合线，将造瘘管移回膀胱壁，充气固定球囊。Lowsley 拉钩直视放置可避免导管放置在膀胱外，并有助于避免经皮耻骨上造瘘管置入时可能发生的腹腔脏器的潜在损伤[6]。

（三）外科手术放置耻骨上造瘘管

外科手术放置耻骨上造瘘管置入适用于既往有腹部手术史肠管损伤风险高的患者，以及尿道断裂、严重尿道狭窄、创伤[7]致尿道无法进入的患者。患者知情同意后，手术在全身麻醉下进行。术前应根据医院和指南要求使用抗生素。下腹和生殖器使用碘伏或氯己定消毒。最佳体位为背侧截石位，也可以采用仰卧位。此外，也可以取Trendelenburg位，以帮助排便远离膀胱。使用电刀自耻骨联合沿中线做一个4～5cm小垂直切口。分离皮下脂肪和腹前壁下部浅筋膜和深筋膜显露腹直肌筋膜，水平或垂直切开腹直肌筋膜。剥离腹直肌，显露出下方的腹横筋膜及膀胱。理想情况下，膀胱应该是充盈的，此时可以使用腰穿针连接注射器抽取尿液确认。确认无误后在膀胱中线两侧用3-0可吸收缝合线垂直缝合固定。膀胱可以用Allis钳固定。为避免导管在切口内闭合，可在切口外侧单独切开形成一个独立切口，将导管穿过独立的导管切口通道。使用电刀或手术刀做小膀胱切开术。然后将导管直接插入膀胱小切口注射无菌水固定导管球囊并拉紧，使气球悬浮在膀胱腔内，而不是靠在三角区或膀胱颈上。然后在导管插入口周围用3-0可吸收缝合线荷包缝合膀胱切口。围绕导管逐层关闭筋膜、皮下组织和皮肤，最后导管用丝线或尼龙线缝合固定。应至少6周后首次置换导管，以便瘘管成形良好，建议早期由泌尿外科医生更换导管，后期由护理人员或患者更换导管。

二、膀胱颈闭合术适应证和方法

当其他手术治疗压力性尿失禁无效时，通常可以选择膀胱出口闭合术。顽固性尿失禁最常见的原因是导尿管引起的尿道糜烂、严重的压力性尿失禁、膀胱颈功能不全或困难尿道等情况[8]。虽然膀胱颈闭合术的成功率通常很高，但它被认为是一种永久性和不可逆的手术，并伴有罕见的急性并发症（如膀胱穿孔）[9]。

膀胱颈闭合的术式有多种，包括经阴道、经尿道和经腹（耻骨后），也可能需要几种术式结合。值得注意的是，膀胱颈闭合术的成功需要通过耻骨上造瘘管、回肠膀胱造口术或带导尿口的扩大膀胱成形术来形成低压导尿。在一项回顾性研究中，经阴道和经腹部膀胱颈闭合的术式尿控效果在统计学上相似。经阴道膀胱颈闭合术具有手术时间短、住院时间少和短期并发症更少的特点[10]。对于具体术式的选择应取决于患者个人态度、身体功能状态和家庭经济情况[11]。

（一）经阴道术式

与经尿道入路手术一样，经阴道入路可避免进腹腔。患者建议取膀胱截石位，经阴道膀胱颈闭合术前耻骨上造瘘管或其他尿路改道已形成。使用缝线悬吊双侧阴唇或固定阴式拉钩显露术野。阴道壁注射生理盐水或稀释利多卡因、肾上腺素来分离膀胱阴道间隙。用15号手术刀在阴道前壁做一个宽的倒U形切口。U形顶端起始于近尿道口处并向阴道穹窿方向延伸切开（图13-1A）。阴道前壁可以通过Allis钳和手术剪刀配合分离，分离显露耻骨颈筋膜的正确平面应呈亮白色，出血少。围绕尿道牵拉分离阴道壁，阴道壁分离的顶端是U形切口顶点。此时尿道全长在膀胱颈部位可被完全解剖显露显现（图13-1B）。用剪刀或止血钳充分分离盆腔内筋膜，使膀胱颈脱离耻骨尿道韧带。在膀胱颈水平离断尿道，自黏膜层开始分层缝合，最后缝合膀胱周围筋膜加固，并做水密性试验加以确认（图13-1C）。封闭膀胱颈并于耻骨固定抬高膀胱颈是封闭瘘管形成的首选方法。借助大阴唇脂肪垫转瓣覆盖创面（图13-1D）。最后，用2-0可吸收缝合线将U型阴道皮瓣缝合至创面，并将涂有雌激素乳膏的阴道填充物置于阴道内24h以协助止血[12, 13]。

（二）经尿道术式

与经阴道术式类似，在闭合膀胱颈手术前，必须已行充分膀胱造瘘引流。患者取头低足高截石位。使用缝线悬吊双侧阴唇或固定阴式拉钩显露术野。用15号刀片在尿道周围做一个椭圆形切口，切口需深达阴道黏膜层。将尿道自阴道至膀胱颈充分分离并用组织剪刀撑开分离盆内筋膜，此时，整个尿道和膀胱颈分离至游离状态。离断

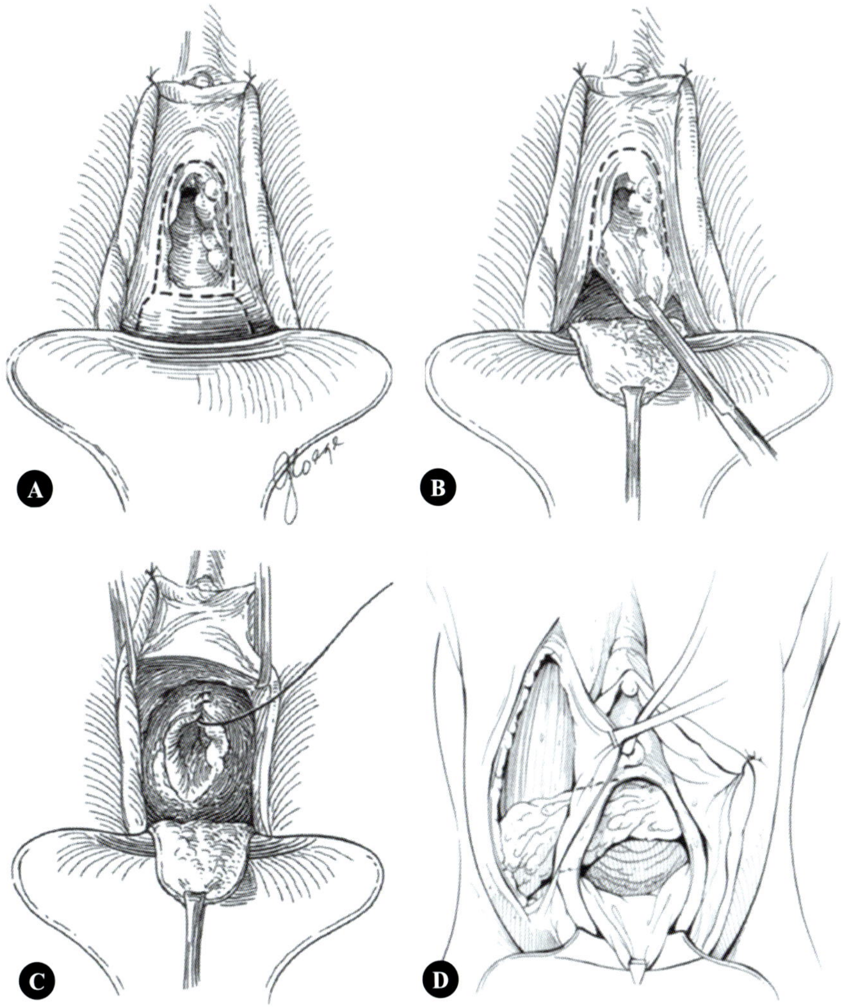

◀ 图 13-1　经阴道膀胱颈闭合术

A. 经阴道做倒 U 形切口；B. 沿膀胱颈外侧分离切开阴道前壁；C. 缝合封闭膀胱颈，第二层对端水平缝合；封闭膀胱颈并于耻骨固定抬高膀胱颈；D. 大阴唇脂肪垫转瓣覆盖创面，提供额外的组织层以防止瘘管形成［（A 至 C）引自 Raz S. Female Urology, 2nd ed. Philadelphia: WB Saunders, 1996. Copyright 1996, with permission from Springer; reprinted in Zimmern P. Vaginal Surgery for Incontinence and Prolapse.（D）引自 Graham SD. Glenn's Urologic Surgery. Philadelphia: Lippincott-Raven, 1998 reprinted in Zimmern P. Vaginal Surgery for Incontinence and Prolapse with permission from Springer）］[14]

远端尿道，然后用 2–0 可吸收缝合线沿尿道断端周围水平褥式荷包缝合，使剩余的尿道倒转膀胱内。此后用 200～300ml 液体灌注膀胱检查缝合水密性[14, 15]。

（三）经腹入路

在经腹入路中，通过膀胱切开术达到膀胱引流目的。患者取低位截石位。腹部和阴道要做好消毒准备。留置 Foley 导尿管。做一个低位横切口。进入腹部后，仔细解剖耻骨后间隙，进入盆内筋膜，用零号可吸收缝线结扎背静脉复合体。尽量充分分离尿道至游离状态后结扎或电灼封闭耻骨尿道韧带。偏远心端横断尿道背侧，一旦 Foley 导尿管显露出来，便向上牵拉导尿管牵引膀胱颈，横切腹侧尿道后分两层闭合尿道。然后沿膀胱颈方向切开膀胱。通过术前静脉注射亚甲蓝或留置输尿管支架管来观察双侧输尿管开口。膀胱颈和膀胱需从膀胱阴道间隙分离充分，后从尿道近端横断膀胱颈。此时可选择耻骨上造瘘管或建立膀胱造瘘管术式。膀胱颈分两层缝合，黏膜层需荷包内翻缝合。膀胱灌注 200～300ml 液体检查水密性。腹膜或网膜可用于覆盖创面以防止瘘管形成。关腹前留置腹腔引流管[14, 15]。

三、尿流改道：适应证和方法

单纯膀胱切除 + 尿道重建

回肠尿流改道（两支输尿管均吻合到一段孤立的回肠，再从前腹壁造口），此种永久性改道术最早由 Bricker 在 20 世纪 50 年代提出并广泛使用至今。难治性膀胱过度活动症 / 急迫性尿失禁患者建议手术治疗，对于某些无法通过尿道或其他通道导尿的患者，应建议行单纯膀胱切除术和尿流改道术，此术式有效性好且应用广泛。由于造瘘口是患者痛苦的重要来源，因此术前造瘘口管理培训，包括更换造瘘袋、造瘘口外形和瘘口皮肤护理等是必需的。考虑到膀胱功能丧失后存在炎症，因此在此手术中膀胱应被切除。既往有膀胱癌病史应行膀胱癌根治的患者禁用。

与膀胱成形术一样，回肠末端因为具有可移动、管径小和血液供应稳定的特点，所以是尿流改道的首选部位。但在某些情况下，肠系膜的牵拉可能会阻止回肠移动出骨盆深处，此时结肠可能是首选。此外，对于有放疗史或既往肠外科手术可能导致回肠大量丢失的患者，可以使用升结肠、横结肠和降结肠。如果使用回肠手术，可导致维生素 B_{12} 吸收不足，故建议在术后 5 年内监测维生素 B_{12} 水平[15, 16]。

单纯膀胱切除术与回肠尿流改道术

(1) 患者取仰卧位（女性取截石位，以便术中操作）（注：考虑术前放置输尿管支架管，以方便术中输尿管识别 / 游离）。术野消毒，留置 Foley 导管。沿脐下中线做切口，如需扩大显露，延至脐以上。

(2) 进腹仔细探查肠道，以确保肠段可被游离。距回盲部 15cm 长末端回肠，短丝线标记末端，（长度适于标识皮肤 / 造瘘口），然后测量 15cm 长回肠用长缝线末端。在输尿管和膀胱切除术后，此段肠管用于形成回肠尿道部。

(3) 左输尿管跨过髂血管，向内侧乙状结肠方向走行。打开腹膜，直角血管钳自肾脏近端至膀胱水平保留输尿管血供并充分游离输尿管（注：输尿管外膜破坏 / 血供受损可增加输尿管肠管吻合口狭窄的风险）。使用外科手术夹在输尿管近膀胱壁入口处夹闭，离断尿管。用 4–0 Vicryl 缝合线在输尿管黏膜 12 点钟方向标记，以便输尿管肠管吻合。右侧输尿管重复同样的手术操作步骤。然而，右侧输尿管因距离回盲部游离肠管侧更近，所以仅需较少游离（注：若术前留置输尿管支架管，则必须夹闭离断输尿管前将其取出）。左输尿管穿过乙状结肠系膜后腹膜间隙，延伸至右侧。

(4) 离断输尿管后，行膀胱切除术。分离耻骨后间隙，分别从两侧腹膜、前筋膜游离膀胱。术前可适量生理盐水灌注充盈膀胱，可有助于游离膀胱。解剖分离膀胱颈或膀胱三角区时可借助缝合线或 Allis 钳适当牵拉协助。膀胱深层游离离断，可使用高频电刀或双极电凝，此时必须避免损伤膀胱后组织（女性的阴道和男性的精囊、直肠）。离断后尿道电凝断端并用 0 号 Vicryl 缝合线封闭膀胱颈。

(5) 选定之前标记的回肠段。牵拉显露肠系膜行透光照射，以确定血管分布走行后用电刀在肠系膜上无血管区建立 2 个开口。在 2 个开口之间放置离断器，离断肠系膜（肠襻）。如有肠系膜出血，应用 3–0 缝合线结扎止血。使用肠管吻合器去管化并重新构造为储尿器（肠管近端、远端折叠吻合，缝合线加固吻合面浆肌层）。盆腔内将去管重塑储尿器与双侧输尿管吻合。

(6) 行回肠肠管侧侧吻合术（也可选端端吻合）。吻合前两个肠襻间可以用 3–0 Vicryl 可吸收缝合线固定（在吻合完成后拆除）。切除肠管近端或远端肠管一角，以便容纳 GIA-75 吻合器。在激发吻合器钉枪之前，务必确认 2 个肠管背肠系膜侧彼此相对。回肠造口术可以避免折叠对缝肠管（使用 Allis 钳或 3–0 Vicryl 缝合线协助完成），选取肠管用 TA 60/90 吻合器切割，用组织剪刀剪去多余组织。沿钉针边缘用 3–0 Vicryl 缝合线加固浆肌层。用 3–0 丝线或 Vicryl 缝合线关闭肠系膜边缘。

(7) 左侧输尿管经乙状结肠肠系膜贯通至右侧盆腔。输尿管肠管吻合术首先要确保两个输尿管走行无扭曲且吻合后无张力。牵拉标记线找到远端肠管，使用爪形肠钳（Babcock clamp）牵拉固定肠管至合适的位置进行输尿管肠管吻合。在肠管合适位置使用电刀 / 手术刀将浆膜层黏膜层切开。用 4–0 线外翻缝合肠黏膜边缘以便于与输尿管吻合。输尿管可以使用组织剪刀按肌腱手术游离。输尿管肠管吻合可根据外科医生的偏好，采用 4–0 Monocryl 缝合线（或任何无编织合成可吸收缝合线）间断或连续缝合。吻合时从输尿管端由外向内进针，肠管由内向外进针，吻合前输尿管置入装有金属丝的单 J 型支架。右侧输尿管吻合口位置选取肠管远端。

(8) 皮肤造口电灼法圆形切开皮肤，逐层穿过皮下组织直达筋膜。使用齿前 Kocher 钳牵拉筋膜以防止闭合过程中的收缩。清除筋膜上的任何皮下脂肪，在前直肌筋膜上做十字切口，切开腹直肌，切开腹直肌后鞘和腹膜。切口应取 2 指宽度，宽度以便肠管轻松通过筋膜。爪形肠钳钳取肠管（Babcock）穿过筋膜切口拉直皮肤切口。务必确保肠管及肠系膜不扭曲且无张力。筋膜层、浆膜肌层、真皮层均选取 4 个点用 2–0 Vicryl 缝合线玫瑰花蕾式固定。肠管外露造瘘口需外翻用 3–0 Vicryl 缝合线固定。

(9) 放置腹腔引流管预防输尿管肠管吻合口瘘，并可在出院前取出。输尿管支架可在术后 4～6 周内取出[15, 16]。

注意：使用结肠段时，造口位置可在右侧或左侧。对于已经有结肠造口、回肠造口的患者，可以首选右侧结肠导管以优化术后造瘘袋问题。

总结

严重的急迫性尿失禁 / 膀胱过度活动可对患者的整体生活质量产生深远影响，应逐步进行治疗（图 13–2）。对于非侵入性治疗（如抗胆碱能

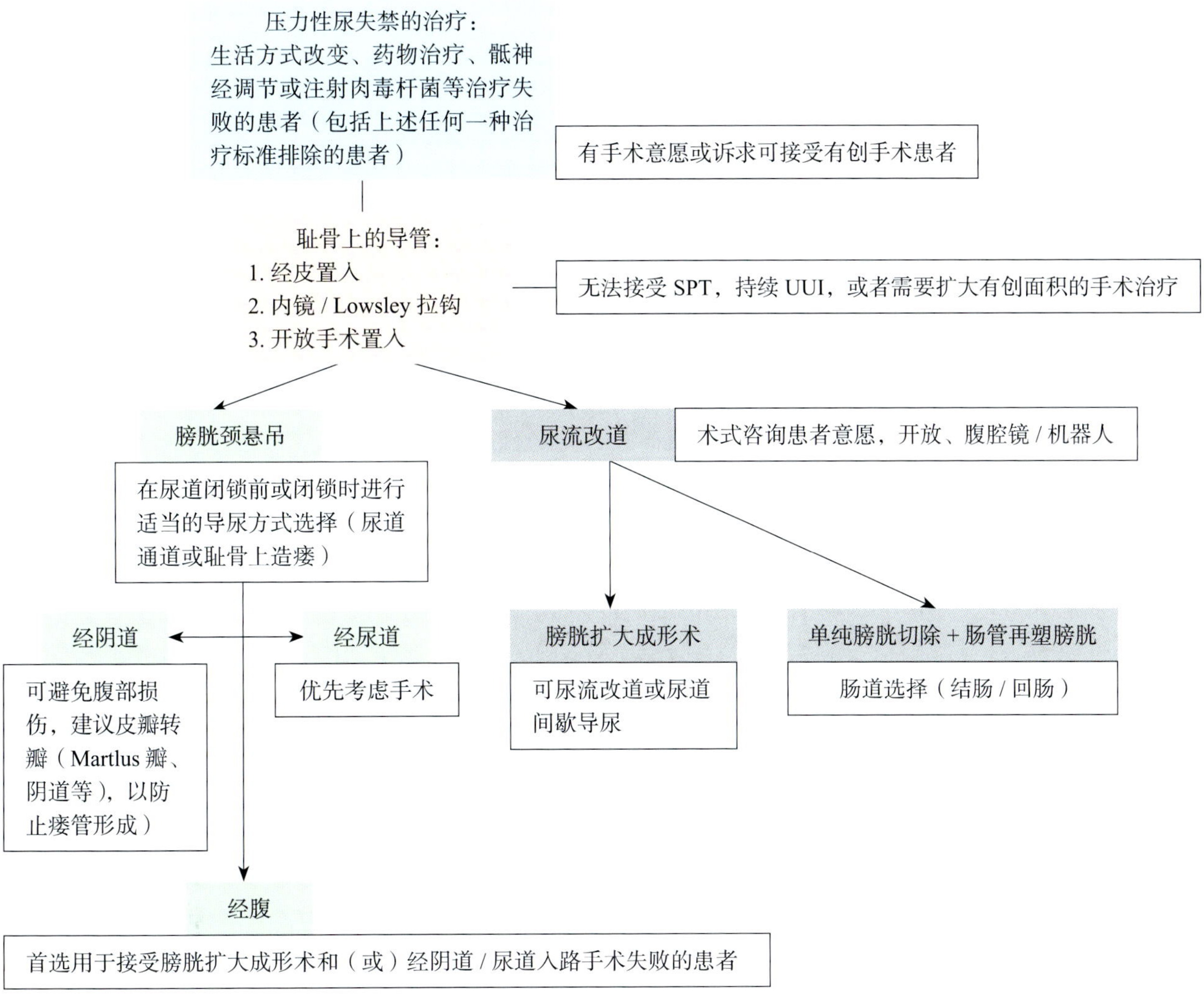

▲ 图 13–2 难治性急尿失禁的治疗算法

SPT. 耻骨上膀胱造瘘；UUI. 急迫性尿失禁

药、β_3受体激动药、膀胱内注射肉毒杆菌毒素或骶神经调节）失败的患者，都可以选择有创手术治疗。术前需详细沟通咨询，以便让患者充分了解可选方案、并发症以及术后日常生活方式改变等。此外，也可多种方式的组合来优化生活质量，其中包括耻骨上造瘘（使用或不使用膀胱内肉毒杆菌）和膀胱颈闭合尿流改道术（耻骨上造瘘、尿流改道）。在极端情况下，应考虑永久的尿流改道方案，包括保留或不保留尿道的膀胱成形术和尿改道。手术方法选择（开腹、腹腔镜/机器人）应由手术医生结合自身技能选择决定。

参考文献

[1] Abrams P, Cardozo L, Fall M, Griffiths D, Rosier P, Ulmsten U, et al. The standardisation of terminology of lower urinary tract function: report from the standardisation sub-committee of the International Continence Society. Neurourol Urodyn. 2002;21(2):167–78.
[2] Lightner DJ, Gomelsky A, Souter L, Vasavada SP. Diagnosis and treatment of overactive bladder (non-neurogenic) in adults: AUA/SUFU guideline amendment 2019. J Urol. 2019;202(3):101097JU0000000000000309–563.
[3] MacLachlan LS, Rovner ES. New treatments for incontinence. Adv Chronic Kidney Dis. 2015;22(4):279–88.
[4] Jr HF. Suprapubic catheterization. In: Hinman, editor. Atlas of urologic surgery. Philadelphia, Pennsylvania: Saunders; 1998. p. 625–9.
[5] Wyner LM. Easy suprapubic tube placement using a Van Buren sound. Urology. 2018;114:245.
[6] Zeidman EJC. Humberto; Alarcon, Antonio; Raz, Shlomo. Suprapubic cystotomy using lowsley retractor. Urology. 1988;32(1):54–5.
[7] Wolter CD, Roger. Suprapubic catheterization. In: Hashim H, AP, Dmochowski R, editors. . London: Springer; 2008. p. 128–31.
[8] Boone TB, Stewart JN, Martinez LM. Additional therapies for storage and emptying failure. In: Wein AJ, Kavoussi LR, Campbell MF, editors. Campbell-Walsh-Wein urology. 12th ed. Philadelphia: Elsevier Saunders; 2012. p. 2889–904.
[9] Ardelt PU, Woodhouse CR, Riedmiller H, Gerharz EW. The efferent segment in continent cutaneous urinary diversion: a comprehensive review of the literature. BJU Int. 2012;109(2):288–97.
[10] Willis H, Safiano NA, Lloyd LK. Comparison of transvaginal and retropubic bladder neck closure with suprapubic catheter in women. J Urol. 2015;193(1):196–202.
[11] Colli J, Lloyd LK. Bladder neck closure and suprapubic catheter placement as definitive management of neurogenic bladder. J Spinal Cord Med. 2011;34(3):273–7.
[12] Rovner ES, Goudelocke CM, Gilchrist A, Lebed B. Transvaginal bladder neck closure with posterior urethral flap for devastated urethra. Urology. 2011;78(1):208–12.
[13] Zimmern PE, Hadley HR, Leach GE, Raz S. Transvaginal closure of the bladder neck and placement of a suprapubic catheter for destroyed urethra after long-term indwelling catheterization. J Urol. 1985;134(3):554–7.
[14] Zimmern PE, et al. In: Zimmern P, editor. Vaginal surgery for incontinence and prolapse [electronic resource]. London: Springer; 2006.
[15] Smith JA Jr, Howards SS, Preminger GM, Dmochowski RR, Smith JA, Howards SS, Preminger GM, Dmochowski RR, editors. Hinman's atlas of urologic surgery. 4th ed. Philadelphia: Elsevier; 2018.
[16] Dmochowski RR, Kavoussi LR, Peters CA. In: Partin AW, Partin AW, Dmochowski RR, Kavoussi LR, Peters C, editors. Campbell-Walsh-Wein urology. 12th ed. Philadelphia: Elsevier; 2020.

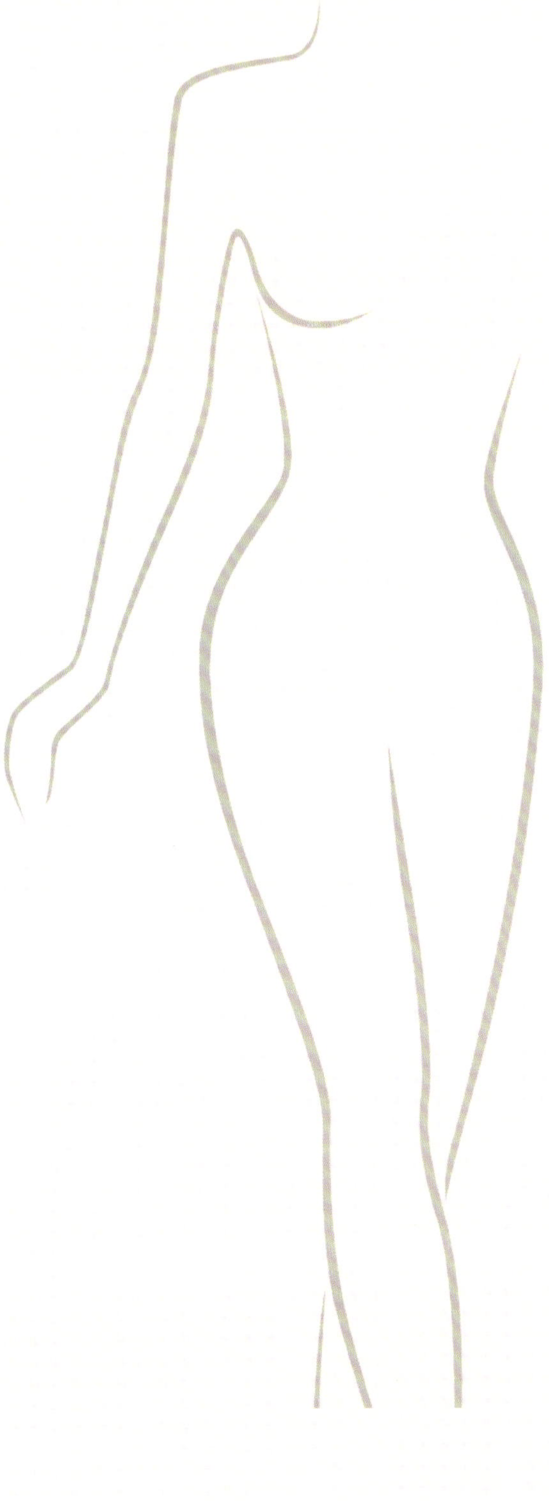

第四篇 女性压力性尿失禁的手术治疗

Surgical Treatment for SUI

第 14 章　尿道填充术
Urethral Bulking Agents

Alexandra L. Tabakin　Siobhan M. Hartigan　著

尿道填充术（UBA）是一种微创治疗方法，可用于治疗原发或其他抗尿失禁失败后的复发性尿失禁。尿道填充术在 20 世纪初首次被引入，并在成分、作用机制和传递方法方面不断发展。在这里，我们讨论了尿道填充术使用的适应证，注射的流程，以及传统和当代的尿道填充术。

一、作用方法

尿道填充术用于治疗尿道内括约肌功能障碍（ISD）患者的压力性尿失禁，该类患者的尿路闭合肌是减弱的。尿道填充术可经尿道或尿道周围组织注射，扩大局部道尿道近端的表面积，增加尿道压力[2]，从而改善尿道接合和尿道出口阻力，防止尿漏。注射尿道填充术也可增加功能性尿道长度[3]。

尿道填充术可以由生物材料或合成材料制成。生物材料的尿道填充术是由去掉细胞膜的自体、同源异体或异源体组织或异种组织制成[4]。合成的尿道填充术可分为颗粒和非颗粒。颗粒尿道填充术由悬浮在可吸收凝胶载体中的微球组成。随着时间的推移，凝胶被重新吸收，周围的宿主组织与剩余的颗粒整合，形成一个庞大的雾化胶囊。颗粒的直径必须至少为 80μm，以防止从注入[5, 6]的原始位置迁移。非颗粒尿道填充术是由均匀、不可吸收的凝胶产生的；对于这些药剂，体积是由薄的纤维网络形成的，这些网络将注入的凝胶固定在宿主组织上[5]。

虽然它们的组成在作用机制上存在显著的差异，但理想的尿道填充术具有相似的关键特征。为了使尿道填充术成功地支持和增强尿道周围组织的重建，因此其应该具备易于注射、不可吸收、无毒和非免疫原性的特点。尿道填充术也应该是脱细胞的，非迁移的，并诱导轻微的磨损纤维化和钙化[7, 8]。

二、患者的选择和适应证

尿道填充术通常用于继发于括约肌功能障碍的压力性尿失禁患者，在尿流动力学方面其腹部薄弱点压力<60cmH_2O。理想的适应者也应缺乏尿道活动过度和特发性逼尿肌收缩[9]。尿道填充术已被证明在每天压力性尿失禁发作少于 2.5 次的女性和 60 岁及以上的女性中最为有效。在老年女性中，尿道填充术的有效性可能归因于较低的基线活动水平，以及通过增加括约肌肌节长度[10]来改善括约肌功能。

虽然尿道填充术在治疗尿道活动过度的压力性尿失禁方面的效果不如金标准的尿道中段悬吊术（MUS）有效，但其具备更有利的不良反应及适应证[11]。对于继发于较多基础疾病、年龄、严重肥胖或不能停止抗凝的患者，可以考虑尿道填充术。尿道填充术推荐用于将来有生育要求的育龄女性，及希望避免全麻手术但接受治愈率较低的女性[12]。尿道填充术也可用于轻度压力性尿失禁、膀胱排空不良的压力性尿失禁，或者压力性尿失禁持续存在[9, 12]，可作为其他抗尿失禁的辅助治疗。尿道填充术注射的禁忌证包括活动性尿路感染（UTI）或对填充剂[12]存在过敏反应。

三、手术方面和注射技术

尿道填充术可以在镇静或局部或全身麻醉下的门诊或手术室内进行注射[13]。注射时患者通常取仰卧截石位，充分显露生殖器并消毒铺无菌单。局部麻醉药或利多卡因可经尿道壁内沉积或在尿道黏膜下层注射。建议医师根据当地抗生素图谱和患者既往尿液培养结果[14]给予单剂量预防性抗生素。尿道填充剂应放置在膀胱颈附近的近端尿道黏膜中[15-17]。本章介绍了 3 种主要的注射方法。

（一）经尿道注射

经尿道注射包括通过膀胱镜的工作通道置入尿道填充剂（图 14–1A）。经尿道方法使临床医生能够直视下进行注射，并选择精确的置入位置。医生也可直视尿道吻合，减少潜在的填充剂使用量。为了获得最佳的吻合，应通过膀胱镜在 3 点钟、9 点钟或 6 点钟[18]方位进行注射。尿道旁弥散和近端尿道注射可获取较好的近期成功率[19]。

（二）尿道周围注射

尿道周围注射包括将尿道填充剂直接放置在尿道周围区域的尿道黏膜中（图 14–1B）。与经尿道法相比，尿道周围注射具有一定的好处（包括减少黏膜渗漏和出血的）[20]。然而，尿道周围注射具有更高的急性尿潴留风险。这可能是由于可视化技术无法应用，导致更大量的填充剂使用[20, 21]。

（三）设备引导注射

一些尿道填充剂需要通过特制的装置进行注射。硅胶粒（Macroplastique，MPQ）™ 置入系统包含一个放置在尿道到膀胱颈水平的注射装置，当尿液通过装置的中央通道时被识别（图 14–2A）。临床医生在远端抽出器械 1cm。然后通过置入装置在 2 点钟、6 点钟和 10 点钟方位[17]将注射针插入尿道黏膜。

水凝胶（Bulkamid）™ 是由它包含一个零度透镜和可视化光纤的输尿管镜进行注射（图 14–2B）。在 6 点钟方位，将一根特制的针插入黏膜下层 1cm。在 2 点钟和 10 点钟方位，或者 3 点钟、9 点钟和 12 点钟方位进行额外的注射。医生应在每次黏膜下注射后观察水泡的形成[15]。

类似地，液体硅橡胶弹性体组合物（Urolastic）™ 是通过一个包含放置在尿道中部的涂抹器的分配枪进行注射的。然后在 2 点钟、5 点钟、7 点钟和 10 点钟方位进行注射，以达到最佳的尿道吻合效果。如果在咳嗽测试后发生持续的渗漏，则可以在 3 点钟或 9 点钟方位放置额外的填充剂[16]。

（四）术后的建议和发现

医生应测量所有术后患者的残余尿量（PVR）[14]。残余尿量大于 100～150ml 的患者可能需要使用 10～12 号 Foley 导管进行单次导尿。建议使用较小的导管，以避免置换最近注射的填充剂。如

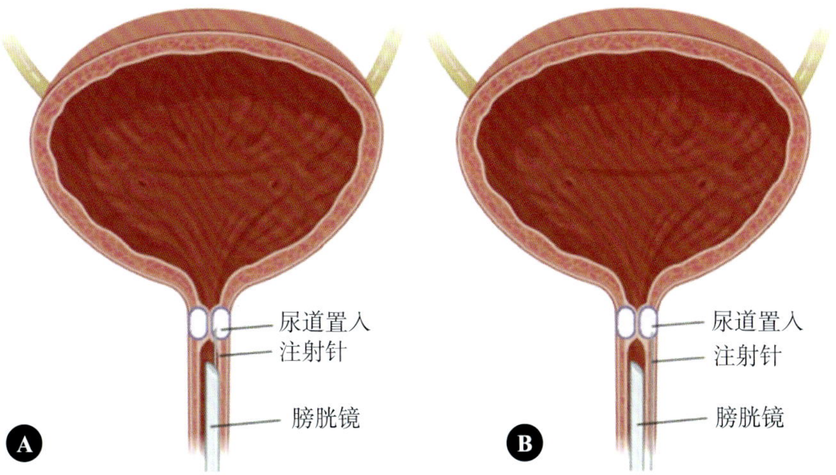

◀ 图 14–1　**A.** 经尿道注射技术，通过膀胱镜的工作通道推进尿道膨胀剂输送通道；**B.** 在尿道周围区域直接放置注射针进行尿道周围尿道填充术的技术

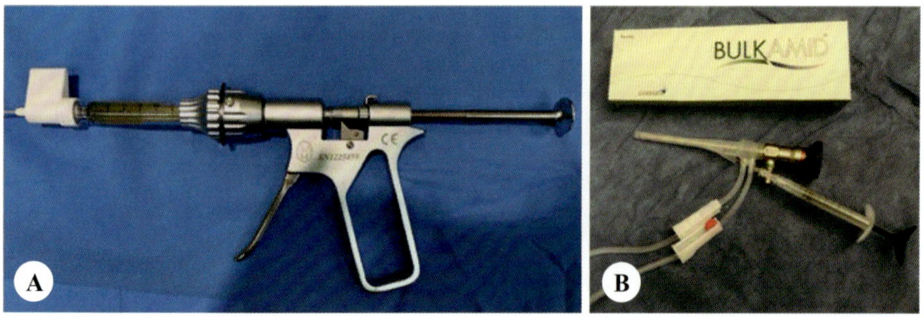

◀ 图 14—2　设备引导的注射器

A. 硅胶粒™ 置入系统包含一个注射装置，放置在尿道至膀胱颈水平，以最佳定位注射部位[90]；B. 水凝胶™ 可旋转鞘在直接可视化下通过尿道，之后临床医生可以注射[15]

果尿潴留持续存在，应教患者进行清洁的间歇性导尿。全麻后 24h 活动局麻当天患者可恢复工作[15, 16]。如果有的话，导尿后通常需要最低限的镇痛药。

值得注意的是，填充剂可以在计算机断层扫描（CT）或磁共振成像（MRI）上看到，并可能与尿道肿块相混淆。有些填充剂也是不透射线的[羟基磷灰石钙(Coaptite)，热解碳(Durasphere)]，因此在肾脏、输尿管和膀胱 X 线检查（KUB）中会被误认为膀胱结石（图 14-3）。最近的一项回顾性研究显示，压力性尿失禁[22]患者的尿道周围填充剂偶尔会被误诊。在本研究中，腹部或盆腔影响检查中很少提及尿道情况。在罕见的病例中，超过 60% 患者的尿道填充剂被误认为泌尿生殖系的病理状态，如盆腔包块或尿道憩室[22]。

（五）注射方法比较

每种注射方法的优缺点已被描述，但没有证据表明在临床成功率方面，一种方法优于另一种方法。一项研究比较了经尿道（n=24）和尿道周围的研究（n=21）注射胶原在 6 个月后治愈率、症状改善率或并发症发生率方面并无统计学差异。然而，与尿道周围组相比，经尿道组的胶原蛋白注射量更低（4.7ml vs. 10.1ml）[21]。

这些结果被 40 例急迫性尿失禁或混合性尿失禁（MUI）女性的分析证实，她们随机接受尿道周围或经尿道注射葡聚糖共聚物。在 1 个月、3 个月、6 个月或 12 个月时，干燥率或主观平均症状改善率没有显著差异。压力性尿失禁的主要原因（ISD vs. OAB）与临床结果无显著关系。重要的是，与经尿道组相比，尿道周围组的尿潴留发生

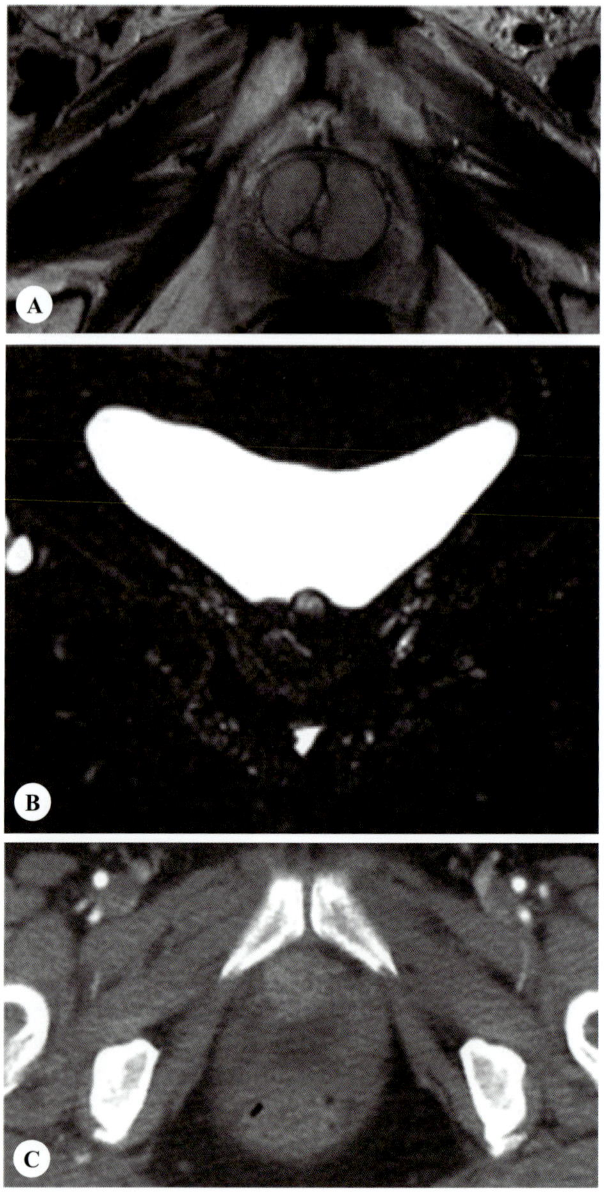

▲ 图 14-3　在各种成像方式上识别的尿道填充术很容易被误解

A. 胶原填充剂的轴位磁共振成像，在影像学读取上被正确解释；B. 胶原填充剂的冠状面磁共振成像，影像学解释为“可能的尿道憩室”；C. 硅胶粒™ 膨胀剂的轴位计算机断层扫描，放射学解释为“软组织衰减增加”

率明显高于经尿道组（分别为 30% 和 5%）。虽然总体上尿道填充剂的注射量没有差异，但尿道周围组发生尿潴留的患者的填充剂沉积量明显大于经尿道组（5.1ml vs. 3.4ml）[20]。

四、女性尿道填充剂的总结：安全性和有效性

（一）传统填充剂

传统尿道填充剂见表 14–1。

1. 硬化剂

鱼肝油酸钠是一种硬化剂，是最早有记录的尿道填充剂。1938 年首次报道，Murless 在阴道前壁注射鱼肝油酸钠，刺激尿道周围组织瘢痕化，以防止尿道过度活动。虽然部分病例成功了，但一些严重的不良反应也随之而来（包括肺栓塞和心搏骤停）[23, 24]。1963 年，Sachse 在女性和男性的尿道中注射了另一种硬化剂，即颗粒醇油。虽然患者的一些症状确实有所改善，但有些病例发生了肺栓塞和尿道黏膜脱落[25]。

2. 聚四氟乙烯（Tefon™）

聚四氟乙烯或 Tefon™，包含大小从小于 50μm 到 300μm[26] 的微粒。它在 20 世纪 70 年代和 80 年代被使用，成功率高达 75%[27]，由于与远端部位粒子移动相关的严重不良反应和潜在致癌性，从未被批准使用[23, 28]。此外，还有一些病例报告了使用聚四氟乙烯相关的排异、尿道周围脓肿、憩室和肉芽肿形成等问题[23, 29]。

3. 自体脂肪

早在 1989 年，几个研究团队就试图从尿道周围注射腹壁[30] 获得的自体脂肪。一项比较经尿道周围注射自体脂肪或生理盐水安慰剂的随机双盲试验被认为是一种易于获取和生物相容性的合适材料，但未能证明治愈率的显著差异。1 例患者甚至并发了肺脂肪栓塞[31]，这进一步阻碍了其作为尿道填充剂的使用。自体脂肪移植物的持久性是有限的，因为移植物在 6 个月时损失会高达 55% 的体积[32]。

4. 戊二醛交联（GAX）胶原蛋白（胶原™）

1993 年，GAX 牛胶原蛋白在磷酸盐缓冲盐水中，作为胶原™（CR Bard, Murray Hill, New Jersey, USA），被美国食品药品管理局（FDA）批准为尿道填充剂。通常在约 3 次注射后，最初的症状改善率为 68%～90%，但随着时间的推移，改善率下降[33, 34]。由 95% 的 Ⅰ 型胶原和 1%～5% 的 Ⅲ 型胶原组成，接受胶原注射的女性在手术前 30 天需要进行皮肤测试，由于其抗原性质，该注射会导致 4% 的患者产生过敏反应。其他不良事件包括尿路感染、血尿、新生急症、关节痛、肺栓塞和无菌脓肿形成[35]。2011 年，制造商停止生产胶原。

表 14–1 传统尿道填充术

尿道填充术	商品名	分 类	相关并发症
Sodium morrhuate	N/A	硬化剂	肺栓塞，心搏骤停
Granugenol oil/Dondren	N/A	硬化剂	肺栓塞，尿道脱落
聚四氟乙烯	Teflon™	微球微粒填充剂	颗粒迁移、挤压、尿道周围脓肿、尿道憩室、肉芽肿形成，可能的致癌因子
自体脂肪	N/A	自体脂肪	肺脂肪栓塞
戊二醛交联（GAX）胶原蛋白	胶原™	牛胶原蛋白	过敏反应、肺栓塞、无菌脓肿
乙烯醇	Uryx™，Tegress™	无颗粒的共聚物	尿道侵蚀
右旋糖酐与透明质酸	Zuidex™，Deflux™	微球微粒填充剂	无菌性脓肿，注射部位肿块和假性囊肿形成

5. 乙烯乙烯醇（Uryx™, Tegress™）

乙烯乙烯醇（EVA）是一种悬浮在二甲亚砜（DMSO）中的共聚物，也被称为Uryx™（GenyxMedical, Inc., Aliso Viejo, CA/C.R. Bard, Murray Hill, NJ, USA）或出口者™（CR Bard, Murray Hill, NJ, USA）。2004年，FDA批准乙烯乙烯醇作为尿道填充剂使用。当注射并显露在体温下的血液或细胞外积液时，二甲亚砜溶解，乙烯乙烯醇形成海绵状肿块，形成尿道块[36]。与胶原蛋白注射剂相比，乙烯乙烯醇注射有更高的治愈率和症状改善率[37]。然而，由于包括严重的尿道侵蚀和瘘管形成[38]等多种不良反应，最终于2007年退出市场。

6. 含透明质酸的聚糖酐（Zuidex™, Defux™）

Zuidex™（Q-MedAB, Uppsala, Sweden）或Defux™（Oceana Therapeutics Inc., Edison, New Jersey, USA）是含有悬浮在透明质酸中的二聚体微球的凝胶。随着透明质酸凝胶的溶解，微球会持续存在4年，促进结缔组织的生长。这些药物通常被批准用于儿童膀胱输尿管复位的内镜治疗。

一项多中心研究对142例接受侵入性治疗的压力性尿失禁患者进行了Zuidex注射，1年后显示了77%的阳性反应，漏尿的激发试验减少率≥50%。24h尿垫试验和每日尿失禁发作次数也有显著减少。大多数不良事件是短暂的，其中包括尿潴留、尿路感染、注射部位反应、尿急、阴道不适、排尿困难、疼痛、假性囊肿形成和注射部位感染[39]。

随后的一项非劣效性试验比较了压力性尿失禁患者的结果，这些患者随机接受经尿道注射Zuidex（n=227）或膀胱颈注射胶原（n=117）。那些接受胶原注射的患者有更高的干反应率和阳性反应率，也被认为是≥在激发试验漏尿方面减少≥50%。虽然两组患者的尿潴留率相同（28%），但Zuidex组经历了更多的并发症，包括无菌脓肿、注射部位肿块和假性囊肿形成[40]，导致其作为压力性尿失禁的尿道填充剂停用。

（二）现代填充术

现代尿道填充术见表14–2。

1. 猪胶原蛋白

猪胶原蛋白（Permaco™）（Covidien，Gosport，United Kingdom）来自交联的猪真皮。在加工过程中，细胞、DNA和RNA被去除，从而使胶原蛋白基质保持其微观结构[41]。这种基质类似人的真皮，可以与宿主组织和血管结合，对比之下，其不需要在植入前进行过敏测试[42]。关于猪胶原蛋白疗效的数据大多局限于一项试验，该试验将患有压力性尿失禁的女性随机分成两组，一组注射猪胶原蛋白（n=25），一组注射交联聚二甲硅氧烷（n=5）。注射6周后，猪胶原蛋白患者的干率无显著提高（60% vs. 41.6%）。6个月时，62.5%的猪胶原蛋白患者保持干燥，而交联聚二甲硅氧烷患者的这一比例为37.5%。此外，猪胶原蛋白患者更少出现术后短暂尿潴留（8 vs. 12%）[42]。

2. 羟磷灰石钙

羟磷灰石钙（Coaptite™）（Bioform Medical Inc., San Mateo, California, USA）是一种合成尿道填充术，由羟基磷灰石钙微球悬浮在羧甲基纤维素凝胶载体中组成。微球颗粒的大小范围为75～125μm。凝胶最初提供了膨胀效果，但随着时间的推移会降解，使原生组织在颗粒周围生长，最终也会溶解[43]。3个月后，羟磷灰石钙。沉积体积减小约40%，保留更多体积的患者更有可能持续改善症状[44]。

支持羟磷灰石钙疗效的主要数据来自一项多中心前瞻性随机对照试验。在这项非不正规性研究中，患有继发于括约肌功能障碍且无尿道过度运动的压力性尿失禁的女性接受了羟磷灰石钙或对照剂的注射。1年后，患者成功的改善不显著，定义为至少一个标准分级的改善，有利于羟磷灰石钙组（63.4% vs. 57.0%）。羟磷灰石钙或对照剂组的1年治愈率（39% vs. 37%）和24h衬垫重量至少减少50%的参与者百分比（62% vs. 54%）也没有差异。此外，羟磷灰石钙组更多患者只需要

表 14-2 当代尿道膨化剂（2021 年 1 月更新）

尿道膨化剂		商品名称	构 成	作用机制	颗粒大小	PDA 批准年份
颗粒剂	碳涂层锆	Durasphere™	碳包覆锆颗粒溶于 2.8% β- 葡聚糖水凝胶		212～500μm	1999 年
	羟基磷灰石钙	Coaptite™	羟磷灰石钙微球溶于羧甲基纤维素凝胶	水凝胶随着时间的推移会降解，包裹的颗粒则保留下来起到膨胀的作用	75～125μm	2005 年
	交联聚二甲基硅氧烷	Macroplastique™	交联聚二甲基硅氧烷弹性体颗粒在聚乙烯吡咯烷酮水凝胶载体中的应用		110μm	2006 年
非颗粒剂	猪胶原蛋白	Permacol™	交联猪真皮	注射的胶原基质与宿主组织和血管结合	无	2004 年
	聚丙烯酰胺水凝胶	Bulkamid™, Aquamid™	水凝胶含有 97.5% 的非热原水和 2.5% 的交联聚丙烯酰胺	水凝胶被巨噬细胞和巨细胞入侵，允许与宿主组织整合	无	2020 年
	聚二甲基硅氧烷	Urolastic™	乙烯基二甲基端封聚二甲基硅氧烷聚合物、四丙氧基硅氧烷交联材料、铂二乙烯基四甲基硅氧烷络合催化剂	以液体的形式注射，然后硬化，包裹在瘢痕组织中	无	待定

单次注射[43]。

尽管羟磷灰石钙组发生急迫性尿失禁的风险明显较低（5.7% vs. 12%），但两组之间在大多数与手术相关的轻微不良事件方面没有差异（包括排尿困难或尿潴留）。羟磷灰石钙组报道了两种主要并发症，特别是阴道壁侵蚀到尿道远端和膀胱三角区下的组织损伤剥脱。这些严重的损伤归因于注射技术和大颗粒对宿主组织造成的压力[43]。据报道，羟磷灰石钙的其他罕见不良反应包括尿道脱垂和需要手术矫正的肉芽肿形成[45, 46]。

3. 碳涂层锆

碳涂层锆（Durasphere™）（Carbon Medical Technologies, St. Paul, Minnesota, USA）含有不可降解的碳包覆锆颗粒，悬浮在可溶解的 2.8% β-葡聚糖水凝胶载体中。相对较大的颗粒为 212～500μm[47]，这可能使注射更加困难，因为增加了阻力[5]。1999 年，FDA 批准其用于尿道填充术[48]。

在一项多中心试验中，碳涂层锆被证明与胶原蛋白注射剂的疗效相当。该研究将 355 例继发于括约肌功能障碍的压力性尿失禁女性随机分为两组，分别注射碳涂层锆和牛胶原蛋白。临床医生在注射过程中使用的碳涂层锆的剂量明显低于胶原蛋白（分别为 4.83ml 和 6.23ml）。注射 1 年后，尿垫重量没有变化，尿失禁程度也没有改善。1 年和 2 年后，骨盆 X 线片上均未观察到颗粒迁移的证据[48]。然而，24 个月后，碳涂层锆的客观效益降低了[49]。在不良事件方面，碳涂层锆组的患者经历了明显更多的尿急和短暂急性尿潴留。除此之外，并发症情况与牛胶原蛋白组相似[48]。虽然大多数不良反应是自限性的，但其他严重的并发症包括颗粒迁移到淋巴结组织[50]，尿道周围脓肿形成，尿道脱垂[51]，以及阴道黏膜可见染色/文身，因为产品是黑色的。

碳涂层锆也可与胶原蛋白结合使用。在一项研究中，比较了联合使用碳涂层锆被证明与胶原蛋白注射液的女性（n=33）和单独使用碳涂层锆的女性（n=33），两周后，联合组的治愈率明显更高（72.7% vs. 39.2%）。疗效没有持续，6 个月后的干燥率在联合组和单独组之间是相同的（33.3% vs. 29.4%）。两组之间在需要后续的抗失禁治疗方面无差异[52]。

4. 交联聚二甲硅氧烷

交联聚二甲硅氧烷（Macroplastique™）（Cogentix Medical, Orangeburg, New York, USA），是含有交联聚二甲基硅氧烷弹性体粒子的有机硅聚合物悬浮在聚乙烯吡咯烷酮水凝胶载体中。注射后，交联聚二甲硅氧烷沉积物被包裹在纤维蛋白囊中，其中渗透着胶原蛋白，水凝胶被肾脏吸收并排出体外[53]。凝胶载体溶解后，约 110μm 大小的不可降解颗粒仍保留在原位[5, 54]。

证明交联聚二甲硅氧烷疗效的最令人信服的数据来自一项对 247 例继发于括约肌功能障碍的压力性尿失禁女性的试验，她们被随机分配接受经尿道注射交联聚二甲硅氧烷或对照剂。12 个月时交联聚二甲硅氧烷组的干率明显高于对照组（36.9% vs. 24.8%）。在交联聚二甲硅氧烷组队列中，更多的患者也至少改善了一个有效分级（61.5% vs. 48%）。两组患者的尿损失均较基线有所减少，尽管两者尿道膨胀剂没有明显的区别。两组之间的注射次数和剂量也相当。两组治疗相关不良事件发生率相似。最常见的不良反应包括尿路感染、下尿路症状、尿潴留和着床部位疼痛。3 例患者出现尿道糜烂（交联聚二甲硅氧烷组 2 例，对照组 1 例）[54]。经过两年的随访，84% 的患者报告他们的治疗持续改善，其中 67% 的患者是干燥的。尿失禁生活质量（I-QoL）评分和平均尿垫重量也比基线有显著改善。随访期间无治疗相关不良事件发生[53]。

随后的系统综述结合了 958 例交联聚二甲硅氧烷注射的压力性尿失禁患者的数据，显示短期、中期和长期干燥率分别为 43%、37% 和 36%，改善率分别为 75%、73% 和 64%。中位再注射率为 30%，其中 63% 的患者报告压力性尿失禁后症状有所改善。不良事件均为轻微，如短暂性尿潴留、急迫性尿失禁、尿路感染、排尿困难、血尿[55]，然而，尽管总体并发症情况良好，但仍有一些罕见而严重的并发症被描述，其中包括疑似免疫反应继发挤压、膀胱颈和尿道糜烂，以及尿道下、阴道和膀胱肿块形成[56-60]。其他几项研究已经证明了交联聚二甲硅氧烷的持久疗效，2～3 年后的治愈率为 47%～49%。虽然许多患者需要多次注射，但大多数客观改善率在 6 个月后保持稳定。在数年的随访后，每日垫重也持续下降[61-63]。

在子宫切除术后的压力性尿失禁患者中，交联聚二甲硅氧烷也可能是有用的。在一项对 24 例接受根治性子宫切除术并导致压力性尿失禁的宫颈癌患者的研究中，交联聚二甲硅氧烷注射在 1 年后的干性率和改善率分别为 42% 和 42%。手术失败与尿道过度活动有关[64]。

5. 聚丙烯酰胺水凝胶

聚丙烯酰胺水凝胶（Bulkamid™ 和 Aquamid™）（Contura International A/S, Soeborg, Denmark）由含有 97.5% 非致热水和 2.5% 交联聚丙烯酰胺的不可降解水凝胶制成[7]。聚丙烯酰胺水凝胶的黏弹性和亲水性使其能够与周围的宿主组织基质交换水分子、营养物质和废物[5]。若干年后，水凝胶被巨噬细胞和巨细胞入侵，然后被纤维和血管组成的永久性网络所取代[65]，以防止迁移[66]。

聚丙烯酰胺水凝胶的效果已经在包括压力性尿失禁，混合性尿失禁和易受伤害患者在内的许多环境中进行了研究。关于压力性尿失禁和混合性尿失禁的治疗，一项主要观察性研究的系统综述显示，聚丙烯酰胺水凝胶注射后，尿失禁发作次数、漏尿次数和生活质量均有所改善。总的重返注射量为 24.3%。并发症大多较轻，其中包括注射部位疼痛、尿路感染、血尿，以及短暂性急性尿潴留[67]。罕见的严重不良事件包括注射部位脓肿形成和尿道黏膜破裂[67-69]，唯一纳入的随机双盲研究是一项多中心试验，证明聚丙烯酰胺水凝胶在治疗压力性尿失禁或应力主导型混合性尿失禁方面的非劣性。注射 1 年后，聚丙烯酰胺水凝胶组和对照组的治愈 / 改善率分别为 77.1% 和 70%。两组间的并发症发生率无差异，主要局限于轻微、短暂的下尿路症状、尿潴留和新生失禁。在聚丙烯酰胺水凝胶组中，仅有一种严重的治疗相关不良反应，即短暂性血尿[8]。研究分析显示，60 岁以上女性的治疗有效率为 90%，治愈率为 38%，而年轻女性的治愈率仅为 13%[10]。

除了改善失禁，聚丙烯酰胺水凝胶还被证明对性行为有积极作用。Leone Roberti Maggiore 等描述了聚丙烯酰胺水凝胶注射液对 29 例压力性尿失禁女性性功能的影响。经过一年的随访，23 例之前性活跃的患者在注射后都能恢复性活动。这些女性报告在性交过程中尿失禁或对尿失禁的恐惧减少，性欲、性高潮和性生活满意度提高。其余 6 例性行为不活跃的女性也能够重新建立性行为[70]。

聚丙烯酰胺水凝胶也已成功应用于一些特殊人群，包括八旬老人和放射后患者[71, 72]。Vecchioli-Scaldazza 等在一组 20 例平均年龄 84.5 岁的 80 岁老人中发现，在注射聚丙烯酰胺水凝胶 2 年后，通过咳嗽压力测试和所需垫的数量，尿丢失显著减少。生活质量评分和尿流动力学参数，其中包括腹漏点压力、尿道闭合平均压力和尿道长度也有所改善[72]。Krhut 等将聚丙烯酰胺水凝胶应用于 46 例有妇科癌症病史的女性，这些女性在接受或不接受盆腔放疗后发生压力性尿失禁。注射后放疗组和非放疗组治愈率分别为 25% 和 36.4%，未见严重不良事件报道[71]。综上所述，这些发现强调了聚丙烯酰胺水凝胶是如何以最小的风险成为尿失禁易感患者的有用工具。

6. 聚二甲硅氧烷（Urolastic™）

聚二甲硅氧烷（Urolastic™）（Urogyn BV, Nijmegen, The Netherlands）是一种合成化合物，包含乙烯基二甲基端聚二甲基硅氧烷聚合物、四丙氧基硅氧烷交联材料和铂二乙烯基四甲基硅氧烷配合物催化剂。二氧化钛的加入使这种膨胀剂不透明[73]。与聚丙烯酰胺水凝胶不同，聚二甲硅氧烷沉积物不含任何颗粒，以液体的形式注入。一旦液体变硬，它就被包裹在瘢痕组织中，不会随着时间的推移而降解、丢失体积或迁移[74]。目前，聚二甲硅氧烷只被批准在欧洲使用。

聚二甲硅氧烷治疗压力性尿失禁的疗效和并发症已经在几个小系列中进行了描述[73-77]。Zajda等报道了20例接受聚二甲硅氧烷注射的压力性尿失禁女性，其中35%的患者需要第二次注射。12个月和24个月的随访后，68%和45%的患者分别保持干燥状态。89%的患者在12个月后自制力得到改善，而在两年后下降到66%[74, 77]。30%的患者出现轻微并发症，其中包括血肿形成、尿潴留、性交困难或阴道疼痛，以及需要清除沉淀物[74]。24个月时，随访分析的18例患者中有4例因性交困难和干燥不佳而进行了种植体移除[77]。同样，Futyma等对105例原发性或复发性压力性尿失禁的女性进行了聚二甲硅氧烷注射。12个月后，客观成功率（定义为尿垫和咳嗽压力测试阴性）在原发性组和复发组分别为71.4%和59.3%。总重复注射率为17%。10例患者中有4例尿潴留患者需要种植体切除[75]。24个月后，复发性压力性尿失禁患者的治愈率为22.4%，32.7%报告客观成功（治愈或改善）[76]。

聚二甲硅氧烷也在医学上不适合手术的女性身上进行了试验。Kowalik等对20例不适合进行尿道中段悬吊术的女性进行了尿片尿道周注射的效果评估。5例患者因持续性尿失禁需要第二次注射，其中3例需要从第一次注射中去除膨体剂。注射后6个月，90%的患者报告主观症状改善，65%的患者咳嗽压力测试呈阴性。通过泌尿生殖窘迫量表（UDI-6）和尿失禁影响问卷（IIQ-7）测量，健康相关的生活质量评分在所有领域都有显著改善。围术期并发症包括血肿形成、疼痛、上皮表面注射尿道填充术需要切除。报道的不良事件均在门诊处理，其中包括注射后立即尿潴留、膨化物质显露和膨化物质自发丢失[73]。

聚二甲硅氧烷的长期成功似乎可以与其他膨胀剂相媲美。在随访6～24个月的系统回顾中，客观治愈率为32.7%～67%，总治愈率为57%。综合主观改善率为84%。16.7%～35%的研究队列需要第二次注射。合并并发症发生率为36%，最常见的并发症为急诊、空腔后残留>150ml、显露或糜烂[78]。最终高达18%的患者可能因持续疼痛、显露或糜烂而需要切除聚二甲硅氧烷[79]。

五、尿道填充术与其他治疗尿失禁方法的比较

管理压力性尿失禁的实践在临床医生之间差别很大，因为没有公认的标准化算法。2017年美国泌尿协会/泌尿动力学、女性盆腔医学和泌尿生殖重建学会（AUA/SUFU）。压力性尿失禁指南指出，对于考虑手术治疗的指数型压力性尿失禁患者，临床医生可以提供尿道填充术、合成尿道中段悬吊术、自体筋膜阴部阴道悬吊或Burch阴道悬吊。该指南还指出，除了耻骨后尿道中段悬吊术和耻骨阴道吊具外，可向非索引型内括约肌功能障碍患者提供尿道填充术。虽然讨论声明确实表示，应该向希望进行微创手术的患者提供尿道填充术，并承认重复注射是常见的，但对于这些治疗方案的试验顺序，没有给出任何建议[80]。同样，欧洲泌尿学协会（EAU）2018年尿失禁指南指出，如果患有压力性尿失禁的女性希望接受低风险的手术，并知道可能需要重复注射，应向她们提供膨胀剂[81]。

尿道填充术应该具体存在压力性尿失禁手术管理决策的精确位置是未知的。这种歧义可能是由于缺乏将尿道填充术与其他抗失禁手术进行比较的随机前瞻性研究[82]。

在2015年的一项系统综述和Meta分析中，作者仅确定了三项将尿道填充术与其他抗失禁手术进行比较的研究，其中只有两项是随机对照试验。分析得出结论，与其他抗尿失禁手术（包括阴部阴道悬吊、尿道中段悬吊术、膀胱颈悬吊和Burch阴道悬垂）相比，尿道填充术与原发性和复发性压力性尿失禁的客观复发率显著较高相关。尿道填充术与较少的排尿功能障碍相关。然而，该Meta分析的规模较小，以及其他许多限制突出了需要更多的比较数据[82]。

最近，一项试验随机选择了224例原发性压

力性尿失禁患者接受无张力阴道胶带（n=111）或聚丙烯酰胺水凝胶注射（n=113）。在一年的随访后，与接受聚丙烯酰胺水凝胶注射的患者相比，接受尿道中段悬吊术治疗的患者报告了更高的患者满意度得分和更高的干燥率（通过阴性咳嗽压力测试测量）。两组女性的性功能和与健康有关的生活质量都有所改善，特别是在身体和社会功能方面。然而，尿道中段悬吊术与较高的围术期并发症和再手术率相关[11, 83]。因此，就这两种选择向压力性尿失禁患者提供建议是很重要的，因为一些患者可能愿意在尿道填充术较低的治愈率和与尿道中段悬吊术相关的较高并发症发生率之间进行权衡[84]。最终，需要更多前瞻性的数据来比较尿道填充术与其他抗尿失禁治疗在不同患者环境下的评估，以明确定义尿道填充术在治疗原发性和复发性压力性尿失禁中的作用。

六、尿道填充术作为失败的尿道中段悬吊术后的补救方式

目前，对于失败的尿道中段悬吊术后理想的治疗技术还没有现成的金标准或共识[66]。在国际泌尿妇科协会成员的一项调查中，尿道填充术被报道为无尿道过度运动患者的首选挽救手术[85]。尽管一些外科医生倾向于试验尿道填充术治疗吊带后复发性压力性尿失禁，尿道填充术作为尿道中段悬吊术失败后复发性压力性尿失禁挽救手术的疗效和持久性仅限于小型回顾性报道，缺乏高质量的证据。

一项包括 23 例在尿道中段悬吊术失败后接受交联聚二甲硅氧烷或碳涂层锆挽救性注射的女性的研究显示，尽管 I-QoL 评分有所改善，92% 的治疗感觉受益，但仅 10 个月后治愈率为 34.8%[86]。同样，Dray 等检查了 73 例在尿道中段悬吊术放置后复发的压力性尿失禁患者，这些患者接受了交联聚二甲硅氧烷或胶原蛋白的挽救性注射。平均 2.6 次注射后，71% 的患者报告症状改善，其中 24.7% 的患者压力性尿失禁完全缓解。在平均 39.5 个月的长期随访信息中，40 例女性中只有 2 例报告压力性尿失禁完全缓解，尽管在密歇根失禁症状指数（M-ISI）的大多数领域都有显著改善[18]。在一项对 17 例女性的分析中，Clark 等在尿道中段悬吊术失败后注射了 2ml 聚丙烯酰胺水凝胶，报告了 42% 的再注射率（发生在首次注射后 10～46 个月），但感知获益率为 71%[87]。Zivanovic 等对 60 例难治性压力性尿失禁或混合性尿失禁患者进行了回顾性观察分析，这些患者在尿道中段悬吊术失败后注射了 1～3ml 聚丙烯酰胺水凝胶。1 个月后，93.3% 的患者治愈或症状改善，6 个月时为 88.3%，12 个月时为 83.6%。最常见的不良事件是持续的急迫性尿失禁，分别在 1 个月、6 个月和 12 个月后分别占 20%、16.7% 和 20%。少数患者出现了其他不良事件，包括排尿功能障碍、尿路感染、新生紧急症、血尿、注射部位撕裂伤和血肿[66]。

只有一项分析直接比较了重复尿道中段悬吊术（n=98）与尿道填充术（n=67）在失败的尿道中段悬吊术后使用对照组、羟磷灰石钙或交联聚二甲硅氧烷作为补救措施。随访 1 年后，接受尿道填充术注射的患者与重复注射的尿道中段悬吊术患者相比，失败的风险明显更高（分别为 38.8% vs. 11.2%），尽管两者的并发症发生率没有差异[88]。

尿道填充术也被用作尿道中段悬吊术移除后的补救技术。Rodriguez 等评估了 70 例在切除失败的尿道中段悬吊术后使用交联聚二甲硅氧烷注射尿道填充术的女性。他们的总体成功率为 69%，主观改善率为 83%，尿垫使用减少了 78%[89]。虽然这些研究规模较小，但当作为辅助救助方法或切除尿道中段悬吊术后，多种类型的尿道填充术似乎对许多女性提供了主客观的症状缓解效果，尽管效果随着时间的推移而减少，可能需要重新注射。

总结

尿道填充术是泌尿科医生治疗压力性尿失禁的重要工具。对于那些不需要做手术或希望避免全身麻醉的女性来说，它们尤其有用。虽然对

比其他治疗方式治愈率较低。尿道填充术展示了更有利的并发症概况。需要更多的前瞻性随机数据来阐明尿道填充术的最佳组合方案和长期疗效。

参考文献

[1] D'Ancona C, Haylen B, Oelke M, et al. The International Continence Society (ICS) report on the terminology for adult male lower urinary tract and pelvic floor symptoms and dysfunction. Neurourol Urodyn. 2019;38(2):433–77.

[2] Radley SC, Chapple CR, Lee JA. Transurethral implantation of silicone polymer for stress incontinence: evaluation of a porcine model and mechanism of action in vivo. BJU Int. 2000;85(6):646–50.

[3] Wasenda EJ, Kirby AC, Lukacz ES, et al. The female continence mechanism measured by high resolution manometry: urethral bulking versus midurethral sling. Neurourol Urodyn. 2018;37(5):1809–14.

[4] Davis NF, Kheradmand F, Creagh T. Injectable biomaterials for the treatment of stress urinary incontinence: their potential and pitfalls as urethral bulking agents. Int Urogynecol J. 2013;24(6):913–9.

[5] Chapple C, Dmochowski R. Particulate versus non-particulate bulking agents in the treatment of stress urinary incontinence. Res Rep Urol. 2019;11:299–310.

[6] Kirchin V, Page T, Keegan PE, et al. Urethral injection therapy for urinary incontinence in women. Cochrane Database Syst Rev. 2017;7:CD003881.

[7] Lose G, Mouritsen L, Nielsen JB. A new bulking agent (polyacrylamide hydrogel) for treating stress urinary incontinence in women. BJU Int. 2006;98(1):100–4.

[8] Sokol ER, Karram MM, Dmochowski R. Efficacy and safety of polyacrylamide hydrogel for the treatment of female stress incontinence: a randomized, prospective, multicenter North American study. J Urol. 2014;192(3):843–9.

[9] Kocjancic E, Mourad S, Acar O. Complications of urethral bulking therapy for female stress urinary incontinence. Neurourol Urodyn. 2019;38(Suppl 4):S12–20.

[10] Elmelund M, Sokol ER, Karram MM, et al. Patient characteristics that may influence the effect of urethral injection therapy for female stress urinary incontinence. J Urol. 2019;202(1):125–31.

[11] Itkonen Freitas AM, Mentula M, Rahkola-Soisalo P, et al. Tension-free vaginal tape surgery versus polyacrylamide hydrogel injection for primary stress urinary incontinence: a randomized clinical trial. J Urol. 2020;203(2):372–8.

[12] Mamut A, Carlson KV. Periurethral bulking agents for female stress urinary incontinence in Canada. Can Urol Assoc J. 2017;11(6Suppl2):S152–S4.

[13] Corcos J, Collet JP, Shapiro S, et al. Multicenter randomized clinical trial comparing surgery and collagen injections for treatment of female stress urinary incontinence. Urology. 2005;65(5):898–904.

[14] Li H, Westney OL. Injection of urethral bulking agents. Urol Clin North Am. 2019;46(1):1–15.

[15] Bulkamid standard operating procedure: Contura; Available from: https://bulkamid.com/wp-content/ uploads/2019/03/BULK_2018_041.2_SOP_12.04.18.pdf.

[16] Urolastic instructions for use: Urogyn BV; Available from: https://www.urogynbv.com/wp-content/ uploads/2015/09/Urolastic-IFU- EN-rev6– 06OCT2014. pdf.

[17] Tamanini JT, D'Ancona CA, Tadini V, et al. Macroplastique implantation system for the treatment of female stress urinary incontinence. J Urol. 2003;169(6):2229–33.

[18] Dray EV, Hall M, Covalschi D, et al. Can urethral bulking agents salvage failed slings? Urology. 2019;124:78–82.

[19] Hegde A, Smith AL, Aguilar VC, et al. Three-dimensional endovaginal ultrasound examination following injection of Macroplastique for stress urinary incontinence: outcomes based on location and periurethral distribution of the bulking agent. Int Urogynecol J. 2013;24(7):1151–9.

[20] Schulz JA, Nager CW, Stanton SL, et al. Bulking agents for stress urinary incontinence: short-term results and complications in a randomized comparison of periurethral and transurethral injections. Int Urogynecol J Pelvic Floor Dysfunct. 2004;15(4):261–5.

[21] Faerber GJ, Belville WD, Ohl DA, et al. Comparison of transurethral versus periurethral collagen injection in women with intrinsic sphincter deficiency. Tech Urol. 1998;4(3):124–7.

[22] Gaines N, Gupta P, Khourdaji AS, et al. Radiographic misdiagnoses after Periurethral bulking agents. Female Pelvic Med Reconstr Surg. 2018;24(4):312–4.

[23] Hussain SM, Bray R. Urethral bulking agents for female stress urinary incontinence. Neurourol Urodyn. 2019;38(3):887–92.

[24] Murless BC. The injection treatment of stress incontinence. J Obstet Gynaecol Br Emp. 1938;45:67–73.

[25] Sachse H. Treatment of urinary incontinence with sclerosing solutions. Indications, results, complications. Urol Int. 1963;15:225–44.

[26] Taylor AK, Dielubanza E, Hairston J. Use of injectable urethral bulking agents in the management of stress urinary incontinence. Curr Bladder Dysfunct Rep. 2011;6:159(2011).

[27] Politano VA. Periurethral polytetrafluoroethylene injection for urinary incontinence. J Urol. 1982;127(3):439–42.

[28] Malizia AA Jr, Reiman HM, Myers RP, et al. Migration and granulomatous reaction after periurethral injection of polytef (Teflon). JAMA. 1984;251(24):3277–81.

[29] Kiilholma PJ, Chancellor MB, Makinen J, et al. Complications of Teflon injection for stress urinary incontinence. Neurourol Urodyn. 1993;12(2):131–7.

[30] Santiago Gonzalez de Garibay AM, Castro Morrondo J, Castillo Jimeno JM, et al. Endoscopic injection of autologous adipose tissue in the treatment of female incontinence. Arch Esp Urol. 1989;42(2):143–6.

[31] Lee PE, Kung RC, Drutz HP. Periurethral autologous fat injection as treatment for female stress urinary incontinence: a randomized double-blind controlled trial. J Urol. 2001;165(1):153–8.

[32] Horl HW, Feller AM, Biemer E. Technique for liposuction fat reimplantation and long-term volume evaluation by magnetic resonance imaging. Ann Plast Surg. 1991;26(3):248–58.

[33] Dmochowski RR, Appell RA. Injectable agents in the treatment of stress urinary incontinence in women: where are we now? Urology. 2000;56(6 Suppl 1):32–40.

[34] Winters JC, Appell R. Periurethral injection of collagen in the treatment of intrinsic sphincteric deficiency in the female patient. Urol Clin North Am. 1995;22(3):673–8.

[35] Sweat SD, Lightner DJ. Complications of sterile abscess formation and pulmonary embolism following periurethral bulking agents. J Urol. 1999;161(1):93–6.

[36] Mukkamala A, Latini JM, Cameron AP. Urethrocutaneous fistula after use of Tegress bulking agent: case report and review of the literature. Can Urol Assoc J. 2013;7(11–12):E833–6.

[37] Dmochowski RR. Tegresstrade mark urethral implant phase III clinical

experience and product uniqueness. Rev Urol. 2005;7(Suppl 1):S22–6.
[38] Hurtado EA, Appell RA. Complications of Tegress injections. Int Urogynecol J Pelvic Floor Dysfunct. 2009;20(1):127; author reply 9.
[39] Chapple CR, Haab F, Cervigni M, et al. An open, multicentre study of NASHA/Dx Gel (Zuidex) for the treatment of stress urinary incontinence. Eur Urol. 2005;48(3):488–94.
[40] Lightner D, Rovner E, Corcos J, et al. Randomized controlled multisite trial of injected bulking agents for women with intrinsic sphincter deficiency: mid-urethral injection of Zuidex via the Implacer versus proximal urethral injection of Contigen cystoscopically. Urology. 2009;74(4):771–5.
[41] Permacol(TM) Surgical implant: Medtronic; 2020. Available from: https://www.medtronic. com/covidien/en-us/ products/hernia-repair/ permacol-surgical- implant. html.
[42] Bano F, Barrington JW, Dyer R. Comparison between porcine dermal implant (Permacol) and silicone injection (Macroplastique) for urodynamic stress incontinence. Int Urogynecol J Pelvic Floor Dysfunct. 2005;16(2):147–50; discussion 50.
[43] Mayer RD, Dmochowski RR, Appell RA, et al. Multicenter prospective randomized 52–week trial of calcium hydroxylapatite versus bovine dermal collagen for treatment of stress urinary incontinence. Urology. 2007;69(5):876–80.
[44] Unger CA, Barber MD, Walters MD. Ultrasound evaluation of the urethra and bladder neck before and after transurethral bulking. Female Pelvic Med Reconstr Surg. 2016;22(2): 118–22.
[45] Lai HH, Hurtado EA, Appell RA. Large urethral prolapse formation after calcium hydroxylapatite (Coaptite) injection. Int Urogynecol J Pelvic Floor Dysfunct. 2008;19(9):1315–7.
[46] Palma PC, Riccetto CL, Martins MH, et al. Massive prolapse of the urethral mucosa following periurethral injection of calcium hydroxylapatite for stress urinary incontinence. Int Urogynecol J Pelvic Floor Dysfunct. 2006;17(6):670–1.
[47] Summary of safety and effectiveness data: Durasphere(TM) Injectable Bulking Agent: United States Food and Drug Administration; 1999. Available from: https://www.accessdata.fda.gov/ cdrh_docs/pdf/ P980053b.pdf.
[48] Lightner D, Calvosa C, Andersen R, et al. A new injectable bulking agent for treatment of stress urinary incontinence: results of a multicenter, randomized, controlled, double-blind study of Durasphere. Urology. 2001;58(1):12–5.
[49] Chrouser KL, Fick F, Goel A, et al. Carbon coated zirconium beads in beta-glucan gel and bovine glutaraldehyde cross-linked collagen injections for intrinsic sphincter deficiency: continence and satisfaction after extended followup. J Urol. 2004;171(3):1152–5.
[50] Pannek J, Brands FH, Senge T. Particle migration after transurethral injection of carbon coated beads for stress urinary incontinence. J Urol. 2001;166(4):1350–3.
[51] Ghoniem GM, Khater U. Urethral prolapse after durasphere injection. Int Urogynecol J Pelvic Floor Dysfunct. 2006;17(3):297–8.
[52] Sokol ER, Aguilar VC, Sung VW, et al. Combined trans- and periurethral injections of bulking agents for the treatment of intrinsic sphincter deficiency. Int Urogynecol J Pelvic Floor Dysfunct. 2008;19(5):643–7.
[53] Ghoniem G, Corcos J, Comiter C, et al. Durability of urethral bulking agent injection for female stress urinary incontinence: 2–year multicenter study results. J Urol. 2010;183(4):1444–9.
[54] Ghoniem G, Corcos J, Comiter C, et al. Cross-linked polydimethylsiloxane injection for female stress urinary incontinence: results of a multicenter, randomized, controlled, single-blind study. J Urol. 2009;181(1):204–10.
[55] Ghoniem GM, Miller CJ. A systematic review and meta-analysis of Macroplastique for treating female stress urinary incontinence. Int Urogynecol J. 2013;24(1):27–36.
[56] Bennett AT, Lukacz ES. Two cases of suspected rejection of polydimethylsiloxane urethral bulking agent. Female Pelvic Med Reconstr Surg. 2017;23(3):e10–e1.
[57] Kulkarni S, Davies AJ, Treurnicht K, et al. Misplaced Macroplastique injection presenting as a vaginal nodule and a bladder mass. Int J Clin Pract Suppl. 2005;(147):85–6.
[58] Rodriguez D, Jaffer A, Hilmy M, et al. Bladder neck and urethral erosions after Macroplastique injections. Low Urin Tract Symptoms. 2020;13:93.
[59] Thompson A, Daborn JP. A vaginal mass and ulceration 8 years following [Macroplastique(R)] injection. Int Urogynecol J. 2015;26(10):1547–8.
[60] Wasenda EJ, Nager CW. Suburethral mass formation after injection of polydimethylsiloxane [Macroplastique(R)] urethral bulking agent. Int Urogynecol J. 2016;27(12):1935–6.
[61] Serati M, Soligo M, Braga A, et al. Efficacy and safety of polydimethylsiloxane injection Macroplastique(R) for the treatment of female stress urinary incontinence: results of a series of 85 patients with >/=3 years of follow-up. BJU Int. 2019;123(2):353–9.
[62] Tamanini JT, D'Ancona CA, Netto NR Jr. Treatment of intrinsic sphincter deficiency using the Macroplastique implantation system: two-year follow-up. J Endourol. 2004;18(9):906–11.
[63] Tamanini JT, D'Ancona CA, Netto NR. Macroplastique implantation system for female stress urinary incontinence: long-term follow-up. J Endourol. 2006;20(12):1082–6.
[64] Plotti F, Zullo MA, Sansone M, et al. Post radical hysterectomy urinary incontinence: a prospective study of transurethral bulking agents injection. Gynecol Oncol. 2009;112(1):90–4.
[65] Christensen LH, Nielsen JB, Mouritsen L, et al. Tissue integration of polyacrylamide hydrogel: an experimental study of periurethral, perivesical, and mammary gland tissue in the pig. Dermatol Surg. 2008;34 Suppl 1:S68–77; discussion S.
[66] Zivanovic I, Rautenberg O, Lobodasch K, et al. Urethral bulking for recurrent stress urinary incontinence after midurethral sling failure. Neurourol Urodyn. 2017;36(3):722–6.
[67] Kasi AD, Pergialiotis V, Perrea DN, et al. Polyacrylamide hydrogel [Bulkamid(R)] for stress urinary incontinence in women: a systematic review of the literature. Int Urogynecol J. 2016;27(3):367–75.
[68] Gopinath D, Smith AR, Reid FM. Periurethral abscess following polyacrylamide hydrogel (Bulkamid) for stress urinary incontinence. Int Urogynecol J. 2012;23(11):1645–8.
[69] Martan A, Masata J, Svabik K, et al. Transurethral injection of polyacrylamide hydrogel [(Bulkamid(R)] for the treatment of female stress or mixed urinary incontinence. Eur J Obstet Gynecol Reprod Biol. 2014;178:199–202.
[70] Leone Roberti Maggiore U, Alessandri F, Medica M, et al. Periurethral injection of polyacrylamide hydrogel for the treatment of stress urinary incontinence: the impact on female sexual function. J Sex Med. 2012;9(12):3255–63.
[71] Krhut J, Martan A, Jurakova M, et al. Treatment of stress urinary incontinence using polyacrylamide hydrogel in women after radiotherapy: 1–year follow-up. Int Urogynecol J. 2016;27(2):301–5.
[72] Vecchioli-Scaldazza CV, Smaali C, Morosetti C, et al. Polyacrylamide hydrogel [Bulkamid(R)] in female patients of 80 or more years with urinary incontinence. Int Braz J Urol. 2014;40(1):37–43.
[73] Kowalik CR, Casteleijn FM, van Eijndhoven HWF, et al. Results of an innovative bulking agent in patients with stress urinary incontinence who are not optimal candidates for mid-urethral sling surgery. Neurourol Urodyn. 2018;37(1):339–45.
[74] Zajda J, Farag F. Urolastic-a new bulking agent for the treatment of women with stress urinary incontinence: outcome of 12 months follow up. Adv Urol. 2013;2013:724082.
[75] Futyma K, Miotla P, Galczynski K, et al. An open multicenter study of

clinical efficacy and safety of Urolastic, an injectable implant for the treatment of stress urinary incontinence: one-year observation. Biomed Res Int. 2015;2015:851823.
[76] Futyma K, Nowakowski L, Galczynski K, et al. Nonabsorbable urethral bulking agent – clinical effectiveness and late complications rates in the treatment of recurrent stress urinary incontinence after 2 years of follow-up. Eur J Obstet Gynecol Reprod Biol. 2016;207: 68–72.
[77] Zajda J, Farag F. Urolastic for the treatment of women with stress urinary incontinence: 24-month follow-up. Cent Eur J Urol. 2015;68(3):334–8.
[78] Capobianco G, Azzena A, Saderi L, et al. Urolastic(R), a new bulking agent for treatment of stress urinary incontinence: a systematic review and meta-analysis. Int Urogynecol J. 2018;29(9):1239–47.
[79] Casteleijn FM, Kowalik CR, Berends C, et al. Patients' satisfaction and safety of bulk injection therapy Urolastic for treatment of stress urinary incontinence: a cross-sectional study. Neurourol Urodyn. 2020;39(6):1753–63.
[80] Kobashi KC, Albo ME, Dmochowski RR, et al. Surgical treatment of female stress urinary incontinence: AUA/SUFU guideline. J Urol. 2017;198(4):875–83.
[81] Burkhard FC, Bosch, JLHR, Cruz F, Lemack GE, Nambiar AK, Thiruchelvam N, Tubaro A, Ambühl D, Bedretdinova DA, Farag F, Lombardo R, Schneider MP. Urinary incontinence 2018. Available from: https://uroweb.org/guideline/urinary-incontinence/.
[82] Leone Roberti Maggiore U, Bogani G, Meschia M, et al. Urethral bulking agents versus other surgical procedures for the treatment of female stress urinary incontinence: a systematic review and meta-analysis. Eur J Obstet Gynecol Reprod Biol. 2015;189:48–54.
[83] Itkonen Freitas AM, Mikkola TS, Rahkola-Soisalo P, et al. Quality of life and sexual function after TVT surgery versus Bulkamid injection for primary stress urinary incontinence: 1 year results from a randomized clinical trial. Int Urogynecol J. 2020;32:595.
[84] Casteleijn FM, Enklaar RA, El Bouyahyaoui I, et al. How cure rates drive patients' preference for urethral bulking agent or mid-urethral sling surgery as therapy for stress urinary incontinence. Neurourol Urodyn. 2019;38(5):1384–91.
[85] Giarenis I, Thiagamoorthy G, Zacche M, et al. Management of recurrent stress urinary incontinence after failed midurethral sling: a survey of members of the International Urogynecological Association (IUGA). Int Urogynecol J. 2015;26(9):1285–91.
[86] Lee HN, Lee YS, Han JY, et al. Transurethral injection of bulking agent for treatment of failed mid-urethral sling procedures. Int Urogynecol J. 2010;21(12):1479–83.
[87] Clark R, Welk B. The use of polyacrylamide hydrogel in the setting of failed female stress incontinence surgery. Can Urol Assoc J. 2018;12(4):95–7.
[88] Gaddi A, Guaderrama N, Bassiouni N, et al. Repeat midurethral sling compared with urethral bulking for recurrent stress urinary incontinence. Obstet Gynecol. 2014;123(6):1207–12.
[89] Rodriguez D, Carroll T, Alhalabi F, et al. Outcomes of Macroplastique injections for stress urinary incontinence after suburethral sling removal. Neurourol Urodyn. 2020;39(3):994–1001.
[90] Macroplastique® Implantation System (MIS): Cogentix Medical; 2021. Available from: https://www.cogentixmedical.com/health-care-professionals/ products/macroplastique/ implantation-system.

第 15 章 Burch 膀胱尿道悬吊术
Burch Colposuspension

Ali Luck　Samantha Raffee　著

20 世纪，直到尿道中段吊带悬吊术的出现前，Burch 膀胱尿道悬吊术是用于矫正尿道过度运动引起的压力性尿失禁（SUI）的“金标准”。1961 年，John C. Burch 在尝试克服实施 Marshall-Marchetti-Krantz（MMK）手术遇到的挑战时首次提出了这种疗法。他发现将膀胱颈连接到 Cooper 韧带上更结实，也能更好地恢复膀胱颈的正常解剖结构[1]。Burch 手术的前身是 MMK 手术。MMK 手术将膀胱颈(尿道膀胱连接处)与耻骨联合骨膜进行悬吊。该术式有时被证明不是一个可靠的悬吊方式，并且有发展为耻骨骨炎的风险。Burch 及其同事发现，与 MMK 相比，Burch 手术有着相似的成功率。当对比后发现疗效相似且发病率较低时，MMK 手术已基本被 Burch 膀胱尿道悬吊术所取代[2]。

自从第一次被描述以来，Burch 膀胱尿道悬吊术经历诸多演变。Emil A. Tanagho 在 1976 年出版的书中对其进行了修改，以便 Burch 手术的规范化[3]。这是目前外科医生采用的最广泛的术式。由于创伤小的尿道中段悬吊术（MUS）的出现，自 2000 年以来 Burch 膀胱尿道悬吊术的使用率逐渐降低[4]。2008 年，美国食品药物管理局（FDA）调查了聚丙烯合成补片在尿道中段悬吊术和盆腔器官脱垂手术中的使用。直到 2013 年，FDA 才宣布多切口吊带手术是安全的，有效率可持续 1 年[5]。在研究合成补片的 5 年里，媒体对合成补片治疗尿道中段悬吊术和脱垂的区别存在混淆。医疗法律实体也参与进来，战略性地将目标锁定在接受了尿道中段悬吊术的患者身上，暂停了最常见的压力性尿失禁手术治疗方式。一些国家甚至禁止使用所有合成网片[6]。患者现在正在寻找替代的非补片手术以纠正压力性尿失禁。也是在这个时候，盆底外科医生开始审视并使用 Burch 膀胱尿道悬吊术。

20 多年来，这种手术已经被证明是安全和有效的。腹腔镜入路或机器人平台下手术均可。使用 Burch 手术的适应证包括提供除外合成补片的另一种选择，并可用于伴随的开放手术，如经腹子宫切除术。

本章将涵盖实施 Burch 膀胱尿道悬吊术的技术，并探讨其如何治疗压力性尿失禁的理论，以及其报道的安全性、有效性和并发症。本章所描述的技术均为开放术式；然而，一旦进入耻骨后间隙，腹腔镜入路的手术原理与开放入路相同。本书的其他章节详细介绍了压力性尿失禁的其他手术治疗和非手术治疗。

一、手术机制

Burch 膀胱尿道悬吊术的确切机制尚未阐明。存在两种对立的理论。第一种理论认为，当膀胱颈被固定在盆底之上，恢复正常解剖结构时，压力传输可以更好地沿尿道分布[7]。第二种理论认为，尿道发生的变化会导致尿道阻力增加，进而导致尿失禁[8]。耻骨后手术从现在的解剖学理论发展而来，解释了 Victor Bonney 医生提出的压力性尿失禁的病因学。1923 年，他发表了一篇论文 *On Diurnal Incontinence of Urine in Women* 描述了压力性尿失禁，并从理论上认为，压力性尿失禁的发生是由于膀胱颈部的支撑功能存在缺陷。引用文章原文“尿失禁似乎是由于耻骨–阴道肌垫前部松弛，因此它在突发的压力下，使膀胱在耻骨联合后面滑落，尿道通过绕耻骨下角旋转向下和向前移动”[9]。Bonney的工作为其他研究人员的跟进奠定了基础。随着20世纪30年代影像学的创新，研究人员使用“watch-chain”膀胱造影来研究压力性尿失禁患者的膀胱颈部，并注意到所谓的“膀胱底漏斗”[10]。由此推断，膀胱颈的漏斗状形成导致膀胱颈薄弱，最终导致压力性尿失禁。引起压力性尿失禁的不一定是阴道和周围尿道周对膀胱的支撑缺陷，而是尿道括约肌本身的问题。

随后，Barnes（1940年）和Enhorning（1960年）利用影像尿流动力学的前身——测压仪进一步研究了缺陷可能是由于尿道括约肌本身所致的观点[10, 11]。他们能够研究尿道内的压力，并注意到压力是如何传递的。他们注意到，当腹腔内压力上升时，这种压力沿尿道的分布很差，而当膀胱颈下垂时，就会出现失禁。这成了压力传递理论的基础。

在此基础上提出了Burch膀胱尿道悬吊术有效的理论依据。Burch膀胱尿道悬吊术将恢复膀胱颈的解剖结构，从而使尿道括约肌的闭合更有效，并使压力沿尿道均匀分布，从而实现控尿。对这一概念的研究始于20世纪80年代初。Hilton和Stanton的研究检查了大小便失禁的女性及其压力传递比（PTR）[12]。压力传递比的计算方法是尿道压力的变化除以膀胱压力的变化，以百分比表示：$\Delta U/\Delta V \times 100\%$。在尿流动力学测试中，在休息和咳嗽刺激时，沿着尿道的长度计算尿道内的压力传输。我们注意到，正常控尿女性在尿道近端有更大的传播维持，其中尿道中段压力传递比最高，接近100%或更高。结果表明，控尿是一种“全或无情况”。而他们的研究发现，接受Burch膀胱尿道悬吊术且被认为成功的患者的压力传递比接近100%或更高这一现象也支持此观点[13]。

Bump等（1988年）仔细研究了压力性尿失禁手术后的压力传递比和并发症[14]。他们的结论是，如果压力传递比接近100%，就实现了控尿；然而，如果超过100%，则可能引起梗阻，并导致逼尿肌不稳定。值得注意的是，这项早期研究的患者群体在压力性尿失禁手术类型方面是小规模和异质性的。Rosenzweig等进一步探讨了控尿压力传递比阈值的概念。他们检查了导致尿失禁的压力传递比的变量，影响压力传递比的患者特征，Burch膀胱尿道悬吊术对压力传递比的影响，以及压力传递比的变化是否预示着手术成功等因素。他们指出，并没有一个百分比来预测控尿，而是依赖于术前和术后压力传递比的变化。术前与术后压力传递比差异越大，说明手术越成功。一些术后可控尿患者压力传递比＜100%，这表明Burch膀胱尿道悬吊术并不需要做到可能引发梗阻就可以达到抗尿失禁的疗效。

20世纪90年代中期，DeLancey描述了“吊床效应”，将解剖学理论和压力传递理论联系在一起[15]。耻骨宫颈筋膜的重建可以提供代偿，通过它尿道可以被压缩，防止腹部压力的异常传递。DeLancey还试图将压力性尿失禁的神经肌肉控制联系起来。通过尸检，他确定耻骨宫颈筋膜插入骨盆腱弓筋膜（ATFP），同时也作为肛提肌的附属结构。在腹内压力增加时，肛提肌被激活，拉起骨盆腱弓筋膜和耻骨宫颈筋膜，以促进尿道的附着。

在20世纪90年代末和21世纪初，一些研究人员提出，阴道悬吊术可能是有效的部分原因是其高尿道阻力。Klutke等（1999年）检查了接受Burch、改良Pereyra和前路修复患者的UDS参数，然后将其绘制在Abrams-Griffiths nomogram（后来命名为膀胱出口梗阻指数，BOOI）[16]上。值得注意的是，Burch组的平均尿道阻力在术前和术后参数之间明显更高。值得注意的是，在被认为“治愈”的患者中，只有50%位于无阻塞区，10%位于阻塞区。这使他们得出结论，Burch手术可能有一种代偿机制。由于可能导致排尿功能障碍，可能不必过度矫正膀胱颈就可以实现控尿。在655例接受Burch膀胱尿道悬吊术或自体悬吊术的女性的大型随机对照试验“尿失禁手术治疗疗效试验

（SISTEr）[17]”中也观察到了这一结果。经 Burch 膀胱尿道悬吊术和自体筋膜悬吊术后 BOOI 较高。自体筋膜吊带具有较高的 BOOI 评分，这可能解释了本组中术后出现排尿功能障碍患者较多的原因。

二、手术技术

（一）解剖学

在进行手术前，了解耻骨后间隙的重要结构是很重要的，以防止血管和神经相关并发症。耻骨后间隙是一个无血管的空间，由耻骨前联合、外侧耻骨支和盆腔肌肉（闭孔内肌、耻尾肌和耻骨直肠肌）和下方尿道近端、中端和腹膜外膀胱所包围形成。腹膜 / 前腹壁是这个空间的顶盖[18]。

膀胱静脉丛是最常见的出血部位。Pathi 等（2009 年）观察了 15 具未经防腐处理的女性尸体，注意到阴道旁结缔组织中与膀胱平行的 2～5 行血管之间存在相互连接。在进入这个间隙之前应该确定的重要结构包括闭孔神经血管束，附属（异常）闭孔血管和髂外血管。闭孔管位于耻骨上支下方约 2cm 处，距耻骨上联合外侧 6cm 处。在尸体解剖研究中，副闭孔静脉的可见率为 52%～70%，副闭孔动脉的可见率为 19%～34%[19, 20]。图 15-1 说明了 Burch 缝合线的解剖结构。

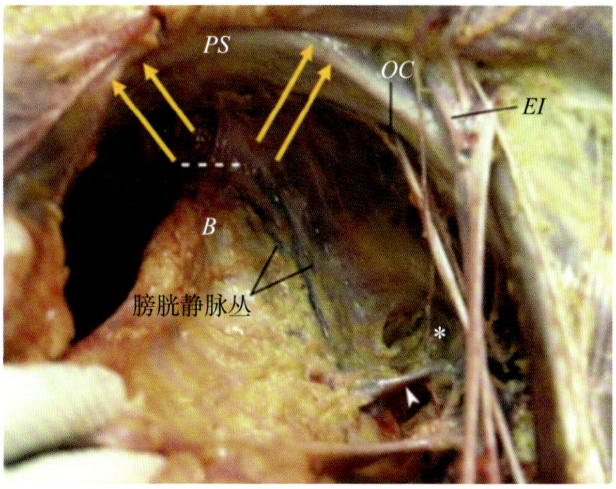

▲ 图 15-1 耻骨后解剖及 Burch 缝合线位置

膀胱颈（PS）耻骨联合处的 Burch 缝合线（黄箭）；右膀胱静脉丛及其与髂内静脉相连的分支的间隙关系（白箭头）；OC. 闭孔管；EI. 髂外血管；B. 膀胱；*. 坐骨棘（经 Elselvier 许可转载，仅做了微小的修改，引自 Pathi et al.[19]）

（二）手术的步骤

与大多数盆底手术一样，最好在膀胱截石位完成。为了达到 Burch 缝合线的最佳位置，外科医生需要一只手在阴道内抬高阴道，另一只手在耻骨后进行缝合线。正因为如此，最好让患者的下肢置于手术靴式腿架（Allen 腿架，Yellowfin 腿架），而不是绑带腿架（candy cane 腿架）。应注意避免膝盖和臀部的过度伸展和屈曲，以及臀部的外展和内旋。由于术中需经阴道及经腹部手术，靴式腿架更容易调整体位以适应手术。术中置入 16 号或 20 号的 French Foley 导尿管并注射 20～30ml 的水囊将有助于在解剖过程中指示膀胱颈部。三腔导尿管虽然非必须，但是可以便于充盈膀胱，在术中是具有帮助作用的。手术缝合后，使用生理盐水稀释亚甲蓝的溶液充盈膀胱可以有助于观察有无膀胱或尿道损伤。术前应使用抗生素和血栓栓塞预防措施。手术开始前进行安全暂停。

1. 进入腹膜后间隙

腹部皮肤切口可由伴随手术（如子宫切除术）决定。有可能需要游离腹直肌，以更好地显露术野。显露的耻骨后间隙是充分显露术野及重要结构的关键。如果单独实施 Burch 膀胱尿道悬吊术，可选择耻骨联合上方 2cm 处的小横切口（6～9cm）以减少创伤。如有必要，可进行 Cherney 或 Maylard 切口以帮助显露耻骨后间隙。如果手术结束时拟重新缝合游离的腹直肌，在耻骨联合的肌腱插入处分离腹直肌的 Cherney 切口是首选。肌腱插入的末端更易接近，且可以作为一个更坚固的锚点，而不是像 Maylard 切口中看到的那样，让缝合线穿过腹直肌本身。当把腹直肌肌腱和锥体肌分开时，要注意腹壁下血管。离耻骨联合最远的外侧结构是闭孔管，距离耻骨联合 5～8cm。当使用拉钩时，要注意髂外血管。

2. 充分显露膀胱颈和耻骨梳韧带（Cooper 韧带）

(1) 触诊并识别闭孔管，以防止在清除耻骨梳韧带上疏松的结缔组织时过于侧向解剖而损伤神经血管束。

(2) 开始将疏松结缔组织从尿道近端和膀胱颈部游离，同时对膀胱施加压力使其朝向头部。操作轻柔，有条理。从中线两侧按压耻骨联合后组织约 2cm 以寻找无血管间隙并向外侧游离。尽量远离中线，因为这是血管最多的区域。你戴着手套的手指，镊子尾端或 Yankauer 吸头有助于分离。

(3) 请阴道助手充盈膀胱，直到膀胱轮廓明显。阴道助手应轻轻将 Foley 球囊拉回膀胱颈部，将手指放在 Foley 球囊和导管的两侧，同时将阴道前壁抬高。这将有助于术者确定何时开始游离组织，直到显露阴道的纤维肌层（盆腔内筋膜）。阴道的纤维肌层自然状态下应该是白色的，甚至有些反光。注意膀胱静脉丛是平行于膀胱的。游离的目标是游离尿道两侧周围约 2cm 的疏松组织，以便可以安全的缝合。可以使用环钳钳夹显影海绵来清除多余的脂肪。以骨盆腱弓筋膜作为向外侧游离到位的标志。

3. 缝合的位置

(1) 在美国泌尿妇科学会和国际泌尿妇科协会关于治疗女性压力性尿失禁的外科手术术语的联合报告（2020 年）中，主张使用延迟可吸收或不可吸收缝合线[21]。首选非编织缝合线，以避免未来窦道形成。作者建议采用 0 号聚丙烯单丝不可吸收缝合线。在 SISTEr 试验[17] 中，使用不可吸收缝合线是标准化选择，且不可吸收缝合线可以降低术后排尿功能障碍的可能性。如果使用延迟可吸收缝线，缝合线张力不应在膀胱颈和耻骨梳韧带之间留下间隙。理论上来说，如果在瘢痕形成之前可吸收线被吸收，那么可能存在阴道悬吊术无效的风险。

(2) 术者将非惯用手置于阴道内，抬高膀胱颈，于尿道近端 1/3，尿道外侧 2cm 处，穿过阴道纤维肌层缝合远端。避免阴道上皮穿孔。将缝线穿过同水平的同侧耻骨梳韧带并留置标记。第二次缝合应位于膀胱颈，尿道外侧 2cm 处，以类似的方式穿过同侧耻骨梳韧带。J. Hamner 等的尸体解剖研究显示（2018），在膀胱颈水平[18]，从尿道周围组织到骨盆腱弓筋膜 2cm 处存在一个“安全区域”。

阴道的纤维肌层应取 8 字缝合，以减少缝合线穿透的风险。为了避免伤到外科医生的手指，可以在外科医生的手指上放一个不锈钢顶针。以类似的方式将缝合线缝合于对侧，并留置标记，直到进行膀胱镜检查。

(3) 应进行膀胱镜检查。在进行膀胱镜检查后，拉紧并打结缝合线，以确认缝合线没有穿孔尿道和膀胱。缝合时，在尿道周围组织和耻骨梳韧带之间留 2～3cm 的缝线桥。该手术的目的是纠正膀胱颈部的过度活动，且避免过度抬高膀胱颈部导致梗阻。更紧并不意味着更好。图 15–1 描绘了缝合线与耻骨后间隙周围重要结构的关系。

(4) 遇到出血时，有几种方法可确保止血。如果在阴道纤维肌层缝线时发生出血，可由助手在穿过耻骨梳韧带之前将缝线打结。最有可能发生的是膀胱静脉丛的静脉出血，此时通过阴道内和腹部的手联合压迫可以帮助止血。如果遇到大量出血，并且认为出血来自膀胱静脉丛，可以行膀胱切开术显露膀胱，以便止血缝线不会损害膀胱或输尿管开口。出血时应在这个部位放置止血药。如果遇到大量出血，并担心在手术结束时出现血肿，可以进行手术引流。

4. 关闭腹部切口

经典的 Cherney 切口关腹时在耻骨联合[23] 处的肌腱插入处重新缝合肌肉。关于重新缝合肌肉是否导致的术后疼痛缺乏相关数据。作者倾向于将肌肉重新缝合于肌腱插入处。用弯钳抓住腹直肌并向耻骨支牵拉。使用延迟可吸收或不可吸收线水平褥式缝合腹直肌前鞘，然后缝合于耻骨联合处切断的肌腱止点进行固定。如果对侧腹直肌分离，也应在对侧直肌上进行类似的缝合。如果联合腹腔内手术，应关闭腹膜。筋膜和皮肤按通常的方式闭合。

5. 膀胱引流

在手术结束时应留置 16Fr Foley 导尿管，并在术后第一天进行排空试验。

三、手术结局

1961 年，随着 Burch 膀胱尿道悬吊术的发展，有着大量关于其疗效和总体结果的长期数据。此外，它已作为一个基准用于和新开发的其他抗尿失禁手术进行对比，如耻骨阴道悬吊和尿道中段悬吊术。2017 年 Cochrane 关于开放性耻骨后阴道悬吊术的综述共纳入了 231 篇文章，最终包括 152 篇（55 项研究）的定性分析报告和 142 篇（50 项研究）的定量分析报道[2]。这篇综述的结论是，治疗后一年内的控尿率为 85%～90%，而 5 年后的控尿率约为 80%[2]。压力性尿失禁手术疗效试验（SISTEr）是一项多中心随机对照试验，比较了 Burch 膀胱尿道悬吊术和筋膜悬吊术。最初发表的报告称，患者对 Burch 膀胱尿道悬吊术和筋膜悬吊术两年期满意度分别为 78% 和 86%[17]。E-SISTEr 试验报告患者对 Burch 膀胱尿道悬吊术的满意度为 73%，接受筋膜悬吊术[24]的患者满意度为 83%。虽然满意率相对较高，但在 2 年随访期时[17]，筋膜悬吊术的压力性尿失禁成功率为 66%，Burch 膀胱尿道悬吊术为 49%。因为他们使用复合结果测量法对成功进行了更严格的定义，而不是使用单一结果测量法，因此这种较低的成功率被认为时次要的。此外，主观和客观结果之间的差异很大，文章指出了影响患者对手术成功的解释的多种因素[17]。Kupasertkul 等报道了来自单一机构的随访 15 年结果，21 例患者中有 3 例再次手术（2 例 Burch，1 例筋膜悬吊术）[25]。Alcalay 等报道了 10～20 年 Burch 膀胱尿道悬吊术后尿失禁的治愈率为 69%[26]。

在 2017 年 Cochrane 评论中[2]，微创吊带手术和腹腔镜 Burch 膀胱尿道悬吊手术与开放式 Burch 膀胱尿道悬吊手术的成功率相似。比较 Burch 膀胱尿道悬吊术与经耻骨后路径和到经闭孔路径的研究报道了术后 2 年及 5 年有相似的主观治愈率[27-29]。然而，一项单一机构 12 年数据的研究确实发现经耻骨后路径和 Burch 膀胱尿道悬吊术的成功率的差异，127 例患者中有 14 例（Burch）和 180 例患者中有 3 例（TVT）的患者接受了再次抗尿失禁手术（$P<0.001$）[30]。此外，一项比较抗尿失禁治疗的随机对照试验的 Meta 分析得出结论，接受尿道中段吊带悬吊术的患者总体（82% vs. 74%）和客观失禁率（79.7% vs. 67.8%）明显高于接受开放 Burch 膀胱尿道悬吊术[31]的患者。因为 Cochrane 综述中最长的随访是一个 5～7 年的小研究，结果支持腹腔镜方法，但没有达到显著性[2]，因此可能需要更多的数据来进一步阐明开放和腹腔镜阴道悬吊术在长期随访中是否存在差异。部分研究结果的摘要见表 15-1。

由于客观治愈率较低，人们已努力了解与不良结果相关的因素。术前体重>80kg，既往膀胱颈部手术史，术中失血量>1000ml，术后逼尿肌不稳定与手术成功率降低有关[27]。此外，对 258 例接受 Burch 膀胱尿道悬吊术的患者的回顾性评估显示，年龄、胎次、绝经状态、使用激素替代疗法、既往子宫切除术和术后并发症的发生对失败率没有显著影响[32]。

传统上，Burch 膀胱尿道悬吊术用于尿道过度活动症的患者。内源性括约肌缺陷（ISD），定义为尿流动力学检查 Valsalva 漏尿点压力<60mmHg，已被证明是手术失败的危险因素[33]。然而，Hsieh 等显示，24 例患者中有 21 例的内源性括约肌缺陷患者对术后进行膀胱测压提示具有自然控尿，认为仅 Valsalva 漏点压低，而没有其他与内源性括约肌缺陷相关的参数（例如，最大尿道闭合压力<20mmHg），并不是手术失败的独立危险因素[34]。

Burch 膀胱尿道悬吊术已被用作失败的抗尿失禁手术的二次治疗方案。一项小型回顾性研究对 16 例在尿道中段悬吊术失败后行腹腔镜 Burch 膀胱尿道悬吊术的患者进行了研究，报道客观治愈率为 54.5%，主观治愈率为 92.9%，中位随访时间为 24.5 个月[35]。Agur 等对复发性压力性尿失禁的管理进行了系统回顾和 Meta 分析，发现 Burch 膀胱尿道悬吊术和耻骨后尿道中段悬吊术之间无显著差异[36]。

表 15-1 Burch 研究结果

研究		研究设计	数量	手术细节	随访时间	结局	不良结局
Burch 膀胱尿道悬吊术 vs. 筋膜吊带悬吊术	Albo 2007	多中心随机对照试验	• 吊带组：326 • Burch 组：328	N/A	24 个月	• 术后成功率：吊带组 66%，Burch 组 49%（$P<0.001$） • 术后满意率：吊带组 86%，Burch 组 78%（$P=0.02$）	• 严重不良事件：吊带组 13%，Burch 组 10%（$P=0.2$） • 不良事件：吊带组 63%，Burch 组 47%（$P<0.001$） • 排尿困难：吊带组 14%，Burch 组 2%（$P<0.001$）
	Brubaker 2012	前瞻性研究	• 吊带组：183 • Burch 组：174	N/A	5 年	• 总体控尿率：Burch 组 24%，吊带组 31%（$P=0.05$） • 满意率：吊带组 83%，Burch 组 73%（$P=0.04$）	• 严重不良事件：无 • 不良事件：吊带组 9%，Burch 组 10%，72/75 不良事件为复发性尿路感染
	Demirci 2001	单中心前瞻性随机对照试验	• 吊带组：23 • Burch 组：23	手术时间：吊带组 60min，Burch 组 54min，无严重手术相关并发症	12 个月	无症状，吊带组 16/17，Bruch 组 15/17	• 再发 DI：吊带组 1 例，Burch 组 1 例 • 耻骨弓疼痛：吊带组 3 例，Burch 0 例 • 脱垂：吊带组 0 例，Burch 组 2 例
	El Barky 2005	单中心前瞻性随机对照试验	• 吊带组：25 • Burch 组：25	手术时间：吊带组 20min，Burch 组 57min	24 个月	治愈率：Burch 组 72%，TVT 组 72%	• 再发尿急：Burch 组 12%，吊带组 8% • 尿潴留：Burch 组 12%，吊带组 20%
Burch 膀胱尿道悬吊术 vs. TVT	Ward 2004	多中心随机对照试验	• 吊带组：137 • Burch 组：108	N/A	24 个月	1h 尿垫试验阴性：Bruch 组 80%，TVT 组 81%	• 术后压力性尿失禁再次手术：TVT 组 1.8%，Burch 组 3.4% • 术后脱垂再次手术：TVT 组 0%，Burch 组 4.8%
	Ward 2008	多中心随机对照试验	• 吊带组：98 • Burch 组：79	N/A	5 年	• 术后满意率 / 非常满意率：Burch 组 90%，TVT 组 91% • 1 小时尿垫试验阴性：Bruch 组 81%，TVT 组 90%	• 术后压力性尿失禁再次手术：TVT 组 2.3%，Burch 组 3.4% • 术后脱垂再次手术：TVT 组 1.8%，Burch 组 7.5%

（续表）

研究		研究设计	数量	手术细节	随访时间	结局	不良结局
Burch 膀胱尿道悬吊术 vs. TOT	Asicioglu 2013	回顾性分析	• 吊带组：272 • Burch 组：498	• 手术时间：Burch 组 41.5min，吊带组 23.7min • 术中出血量：Burch 组 119.3ml，吊带组 52.7ml	5 年	• 主观治愈率：Burch 组 73.9%，吊带组 77.5%（P=0.991） • 客观治愈率：Burch 组 76.8%，吊带组 81.7%（P=0.791）	• 尿潴留：Burch 组 24%，吊带组 7.6%（$P = 0.001$） • 再发尿急：Burch 组 6.7%，吊带组 2.8%（$P = 0.169$） • 长期排尿困难：Burch 组 5.3%（$P = 0.005$）
	Sivaslioglu 2007	前瞻性随机对照试验	• 吊带组：49 • Burch 组：51	• 手术时间：Burch 组 48min，吊带组 23.2min • 术中出血量>100ml，Bruch 组 1 例，吊带组 0 例	24 个月	• 主观治愈率：Burch 组 83.8%，吊带组 87.5%（P=0.6） • 客观治愈率：Burch 组 87%，吊带组 87.5%（P=0.9）	• 再发急迫性尿失禁：Burch 组 5.8%，TOT 组：2%（$P = 0.3$） • 术后第 2 天尿潴留>100ml：Burch 组 5.8%， • TOT 组 2%（$P = 0.3$）
开放 Burch 膀胱尿道悬吊术 vs. 腹腔镜下 Burch 膀胱尿道悬吊术	Carey 2006	多中心随机对照试验	• 开放组：104 • 腹腔镜组：96	• 手术时间：开放组 42min，腹腔镜组 87min（$P<0.001$） • 术中出血：开放组 170ml，腹腔镜组 126ml（P= 0.03）	24 个月	患者满意度（评分>80 分）：开放组 70%，腹腔镜组 58%（P= 0.10）	• 术后频繁尿急：开放组 10% 腹腔镜组 23%（$P = 0.40$）。术后频繁急迫性尿失禁：开放组 10%， • 腹腔镜组：18%（$P = 0.21$）
	Ankardal 2004	对中心前瞻性随机性试验	• 开放组：120 • 腹腔镜组：120	• 手术时间：开放组 60min，腹腔镜组 75min（$P< 0.0001$） • 术中出血：开放组 105 ml，腹腔镜组 35ml（$P< 0.0001$）	12 个月	• 客观症状缓解率：开放组 89%，腹腔镜组 64%（$P<0.001$） • 48h 尿垫试验漏尿量<8g/24h：开放组 92%，腹腔镜组 74%（$P<0.001$）	• 术后 1 个月内尿路感染：开放组 20%，腹腔镜组 10%（NS） • 伤口感染：开放组 3%，腹腔镜组 2%（NS） • 尿潴留>5 天：开放组 26%，腹腔镜组 9%（$P = 0.002$）

四、并发症和不良事件

开放式 Burch 膀胱尿道悬吊术虽然比其他抗尿失禁手术更具侵入性，但并未显示其有显著的发病率或并发症。Dimerci 等描述了涉及阴道旁静脉的错误平面游离继发出血的风险。他们的综述指出输血或血肿的风险为 0.02%～4.8%，其中一项令人惊讶的研究显示输血率为 33%[37]。虽然使用腹腔镜方法可减少失血量，其代价是报道的手术时间较长[38, 39]。在 SISTEr 试验中报道的最常见的严重不良事件包括偶然的膀胱切开术（3%）和需要手术干预的伤口并发症（4%）。总体而言，最常见的不良事件是尿路感染（62%），尽管明显低于接受筋膜吊带术的患者（93%）[17]。

在任何抗尿失禁手术前，必须告知患者的一个重要风险是术后排尿功能障碍。由于对这些症状的定义和考虑的术后时间不同，这可能很难量化。正因为如此，术后尿潴留的范围很大（0%～24%），尽管只有 3% 的报告为需要永久自我导尿[37]。此外，术前尿流动力学检测并不能预测术后排尿功能障碍[40]。

除了排尿困难之外，手术干预后可能会出现新发或加重的尿频、尿急和急迫性尿失禁。据报道，在 Burch 膀胱尿道悬吊术[41]后，3%～8% 的患者会出现复发性逼尿不稳定性。在 E-SISTEr 试验中接受 Burch 膀胱尿道悬吊术并完成 5 年随访的 174 例女性中，29 例有持续性尿失禁，7 例有新发尿失禁[25]。尿失禁复发率与 Ward 等报道的术后 5 年随访数据（4%）相似[42]。

Burch 最初的文章描述了他的阴道悬吊术，尽管发生率很低，暗示了与术后阴道脱垂的发展相关，特别是肠疝[1]。多年来，进一步的研究支持了这一发现。Wiskind 等显示，他们的队列（131 例患者）中 26.7% 的患者[43]术后需要对盆腔脏器脱垂进行手术矫正[26]。另一项 109 例患者的研究显示，在 10～20 年的随访期间，30% 的患者需要进行直肠膨出或肠疝进行手术修复。在一项比较 Burch 膀胱尿道悬吊术术后复发性尿失禁患者与未复发患者的研究中，发现失禁患者术后膀胱和直肠膨出发生率明显较高，而肠疝发生率相似（24%）[44]。当比较 Burch 和尿道中段吊带悬吊术时，发现了类似的结果[42]。

总结

Burch 膀胱尿道悬吊术是一种经过充分研究的治疗过度活动的压力性尿失禁的方法，被证明是安全有效的。这是一个适合的非病态肥胖且不希望使用合成网片患者的替代手术方式。腹腔镜 Burch 手术可能减少疼痛，失血，并更快地恢复日常活动；然而，还需要更多的研究来观察它的长期安全性和有效性。与任何抗尿失禁手术一样，患者应被告知术后可能发生尿频、尿急和急迫性尿失禁的风险。

参考文献

[1] BURCH JC. Urethrovaginal fixation to Cooper's ligament for correction of stress incontinence, cystocele, and prolapse. Am J Obstet Gynecol. 1961;81:281–90.

[2] Lapitan MCM, Cody JD, Mashayekhi A. Open retropubic colposuspension for urinary incontinence in women. Cochrane Database Syst Rev. 2017;7(7):CD002912.

[3] Tanagho EA. Colpocystourethropexy: the way we do it. J Urol. 1976;116(6):751–3.

[4] Jonsson Funk M, Levin PJ, Wu JM. Trends in the surgical management of stress urinary incontinence. Obstet Gynecol. 2012;119(4):845–51. https://doi.org/10.1097/ AOG.0b013e31824b2e3e.

[5] Souders CP, Eilber KS, McClelland L, Wood LN, Souders AR, Steiner V, Anger JT. The truth behind transvaginal mesh litigation: devices, timelines, and provider characteristics. Female Pelvic Med Reconstr Surg. 2018;24(1):21–25.

[6] Zacche MM, Mukhopadhyay S, Giarenis I. Changing surgical trends for female stress urinary incontinence in England. Int Urogynecol J. 2019;30(2):203–9.

[7] Hilton P, Stanton SL. A clinical and urodynamic assessment of the Burch colposuspension for genuine stress incontinence. Br J Obstet Gynaecol. 1983;90(10):934–9.

[8] Klutke JJ, Klutke CG, Bergman J, Elia G. Urodynamics changes in voiding after anti-incontinence surgery: an insight into the mechanism of cure. Urology. 1999;54(6):1003–7.

[9] Bonney V. On diurnal incontinence of urine in women. J Obset Gynaecol Br Emp. 1923;30:358–65.

[10] Barnes A. A method for evaluating the stress of urinary incontinence. Am J Obstet Gynecol. 1940;40:381–90.

[11] Enhorning G. Simultaneously recording of intravesical and intra-urethral pressure: a study on urethral closure in normal and stress incontinent women. Acta Chir Scand. 1961;suppl 276:1–68.
[12] Hilton P, Stanton SL. Urethral pressure measurement by microtransducer: the results in symptom-free women and in those with genuine stress incontinence. Br J Obstet Gynaecol. 1983;90:919–33.
[13] Hilton P, Stanton SL. A clinical and urodynamic assessment of the Burch colposuspension for genuine stress incontinence. Br J Obstet Gynaecol. 1983;90(10):934–9.
[14] Bump RC, Fantl JA, Hurt WG. Dynamic urethral pressure profilometry pressure transmission ratio determinations after continence surgery: understanding the mechanism of success, failure, and complications. Obstet Gynecol. 1988;72(6):870–4.
[15] DeLancey JO. The pathophysiology of stress urinary incontinence in women and its implications for surgical treatment. World J Urol. 1997;15(5):268–74.
[16] Klutke JJ, Klutke CG, Bergman J, Elia G. Urodynamics changes in voiding after anti-incontinence surgery: an insight into the mechanism of cure. Urology. 1999;54(6):1003–7.
[17] Albo ME, Richter HE, Brubaker L, Norton P, Kraus SR, Zimmern PE, Chai TC, Zyczynski H, Diokno AC, Tennstedt S, Nager C, Lloyd LK, FitzGerald M, Lemack GE, Johnson HW, Leng W, Mallett V, Stoddard AM, Menefee S, Varner RE, Kenton K, Moalli P, Sirls L, Dandreo KJ, Kusek JW, Nyberg LM, Steers W. Urinary Incontinence Treatment Network. Burch colposuspension versus fascial sling to reduce urinary stress incontinence. N Engl J Med. 2007;356(21):2143–55.
[18] Hamner JJ, Carrick KS, Ramirez DMO, Corton MM. Gross and histologic relationships of the retropubic urethra to lateral pelvic sidewall and anterior vaginal wall in female cadavers: clinical applications to retropubic surgery. Am J Obstet Gynecol. 2018;219(6):597.e1–597.e8.
[19] Pathi SD, Castellanos ME, Corton MM. Variability of the retropubic space anatomy in female cadavers. Am J Obstet Gynecol. 2009;201(5):524.e1–5.
[20] Kinman CL, Agrawal A, Deveneau NE, Meriwether KV, Herring NR, Francis SL. Anatomical relationships of Burch colposuspension sutures. Female Pelvic Med Reconstr Surg. 2017;23(2):72–4.
[21] Joint report on the terminology for surgical procedures to treat stress urinary incontinence in women. Developed by the Joint Writing Group of the American Urogynecologic Society and the International Urogynecological Association. Int Urogynecol J. 2020;31(3):465–78.
[22] Loughlin KR. The thimble: a useful adjunct to needle suspension procedures for female stress incontinence. Urology. 2000;56(6):1050–1.
[23] CHERNEY LS. Transverse low abdominal incision with detachment of the recti from the pubis: follow-up study of eight hundred cases. J Am Med Assoc. 1955;157(1):23–6.
[24] Brubaker L, Richter HE, Norton PA, Albo M, Zyczynski HM, Chai TC, Zimmern P, Kraus S, Sirls L, Kusek JW, Stoddard A, Tennstedt S. Gormley EA; Urinary Incontinence Treatment Network. 5-year continence rates, satisfaction and adverse events of burch urethropexy and fascial sling surgery for urinary incontinence. J Urol. 2012;187(4):1324–30.
[25] Kuprasertkul A, Christie AL, Lemack GE, Zimmern P. Long-term results of Burch and autologous sling procedures for stress urinary incontinence in E-SISTEr participants at 1 site. J Urol. 2019;202(6):1224–9.
[26] Alcalay M, Monga A, Stanton SL. Burch colposuspension: a 10–20 year follow up. Br J Obstet Gynaecol. 1995;102(9):740–5. Erratum in: Br J Obstet Gynaecol 1996;103(3):290.
[27] Sivaslioglu AA, Caliskan E, Dolen I, Haberal A. A randomized comparison of transobturator tape and Burch colposuspension in the treatment of female stress urinary incontinence. Int Urogynecol J Pelvic Floor Dysfunct. 2007;18(9):1015–9.
[28] El-Barky E, El-Shazly A, El-Wahab OA, Kehinde EO, Al-Hunayan A, Al-Awadi KA. Tension free vaginal tape versus Burch colposuspension for treatment of female stress urinary incontinence. Int Urol Nephrol. 2005;37(2):277–81.
[29] Asıcıoglu O, Gungorduk K, Besımoglu B, Ertas IE, Yıldırım G, Celebı I, Ark C, Boran B. A 5-year follow-up study comparing Burch colposuspension and transobturator tape for the surgical treatment of stress urinary incontinence. Int J Gynaecol Obstet. 2014;125(1):73–7. https://doi.org/10.1016/j.ijgo.2013.09.026. Epub 2013 Dec 14.
[30] Holdø B, Verelst M, Svenningsen R, Milsom I, Skjeldestad FE. Long-term clinical outcomes with the retropubic tension-free vaginal tape (TVT) procedure compared to Burch colposuspension for correcting stress urinary incontinence (SUI). Int Urogynecol J. 2017;28(11):1739–46.
[31] Fusco F, Abdel-Fattah M, Chapple CR, Creta M, La Falce S, Waltregny D, Novara G. Updated systematic review and meta-analysis of the comparative data on Colposuspensions, Pubovaginal slings, and Midurethral tapes in the surgical treatment of female stress urinary incontinence. Eur Urol. 2017;72(4):567–91.
[32] Sun MJ, Ng SC, Tsui KP, Chang NE, Lin KC, Chen GD. Are there any predictors for failed Burch colposuspension? Taiwan J Obstet Gynecol. 2006;45(1):33–8.
[33] Koonings PP, Bergman A, Ballard CA. Low urethral pressure and stress urinary incontinence in women: risk factor for failed retropubic surgical procedure. Urology. 1990;36(3):245–8.
[34] Hsieh GC, Klutke JJ, Kobak WH. Low valsalva leak-point pressure and success of retropubic urethropexy. Int Urogynecol J Pelvic Floor Dysfunct. 2001;12(1):46–50.
[35] De Cuyper EM, Ismail R, Maher CF. Laparoscopic Burch colposuspension after failed sub-urethral tape procedures: a retrospective audit. Int Urogynecol J Pelvic Floor Dysfunct. 2008;19(5):681–5.
[36] Agur W, Riad M, Secco S, Litman H, Madhuvrata P, Novara G, Abdel-Fattah M. Surgical treatment of recurrent stress urinary incontinence in women: a systematic review and meta-analysis of randomised controlled trials. Eur Urol. 2013;64(2):323–36.
[37] Demirci F, Petri E. Perioperative complications of Burch colposuspension. Int Urogynecol J Pelvic Floor Dysfunct. 2000;11(3):170–5.
[38] Carey MP, Goh JT, Rosamilia A, Cornish A, Gordon I, Hawthorne G, Maher CF, Dwyer PL, Moran P, Gilmour DT. Laparoscopic versus open Burch colposuspension: a randomised controlled trial. BJOG. 2006;113(9):999–1006.
[39] Ankardal M, Ekerydh A, Crafoord K, Milsom I, Stjerndahl JH, Engh ME. A randomised trial comparing open Burch colposuspension using sutures with laparoscopic colposuspension using mesh and staples in women with stress urinary incontinence. BJOG. 2004;111(9):974–81.
[40] Lemack GE, Krauss S, Litman H, FitzGerald MP, Chai T, Nager C, Sirls L, Zyczynski H, Baker J, Lloyd K. Steers WD; Urinary Incontinence Treatment Network. Normal preoperative urodynamic testing does not predict voiding dysfunction after Burch colposuspension versus pubovaginal sling. J Urol. 2008;180(5):2076–80.
[41] Sohlberg EM, Elliott CS. Burch Colposuspension. Urol Clin North Am. 2019;46(1):53–9.
[42] Ward KL. Hilton P; UK and Ireland TVT Trial Group. Tension-free vaginal tape versus colposuspension for primary urodynamic stress incontinence: 5-year follow up. BJOG. 2008;115(2):226–33.
[43] Wiskind AK, Creighton SM, Stanton SL. The incidence of genital prolapse after the Burch colposuspension. Am J Obstet Gynecol. 1992;167(2):399–404; discussion 404–5.
[44] Kjølhede P. Genital prolapse in women treated successfully and unsuccessfully by the Burch colposuspension. Acta Obstet Gynecol Scand. 1998 Apr;77(4):444–50.

第 16 章　无张力吊带尿道中段悬吊术的发展历程

The Innovation of Midurethral Slings: Where We've Been and Where We Are Today

Suzette E. Sutherland　Ellen C. Thompson　著

无张力吊带尿道中段悬吊术（MUS）的发展创新彻底改变了近年来对女性压力性尿失禁（SUI）的认识和治疗。如今，尿道中段悬吊术已成为女性压力性尿失禁研究最广泛和实施最多的手术治疗方法，近 20 年来，全球有关此类研究的文献报道数据已超过一千万例。美国妇科泌尿协会（AUGS）、女性盆底医学和泌尿生殖道重建学会（SUFU）、美国泌尿外科协会（AUA）、欧洲泌尿外科协会（EAU）和欧洲妇科泌尿协会（EUGA）等均报道了该手术是迄今为止最安全、最有效的手术治疗方法，国际妇科泌尿协会（IUGA）也发表立场文件宣布 MUS 是女性压力性尿失禁手术治疗的金标准[4, 5, 14, 51, 52]。

尽管该手术严重的并发症不常见，但是已经发生过的相关不良结局所引发的纠纷及社会关注则已经被媒体广泛传播。对于女性压力性尿失禁应用聚丙烯网片的尿道中段悬吊术，美国食品药品管理局（FDA）在 2013 年明确指出“多切口吊带的安全性和有效性已在临床试验中得到充分确立”[35]。虽然网片置入导致自身免疫性疾病[15]和癌症[15, 16, 61, 62]的观念是未经证实的，但是随着反网片置入者不断努力地宣扬，可想而知，有朝一日尿道中段悬吊术可能不再可用。不幸的是，若放弃或禁止尿道中段悬吊术可能会使女性面临更大的手术安全风险。因为无法为压力性尿失禁患者提供高效且微创的手术，从而迫使她们不得不寻求更具侵入性的手术替代方案。

本章内容主要介绍了尿道中段悬吊术应用中不断创新演变的基本原理，包括从最初的经耻骨后路径到经闭孔路径到单切口路径的阴道无张力吊带尿道中段悬吊术的演变，对不同路径手术的尿道中段悬吊术与其他传统尿失禁手术的疗效进行比较分析。当然，本章提供的数据资料所提示的所有这些手术的相关风险、益处均由经验丰富的外科医生执行的结果。

一、压力性尿失禁：理论回顾

事实证明，回顾整个 20 世纪关于压力性尿失禁的病理生理机制的历史演变对我们理解无张力吊带尿道中段悬吊术的理论发展创新历程是有帮助的。我们对尿失禁病理生理学认识的进展与压力性尿失禁外科治疗技术的进步相辅相成。从几代人的发展来看，压力性尿失禁在概念和治疗方面对医生来说都十分具有挑战性[54]。关于压力性尿失禁潜在病因的研究包括：Valsalva 相关动作导致腹压变化、骨盆肌肉和韧带结构的退行性变使盆底失去支撑、尿道括约肌固有特性的改变导致尿道闭合不良、复杂的排尿神经生理因素导致的尿道括约肌功能障碍，当然也包括下表其他因素的相互作用（表 16–1）。

非常早期的手术技术侧重于通过筋膜瓣的方式，用股薄肌或锥体肌环绕尿道来增强尿道括约肌强度[95]。在 20 世纪早期，膀胱镜检查的改进使 Kelly 能够观察和描述尿道内外括约肌的结构，注意到压力性尿失禁患者的内括约肌障碍和随后膀胱颈作用机制的形成过程[55]。他研究出 Kelly 缝合技术[9]，该技术通过将尿道周围和耻骨颈筋膜的中线缝合形成一个狭窄的后尿道膀胱角来加强

表 16-1 摘要：压力性尿失禁治疗的发展创新之路

年 份	创 新	压力性尿失禁治疗
20 世纪初	尿道括约肌缺陷	肌肉“吊带”：股薄肌或锥状肌包裹尿道
20 世纪 10 年代	内括约肌功能缺陷引起膀胱颈漏尿	• Kelly 尿道折叠术 • 尿道周围 / 耻骨宫颈筋膜中线折叠术
20 世纪 20—30 年代	在 Valsalva 动作下，耻骨下尿道膀胱角增大	• Kelly 尿道折叠术 • 阔筋膜耻骨阴道悬吊术
20 世纪 40 年代	盆底肌肉支持	凯格尔锻炼
20 世纪 40—60 年代	压力传递理论	将尿道前部 / 膀胱颈固定于耻骨后的耻骨后尿道固定术 腹直肌筋膜耻骨后膀胱尿道悬吊固定术
20 世纪 60—70 年代	微创技术	耻骨后针刺悬吊术
	加固尿道近端 / 膀胱颈复合体	• 尿道悬吊术 • 针刺悬吊术 • 尿道固定术
20 世纪 80 年代	尿道固有括约肌功能缺陷（ISD）	尿道过度活动患者（UHM）采用 Kelly 尿道悬吊术
	压力性尿失禁病因二分类比较：UHM vs. ISD	尿道固有括约肌功能下降（ISD）采用自体筋膜的耻骨阴道悬吊术
20 世纪 90 年代	吊床理论将肌肉、筋膜、神经系统有机整合	自体筋膜的耻骨阴道悬吊术成为“金标准”，可同时解决尿道过度活动和内在括约肌缺陷的问题
	整体理论考虑到韧带和肌肉支持驱动功能	无张力吊带尿道中段悬吊术（MUS）使尿道中段出现动态的弯曲改变 1996 年提出经耻骨后尿道中段悬吊术（TVT）
21 世纪初	采取避开耻骨后间隙的方法来提高 TVT 手术的安全性	2001 年提出经闭孔尿道中段悬吊术（TOT） 2006 年提出单切口路径尿道中段悬吊术（SIS）
2008 年到 2011 年	FDA 发布的针对压力性尿失禁（SUI）和盆底器官脱垂（POP）的阴道网片安全通知	无张力吊带尿道中段悬吊术（MUS） 自体筋膜的耻骨阴道悬吊术（PVS）
2014 年、2016 年和 2017 年更新	AUGS/SUFU/AUA EAU/EUGA 均发表声明支持无张力吊带尿道中段悬吊术（MUS）网片应用	支持采用耻骨后尿道中段吊带（RPS）完成经闭孔尿道中段悬吊术（TOT）作为“金标准”
	IUGA 全球声明	关于单切口路径尿道中段悬吊术（SIS）的数据尚不成熟
2017 年	SUFU/AUA 关于压力性尿失禁的指南	对于指征明确的患者，建议采用无张力吊带尿道中段悬吊术（MUS） 对于病情复杂的患者，推荐自体筋膜的耻骨阴道悬吊术（PVS），但需要注意相关风险
2018 年	EAU 关于压力性尿失禁的指南	无张力吊带尿道中段悬吊术（MUS）是一线治疗方案 如果无法采用无张力吊带尿道中段悬吊术（MUS），建议选择自体筋膜的耻骨阴道悬吊术（PVS）

AUGS. 美国妇科泌尿协会；SUFU. 女性盆底医学和泌尿生殖道重建学会；AUA. 美国泌尿外科协会；EAU. 欧洲泌尿外科协会；EUGA. 欧洲妇科泌尿协会；IUGA. 国际妇科泌尿协会

近端尿道膀胱颈的支撑。尽管该技术 1 年的失败率高达 30%[46]，但该技术也广泛应用于临床数十年[95]。在 20 世纪 20—30 年代，Bonney 继续研究近端尿道，他指出尿道周围失去支撑和尿道 – 膀胱角度增加会导致压力性尿失禁患者在做 Valsalva 相关动作时膀胱降至耻骨以下[23]。20 世纪 40—50 年代，Kegel 使人们重新认识到盆底肌在盆底物理康复产生的持久影响，现在仍然是尿失禁以及许多其他盆底疾病的非手术治疗的主要方法[54]。在 20 世纪 60 年代，Enhoerning 专注研究腹压增加时压力传递到膀胱和尿道的情况，这似乎验证了通过尝试恢复近端尿道的盆腔位置来防止漏尿的手术技术的可行性[30, 31]。在这段时间内，像采用自体筋膜的耻骨阴道悬吊术（阔筋膜，1933；腹直肌筋膜，1942[2]）和耻骨后膀胱尿道悬吊固定术［Marshall-Marchetti-Krantz（MMK），1949[71]；（Cooper 韧带 Burch 悬吊术，1961）］[12] 通过在耻骨后位置固定近端尿道来控制尿失禁[107]。尝试了侵入性较小的尿道固定术（Pereyra[86]、Stamey 针刺悬吊术[100, 101]、Raz 尿道固定术[89] 和 Raz 四角悬吊术[90]），但因易复发而逐渐被淘汰。Cochrane 的一篇回顾性研究发现针刺悬吊尿道固定术仅 1 年的失败率就接近 30%[46]。

在 20 世纪 80 年代，尿道括约肌的去神经损伤被进一步描述并称为尿道内括约肌功能障碍（ISD）[107]，从而将关于压力性尿失禁的病因学理论分为：解剖学（缺乏支持导致尿道过度活动症）与功能性（去神经损伤导致括约肌功能障碍）。这进一步导致了治疗的二分法，对尿道过度活动患者使用 Kelly 缝合术和 Burch 阴道悬吊术，对伴有括约肌功能障碍的患者使用耻骨阴道悬吊术（如 Blaivas[10] 所述自体筋膜的耻骨阴道悬吊术）[72-74]。DeLancey 在 20 世纪 90 年代的“吊床理论”描述了肌肉、筋膜和神经系统对维持女性尿控的重要性[25, 26]。这一理论进一步表明使用自体筋膜的耻骨阴道悬吊术治疗压力性尿失禁能够解决尿道过度活动症和并发括约肌功能障碍[13]，因 20 世纪 90 年代中后期该手术被认为是压力性尿失禁手术治疗的“金标准”。

后来，Petros 和 Ulmsten[87] 提出的盆底整体理论，促使了尿道中段悬吊术的创新发展。

二、盆底整体理论

虽然早期的手术通过将近端尿道 / 膀胱颈复合体稳定在耻骨后位置来控制尿失禁[107]，但是由 Petros 和 Ulmsten 在 1990 年提出的整体理论、肌弹性理论确定了尿道中段的解剖区域，称为耻骨尿道韧带（PUL）。该 PUL 不是稳定整个尿道，而是用于支撑尿道中段，在腹压增加的 Valsalva 相关动作时充当近端尿道旋转的支点。这使得中尿道可进行动态“弯曲”，从而消除腹压增加、特别是压力性尿失禁相关因素引起的不必要漏尿[87]（图 16–1 和 16–2）。

三、尿道中段悬吊术的演变

这种对中段尿道而不是近端尿道 / 膀胱颈复合体的专注打破了关于女性压力性尿失禁的传统思维方式，为治疗女性压力性尿失禁提供了灵感和创新，从而产生了第一个用于外科手术的合成尿道中段吊带，开启了一种新型的手术方式，即经阴道无张力尿道悬吊术（TVT）[103]。作为“假性耻骨阴道韧带”，合成网片尿道中段吊带旨在恢复或加强尿道中段水平的悬吊尿道和固定尿道外口作用。当组织生长到吊带中，利用常春藤攀爬在网格上形象化的视觉类比，在愈合过程中将吊带固定在适当的位置，从而在腹压增加时为尿道提供支撑。这一机制可以理解对尿道过度活动的患者最有效。

尿道中段吊带的初始入路源于外科医生对耻骨后（RP）间隙的丰富经验。这种耻骨后路径手术在尿道下和沿着尿道外侧形成一个 U 形吊带，网片向上延伸穿过耻骨后（RP）间隙，直接穿过耻骨后面，并通过下腹前壁耻骨上区域的两个小切口穿出固定（图 16–3）。在套管针的帮助下，通过尿道下方的小切口（自下而上）将经耻骨后路径尿道中段吊带置于阴道内。后来的技术发展允许放置尿道中段吊带，套针从腹部开始向下移动到阴道（自上而下）。无论哪种方式，专注于尿道中段通过经阴道入路治疗尿失禁的手术，更加贴合解剖结构，因此侵入性更小。

近 20 年的长期研究数据显示使用合成网片的耻骨后路径尿道中段吊带疗效已得到很好的证实[81]。虽然盲刺套管针通过耻骨后和网片通过时相关的严重并发症不常见，但如果不加以识别，包括像膀胱穿孔等损伤，可能导致膀胱网片滞留，继发泌尿道感染和膀胱结石、肠损伤、严重血管损伤、大出血甚至死亡等严重不良结局。这为 Delormein 2001 年研发第二代吊带技术，即经闭孔路径吊带提供了灵感（图 16–3）[28]。经闭孔路径吊带将网片吊带放置在与耻骨后路径吊带相同的中

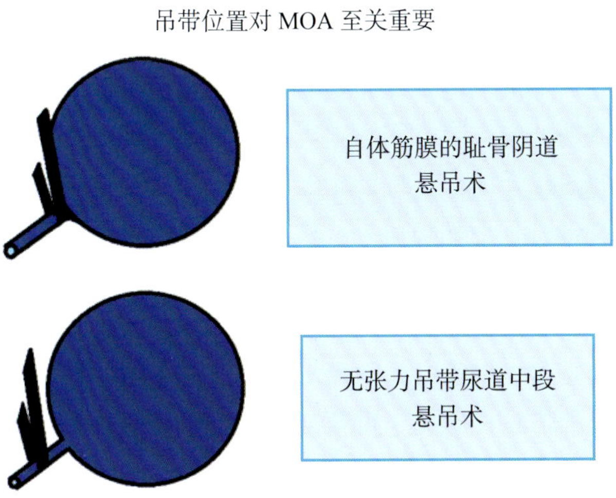

▲ 图 16–1　吊带放置：吊带位置的作用机制（MOA）

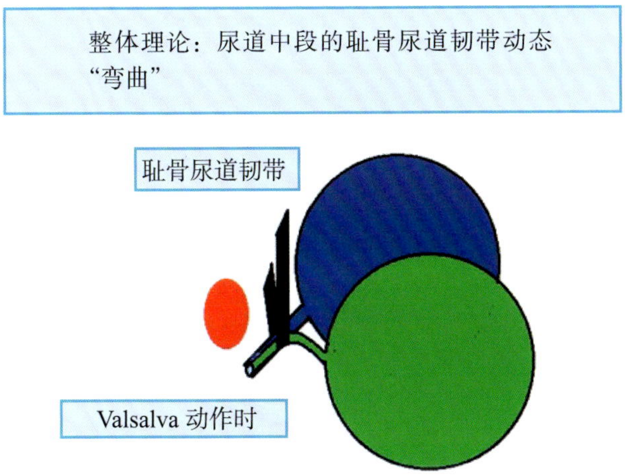

▲ 图 16–2　整体理论做 Valsalva 动作时，耻骨尿道韧带对尿道中段有支撑和悬吊作用

尿道中段悬吊术的作用机制

尿道位置，但不穿过耻骨后间隙。利用螺旋套管针穿过闭孔和双侧耻骨下周围，在闭孔的上方和内侧避开位于闭孔上外侧的闭孔神经、动静脉丛来实现远离耻骨后间隙，理论上可以避免这些严重的并发症。随着经闭孔入路到作为由外向内（闭孔到阴道）或由内向外（阴道到闭孔）的入路演变[27]，开始发现越来越多的腹股沟疼痛和网片相关的性交痛。在适当的高截石位通过识别内收肌长肌腱的位置，避免套管针通过时造成损伤，有助于减少术后腹股沟疼痛的发生率。此外，确保在耻骨下支后面 2 点钟和 10 点钟方位分离阴道间隙可以获得足够的解剖深度和角度，以消除术后因挤压导致网片穿透阴道壁和网片紧贴阴道侧壁可能导致的性交痛风险。

选择适当的手术技术，通过对耻骨后和经闭孔两种路径的吊带张力进行差异性调整，多个 RCT 研究均提示这两种尿道中段悬吊术可达到相当的疗效[8, 19, 24, 37, 43, 59, 66, 91, 97, 104, 109]。

为了避免耻骨后和闭孔间隙基于它们本身设计和套管针盲穿时存在的固有潜在并发症，进一步创新开发了第三代尿道中段悬吊术，即 2006 年首次推出（图 16–3）[76] 的单切口路径悬吊术。单切口路径悬吊术真正创新的方面是锚钉技术，它使网片在组织愈合生长中在适当位置固定更牢固。锚钉垂直放置在与经闭孔路径相同的闭孔肌间区域，不穿过整个闭孔和大腿，从而避免腿部出血、瘀伤、血肿和疼痛的发生。其他优点包括更小的

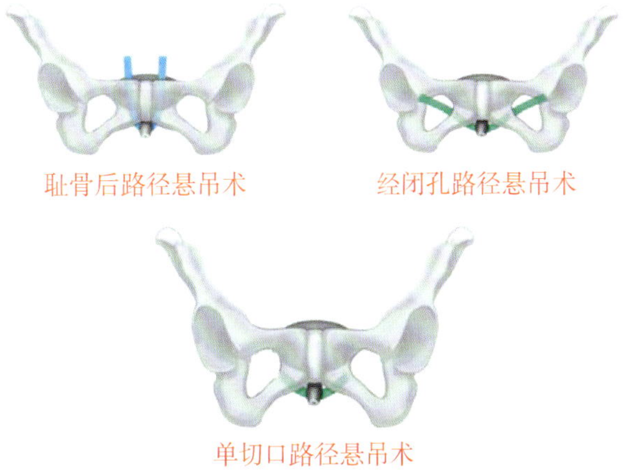

▲ 图 16–3　尿道中段悬吊术的演变

网片残留，仅 1～2cm 的尿道下切口损伤及更窄的套管针，较少的出血和术后不适，可以更快地恢复工作和所有正常活动（包括剧烈运动在内）。单切口路径手术最常使用局部麻醉和静脉镇静相结合方式的麻醉方案，目前，在美国各地的医疗中心，单切口路径手术已经成功地过渡到完全使用局部麻醉即可完成的阶段。

在 2006 年国际妇科泌尿协会（IUGA）会议上第一次提出单切口路径悬吊术，即 TVT-Secur 手术（Gynecare®）[76] 导致无法接受的较高失败率的两个重要原因：①基于简单可吸收线的无效“锚定”方法；②与之前的耻骨后路径悬吊术和经闭孔路径悬吊术相比，不符合更严格的张紧技术。利用适当的张力，从耻骨后路径悬吊术过渡到经闭孔路径悬吊术，然后从其中一种方法过渡到单切口路径悬吊术时，我们已经认识到尊重“学习曲线”的重要性[57, 98, 99]。单切口路径悬吊术需放置并紧贴于中尿道。然而，由于早期的 TVT-Secur 手术的失败案例被媒体广泛宣传，4.5 年的中期失败率高达 70%，该手术在 2012 年以后逐渐在临床上受到了较多的限制[20, 21]。不幸的是，从此开始给单切口路径悬吊术带来了不好的影响。但当改进锚定技术和坚持适当的单切口路径悬吊术（SIS）特定张紧技术后，我们进一步研究发现其疗效与耻骨后路径悬吊术和经闭孔路径悬吊术相当，而且并发症更少[79]。

四、压力性尿失禁外科治疗的比较研究

如前所述，耻骨阴道悬吊术在 20 世纪 90 年代被认为是压力性尿失禁手术治疗的“金标准”。随着尿道中段吊带悬吊术用于治疗压力性尿失禁，耻骨阴道悬吊术的这一地位受到了挑战。2017 年美国泌尿外科协会 / 泌尿动力学、女性盆底医学和泌尿生殖道重建学会（AUA/SUFU）联合发布了压力性尿失禁特定患者的手术治疗指南，其中包括尿道中段悬吊术（合成材料）、耻骨阴道自体筋膜悬吊术、Cooper 韧带（Burch 手术）和尿道填充术（图 16–4）。

任何压力性尿失禁手术治疗的成功率取决于我们对成功的定义。遗憾的是，文献中关于手术成功的定义存在很大差异，这使得研究和治疗之间的充分对比变得复杂[7]。此外，手术成功与否需要进行长期随访研究，这通常比较困难。大多数关于压力性尿失禁手术干预的研究持续时间仅为 1 年，很少超过 3～5 年。对于侵入性外科手术，尤其是仅 1 年的时间间隔不足以向患者提供更有价值的信息，即关于可预期的长期有效性和需要重复手术干预的可能性说明。

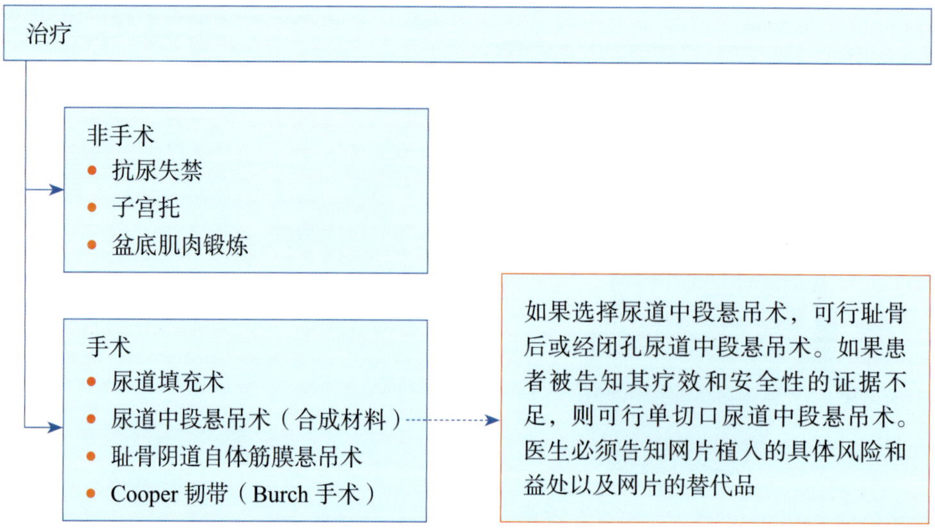

▲ 图 16–4 2017 年 AUA/SUFU 发表的女性压力性尿失禁治疗指南（经许可转载，引自 the AUA；Kobashi KC，et al. J Urol [64]）

五、耻骨后 Cooper 韧带悬吊术（Burch）与自体筋膜的耻骨阴道悬吊术及无张力吊带尿道中段悬吊术的疗效比较

尽管研究结果显示耻骨后 Cooper 韧带悬吊术（Burch）、自体筋膜的耻骨阴道悬吊术（PVS）和无张力吊带尿道中段悬吊术（MUS）在术后 1 年随访时的疗效相似[6, 37, 43, 49, 65, 75]，但 Burch 或耻骨阴道悬吊术与尿道中段悬吊术相比，症状改善的有效维持时间不足。根据 2017 年 Cochrane 数据库中对涉及 Burch 膀胱颈悬吊术的各种资料分析，术后 1 年有效率为 85%～90%，至术后 5 年则下降为 70%[65]。SISter 试验（压力性尿失禁手术治疗疗效试验）是尿失禁治疗网（UITN）中精心设计的 RCT，比较了 Burch 和耻骨阴道悬吊术在治疗后 2 年和 5 年的情况。其中，耻骨阴道悬吊术与 Burch 相比，随着治疗后随访时限的延长，根据症状和体征等因素综合评价标准的要求（压力试验阴性，无压力性尿失禁的自主症状，以及没有任何形式的再治疗），压力性尿失禁的复发率逐渐升高，两者的总体有效率均明显下降：耻骨阴道悬吊术与 Burch 在术后 2 年时的压力性尿失禁复发率分别为 66% 和 49%，至术后 5 年则只有 31% 和 24%[1, 11]。另一项 RCT 研究结果显示，根据泌尿生殖器道压力量表（UDI-6）统计的数据，耻骨阴道悬吊术术中无论选择较短的 10cm 或较长的 21cm（可在耻骨后间隙中形成更广泛附着）聚丙烯悬吊线，均提示远期疗效有限，术后 5 年患者主观压力性尿失禁症状复发率为 49% 和 57%[60]。

与尿道中段悬吊术相比，Burch 在长期疗效和安全性方面明显逊色[43, 82]。然而，在一些术后随访长达 5 年的研究中，耻骨阴道悬吊术似乎显示出与尿道中段悬吊术相当的功效。在最近一项纳入超过 10 000 例患者（n=15 855）并进行长期随访（至少 60 个月）的 Meta 分析中，相较于耻骨阴道悬吊术与 Burch 手术，尿道中段悬吊术具有更可靠的有效率和安全性[43]。尽管研究显示耻骨阴道悬吊术在术后 5 年时的有效率与尿道中段悬吊术相似，但仍缺乏长期（>5 年）随访数据支持。

六、无张力吊带尿道中段悬吊术不同手术路径的疗效比较（经耻骨后路径、经闭孔路径和单切口路径）

自 20 世纪 90 年代末至 21 世纪初以来，采用“全长”网片的经耻骨后路径悬吊术和经闭孔路径悬吊术（TOT）受到广泛关注与研究。作为迄今为止随访时限最长的研究，Nilsson 对最初的无张力性阴道悬吊术患者进行了 17 年的随访，并指出客观检查和主观症状的改善率分别为 91% 和 87%[81]。近期，有关耻骨后路径悬吊术和闭孔路径悬吊术研究的系统评价和 Meta 分析也证明了其显著的长期疗效[67]。此外，针对耻骨后路径悬吊术与闭孔路径悬吊术疗效比较的 RCT 研究受到广泛关注，大多数研究均得出两种手术路径具有相似功效的结论[8, 19, 24, 43, 59, 66, 91, 97, 104, 109]。一项纳入 55 项研究的 Meta 分析显示，耻骨后路径悬吊术与闭孔路径悬吊术相比，术后随访 5 年的客观检查和主观症状的改善率相似：其中耻骨后路径悬吊术的客观检查改善率为 87%，而闭孔路径悬吊术为 86%；耻骨后路径悬吊术的主观症状改善率为 71%～97%，而闭孔路径悬吊术为 62%～98%[37]。尿道中段悬吊试验（TOMUS 试验）进一步验证，术后 5 年时随访，耻骨后路径悬吊术的有效维持率仅略高于闭孔路径悬吊术[59]。然而，在明确合并括约肌功能障碍的情况下，耻骨后路径悬吊术的远期疗效似乎确实优于闭孔路径悬吊术。术后 3 年，耻骨后路径悬吊术仅有 1.4% 需要再治疗，而闭孔路径悬吊术为 20%[38, 94]。总体而言，与闭孔路径悬吊术相比，尽管耻骨后路径悬吊术在压力性尿失禁手术路径选择中，远期有效率略高，但同时需要面临更高的术中并发症和术后排尿功能障碍的发生率[43]。

相比前两种手术路径，单切口路径悬吊术的出现要晚得多。根据目前较新的数据，2017 年 Cochrane 评价指出，已发表文献中的长期随访数据不足，无法将单切口路径悬吊术与更传统的采

用“全长”网片的耻骨后路径悬吊术和闭孔路径悬吊术[80]进行充分比较。与不受年龄、体重指数或产科病史影响的耻骨后路径悬吊术和闭孔路径悬吊术相比，单切口路径悬吊术的短期（12～24个月）疗效和安全性得到了证实[3, 42, 78, 79, 85]。2014年的一项比较评估单切口路径悬吊术（不包括单切口路径经阴道经闭孔尿道中段悬吊术，TVT-S）与“全长”网片（耻骨后路径悬吊术和闭孔路径悬吊术）的疗效和安全性的RCT Meta分析指出，平均随访18个月，对生活质量或性功能而言，不论客观检查有效率（88% vs. 90%），还是主观症状改善率均没有显著性差异（83% vs. 90%）[79]，但仍缺乏长期数据。因此，2017年美国泌尿外科学会/泌尿动力学、女性盆底医学和泌尿生殖道重建学会指南小组关于压力性尿失禁手术治疗的声明则重新提出了这样的建议，即在做出关于采用单切口路径悬吊术手术路径的更强有力的声明之前需要更长期可靠的数据支持[64]。

最近，有许多较大规模的RCT、比较试验和系统评价以及Meta分析来支持这些初步发现，即单切口路径悬吊术与耻骨后路径悬吊术和闭孔路径悬吊术相比具有相对可比的疗效和安全性[3, 41, 69, 70, 105]。一项FDA授权的522项上市后批准研究将单切口路径悬吊术与闭孔路径悬吊术进行了比较，指出术后3年的可比综合有效率（客观和主观）分别为90.4%和88.9%[105]。部分RCT研究注意到术后3年随访，单切口路径悬吊术与闭孔路径悬吊术之间的有效率具有相似结果，单切口路径悬吊术的客观和主观有效率分别为89%和86%，而闭孔路径悬吊术分别为88%和87%；第1年、第2年与第3年之间没有发现明显差异[93]。总体而言，并发症的风险非常低，但单切口路径悬吊术术后疼痛的发生率则显著降低。同样，据报道，单切口路径悬吊术术后3年的主观和客观治愈率分别为83%和88%术后5年则为85%和80%[69, 70]。甚至最近，一项对60例单切口路径悬吊术患者进行的为期10年的回顾性研究发现，与2年到10年相比，疗效没有随着时间的推移而降低，客观和主观治愈率分别为86%和88%[41]。

由于治疗并改善了压力性尿失禁患者的主观症状及客观检查，在选择单切口路径悬吊术（Solyx）或闭孔路径悬吊术（Obtryx Ⅱ）的两组手术病例中，用于评价对性功能的短期和长期（6～36个月）影响的盆腔器官脱垂尿失禁性功能问卷（PISQ-12）得分均有明显改善。此外，在术后36个月内新发性交痛是十分罕见的并发症（单切口路径悬吊术的141例患者中有1例，闭孔路径悬吊术的141例患者中无患者，P=1.00）[106]。对各种路径的无张力吊带尿道中段悬吊术的随机对照试验的Meta分析表明，与传统的尿道中段悬吊术相比，单切口路径悬吊术显著改善性功能（PISQ-12）并降低术后疼痛的发生率[33]。

七、网片相关并发症

经过长期随访观察证实，选择合成材料的尿道中段悬吊术是全球患压力性尿失禁女性最常选择的外科手术方案。2017年一项来源于Cochrane的综述对尿道中段悬吊术的疗效评价指出：“尿道中段悬吊术是研究最广泛的女性压力性尿失禁手术治疗，具有良好的安全性。不论选择何种路径的手术，其短期和中期的疗效都非常显著，并且越来越多的证据表明此类手术的长期有效率也是十分可靠的”[37]。然而，在阴道中使用合成网片仍然存在很多争议，主要是由于担心网片相关并发症，如网片显露（穿透阴道壁）、网片侵蚀（侵犯邻近脏器）、感染愈合不良、性交困难和疼痛等。据报道，尽管存在这些担忧，但采用网片完成尿失禁手术后，真正出现严重并发症的风险还是非常低的。正如在20多年前就开始（1997—2016年）进行的一项基于苏格兰人群调查中所指出的那样，与所有其他非网片抗尿失禁手术相比，选择网片的尿道中段悬吊术的短期和长期（5年）并发症发生率均较低[77]。具体而言，长达5年的随访数据显示，选择耻骨后路径悬吊术（RPS），与非网片手术的效果相当，但耻骨后路径悬吊术术后即刻并发症的相对风险则比其他非网片手术低50% 左右。这项超过 20 年的研究数据证实了尿道中段悬吊术的安全性和有效性。而对于不同路径的尿道中段悬吊术手术而言，耻骨后路径悬吊术会导致更高的术后梗阻和排尿功能障碍发生率，包括需要后续干预的新发尿急和急迫性尿失禁[58]。耻骨后路径悬吊术引起的术后并发症主要为邻近血管或内脏损伤、膀胱或尿道穿孔及耻骨上疼痛等，而闭孔路径悬吊术则会出现更多有关腹股沟和腿部不适的并发症，包括出血和疼痛[37, 102]。相比之下，与耻骨后路径悬吊术和闭孔路径悬吊术相比，单切口路径悬吊术的术中损伤风险更低、术后短期和长期疼痛更少，性功能评分更高[33, 36, 79, 92, 96, 108]。

随着时间的推移，网片材料及工艺不断改进，与尿道中段悬吊术相关的术中和术后并发症均有所减少。同时，手术医生从中获得了更多的手术经验，也提高了对于术后患者潜在并发症的预防意识。

网片相关并发症和再手术率的相关报道最常见于术后网片出现阴道壁穿透。再次手术往往仅需要切除显露的网片，手术范围相对局限。因为显露的网片很容易在阴道内探查到，所以，条件允许的情况下，可以在门诊或门诊手术室完成治疗。如果显露的范围比较小（<1cm），对于性生活不活跃的女性，可以随访观察或阴道局部使用雌激素治疗[48]。当然，因为术中操作不当或术后伤口愈合不良甚至出现更严重的并发症，可能需要取出网片再治疗，但这类严重并发症并不常见。当然，由于多种原因，早期对于网片并发症的报道明显高于目前使用网片的手术，大多数网片相关并发症都由于网片穿透阴道壁所引起。尽管如此，术后网片穿透显露的发生率还是非常低的（<5%），对没有其他症状的患者而言，大多数情况下仅需要通过简单切除显露的网片或期待治疗即可[48, 68]。因此，网片相关并发症所导致的再手术率是非常低的。根据最近一项基于人群的大规模临床研究，从 2006 年至 2015 年，对超过 90 000 例在英格兰接受尿道中段悬吊术的女性进行回顾性研究发现，在术后 9 年内取出 / 剪除网片（部分或全部）和压力性尿失禁复发再手术的比例非常低，仅为 6.9%；仅取出 / 剪除网片（部分或全部）的比例为 3.3%；仅压力性尿失禁复发再手术的比例为 4.5%[47]。

目前的证据表明，在评估长期（>5 年）疗效和安全性时，尿道中段悬吊术在治疗合并尿道过度活动症的压力性尿失禁患者方面优于 Burch 和耻骨阴道悬吊术。虽然尿道中段悬吊术和耻骨阴道悬吊术的长期疗效（5 年）均十分可靠，但目前仍缺乏关于耻骨阴道悬吊术术后更久随访期疗效的研究数据。与尿道中段悬吊术相比，耻骨阴道悬吊术可能更容易引起术后排尿功能障碍和腹直肌筋膜损伤相关症状。

根据膀胱颈的相关作用机制，耻骨阴道悬吊术被巧妙地设计用于解决更困难的括约肌功能障碍相关压力性尿失禁[10]。相比较而言，Burch 则疗效欠佳，且会增加经腹手术相关并发症的发生率，建议仅在抢救情况下或在因其他疾病需经腹手术时同时完成[88]。

对于以上 3 种路径的尿道中段悬吊术手术而言，耻骨后路径悬吊术、闭孔路径悬吊术和单切口路径悬吊术三者在术后 5 年内的疗效相似。对于这 3 种路径，与手术相关的网片并发症都很低。而随着时间的推移，耻骨后路径悬吊术的长期有效率更稳定，但代价是术中并发症（膀胱和阴道穿孔）以及术后疼痛和排尿功能障碍的发生率更高。而采取闭孔路径悬吊术，则腹股沟疼痛、阴道网片显露和网片相关的性交困难发病率更高；相对而言，单切口路径悬吊术的术后并发症发病率较低。

八、尿道填充术的疗效与安全性

根据尿道填充术的作用机制，由于其注射后可使尿道腔变窄、拉长以提高尿道阻力，因此传统上常被用于治疗与括约肌功能障碍相关的压力性尿失禁[63]。尿道中段填充剂注射常在门诊膀胱镜检查过程中即可完成治疗，而且相关并发症的发病率较低，受到了医患双方的广泛认可[18]。

一种新的填充剂 Bulkamid®（聚丙烯酰胺水凝胶）自 2006 年以来在欧洲得到广泛使用，与其他尿道填充术相比，此产品具有良好的长期效果，并于 2020 年 1 月进入美国市场[84]。目前认为，与其他尿道填充术相比，此产品的新颖性和优势在于其是完全不可再吸收的，从而使疗效持续时间更久。和其他尿道填充术相比，此产品用于轻度及中度压力性尿失禁患者时，可获得更明显的长期疗效[29]。尽管以固化速率为标准的完全临床缓解率并不高，但至少 80% 患者认为临床症状得到了满意的缓解和改善。鉴于采用新的填充剂进行尿道中段注射手术后出现相关不良事件的风险非常低，有些学者指出，对于那些希望避免网片相关并发症的患者，以往将尿道中段悬吊术手术方案作为压力性尿失禁患者首选治疗的地位受到了来自 Bulkamid® 的挑战。然而，在最近一项针对原发性压力性尿失禁的头对头随机对照试验中，在术后 1 年的疗效评价时，客观指标以压力试验和尿垫试验均阴性作为评价标准，无张力性阴道悬吊术有效率为 95%，Bulkamid® 为 66%；主观指标以患者满意度作为评价标准，无张力性阴道悬吊术有效率为 95%，而 Bulkamid® 为 60%。其中，大约有 53% 接受 Bulkamid® 治疗的患者由于初次治疗效果不理想而接受了第二次注射治疗。因此，Bulkamid® 与尿道中段悬吊术相比，尿道中段悬吊术在治疗后 1 年时的疗效优势更显著。尽管有许多人认为因患者注射后效果不满意而需要重复手术属于治疗后“并发症”，但目前尚未发现有关 Bulkamid® 注射后需再次手术干预的相关不良事件报道。当然，在无张力性阴道悬吊术组患者中，有关网片相关并发症需要再次手术干预的不良事件发生率也非常低。由于无张力性阴道悬吊术与 Bulkamid® 在临床治愈率和患者满意度方面的优势均得到广泛肯定，因此，有观点认为：“对于希望通过初次治疗即获得完全治愈的女性，应推荐无张力阴道网片尿道中段悬吊术作为一线治疗——患者愿意并接受网片相关并发症风险”[50]。对于那些希望避免使用网片，同时又愿意接受稍逊疗效的患者而言，Bulkamid® 是一种很好的微创治疗方案。

九、国际压力性尿失禁治疗标准及现行指南

根据 2017 年 AUA/SUFU 最新发布的压力性尿失禁指南建议手术治疗方案选择主要包括：尿道中段悬吊（合成材料）、耻骨阴道自体筋膜悬吊、Burch 手术和尿道填充术（强烈推荐；证据等级：A 级）。对于选择尿道中段悬吊术的患者，医师应提供耻骨后或经闭孔尿道中段悬吊（中等推荐；证据级别：A 级），对于单切口悬吊术后的注意事项是“需告知患者其有效性和安全性的证据尚不充分”（有条件的推荐；证据级别：B 级）（图 16–4）[64]。

截至 2021 年，包括 FDA 授权的 522 项研究的结果在内的高质量长期随访数据显示，单切口路径悬吊术与闭孔路径悬吊术相比，在术后 3 年或更长时间具有相似且稳定的有效率和更高的安全性[105]。

值得注意的是，多个有关妇科泌尿领域的国内和国际专业学术团体都发表了正式的立场声明，支持 MUS 的整体安全性和有效性。美国妇科泌尿学会 / 泌尿动力学、女性盆底医学和泌尿生殖道重建学会（AUGS/SUFU）在联合立场声明中写道：“本立场声明的目的是支持在外科手术中使用无张力阴道网片进行尿道中段悬吊术来实现对压力性尿失禁的有效治疗”。同时，AUGS/SUFU 还指出：“聚丙烯网片为材料的尿道中段悬吊术是全球公认的压力性尿失禁手术治疗标准。该方案安全、有效，同时显著改善了数百万女性的生活质量”。美国妇产科医师学会（ACOG）、妇科医师协会（SGS）、国际妇科泌尿学会（IUGA）、美国尿失禁协会（NAFC）和美国妇科腹腔镜医师协会（AAGL）及美国泌尿学会（AUA）的立场声明同样倡导尿道中段悬吊术，并承认其相关的风险及获益。AUA 所宣称的意见是：“任何限制

使用合成聚丙烯网片进行尿道下悬吊术的行为都会对那些选择手术治疗压力性尿失禁的女性造成伤害"[5]。

在欧洲，欧盟新兴及新鉴定健康风险科学委员会（SCENIHR）得出结论："采用合成吊带材料的压力性尿失禁手术是一种公认的手术，由经验丰富的受过适当培训的外科医生来完成的话，在大多数中度至重度压力性尿失禁患者中被证明是有效和安全的。因此，SCENIHR 支持继续在压力性尿失禁中使用合成吊带，但同时也强调了手术需由经过适当培训的外科医生来操作，以及相关风险益处需向患者提供详细咨询的重要性。目前，有超过 2000 篇高水平文献提供的证据支持使用尿道中段悬吊术，从而使这种手术成为压力性尿失禁患者最受关注和认可的治疗方案"[32]。

与此同时，欧洲泌尿外科协会（EAU）和欧洲妇科泌尿协会（EUGA）的共识指南（2017 年修订）也认可尿道中段悬吊术对整个欧洲女性的生活质量产生了深远的积极影响，并推荐其作为普通压力性尿失禁患者的首选手术方案，同时推荐耻骨阴道悬吊术用于那些不适合尿道中段悬吊术的患者[14]。1998—2007 年，丹麦的一项全国性研究评估了 5820 例因压力性尿失禁选择尿道中段悬吊术手术治疗的患者，即使是由于合成网片尿道中段悬吊术术后再复发压力性尿失禁的情况下（5 年时仅为 6%），尿道中段悬吊术以其出色的长期疗效[39, 40]、易于操作性和安全性，使得再次手术治疗仍选择重复尿道中段悬吊术的比例高达 45.5%。

在已经得到 53 个国际妇科泌尿学会认可的全球立场声明中，国际妇科泌尿协会（IUGA）进一步认可聚丙烯网片的尿道中段悬吊术与传统手术相比不仅具有同等疗效，同时具有手术和住院时间更短等临床优势，并且手术并发症更少，恢复正常生活更快。正是这种非常有利的风险收益比"促使尿道中段悬吊术成为欧洲、亚洲、南美洲、南非、大洋洲和北美地区治疗压力性尿失禁的首选手术，目前全球范围内已有超过数百万例患者接受了此类手术"（IUGA 2014 全球立场陈述）。

总结

尽管围绕着阴道内是否可以使用网片的话题仍争论不休，但不可否认的是，迄今为止，采用无张力阴道网片尿道中段悬吊术仍然是治疗尿道过度活动相关压力性尿失禁的主要手术治疗方法。自尿道中段悬吊术问世以来，全球压力性尿失禁手术治疗的病例数量明显增加[45, 56, 83]。在美国，2000—2009 年的 10 年间，压力性尿失禁的手术治疗量大约增加了 27%。促使这一现象的原因可能是，和其他传统的手术方案（Burch、PVS、尿道填充术等）相比，尿道中段悬吊术在治疗压力性尿失禁方面具有侵入性损伤较小而疗效更好的优势[53]。尿道中段悬吊术是迄今为止研究最广泛的抗压力性尿失禁手术方案，和其他方案相比，尿道中段悬吊术具有长期（>5 年和长达 17 年）疗效更稳定而短期、中期及长期并发症发生率均较低的优势[37, 50]。因此，尿道中段悬吊术被美国泌尿学会 / 泌尿动力学、女性盆底医学和泌尿生殖道重建学会（AUA/SUFU）、美国妇科泌尿协会（AUGS）、欧洲泌尿学会（EAU）、欧洲妇科泌尿协会（EUGA）及国际妇科泌尿协会（IUGA）等多个学会组织认定为压力性尿失禁手术治疗的"金标准"[22]。

截至 2021 年，采用合成网片的尿道中段悬吊术仍然是全球治疗女性压力性尿失禁最常用的手术。虽然使用阴道网片仍存在争议和相关的医疗纠纷，但大多数医生仍然愿意继续选择尿道中段悬吊术作为女性压力性尿失禁的主要手术方案。即使在 2011 年 FDA[34] 发布了关于使用经阴道网片的安全警告后不久，99% 的美国泌尿妇科协会（AUGS）成员仍愿意选择尿道中段悬吊术作为压力性尿失禁的首选手术方案[17]。与此同时，多国医生均支持继续使用阴道网片来治疗女性压力性尿失禁。根据国际妇科泌尿协会（IUGA）的一项针对协会会员的调查报告显示，综合既往的治疗病史、与尿失禁手术同时完成的其他手术及术前相关检查评估的结果，多数医生仍将尿道中段悬吊术作为治疗压力性尿失禁的首选方法[44]。目前，越来越多的医生按照循证医学的原则来指导自己的临床工作，目的是为了可以给患者提供更好的医疗服务。因此，只有经过规范培训的医生才能够更精准的评估患者的病情，从而更加安全地选择尿道中段悬吊术来治疗压力性尿失禁。这样既可以获得满意的治疗效果，又可以控制阴道网片相关并发症的发生率，有利于尿道中段悬吊术手术的临床应用并使患者获益最大化。

参考文献

[1] Albo ME, Richter HE, Brubaker L, et al. Burch colposuspension versus fascial sling to reduce urinary stress incontinence. N Engl J Med. 2007;356:2143.
[2] Aldridge AH. Transplantation of fascia for relief of urinary stress incontinence. Am J Obstet Gynecol. 1942;44(3):398–411.
[3] Alexandridis V, Rudnicki M, Jakobsson U, Teleman P. Adjustable mini-sling compared with conventional mid-urethral slings in women with urinary incontinence: a 3-year follow-up of a randomized controlled trial. Int Urogynecol J. 2019;30(9):1465–73.
[4] American Urogynecologic Society (AUGS) and the Society for Urodynamics and FPMRS (SUFU). Position statement: mesh mid-urethral slings for stress urinary incontinence. https:// sufuorg.com/docs/guidelines/augs-sufu-mus-position-statement.aspx . Adopted 2014; Last revised 2017. Accessed March 2021.
[5] American Urological Association. AUA position statement on the use of vaginal mesh for the surgical treatment of stress urinary incontinence (SUI). https://www.auanet.org/guidelines/ guidelines/use-of-vaginal-mesh-for-the-surgical-treatment-of-stress-urinary-incontinence . Adopted 2011; Last revised 2019. Accessed March 2021.
[6] Bai SW, Sohn WH, Chung DJ, et al. Comparison of the efficacy of Burch colposuspension, pubovaginal sling, and tension-free vaginal tape for stress urinary incontinence. Int J Gynaecol Obstet. 2005;91:246.
[7] Bakali E, Buckley BS, Hilton P, et al. Treatment of recurrent stress urinary incontinence after failed minimally invasive synthetic suburethral tape surgery in women. Cochrane Database Syst Rev. 2013;2:CD009407.
[8] Ballester M, Bui C, Frobert JL, et al. Four-year functional results of the suburethral sling procedure for stress urinary incontinence: a French prospective randomized multicenter study comparing the retropubic and transobturator routes. World J Urol. 2012;30(1):117–22.
[9] Barnett RM. The modern Kelly plication. Obstet Gynecol. 1969;34(5):667–9.
[10] Blaivas JG, Jacobs BZ. Pubovaginal fascial sling for the treatment of complicated stress urinary incontinence. J Urol. 1991;145(6):1214–8.
[11] Brubaker L, Richter HE, Norton PA, et al. Five year continence rates, satisfaction and adverse events of burch urethropexy and fascial sling surgery for urinary incontinence. J Urol. 2012;187(4):1324–30.
[12] Burch JC. Urethrovaginal fixation to Cooper's ligament for correction of stress incontinence, cystocele, and prolapse. Am J Obstet Gynecol. 1961;81:281–90.
[13] Chaikin DC, Rosenthal J, Blaivas JG. Pubovaginal fascial sling for all types of stress urinary incontinence: long-term analysis. J Urol. 1998;160:1312.
[14] Chapple CR, Cruz F, Deffieux X, et al. Consensus statement of the European Urology Association and the European Urogynaecological Association on the use of implanted materials for treating pelvic organ prolapse and stress urinary incontinence. Eur Urol. 2017;72(3):424–31.
[15] Chughtai B, Sedrakyan A, Mao J, et al. Is vaginal mesh a stimulus of autoimmune disease? Am J Obstet Gynecol. 2017a;216(5):495.
[16] Chughtai B, Sedrakyan A, Mao J, et al. Challenging the Myth: transvaginal mesh is not associated with carcinogenesis. J Urol. 2017b;198(4):884–9.
[17] Clemons JL, Weinstein M, Guess MK, et al. Impact of the 2011 FDA transvaginal mesh safety update on AUGS members' use of synthetic mesh and biologic grafts in pelvic reconstructive surgery. Female Pelvic Med Reconstr Surg. 2013;19(4):191–8.
[18] Corcos J, Collet JP, Shapiro S, et al. Multicenter randomized clinical trial comparing surgery and collagen injections for treatment of female stress urinary incontinence. Urology. 2005;65:898.
[19] Costantini E, Kocjancic E, Lazzeri M, et al. Long-term efficacy of the trans-obturator and retropubic mid-urethral slings for stress urinary incontinence: update from a randomized clinical trial. World J Urol. 2016;34(4):585–93.
[20] Cornu JN, Sebe P, Peyrat L, et al. Midterm propective evaluation of TVT-Secur reveals high failure rate. Eur Urol. 2010;58(1):157–61.
[21] Cornu JN, Lizee D, Sebe P, et al. TVT SECUR single-incision sling after 5 years of followup: the promises made and the promises broken. Eur Urol. 2012;62(4):737–8.
[22] Cox A, Hershorn S, Lee L. Surgical management of female SUI: Is there a gold standard? Nat Rev Urol. 2013;10(2):78–89.
[23] Cundiff GW. The pathophysiology of stress urinary incontinence: a historical perspective. Rev Urol. 2004;6 Suppl 3(Suppl 3):S10–8.
[24] Deffieux X, Daher N, Mansoor A, et al. Transobturator TVT-O versus retropubic TVT: results of a multicenter randomized controlled trial of 24 months follow-up. Int Urogynecol J. 2010;21:1337.
[25] DeLancey JO. Stress urinary incontinence: where are we now, where should we go? Am J Obstet Gynecol. 1996;175(2):311–9.
[26] DeLancey JO, Trowbridge ER, Miller JM, et al. Stress urinary incontinence: relative importance of urethral support and urethral closure pressure. J Urol. 2008;179:2286.
[27] de Leval J. Novel surgical technique for the treatment of female stress urinary incontinence: transobturator vaginal tape insideout. Eur Urol. 2003;44(6):724–30.
[28] Delorme E. Transobturator urethral suspension: mini-invasive procedure in the treatment of stress urinary incontinence in women. Prog Urol. 2001;11(6):1306–13.
[29] Elmelund M, Sokol ER, Karra MM, et al. Patient characteristics that may influence the effect of urethral injection therapy for female stress urinary incontinence. J Urol. 2019;202:125–31.
[30] Enhoerning G. Simulateous recording of intravesical and intra-urethral pressure. A study on urethral closure in normal and stress incontinent women. Acta Chir Scand Suppl. 1961;Suppl 276:1–68.
[31] Enhoerning G, Miller ER, Hinman F Jr. Urethral closure studied with cineroentgenography and simultaneous bladder-urethra pressure recording. Surg Gynecol Obstet. 1964;118:507–16.
[32] European Commission Scientific Committee on Emerging and Newly Identified Health Risks. Opinion on the safety of surgical meshes used in urogynecological surgery. 2015. Available at: http://ec.europa.eu/health/scientific_committees/emerging/Opinions/index_en.htm.
[33] Fan Y, Huang Z, Yu D. Incontinence-specific quality of life measures

used in trials of sling procedures for female stress urinary incontinence: a meta-analysis. Int Urol Nephrol. 2015;47(8):1277–95.
[34] FDA, FDA safety communication: UPDATE on serious complications associated with transvaginal placement of surgical mesh for pelvic organ prolapse. 2011. http://wayback.archive-it.org/7993/20170722150848/https://www.fda.gov/MedicalDevices/Safety/AlertsandNotices/ uc m262435.htm.
[35] FDA, Considerations about surgical mesh for SUI. 2013. http://www.fda.gov/MedicalDevices/ ProductsandMedicalProcedures/ImplantsandProsthetics/UroGynSurgicalMesh/ ucm345219.htm.
[36] Foote A. Randomized prospective study comparing Monarc and Miniarc suburethral slings. J Obstet Gynaecol Res. 2015;41:127.
[37] Ford AA, Rogerson L, Cody JD, et al. Mid-urethral sling operations for stress urinary incontinence in women. Cochrane Database Syst Rev. 2017;7(7):CD006375.
[38] Ford AA, Ogah JA. Retropubic or transobturator mid-urethral slings for intrinsic sphincter deficiency-related stress urinary incontinence in women: a systematic review and meta-analysis. Int Urogynecol J. 2016;27(1):19–28.
[39] Foss Hansen M, Lose G, Schioler Kesmodel U, Gradel KO. Reoperation for urinary incontinence: a nationwide cohort study, 1998–2007. Am J Obstet Gynecol. 2016a;214(2):263.e1.
[40] Foss Hansen M, Lose G, Schioler Kesmodel U, Gradel KO. Repeat surgery after failed midurethral slings: a nationwide cohort study, 1998–2007. Int Urogynecol J. 2016b;27:1013–19.
[41] Frigerio M, Milani R, Barba M, et al. Single-incision slings for the treatment of stress urinary incontinence: efficacy and adverse effects at 10–year follow-up. Int Urogynecol J. 2021;32(1):187–91. https://doi.org/10.1007/s00192–020–04499–8. Epub 2020 Sep 9.
[42] Frigerio M, Regini C, Manodoro S, et al. Mini-sling efficacy in obese versus non-obese patients for treatment of stress urinary incontinence. Minerva Ginecol. 2017;69(6):533–7.
[43] Fusco F, Abdel-Fattah M, Chapple CR, et al. Updated systematic review and meta-analysis of the comparative data on Colposuspensions, Pubovaginal slings, and Midurethral tapes in the surgical treatment of female stress urinary incontinence. Eur Urol. 2017;72(4):567–91.
[44] Ghoniem G, Hammett J. Female pelvic medicine and reconstructive surgery practice patterns: IUGA member survey. Int Urogynecol J. 2015;26(10):1489–94.
[45] Gibson W, Wagg A. Are older women more likely to receive surgical treatment for stress urinary incontinence since the introduction of the mid-urethral sling? An examination of Hospital Episode Statistics data. BJOG. 2016;123:1386–92.
[46] Glazener CM, Cooper K. Bladder neck needle suspension for urinary incontinence in women. Cochrane Database Syst Rev. 2004;2:CD003636.
[47] Gurol-Urganci I, Geary RS, Mamza JB, et al. Long-term rate of mesh sling removal following Midurethral mesh sling insertion among women with stress urinary incontinence. JAMA. 2018;320(16):1659–69.
[48] Illiano E, Giannitsas K, Li Marzi V, et al. No treatment required for asymptomatic vaginal mesh exposure. Urol Int. 2019:1–5.
[49] Mari I, Jemma H, Wallace Sheila A, et al. Surgical interventions for women with stress urinary incontinence: systematic review and network meta-analysis of randomised controlled trials. BMJ. 2019;365:l1842.
[50] Itkonen Freitas AM, Mentula M, Rahkola-Soisalo P, et al. Tension-free vaginal tape surgery versus polyacrylamide hydrogel injection for primary stress urinary incontinence: a randomized clinical trial. J Urol. 2020;203(2):372–8.
[51] IUGA. Position statement on mid-urethral slings for stress urinary incontinence. http://www. iuga.org/?page=mus&hSearchTerms=%22midurethral+and+slings%22.
[52] IUGA. Statement in support of midurethral slings for stress urinary incontinence – on behalf of the International Urogynecological Community. http://www.iuga.org/urogynglobal.com.
[53] Jonsson Funk M, Levin PJ, Wu JM. Trends in the surgical management of stress urinary incontinence. Obstet Gynecol. 2012;119(4):845–51.
[54] Kegel AH. The physiologic treatment of poor tone and function of the genital muscles and of urinary stress incontinence. West J Surg Obstet Gynecol. 1949;57(11):527–35.
[55] Kelly HA, Dumm WM. Urinary incontinence in women, without manifest injury to the bladder. 1914. Int Urogynecol J Pelvic Floor Dysfunct. 1998;9(3):158–64.
[56] Keltie K, Elneil S, Monga A, et al. Complications following vaginal mesh procedures for stress urinary incontinence: an 8 year study of 92,246 women. Sci Rep. 2017;7:12015.
[57] Kennelly MJ, Moore R, Nguyen JN, et al. Prospective evaluation of a single incision sling for stress urinary incontinence. J Urol. 2010;184(2):604–9.
[58] Kenton K, Richter H, Litman H, et al. Risk factors associated with urge incontinence after continence surgery. J Urol. 2009;182:2805.
[59] Kenton K, Stoddard AM, Zyczynski H, et al. 5–year longitudinal followup after retropubic and transobturator mid urethral slings. J Urol. 2015;193:203.
[60] Khan ZA, Manbiar A, Morley R, et al. Long-term follow-up of a multicenter randomized controlled trial comparing tension-free vaginal tape, xenograft and autologous fascial slings for the treatment of stress urinary incontinence in women. BJU Int. 2015;115(6):968–77.
[61] King AB, Zampini A, Vasavada S, et al. Is there an association between polypropylene midurethral slings and malignancy? Urology. 2014;84(4):789–92.
[62] King AB, Goldman HB. Current controversies regarding oncologic risk associated with polypropylene midurethral slings. Curr Urol Rep. 2014;15(11):453.
[63] Klarskov N, Lose G. Urethral injection therapy: what is the mechanism of action? Neurourol Urogy. 2008;27:789.
[64] Kobashi KC, Albo ME, Dmochowski RR, et al. Surgical treatment of female stress urinary incontinence: AUA/SUFU guideline. J Urol. 2017;198(4):875–83. https://www.auanet.org/ guidelines/guidelines/stress-urinary-incontinence-(sui)–guideline.
[65] Lapitan MCM, Cody JD, Mashayekhi A. Open retropubic colposuspension for urinary incontinence in women. Cochrane Database Syst Rev. 2017;2017:1–235.
[66] Laurikainen E, Valpas A, Aukee P, et al. Five-year results of a randomized trial comparing retropubic and transobturator midurethral slings for stress incontinence. Eur Urol. 2014;65:1109.
[67] Leone Roberti Maggiore U, Finazzi Agro E, Soligo M, et al. Long-term outcomes of TOT and TVT procedures for the treatment of female stress urinary incontinence: a systematic review and meta-analysis. Int Urogynecol J. 2017;28(8):1119–30.
[68] Linder B, El-Nashar SA, Carranza Leon DA, Trabuco E. Predictors of vaginal mesh exposure after midurethral sling placement: a case-control study. Int Urogynecol J. 2016;27(9): 1321–6.
[69] Lo TS, Chua S, Kao CC, et al. Five-year outcome of MiniArc single-incision sling used in the treatment of primary urodynamic stress incontinenc. J Minim Invasive Gynecol. 2018a;25(1):116–23.
[70] Lo TS, Chua S, Tan YL, et al. Ultrasonography and clinical outcomes following antiincontinence procedures (Monarc vs MiniArc): a 3–year post-operative review. PLoS One. 2018b;13(12):e0207375.
[71] Marshall VF, Marchetti AA, Krantz KE. The correction of stress incontinence by simple vesicourethral suspension. Surg Gynecol Obstet. 1949;88(4):509–18.
[72] McGuire EJ, Lytton B. Pubovaginal sling procedure for cure of stress incontinence. J Urol. 1978;119:82–4.
[73] McGuire EJ, Cespedes RD, O'Connell HE. Leak-point pressures. Urol

Clin North Am. 1996;23(2):253–62.
[74] McGuire EJ. Pathophysiology of stress urinary incontinence. Rev Urol. 2004;6 Suppl 5:S11.
[75] Mock S, Angelle J, Reynolds WS, et al. Contemporary comparison between retropubic midurethral sling and autologous pubovaginal sling for stress urinary incontinence after the FDA advisory notification. Urology. 2015;85(2):321–5.
[76] Molden SM, Lucente VR. New minimally invasive slings: TVT secur. Curr Urol Rep. 2008;9(5):358–61.
[77] Morling JR, McAllister DA, Agur W, et al. Adverse events after first, single, mesh and non-mesh surgical procedures for stress urinary incontinence and pelvic organ prolapse in Scotland, 1997–2016: a population-based cohort study. Lancet. 2017;389(10069):629–40.
[78] Mostafa A, Agur W, Abdel-All M, et al. Multicenter prospective randomized study of singleincision mini-sling vs tension-free vaginal tape-obturator in management of female stress urinary incontinence: a minimum of 1-year follow-up. Urology. 2013;82:552.
[79] Mostafa A, Lim CP, Hopper L, Madhuvrata P, Abdel-Fattah M. Single-incision mini-slings versus standard midurethral slings in surgical management of female stress urinary incontinence: an updated systematic review and meta-analysis of effectiveness and complications. Eur Urol. 2014;65(2):402–27.
[80] Nambiar A, Cody JD, Jeffery ST, Aluko P. Single-incision sling operations for urinary incontinence in women. Cochrane Database Syst Rev. 2017;7(7):CD008709.
[81] Nilsson CG, Palva K, Aarnio R, et al. Seventeen years' follow up of the tension-free vaginal tape procedure for female stress urinary incontinence. Int Urogynecol J. 2013;24:1265.
[82] Novara G, Artibani W, Barber M, et al. Updated systematic review and meta-analysis of the comparative data on colposuspensions, pubovaginal slings, and midurethral tapes in the surgical treatment of female stress urinary incontinence. Eur Urol. 2010;58(2):218–38.
[83] Oliphant SS, Wang L, Bunker CH, et al. Trends in stress urinary incontinence inpatient procedures in the United States, 1979–2004. Am J Obstet Gynecol. 2009;200:521.
[84] Pai A, Al-Singary W. Durability, safety and efficacy of polyacrylamide hydrogel (Bulkamid(®)) in the management of stress and mixed urinary incontinence: three year follow up outcomes. Cent European J Urol. 2015;68(4):428–33.
[85] Palmieri S, Frigerio M, Spelzini F, et al. Risk factors for stress urinary incontinence recurrence after single-incision sling. NeurourolUrodyn. 2018;37(5):1711–6.
[86] Pereyra AJ. A simplified surgical procedure for the correction of stress incontinence in women. West J Surg Obstet Gynecol. 1959;67(4):223–6.
[87] Petros PE, Ulmsten UI. An integral theory of female urinary incontinence. Experimental and clinical considerations. Acta Obstet Gynecol Scand Suppl. 1990;153:7–31.
[88] Rashid TG, De Ridder D, Van der Aa F. The role of bladder neck suspension in the era of miurethral sling surgery. World J Urol. 2015;33:1235–41.
[89] Raz S. Modified bladder neck suspension for female stress incontinence. Urology. 1981;17(1):82–5.
[90] Raz S, Klutke CG, Golomb J. Four-corner bladder and urethral suspension for moderate cystocele. J Urol. 1989;142(3):712–5.
[91] Richter HE, Albo ME, Zyczynski HM, et al. Retropubic versus transobturator midurethral slings for stress incontinence. N Engl J Med. 2010;362:2066.
[92] Schellart RP, Oude Rengerink K, Van der Aa F, et al. A randomized comparison of a singleincision midurethral sling and a transobturator midurethral sling in women with stress urinary incontinence: results of 12-mo follow-up. Eur Urol. 2014;66:1179.
[93] Schellert RP, Zwolsman SE, Lucot JP, et al. A randomized, nonblinded extention study of single-incision versus transobturator midurethral sling in women with stress urinary incontinence. Int Urogynecol J. 2018;29:37–44.
[94] Schierlitz L, Dwyer PL, Rosamilia A, et al. Three-year follow-up of tension-free vaginal tape compared with transobturator tape in women with stress urinary incontinence and intrinsic sphincter deficiency. Obstet Gynecol. 2012;119:321.
[95] Schreiner G, Beltran R, Lockwood G, Takacs EB. A timeline of female stress urinary incontinence: how technology defined theory and advanced treatment. NeurourolUrodyn. 2020;39(6):1862–7.
[96] Schweitzer KJ, Milani AL, Van Eijndhoven HW, et al. Postoperative pain after adjustable single-incision or transobturator sling for incontinence: a randomized controlled trial. Obstet Gynecol. 2015;125:27.
[97] Shirvan MK, Rahimi HR, Darabi Mahboub MR, et al. Tension-free vaginal tape versus transobturator tape for treatment of stress urinary incontinence: a comparative randomized clinical trial study. Urol Sci. 2014;25:54.
[98] Spelzini F, Frigerio M, Regini C, et al. Learning curve for the single-incision suburethral sling procedure for female stress urinary incontinence. Int J Gynaecol Obstet. 2017;139(3):363–7.
[99] Spelzini F, Cesana MC, Verri D, et al. Three-dimensional ultrasound assessment and middle term efficacy of a single-incision sling. Int Urogynecol J. 2013;24(8):1391–7.
[100] Stamey TA. Endoscopic suspension of the vesical neck for urinary incontinence. Obstet Gynecol Surv. 1973;28(10):762–4.
[101] Stamey TA. Endoscopic suspension of the vesical neck for urinary incontinence in females. Report on 203 consecutive patients. Ann Surg. 1980;192:465.
[102] Sun X, Yang Q, Sun F, et al. Comparison between the retropubic and transobturator approaches in the treatment of female stress urinary incontinence: a systematic review and meta-analysis of effectiveness and complications. Int Braz J Urol. 2015;41:220.
[103] Ulmsten U, Henriksson L, Johnson P, Varhos G. An ambulatory surgical procedure under local anesthesia for treatment of female urinary incontinence. Int Urogynecol J Pelvic Floor Dysfunct. 1996;7(2):81–5.
[104] Wadie BS, Elhefnawy AS. TVT versus TOT, 2-year prospective randomized study. World J Urol. 2013;31:645.
[105] White AB, Kahn B, Gonzalez R, et al. Prospective study of a single-incision sling versus transobturator sling in women with stress urinary incontinence: 3-year results. Am J Obtet Gynecol. 2020;223(4):545.e1–545.e11. https://doi.org/10.1016/j.ajog.2020.03.008. Epub 2020 Mar 14.
[106] White AB, Anger JT, Eilber K, et al. Female sexual function following sling surgery: a prospective parallel multi-center study of the Solyx single incision sling system versus the Obtryx II sling system (FDA-mandated 522 results at 36 months). J Urol. 2021:101097JU0000000000001830. https://doi.org/10.1097/JU.0000000000001830. Online ahead of print.
[107] Whiteside J, Walters M. Pathophysiology of stress urinary incontinence. In: Urogynecology and Reconstructive pelvic surgery. 4th ed; 2015. p. 215–23.
[108] Zhang P, Fan B, Zhang P, et al. Meta-analysis of female stress urinary incontinence treatments with adjustable single-incision mini-slings and transobturator tension-free vaginal tape surgeries. BMC Urol. 2015;15:64.
[109] Zhu L, Lang J, Hai N, et al. Comparing vaginal tape and transobturator tape for the treatment of mild and moderate stress incontinence. A prospective randomized controlled study. Int J Gynecol Obstet. 2007;99:14.

第 17 章　自体筋膜悬吊术

Autologous Fascial Sling

Annah Vollstedt　Priya Padmanabhan　著

一、历史回顾

20 世纪初，德国外科医生首次描述了经耻骨阴道悬吊术。1910 年，Goebel 描述了通过旋转锥形肌来治疗儿童尿失禁，使锥形肌插入耻骨后的位置得以保留，但两末端在膀胱颈和尿道下方相接[1]。1914 年，Frangenheim 改进了 Goebel 的手术方法，将腹直肌膜与锥形肌一起进行悬吊[2]。此后不久，Stoeckel 首次描述了放置耻骨阴道筋膜吊带的经腹和阴道入路[3]。在这些早期技术的基础上，McGuire 在 20 世纪 70 年代首次描述了现代版本的耻骨阴道悬吊术（PVS），使用在一侧保持横向附着的腹直肌筋膜条[4]。Blaivas 和 Jacobs 于 1991 年发明了从腹直肌筋膜上获取游离移植物的当代技术，使其能够调节耻骨阴道悬吊的张力[5]。

自 1998 年获批准以来，合成网片尿道中段悬吊术取代自体筋膜悬吊术和穿刺悬吊术，成为压力性尿失禁（SUI）最常用的治疗方法[6]。然而，在 2001 年和 2008 年美国食品药品管理局发布关于经阴道网片治疗盆腔器官脱垂疾病的公共卫生通知后，用于治疗压力性尿失禁的合成网状悬吊的使用有所减少，自体筋膜悬吊的放置又有所增加[7]。

二、适应证

耻骨阴道吊带的基本机制是纠正尿道过度活动及改变因腹内压增加而引起的压力传导[8]。除了纠正尿道过度活动外，耻骨阴道吊带也适用于治疗先天性尿道固有括约肌功能障碍（ISD）。尿道固有括约肌功能障碍是指尿道固有括约肌的功能缺陷，曾经需要通过严格的尿流动力学标准才能诊断，当腹压漏尿点压低于 60mmH_2O[9] 和（或）最大尿道闭合压力低于 20cmH_2O 才能诊断为括约肌功能障碍[10]。尽管仍有临床意义，但近年来括约肌功能障碍的定义已逐渐演变为不够精确的主观诊断。国际尿控协会（ICS）现在将尿道固有括约肌功能障碍定义为“尿道闭合功能薄弱”[11]。

耻骨阴道悬吊术的其他适应证包括尿道中段悬吊失败后复发性压力性尿失禁，与神经疾病相关的压力性尿失禁或无感觉性尿失禁，尿道瘘或憩室修复后的组织加固，或者因合成材料侵蚀、长期居家导尿造成近端尿道创伤性缺损后的尿道重建。自体筋膜悬吊术可能在各种尿道重建术中发挥重要作用，包括延迟分娩、侵袭性经尿道电切术或膀胱颈破裂、骨盆创伤、肿瘤和放疗引起的尿道损伤[12]。

三、尿道力学

女性压力性尿失禁是由于尿道过度活动和（或）括约肌功能障碍所致。曾经这两者被认为是两个独立的事件，而现在我们认为这二者间存在关联[13]。据证实，失去结构性尿道支撑会导致膀胱颈和尿道下降，从而引起尿道活动过度。在具有正常解剖支撑的膀胱颈和近端尿道中，腹内压力的增加会均匀地传递到膀胱和尿道。而失去这种支撑时，腹内压力就会不均衡地传递到膀胱和尿道。在通过“压力动作”（如咳嗽、打喷嚏和大笑）增加腹内压的过程中，尿道后壁错位滑动，导致膀胱颈打开（图 17-1）。这种不均衡压力的传递和膀胱颈的打开使得压力性尿失禁发生[13]。正常尿道即使在过度活动中仍能保持闭合状态，而括约肌功能障碍的情况下，无论解剖位置如何，尿道本身都存在固有缺陷，因此尿道无法紧密贴近并保持闭合状态，尿液无法正常储存在膀胱中引起尿失禁[12]。

尿道过度活动和括约肌功能障碍的概念对于理解耻骨阴道悬吊术的作用机制很重要。耻骨阴道悬吊术位于膀胱颈，其目的是在腹部发生压力动作时压迫近端尿道，避免尿失禁的发生。如图所示，当尿道充分贴合时，可以保持正常的尿控能力[12]。当腹内压增加时，吊带向前拉动，通过向后下方旋转膀胱底和"缠紧"尿道后壁增加膀胱出口阻力，从而减少尿液漏出（图 17–2）[14]。

四、术前评估

术前评估应该尽可能详细地询问病史并进行彻底的体格检查。尤其是术者应询问与排尿相关的症状，其中包括压力性漏尿和储尿障碍情况，是否在咳嗽、打喷嚏、大笑等腹压增加后有尿液溢出，是否存在尿频、尿急、急迫性尿失禁等储尿障碍症状。同时应告知患者，这些储尿障碍症状在术后可能不会明显改善，甚至可能会加重。应注意到的是，1/3 的患者会有持续的急迫性尿失禁（UUI），约 10% 的患者会新发急迫性尿失禁[15]。同时需要详细询问的是手术史，包括所有的腹部和经阴道手术。另外需要注意，曾经接受过放射治疗可能会影响膀胱和阴道组织的质地以及括约肌功能障碍（尿道固有括约肌缺陷）的程度。

查体需要进行完整的腹部及盆腔检查，并记录既往的手术瘢痕。此外，需要注意是否存在尿道过度活动。尿道过度活动可以通过棉签试验（Q-tip）或大体可视化（以肉眼观察）来检查。进行咳嗽负荷测试，注意有无漏尿和相对充盈的膀胱。此外，还需要关注阴道组织的质地，盆腔器官是否存在脱垂，或者发现任何既往手术放置的显露的网片。由于阴道前壁的脱垂可能会导致后期发生尿路梗阻，所以对于阴道前壁脱垂的评估非常重要，需要在放置吊带的同时进行阴道前壁脱垂的修复。

应行膀胱残余尿检测。根据 2017 年美国泌尿协会 / 泌尿动力学、女性盆底医学和泌尿生殖重建学会（AUA/SUFU）的建议，对"指示病例"即

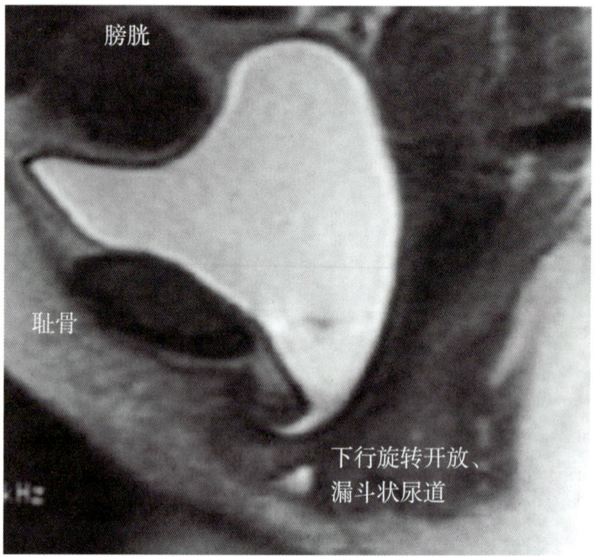

▲ 图 17–1　压力性尿失禁患者增加腹压时的矢状位 T_2 加权 MRI。腹压增加导致尿道向下旋转下降，以及膀胱颈漏斗状，导致尿道开放，继而出现漏尿

经许可转载，引自 Atlas of Vaginal Reconstructive Surgery, Raz, 2015, Springer Figure 2.7b

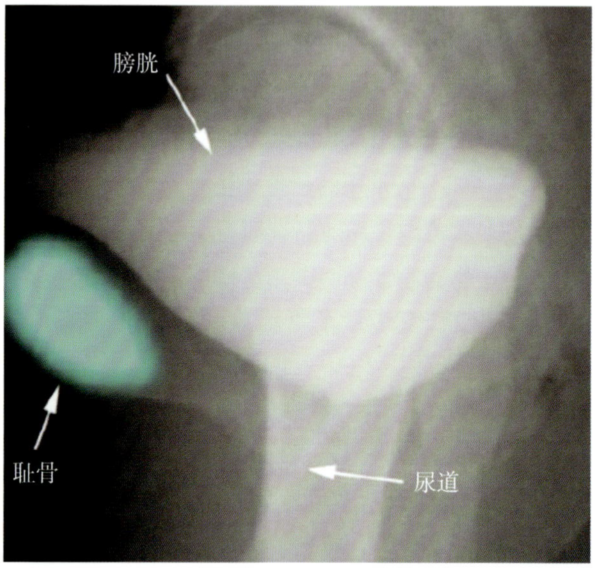

▲ 图 17–2　吊带放置后患者的侧膀胱造影。这个吊带防止尿道向下旋转和漏斗状引流。吊带可以在绷紧时正确传递腹部压力

经许可转载，引自 Atlas of Vaginal Reconstructive Surgery, Raz, Springer, 2015, Figure 2.8

既往未经历过压力性尿失禁手术治疗的单纯性压力性尿失禁和（或）以压力性尿失禁为主的混合性尿失禁（MUI）的其他方面正常的女性患者，不推荐常规进行尿流动力学检查（UDS）[16]。对于病情更加复杂的患者，可以考虑行尿流动力学检查，特别是当怀疑逼尿肌收缩功能受损或梗阻的患者。术前尿流动力学检查还可以检测到逼尿肌过度活动（DO）。通常，自体筋膜悬吊术用于治疗复发的压力性尿失禁。在这些患者中，术前通常需要进行尿流动力学检查。同时，除非担心尿路异常，否则不建议对常规在术前进行膀胱镜检查[16]。

术前应常规进行尿培养，如果发现尿路感染且还未经过正规抗感染治疗，则手术应该暂缓。

麻醉方式可以采用全身麻醉或腰麻。手术切皮前 1h 开始给予抗生素预防感染，建议选择一代或二代头孢菌素类药物。根据 2019 年美国泌尿协会（AUA）实践声明、泌尿外科手术和抗菌预防，在选择经阴道手术的预防感染方案时，应考虑覆盖厌氧菌，最常使用二代头孢菌素如头孢西丁[17]。阴道手术病例可增加甲硝唑覆盖厌氧菌和抗真菌药，尤其对于高危患者[17]。

五、手术技巧

（一）患者体位

麻醉诱导前，应在下肢放置续惯加压装置（SCD）。然后患者取膀胱截石位。术前患者的阴道一直向头侧至脐部均需做消毒准备。作者习惯使用一种 Scherbak 阴道重锤拉钩来拉开阴道后壁。膀胱放置一根 16F 的导尿管。术中将患者体位放置于适度的头低位，有利于更好显露和观察阴道前壁。可以使用阴道环形拉钩（如一次性 Lone Star® 牵开器）来进行阴唇的牵开和显露，或者也可以将大阴唇用缝线缝合到大腿内侧。

（二）获取腹直肌筋膜移植物

于耻骨联合上方约两横指处行 5～7cm 的横切口（Pfannenstiel 切口），向下分离至腹直肌筋膜水平（图 17-3A）。应用自动牵引器，如 Alexis® 切口保护器，可用于帮助牵拉皮下组织和提供良好的视野。用记号笔或者电刀在腹直肌前鞘表面做好长 8cm、宽 2cm 的边界标记。Allis 钳横向夹持固定后将用电刀将筋膜从腹直肌表面分离。切下的筋膜作为移植物放置在生理盐水中。然后在 CTX 锥形针上用 1 号聚二氧烷酮（PDS）线连续或间断重新缝合筋膜。

移植物表面的脂肪需要清理干净。移植物两端需要各缝合固定一针 1 号 PDS 缝合线，用于移植物的放置和拉紧。注意两侧的针脚要缝合均匀。将针脚锁紧，缝线留长。

（三）分离阴道

向阴道膀胱间隙注入阴道前壁生理盐水或局麻药形成阴道前壁水垫。使用 5 号刀片于阴道前壁做倒 U 形切口或正中垂直切口，切口最远端部分距尿道口约 2cm（图 17-4）。Allis 钳夹远端切口阴道壁切缘以利于反向牵引至切口最远端做标记。用手指触及导尿管球囊确定膀胱颈水平。使用 Metzenbaum 剪从尿道旁和膀胱宫颈筋膜锐性分离直至剪刀尖端能及坐骨支。排空膀胱后，组织剪向

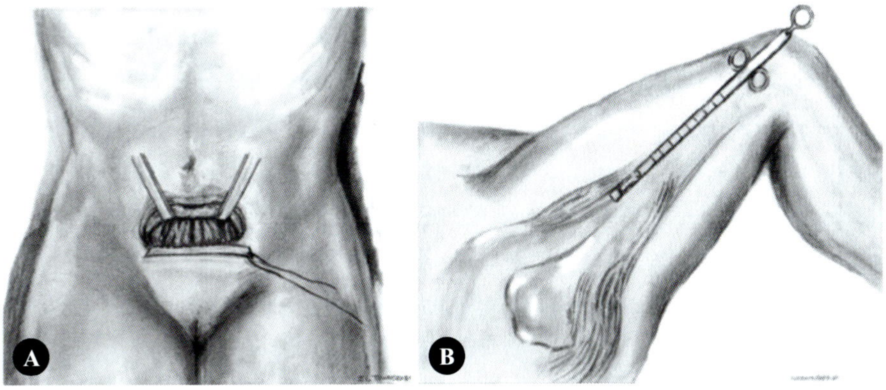

◀ 图 17-3 A. 获取腹直肌筋膜；B. 获取阔筋膜

上朝向同侧肩部，穿刺突破盆内筋膜（图 17–5）。张开剪刀向耻骨后间隙继续扩大分离面，然后示指插入切口进一步钝性分离（图 17–6）以贯通耻骨下和耻骨后间隙，从而完全游离膀胱颈，此时可触及内侧的膀胱壁，但应注意避免向膀胱侧暴力操作损伤膀胱。

（四）吊带放置和固定

穿刺前应充分排空膀胱。对于吊带的放置，作者更倾向于使用 15°Stamey 针。部分外科医生也使用过长钳，如扁桃体夹钳或 Raz 穿刺针。通过之前做的耻骨上切口，Stamey 针从耻骨后通过，紧贴耻骨后下行（图 17–7）。一只手的示指置于之前分离的同侧阴道切口内接应针尖，以控制远端针尖，引导其通过耻骨后间隙，穿过盆底筋膜，从阴道前壁切口穿出。注意当穿刺时针头和示指之间不应触及组织，如果在手指和针头之间感觉到较厚一层组织，可能为膀胱。在这种情况下，需要进一步仔细分离，以避免膀胱损伤。

穿刺针通过后，需要用 30° 或 70° 硬性膀胱镜进行检查，以排除膀胱或尿道损伤。为避免发生膀胱延迟性损伤，笔者认为这一步骤不可省。2010 年 AUA 尿失禁手术治疗指南更新指出，术中膀胱尿道镜检查被认为是标准治疗[15]。如果发现

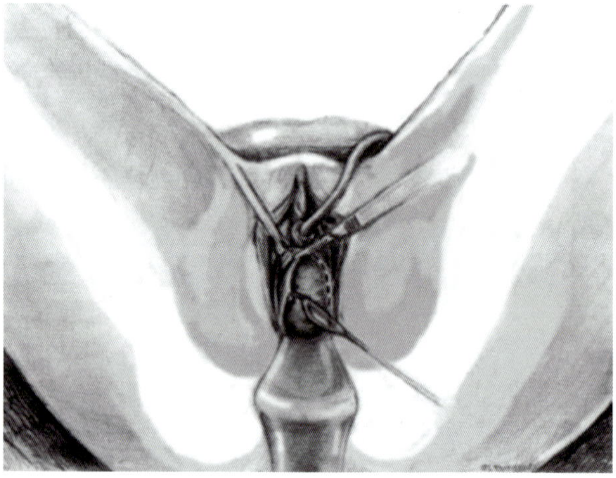

▲ 图 17–4　阴道前壁的倒 U 形切口
引自 Dmochowski et al.[12]

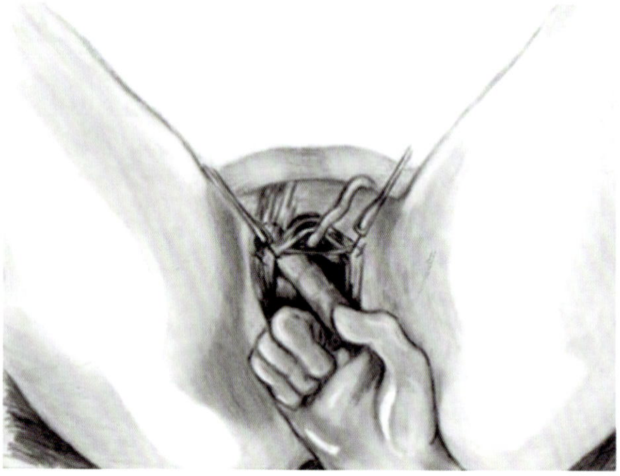

▲ 图 17–6　钝性分离耻骨后间隙
引自 Dmochowski et al.[12]

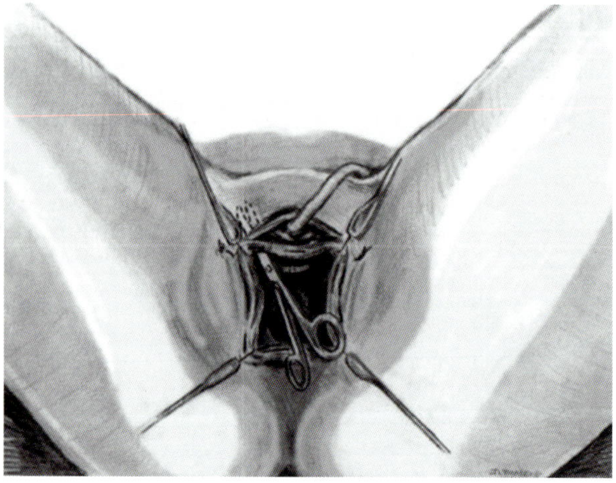

▲ 图 17–5　盆腔内筋膜穿刺
引自 Dmochowski et al.[12]

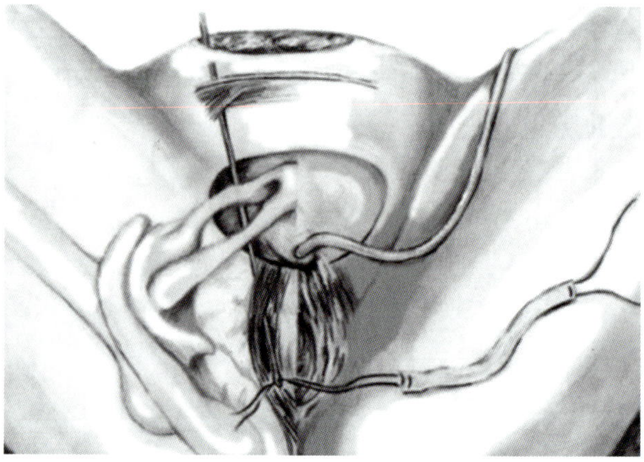

▲ 图 17–7　**Stamey** 针从耻骨后穿过，通过阴道切口从膀胱和尿道外侧穿出
引自 Dmochowski et al.[12]

膀胱损伤，退出 Stamey 针，排空膀胱后重新选择穿刺方向。一旦 Stamey 针就位，退出导尿管并再次行膀胱镜检查。确定无膀胱穿孔，导针位置合适，无尿道损伤后，即可将吊带牵引线穿入针孔中，退出穿刺器将悬吊线穿出腹直肌前鞘，穿刺器通过腹部切口向上拉，通过腹部切口取出缝线末端，并用止血钳固定缝合线。吊带长度应足够长，使其可完全穿透进入耻骨后间隙（图 17-8）。使用两根单股 4-0 合成可吸收缝合线将吊带的中点缝合到尿道的近端 1/3 处。

作者的经验是在调整吊带张力前关闭阴道切口并取出阴道重锤拉钩，以消除可能影响最终吊带松紧度的因素。冲洗阴道切口并检查止血情况，然后使用连续 2-0 合成可吸收缝合线闭合阴道切口。

PDS 吊带牵引线打结应在腹直肌筋膜上方以提供给吊带张力。部分术者调整吊带张力时会使用 30° 硬性膀胱镜直接观察近端尿道的顺应性。作者的做法是在导尿管在位的情况下进行拉紧（图 17-9）。最后，缝线在腹直肌筋膜上方的中心打结，腹直肌筋膜和缝线结之间应能容 1～2 根手指宽度以保证充足的松弛度。然而，张力的大小可能因患者的解剖结构、尿道活动度，以及是否引起尿潴留或闭合膀胱出口的手术而异。没有标准化的手段来确定吊带的合适张力。

在某些情况下，可能需要使用闭塞筋膜吊带完全闭合膀胱出口，如难治性压力性尿失禁、尿道糜烂和膀胱出口功能不全，通常同时进行经腹膀胱增容术或耻骨上膀胱造瘘。膀胱颈筋膜吊带术可能优于膀胱颈闭合术，因为紧急情况下仍可使用导管进入膀胱。应避免吊带过度拉紧，防止尿道侵蚀或损伤。

冲洗腹壁切口并充分止血后，逐层闭合切口，以降低形成血肿的风险。留置尿管，阴道内填塞纱布卷。

（五）阔筋膜吊带注意事项

如果肥胖症患者或接受过多次腹部手术的患者，尤其是腹壁成形术或疝修补术，选择阔筋膜会优于腹直肌筋膜（图 17-10）。为了获取阔筋膜，应将大腿内旋内收，消毒大腿前外侧，铺巾范围为股骨大转子至髌骨远端。触诊并标记股骨大转子和股骨外侧髁（表示阔筋膜的内侧和外侧附着点）。在髌骨正上方髂胫束做 3cm 横向切口，向下游离脂肪层至阔筋膜水平。在阔筋膜上做两个垂直于皮肤切口、沿筋膜纤维方向、相距 2cm 的平行切口，钝性分离筋膜与筋膜下肌肉，避免损伤肌纤维。然后将两个平行切口连接起来，并

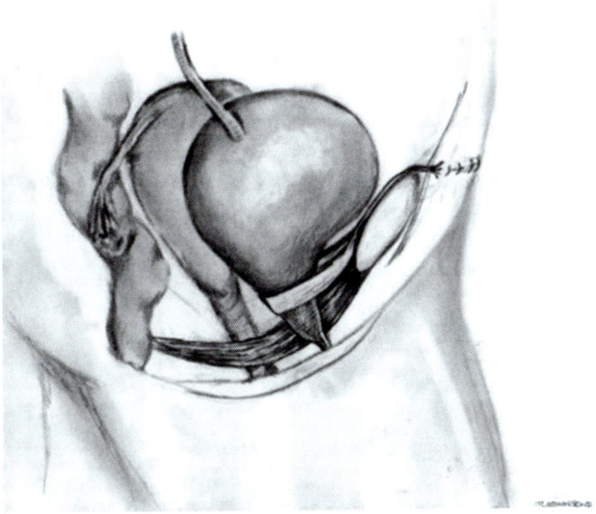

▲ 图 17-8　筋膜吊带在位的矢状面，位于耻骨后间隙及膀胱颈部
引自 Dmochowski et al.[12]

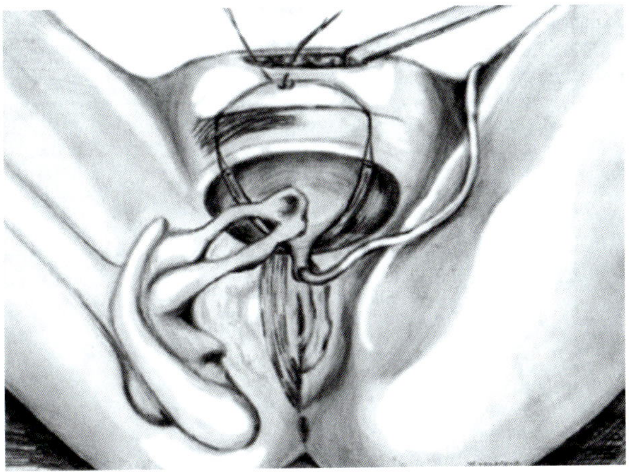

▲ 图 17-9　吊带的拉紧和固定
引自 Dmochowski et al.[12]

使用2-0不可吸收单股缝合线水平褥式缝合固定该端游离阔筋膜。在准备切取的部分阔筋膜正下方放置可延伸牵开器，使其与下方肌肉分离。将Crawford剥离器伸入切口，向上推进至所需长度[18]（图17-3B）。如果没有Crawford剥离器，可以通过在髌骨上约3指横向4cm切开皮肤，“徒手”剥离约6cm×2cm的阔筋膜。可以间隔1cm通过电刀标记移植物的边界。

经过冲洗和严格止血后，不用修补筋膜缺损，直接缝合皮下组织和皮肤，伤口表面放置加压绷带。加压敷料应保留至少8h或直至术后第1天早晨，鼓励患者早期下床活动[19]。

（六）术后护理

术后第1天取出阴道内填塞的纱布，拔除导尿管。患者可在确认正常排尿且未见残余尿后出院。如果排尿后残余尿较高，则再次留置尿管5天内重复排尿试验或可教授患者行间歇性自导尿。应指导患者术后3个月内不得做重体力活动，避免搬重物等增加腹压的活动。术后2个月内禁止阴道内用药及性生活，性生活可在2个月后复查无殊后恢复。

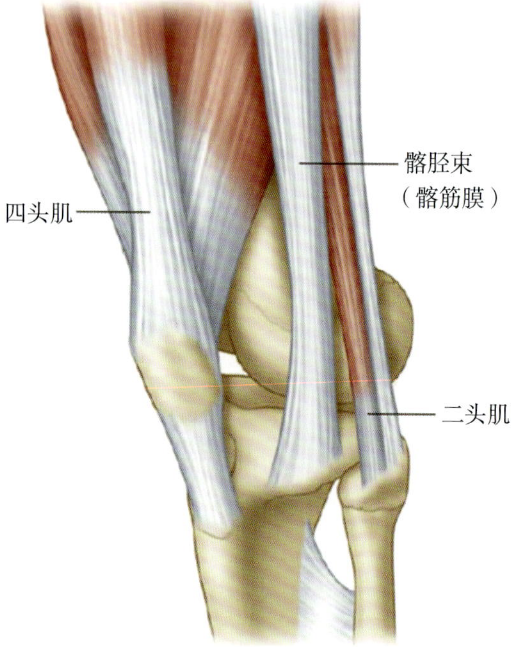

▲ 图17-10 阔筋膜张肌和臀大肌形成一个延伸到胫骨的腱膜，称为髂胫束，它下方附着于胫骨外侧髁

经许可转载，引自Atlas of Vaginal Reconstructive Surgery, Raz, Spring, 2015, Figure 2.66

六、结局和并发症

（一）治愈率/改善率

McGuire对自体耻骨阴道吊带的原始研究显示，他的52例患者中有50例的压力性尿失禁有改善。之后，Blaivas等报道了成功率为82%[4, 5]。在更近期的研究中，根据对治愈率的定义不同，治愈率为31%～100%[12, 20]。困难在于尿失禁手术后改善或治愈的客观和主观测量之间缺乏直接的相关性。根据美国泌尿学会2010年关于压力性尿失禁手术治疗的综述，未进行脱垂手术的自体筋膜吊带的治疗/干化率在12～23个月时为90%，48个月或更长时间时为82%[15]。其他一些回顾性和队列研究已经发表，表17-1总结了基于现有的随机对照试验的结果数据。

压力性尿失禁手术治疗疗效试验（SISTEr）于2012年发表，将655例患者随机分为两组，一组采用自体筋膜悬吊，另一组采用Burch阴道悬吊。主要结果是术后24个月的总体尿失禁（包括自我报告症状、尿垫称重试验和尿失禁的进一步药物或手术治疗）和特异性压力测量（包括自我报告症状和阴性压力测试）。自体筋膜吊带对混合性尿失禁（47% vs. 38%，P=0.01）及压力性尿失禁（66% vs. 49%，P<0.001）[22]都有较好的疗效。然而，Burch阴道镜悬吊组的尿路感染率（32% vs. 48%）和术后排尿功能障碍率（2% vs. 14%）较低（P<0.001）。为减少排尿症状或改善尿潴留而进行的所有后续手术仅在PVS组，其中19例患者共接受了20次手术[22]。5年SISTEr扩展研究的结果表明，尽管排尿障碍发生率高，接受自体筋膜悬吊手术的女性仍具有较高的满意度[23]。

2017年，一项Cochrane评价显示，使用自体筋膜手术的患者压力性尿失禁症状在1年内和1年后都有明显的改善。没有证据表明自体筋膜与其他材料在围术期并发症或术后发病方面存在差

表 17-1 涉及筋膜吊带的随机对照试验结果总结

研 究	结局评估方法	跟进时间	研究设计和结果		
			设 计	患者数目	疗 效
Albo, 2007[22] (SISTEr trial)	垫重、压力试验、排尿日记	24 个月	腹直肌筋膜悬吊术	326	66%
			Burch 手术	329	49%
Wadie, 2005[26]	压力试验，完全干燥，不使用垫	9 个月	腹直肌筋膜悬吊术	15	92%
			TVT	17	92.9%
Al-Azzawi, 2014[60]	患者感觉干燥，压力试验，Q_{max}＞15ml/s	1 年	腹直肌筋膜悬吊术	40	98%
			TOT	40	95%
Basok, 2008[61]	尿垫试验，患者问卷	12 个月	悬吊阔筋膜	67	79%
			阴道内吊带成形术	72	70.8%
Khan, 2015[62]	患者报告“完全干燥”或“改善”	10 年	自体悬吊术	61	75.4%
			异种移植悬吊术	38	73%
			TVT	63	58%
Bai, 2005[63]	无压力性尿失禁的患者报告，压力试验	12 个月	腹直肌筋膜悬吊术	28	92.8%
			TVT	31	87%
			Burch 手术	33	87.8%
Tcherniakovsky, 2009[64]	尿流动力学，压力测试	12 个月	腹直肌筋膜悬吊术	20	95%
			TOT	21	90.5%
Culligan, 2003[65]	应力试验，垫重	73 个月	悬吊术	17	100%
			Burch 手术	19	82%
Amaro, 2009[a][66]	完全干燥，不使用垫	44 个月	腹直肌筋膜悬吊术	21	57%
			TVT	20	65%
Guerrero, 2010[67]	患者报告完全干燥或好转	12 个月	腹直肌筋膜悬吊术	79	90%
			TVT	72	93%
			同种异体移植物悬吊术	50	61%
Sharifiaghdas, 2008[68]	压力试验	40 个月	腹直肌筋膜悬吊术	36	83%
			TVT	25	80%
Sharifiaghdas, 2017[69]	压力试验	10.5 年	腹直肌筋膜悬吊术	36	84%
			TVT	25	80%
Sharma, 2020[70]	失禁问题国际咨询问卷得分	6 个月	腹直肌筋膜悬吊术	15	100%
			TOT	15	100%
Kuprasertkul, 2019[71]	无须再次手术时间	15.1 年	腹直肌筋膜悬吊术	15	90%
			Burch 手术	14	80.8%

PVS 在术后疗效及随访问卷等评价指标中均不如对照组。上表为 TVT、PVS、Burch 术、TOT 术后在压力性尿失禁、尿流动力学、失禁问题国际咨询问卷得分中的比较

异[24]。然而，这些研究规模较小，随访时间短，尤其未比较与网片相关的并发症。此外，这些研究没有根据压力性尿失禁的术前严重程度对结果进行分层。

一项大型队列研究比较了79例筋膜悬吊患者（由泌尿科医生进行）和163例合成网尿道中悬吊患者（由妇科医生进行）的3年结果。合成网片组在任何尿失禁、严重尿失禁和压力性尿失禁的治疗成功率均高于自体筋膜吊带组。并发症方面无差异；然而，自体筋膜组有较高的尿潴留发生率，需要清洁的间歇导尿、尿道松解术或长期使用耻骨上膀胱造瘘[25]。在53例患者的随机试验中，自体筋膜组和TVT的治愈率没有差异[26]。

（二）排尿功能障碍/尿急迫/尿潴留

术后排尿功能障碍是自体筋膜悬吊术后最重要的并发症。排尿功能障碍可表现为一系列症状，从尿急到尿潴留。新发的急迫性尿失禁率为3%～20%，术后急迫性尿失禁率为8%～25%[15, 18, 27]。美国泌尿学会2010年的Meta分析报道称，在术前有急迫性尿失禁（UUI）患者中，33%的患者在压力性尿失禁症状[15]消退的情况下仍持续存在急迫性尿失禁。

据报道，与Burch手术和合成网片尿道中悬吊相比，自体筋膜悬吊的排尿功能障碍发生率更高。SISTEr试验报告显示，筋膜悬吊组有14%的患者出现排尿障碍，而Burch手术组只有2%出现排尿障碍（$P<0.001$）[22]。

Athnan Scpoulos等的另一项研究报道，超过260例接受筋膜悬吊术的患者，10%出现术后排尿功能障碍[27]。大多数2个月后缓解，但5例（1.9%）的患者需要行尿道松解术[27]。

逼尿肌过度活动和逼尿肌收缩功能受损（膀胱活动不足）也可能加剧筋膜吊带引起的医源性出口梗阻。虽然术后尿急和急迫性尿失禁与手术失败密切相关，但目前还没有研究对筋膜吊带术的术前危险因素的共识。先前的研究表明，膀胱残余尿量>100ml或Q_{max}≤20ml/s可能导致长时间清洁间歇导尿的风险更高，但这些尿流动力学因素还没有达到统计意义[28]。同样，Nager等分析了参与SISTEr试验的患者的术前和术后尿流动力学数据，发现逼尿肌过度活动和Valsalva漏点压力水平不能预测术后排尿功能障碍或接受筋膜悬吊术[29]的患者的手术修补风险。

术后尿潴留被定义为持续时间超过1个月或需要干预。在未同时进行脱垂治疗的情况下术后尿潴留率估计为8%，低于术后尿急或急迫性尿失禁。在同时进行脱垂治疗的情况下为5%。医源性梗阻的风险最可能与手术技术有关。吊带张力过高时，膀胱颈过度向耻骨抬高，导致尿道膀胱角[12]“过度悬吊”或过度矫正。

正确拉紧吊带是手术中最复杂的部分，不同的外科医生使用不同的技术。在Preece等最近的一项研究中，当缝线在直肌筋膜上方打结时，调节悬吊的高度可以预测术后排尿功能障碍。作者表明，悬吊高度<40mm的松弛悬吊与术后潴留的高风险相关，需要间歇性自我导尿和尿道松解术[30]。

最重要的临床因素是吊带放置和出现排尿症状之间的时间关系。体格检查可发现尿道角度异常或尿道不活动。应该记录残余尿量，尽管对于“正常”值的特定（ut-off值）没有达成共识。膀胱镜检查可能有助于排除膀胱病变、吊带侵蚀和尿道过度悬吊。可视尿流动力学也有助于评估梗阻、逼尿肌过度活动或活动不足。然而，也有研究表明，当排尿症状或尿潴留是吊带放置后干预的主要指征时，尿流动力学结果不能预测解除梗阻[31]干预后的结果。

尚无对于术后排尿功能障碍的处理共识。短暂性尿潴留是常见的，大多数患者在最初10天内恢复自主排尿。因此，如果排尿后残余尿仍然很高，或者患者出现新的或加重的尿急或急迫性尿失禁，在决定行尿道松解前，作者建议通过定时排尿、二次排尿、生物反馈、盆底肌训练、抗毒蕈碱药物和清洁间歇导尿3个月来处理。筋膜吊带术后梗阻的手术处理包括经耻骨后、经阴道或经尿道上入路的尿道松解术，成功率为45%～100%[12]。持续性或反复性梗阻、逼尿肌过度活动、逼尿肌收缩功能受损或习得性排尿功能障碍均可导致尿道松解术[12]失败。然而，最常见的原因是尿道的不完全松解。在一项对 24 例患者的小型研究中，患者接受了重复的尿道松解术，外科医生通过经阴道或耻骨后入路对所有 24 例患者进行了“积极的”尿道松解术。24 例患者中有 22 例尿潴留得到缓解。然而，只有 12% 的情况下急迫性尿失禁得到了完全解决。作者的结论是，在第一次失败后或初次尿道松解术的情况未知时，考虑再次尿道松解术是合理的[33]。可以理解的是，患者可能会担心尿道松解术后压力性尿失禁复发的风险；然而，据报道，这一比率相对较低（0%～34%）[12, 33]。

（三）侵蚀和挤压

与合成网片材料相比，自体筋膜耻骨阴道吊带后尿道侵蚀及阴道挤压极为罕见。Leach 等研究显示，接受自体和同种异体移植[34]吊带的患者尿道侵蚀率为 0.003%，阴道挤压率为 0.0001%。导致自体筋膜吊带尿道糜烂的原因通常是围术期的技术，包括不正确的吊带通道的穿刺技术，吊带的位置，过紧的张力，或者术后立即插导尿管。处理包括切除被侵蚀的部分吊带和尿道闭合[35]。

（四）其他并发症

总体围术期尿路感染率为 11%～48%[15, 22]。耻骨后穿刺不当导致膀胱损伤的比例为 4%[15]。据报道，伤口并发症发生率为 8%[15]。2015 年的一项 Meta 分析比较了合成材料尿道中段悬吊术（MUS）和自体筋膜吊带，发现尿道中段悬吊术有更高的侵蚀率、盆腔疼痛和新发的膀胱过度尿道中段悬吊术综合征，而自体筋膜吊带术有增加伤口感染的风险[36]。最近的一项系统综述和 Meta 分析比较了不同压力性尿失禁治疗方法，结果显示，与 Burch 膀胱尿道悬吊术[37]相比，自体筋膜悬吊术可降低伤口感染、膀胱或阴道穿孔和肠道损伤的发生率。

七、合成网片悬吊术后的自体筋膜悬吊

自体筋膜悬吊可用于治疗经合成网片尿道中段悬吊术后复发或症状持续的压力性尿失禁患者。Petrou 等对 21 例尿道中段悬吊术失败后进行自体筋膜悬吊的患者进行至少持续 36 个月随访的一项回顾性研究，该研究发现约 3/4 的患者术后症状改善，术后无尿失禁表现或仅有轻度尿失禁，总体而言，86% 的患者表示满意并愿意向其他患者推荐[38]。同样的，Milose 等在对 16 例前次吊带手术失败后接受挽救自体筋膜悬吊术的单纯压力性尿失禁患者随访中发现有 70% 的治愈率[39]。

一篇关于 SISTEr 和尿道中段悬吊术（TOMUS）的二次分析文献显示，自体筋膜悬吊的再治疗率为 5%，而 Burch 膀胱尿道悬吊术为 10%，经闭孔尿道中段悬吊术为 6%，耻骨后尿道中段悬吊术为 4%。绝大多数的患者采取自体筋膜悬吊作为补救治疗措施[40]。

如何及何时移除原先放置的尿道中段吊带网片目前尚无定论[39]。某些术者选择移除吊带并一次性进行自体筋膜悬吊手术，而另一些术者选择分次手术。Parker 等在近期一项比较自体筋膜悬吊作为首选 / 尿道中段悬吊术失败后的补充治疗方式的前瞻性研究中发现：尿道中段悬吊失败原因包括复发性压力性尿失禁、吊带挤压或梗阻；在中位随访时间 15 个月中，两组在尿垫使用数目和患者疗效评估问卷调查方面均有明显改善；两组并发症发生率没有差异；尿道中段悬吊术尿潴留的发生率（8.5%）较首选自体筋膜悬吊组（3.1%）更高；尿道中段悬吊术术后进行自体筋膜悬吊组需要额外尿失禁治疗的发生率为 13.6%，而首选自体筋膜悬吊组的为 3.5%[41]。

自体筋膜悬吊不是治疗尿道中段悬吊术术后复发压力性尿失禁的唯一选择。某些术者选择进行二次尿道中段悬吊术。Aberger 等对 224 例尿道中段悬吊术失败后接受耻骨后尿道中段悬吊术（153 例或 68.3%）和自体筋膜悬吊术（ARFS）（71 例或 31.6%）的患者进行中位随访时间为 29 个月

（最少 12 个月）的回顾性比较中发现，尿道中段悬吊组的总治愈率为 61.4%，自体筋膜悬吊术组为 66.1%，两组无统计学差异[42]。

八、腹直肌筋膜 / 阔筋膜

许多泌尿专家由于更为熟悉腹壁解剖从而倾向使用腹直肌筋膜，此外，许多人认为获取腹直肌筋膜而造成的腹壁切口比在大腿侧面取阔筋膜更隐蔽。切取阔筋膜的优点则包括潜在的低术后疼痛率、更低的血肿、切口疝发生率和获得更强韧的移植物。一项研究发现阔肌筋膜的拉伸强度是腹直肌筋膜的 4 倍，阔肌筋膜的纵向纤维可能比腹直肌筋膜的水平纤维更具支撑力[43, 44]。此外，有腹部广泛手术史的患者获取阔筋膜较获取腹直肌筋膜可能更为容易。使用阔筋膜的缺点包括定位难度及第二切口的并发症。

最近一项通过比较 21 例使用阔筋膜和 84 例腹直肌筋膜患者的手术结果的回顾性研究发现：两组手术时间相似；阔肌筋膜组的估计失血量较腹直肌筋膜组低，是唯一具有统计学意义的差异；阔筋膜组的住院时间更短，伤口并发症更少，Clavien 2 级及以上的并发症更少，但围术期结局无统计学差异；两组在 1 个月、1 年和最后一次随访时的干燥率相似[45]。

九、自体移植与同种异体移植的比较

为了减少手术时间、术后病率、疼痛和住院时间，使用同种异体材料（取自另一个人的组织）变得越来越流行。相较于同种异体材料，自体材料具有完全的生物相容性。自体筋膜悬吊后的组织学检查结果显示广泛的成纤维细胞浸润和新生血管形成，炎症反应最小[46]。

研究表明，对于取材自尸体的同种异体移植材料的处理可能会破坏移植物的完整性，从而导致较高的远期失败率。移植物特殊的处理技术的也会影响组织的完整性，不同于溶剂脱水，组织冷冻会导致冰晶形成而破坏胶原基质，从而削弱组织[47]。移植物进行冷冻或冻干处理其失败率为 6.0%～38%[12]。因此，在同种异体移植材料的处理中，溶剂脱水占主导。

在使用同种异体材料进行移植时，术者必须考虑材料中 DNA 和蛋白质移植进而增加传染病传播的风险。理论上同种异体移植有由朊病毒导致感染的可能，而其相关的人类免疫缺陷病毒的传播可能发生在 1/800 万的病例中[48-50]。术前告知同种异体移植材料来自人体组织是必需的，某些患者由于宗教信仰或道德认知反对使用来自他人的组织材料。

研究者对使用自体筋膜与同种异体筋膜进行经阴道悬吊手术的效果进行了比较。文献结论不一致。一些文献报道了两者具有同样的高成功率，且在并发症方面没有差异，认为使用同种异体材料移植减少手术时间和降低发病率[51, 52]。另一些文献则提示使用同种异体材料效果差于自体筋膜，导致复发和较高的再次手术率[53-56]。我们需要进行更大规模的长期的随机性前瞻性研究，进行使用自体筋膜和溶剂脱水尸体同种异体筋膜手术效果的比较。表 17-2 概述了同种异体移植与自体移植的优缺点。

表 17-2　自体移植与同种异体移植的比较

	同种异体移植	自体移植
优点	• 较小的耻骨上切口 • 缩短手术时间 • 减少手术疼痛	• 完全的生物相容性 • 最小的组织反应
缺点	• 成本增加 • 抗拉强度较低 • 传播传染病的风险，如艾滋病病毒和朊病毒	• 延长手术时间 • 需要术前定位[a] • 耻骨上血肿的风险[b] • 耻骨上切口疝的风险[b]

a. 特指阔肌筋膜的获取
b. 特指腹直肌筋膜的获取

十、应用自体筋膜经闭孔悬吊

目前，应用自体筋膜经闭孔悬吊引起了关注。在埃及的一项研究中，研究者使用一条中间有自体筋膜、侧面有 2 条聚丙烯臂的材料经闭孔悬吊，1 年后显示主观治愈率的 90.5%，由咳嗽压力试验阴性作为治愈标准的客观治愈率为 93%[57]。2020 年的一项研究中，2 例尿道憩室治疗后的患者放置了类似的材料，结果显示术后 6 个月 2 例患者均无压力性尿失禁[58]。也许最大的研究来自 Cubuk 等，研究者对 36 例接受了自体筋膜经闭孔悬吊术的患者与 81 例传统的经闭孔悬吊术的患者进行了比较，发现在 12 个月时两组的主观或客观治愈率没有差异[59]。目前需要更大规模、随访时间更长的随机试验来进一步评估自体筋膜在经闭孔悬吊术中的应用。

参考文献

[1] Zacharin RF. Abdominoperineal urethral suspension in the management of recurrent stress incontinence of urine- a 15-year experience. Obstet Gynecol. 1983;62(5):644–54.
[2] Frangenheim P. Zur operativen Behandlung der Inkontinenz der männlichen Harnröhre. Verh Dtsch Ges Chir. 1914;43:149–56.
[3] Stoeckel W. Über die Verwendung der Musculi pyramidales bei der operativen Behandlung der Incontinentia urinae. Zentralbl Gynak. 1917;41:11–9.
[4] McGuire EJ, Lytton B. Pubovaginal sling procedure for stress incontinence. J Urol. 1978;119(1):82–4.
[5] Blaivas JG, Jacobs BZ. Pubovaginal fascial sling for the treatment of complicated stress urinary incontinence. J Urol. 1991;145(6):1214–8.
[6] Geller EJ, Wu JM. Changing trends in surgery for stress urinary incontinence. Curr Opin Obstet Gynecol. 2013;25(5):404–9.
[7] Rac G, et al. Stress urinary incontinence surgery trends in academic female pelvic medicine and reconstructive surgery urology practice in the setting of the food and drug administration public health notifications. Neurourol Urodyn. 2017;36(4):1155–60.
[8] Blaivas JG, Olsson CA. Stress incontinence: classification and surgical approach. J Urol. 1988;139(4):727–31.
[9] Wan J, et al. Stress leak point pressure: a diagnostic tool for incontinent children. J Urol. 1993;150(2 Pt 2):700–2.
[10] McGuire EJ. Urodynamic findings in patients after failure of stress incontinence operations. Prog Clin Biol Res. 1981;78:351–60.
[11] D'Ancona CD, Haylen B, Oelke M, Herschorn S, Abranches-Monteiro L, Arnold EP, Goldman HB, Hamid R, Homma Y, Marcelissen T, Rademakers K, Schizas A, Singla A, Soto I, Tse V, de Wachter S. An International Continence Society (ICS) report on the terminology for adult male lower urinary tract and pelvic floor symptoms and dysfunction. Neurourol Urodyn. 2019.
[12] Dmochowski RR, Padmanabhan P, Scarpero HM. Slings: autologous, biologic, synthetic, and midurethral. In: Kavoussi LR, Wein AJ, Novick AC, editors. Campbell-Walsh urology. 10th ed. Philadelphia: Elsevier-Saunders; 2012. p. 2115–67.
[13] Chapple CR, Milson I. Urinary incontinence and pelvic prolapse: epidemiology and pathophysiology. In: Wein A, editor. Campbell-Walsh urology. Philadelpia: Elsevier; 2012.
[14] Plagakis S, Tse V. The autologous pubovaginal fascial sling: an update in 2019. Low Urin Tract Symptoms. 2020;12(1):2–7.
[15] Dmochowski RR, et al. Update of AUA guideline on the surgical management of female stress urinary incontinence. J Urol. 2010;183(5):1906–14.
[16] Kobashi KC, et al. Surgical treatment of female stress urinary incontinence: AUA/SUFU guideline. J Urol. 2017;198(4):875–83.
[17] Lightner DJ, et al. Best practice statement on urologic procedures and antimicrobial prophylaxis. J Urol. 2020;203(2):351–6.
[18] Blaivas JG, et al. Surgery for stress urinary incontinence: autologous fascial Sling. Urol Clin North Am. 2019;46(1):41–52.
[19] Dwyer NT, et al. Fascia lata sling. In: Raz LVRS, editor. Female urology. W.B. Saunders; 2008. p. 406–14.
[20] Mahdy A, Ghoniem GM. Autologous rectus fascia sling for treatment of stress urinary incontinence in women: a review of the literature. Neurourol Urodyn. 2019;38 Suppl 4:S51–8.
[21] Padmanabhan P, Nitti VW. Female stress urinary incontinence: how do patient and physician perspectives correlate in assessment of outcomes? Curr Opin Urol. 2006;16(4):212–8.
[22] Albo ME, et al. Burch colposuspension versus fascial sling to reduce urinary stress incontinence. N Engl J Med. 2007;356(21):2143–55.
[23] Brubaker L, et al. 5-year continence rates, satisfaction and adverse events of burch urethropexy and fascial sling surgery for urinary incontinence. J Urol. 2012;187(4):1324–30.
[24] Rehman H, et al. Traditional suburethral sling operations for urinary incontinence in women. Cochrane Database Syst Rev. 2017;7(7):Cd001754.
[25] Trabuco EC, et al. Medium-term comparison of continence rates after rectus fascia or midurethral sling placement. Am J Obstet Gynecol. 2009;200(3):300.e1–6.
[26] Wadie BS, Edwan A, Nabeeh AM. Autologous fascial sling vs polypropylene tape at short-term followup: a prospective randomized study. J Urol. 2005;174(3):990–3.
[27] Athanasopoulos A, Gyftopoulos K, McGuire EJ. Efficacy and preoperative prognostic factors of autologous fascia rectus sling for treatment of female stress urinary incontinence. Urology. 2011;78(5):1034–8.
[28] Mitsui T, et al. Clinical and urodynamic outcomes of pubovaginal sling procedure with autologous rectus fascia for stress urinary incontinence. Int J Urol. 2007;14(12):1076–9.
[29] Nager CW, et al. Urodynamic measures do not predict stress continence outcomes after surgery for stress urinary incontinence in selected women. J Urol. 2008;179(4):1470–4.
[30] Preece PD, et al. Optimising the tension of an autologous fascia pubovaginal sling to minimize retentive complications. Neurourol Urodyn. 2019;38(5):1409–16.
[31] Aponte MM, et al. Urodynamics for clinically suspected obstruction after anti-incontinence surgery in women. J Urol. 2013;190(2):598–602.
[32] Cross CA, Cespedes RD, McGuire EJ. Our experience with pubovaginal slings in patients with stress urinary incontinence. J Urol. 1998;159(4):1195–8.
[33] Scarpero HM, Dmochowski RR, Nitti VW. Repeat urethrolysis after failed urethrolysis for iatrogenic obstruction. J Urol. 2003;169(3):1013–6.
[34] Leach GE, et al. Female Stress Urinary Incontinence Clinical Guidelines Panel summary report on surgical management of female stress urinary incontinence. The American Urological Association. J Urol. 1997;158(3 Pt 1):875–80.

[35] Blaivas JG, Sandhu J. Urethral reconstruction after erosion of slings in women. Curr Opin Urol. 2004;14(6):335–8.
[36] Blaivas JG, et al. Safety considerations for synthetic sling surgery. Nat Rev Urol. 2015;12(9):481–509.
[37] Schimpf MO, et al. Sling surgery for stress urinary incontinence in women: a systematic review and metaanalysis. Am J Obstet Gynecol. 2014;211(1):71.e1–71.e27.
[38] Petrou SP, et al. Salvage autologous fascial sling after failed synthetic midurethral sling: greater than 3-year outcomes. Int J Urol. 2016;23(2):178–81.
[39] Milose JC, et al. Success of autologous pubovaginal sling after failed synthetic mid urethral sling. J Urol. 2015;193(3):916–20.
[40] Zimmern PE, et al. Management of recurrent stress urinary incontinence after burch and sling procedures. Neurourol Urodyn. 2016;35(3):344–8.
[41] Parker WP, Gomelsky A, Padmanabhan P. Autologous fascia pubovaginal slings after prior synthetic anti-incontinence procedures for recurrent incontinence: a multi-institutional prospective comparative analysis to de novo autologous slings assessing objective and subjective cure. Neurourol Urodyn. 2016;35(5):604–8.
[42] Aberger M, Gomelsky A, Padmanabhan P. Comparison of retropubic synthetic mid-urethral slings to fascia pubovaginal slings following failed sling surgery. Neurourol Urodyn. 2016;35(7):851–4.
[43] Govier FE, et al. Pubovaginal slings using fascia lata for the treatment of intrinsic sphincter deficiency. J Urol. 1997;157(1):117–21.
[44] Choe JM, et al. Autologous, cadaveric, and synthetic materials used in sling surgery: comparative biomechanical analysis. Urology. 2001;58(3):482–6.
[45] Peng M, et al. Rectus fascia versus fascia lata for autologous fascial pubovaginal sling: a single-center comparison of perioperative and functional outcomes. Female Pelvic Med Reconstr Surg. 2020;26(8):493–7.
[46] Woodruff AJ, et al. Histologic comparison of pubovaginal sling graft materials: a comparative study. Urology. 2008;72(1):85–9.
[47] Lemer ML, Chaikin DC, Blaivas JG. Tissue strength analysis of autologous and cadaveric allografts for the pubovaginal sling. Neurourol Urodyn. 1999;18(5):497–503.
[48] Buck BE, Malinin TI. Human bone and tissue allografts. Preparation and safety. Clin Orthop Relat Res. 1994;303:8–17.
[49] Wilson TS, Lemack GE, Zimmern PE. Management of intrinsic sphincteric deficiency in women. J Urol. 2003;169(5):1662–9.
[50] Bayrak Ö, et al. Pubovaginal sling materials and their outcomes. Turk J Urol. 2014;40(4):233–9.
[51] Flynn BJ, Yap WT. Pubovaginal sling using allograft fascia lata versus autograft fascia for all types of stress urinary incontinence: 2-year minimum followup. J Urol. 2002;167(2 Pt 1):608–12.
[52] Elliott DS, Boone TB. Is fascia lata allograft material trustworthy for pubovaginal sling repair? Urology. 2000;56(5):772–6.
[53] Dora CD, et al. Time dependent variations in biomechanical properties of cadaveric fascia, porcine dermis, porcine small intestine submucosa, polypropylene mesh and autologous fascia in the rabbit model: implications for sling surgery. J Urol. 2004;171(5):1970–3.
[54] McBride AW, et al. Comparison of long-term outcomes of autologous fascia lata slings with suspend Tutoplast fascia lata allograft slings for stress incontinence. Am J Obstet Gynecol. 2005;192(5):1677–81.
[55] Simsiman AJ, et al. Suburethral sling materials: best outcome with autologous tissue. Am J Obstet Gynecol. 2005;193(6):2112–6.
[56] Soergel TM, Shott S, Heit M. Poor surgical outcomes after fascia lata allograft slings. Int Urogynecol J Pelvic Floor Dysfunct. 2001;12(4):247–53.
[57] El-Gamal O, et al. Use of autologous rectus fascia in a new transobturator hybrid sling for treatment of female stress urinary incontinence: a pilot study. Scand J Urol. 2013;47(1):57–62.
[58] Ito WE, et al. Hybrid Sling for the treatment of concomitant female urethral complex diverticula and stress urinary incontinence. Res Rep Urol. 2020;12:247–53.
[59] Cubuk A, et al. Modified autologous transobturator tape surgery – a prospective comparison with transobturator tape surgery. Urology. 2020.
[60] Al-Azzawi IS. The first Iraqi experience with the rectus fascia sling and transobturator tape for female stress incontinence: a randomised trial. Arab J Urol. 2014;12(3):204–8.
[61] Basok EK, et al. Cadaveric fascia lata versus intravaginal slingplasty for the pubovaginal sling: surgical outcome, overall success and patient satisfaction rates. Urol Int. 2008;80(1):46–51.
[62] Khan ZA, et al. Long-term follow-up of a multicentre randomised controlled trial comparing tension-free vaginal tape, xenograft and autologous fascial slings for the treatment of stress urinary incontinence in women. BJU Int. 2015;115(6):968–77.
[63] Bai SW, et al. Comparison of the efficacy of Burch colposuspension, pubovaginal sling, and tension-free vaginal tape for stress urinary incontinence. Int J Gynaecol Obstet. 2005;91(3):246–51.
[64] Tcherniakovsky M, et al. Comparative results of two techniques to treat stress urinary incontinence: synthetic transobturator and aponeurotic slings. Int Urogynecol J Pelvic Floor Dysfunct. 2009;20(8):961–6.
[65] Culligan PJ, Goldberg RP, Sand PK. A randomized controlled trial comparing a modified Burch procedure and a suburethral sling: long-term follow-up. Int Urogynecol J Pelvic Floor Dysfunct. 2003;14(4):229–33. discussion 233.
[66] Amaro JL, et al. Clinical and quality-of-life outcomes after autologous fascial sling and tension-free vaginal tape: a prospective randomized trial. Int Braz J Urol. 2009;35(1):60–6. discussion 66–7.
[67] Guerrero KL, et al. A randomised controlled trial comparing TVT, Pelvicol and autologous fascial slings for the treatment of stress urinary incontinence in women. BJOG. 2010;117(12):1493–502.
[68] Sharifiaghdas F, Mortazavi N. Tension-free vaginal tape and autologous rectus fascia pubovaginal sling for the treatment of urinary stress incontinence: a medium-term follow-up. Med Princ Pract. 2008;17(3):209–14.
[69] Sharifiaghdas F, et al. Long-term results of tension-free vaginal tape and pubovaginal sling in the treatment of stress urinary incontinence in female patients. Clin Exp Obstet Gynecol. 2017;44(1):44–7.
[70] Sharma JB, et al. A comparative study of autologous rectus fascia pubovaginal sling surgery and synthetic transobturator vaginal tape procedure in treatment of women with urodynamic stress urinary incontinence. Eur J Obstet Gynecol Reprod Biol. 2020;252:349–54.
[71] Kuprasertkul A, et al. Long-term results of burch and autologous aling procedures for stress urinary incontinence in E-SISTEr participants at 1 site. J Urol. 2019;202(6):1224–9.

第 18 章 压力性尿失禁手术治疗后并发症的处理

Managing Complications After Surgical Treatment of Stress Urinary Incontinence

Alyssa K. Gracely 著

随着人口老龄化，压力性尿失禁（SUI）的年发病率据报道为 4%～10%[1]，一些研究报告显示中老年女性的年发病率高达 14.9%[2]。因为压力性尿失禁发病呈稳步上升趋势，所以不仅需要迫切的对压力性尿失禁进行管理方案研究，而且需要对每种治疗方案可能出现的潜在并发症进行探讨。通过对潜在的较高并发症发生率的比较发现，手术治疗增加的成功率与侵入性较小的治疗方案增加的成功率相比是一样的。压力性尿失禁的手术治疗方案选择包括耻骨后悬吊术、经阴道缝合悬吊术、耻骨阴道吊带和尿道中段悬吊术（MUS）。虽然所有手术方案都有许多并发症，但也有一些并发症是特定于某类手术的。本章将讨论在压力性尿失禁手术治疗后可能出现的并发症，特别关注与"金标准"尿道中段悬吊术相关的并发症，因为其引起了媒体和监管机构的广泛关注。虽然前几章重点介绍了压力性尿失禁的术前评估、手术决策、手术技术和术中并发症，本章特别关注术后并发症及并发症相关的处理。

一、评估与诊断

对于压力性尿失禁手术治疗后，当患者在术后出现新的排尿症状时，需要对其进行彻底的评估。从了解他们的术前排尿习惯开始，术前和术后症状的变化以及症状发作的时间可以提供信息，观察他们出现排尿不适的病因并帮助指导治疗。回顾术前尿流动力学检查（UDS）可能有助于确定与术后尿潴留相关的因素，其中包括逼尿肌活动不足、Valsalva 排尿或术前梗阻[3, 4]。在最近的一个研究中显示，逼尿肌活动不足或在尿流动力学检查上出现 Valsalva 排尿的女性更多与吊带手术后可能出现术后尿潴留相关。此外，术前残余尿量升高和术前最大尿流率降低有增加术后尿潴留的风险[5]。在新患者转诊的情况下，回顾手术记录是有用的，因为这通常可以揭示并发症的发生原因或揭示不当操作。

在获得与手术干预相关的症状的病史后，应进行尿液分析和残余尿分析。当存在感染时，应提供培养分析来指导治疗并重新评估症状。应进行体格检查，以评估尿道活动度、成角和网片显露。在新发的刺激症状、复发性尿路感染（UTI）或血尿时，应进行膀胱尿道镜检查，以评估网片侵蚀到尿道或膀胱情况。当身体习惯或伴随的盆腔器官脱垂进行盆腔检查困难时，在膀胱尿道镜检查同时进行阴道镜检查有助于评估阴道网片显露情况。如果由于患者的不适、习惯或偏好而无法进行门诊检查或膀胱尿道镜检查，需在手术室进行麻醉和膀胱镜检查。根据怀疑患者的情况及患者咨询，可以在麻醉下进行检查时及时行手术干预，或者分阶段按计划进行干预。

根据患者症状和检查结果，可能需要进行其他的诊断分析。在某些病例中，尿流动力学检查可能会被证明是有用的，特别是对于有尿频、尿不尽症状的女性，或者对那些有复杂手术史的女性，如既往多次的吊带手术或修补。在这些情况下，增加尿镜（影像尿流动力学）或单独排尿膀胱尿道造影有助于确定解剖上梗阻的位置，但并不总是必要的[6]（图 18-1）。

女性尿流动力学检查诊断梗阻可能具有挑战性，现在没有真正的压力和流速截止值[7]。最近，诊断压力性尿失禁手术后膀胱出口梗阻的尿流动力学参数已经被取消，在尿道中段悬吊术放置后排尿功能障碍的女性中，最常见的压力 – 排便模式是正常压力和排便差。对于 Y 压力性尿失禁手术干预后出现新发尿潴留或排空不完全，仅临床怀疑就足以进行干预。偶尔，进一步的影像学研究，如超声检查（US）、计算机断层扫描（CT）或磁共振成像（MRI）可用于识别血肿或脓肿。在下尿路发现钙化应引起对网状侵蚀的怀疑。MRI 被证明是可以用来识别患者出现与网片有关的疼痛或伤口并发症（图 18–2）。经阴道内超声是另一种有用的识别网片位置的工具，尤其是在没有既往的手术记录的情况下，不知道是否放置了网片或已经有网片的患者做了修补手术（图 18–3）。

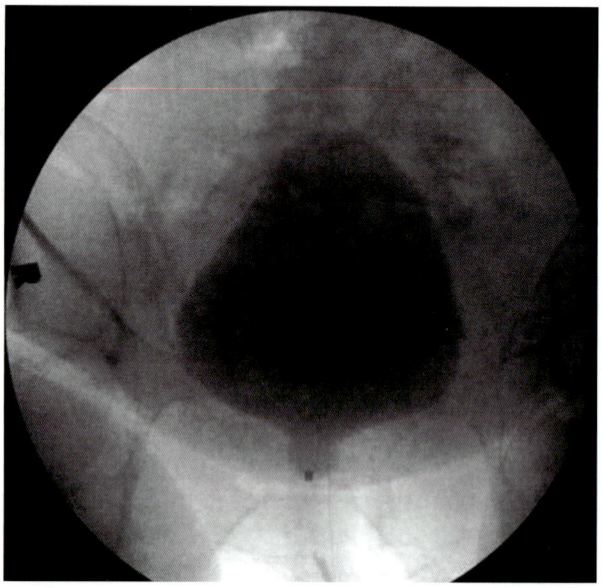

▲ 图 18–1　尿流动力学研究排尿期的透视图像显示了 1 例有尿道中段悬吊术后尿潴留史的女性中尿道梗阻的证据

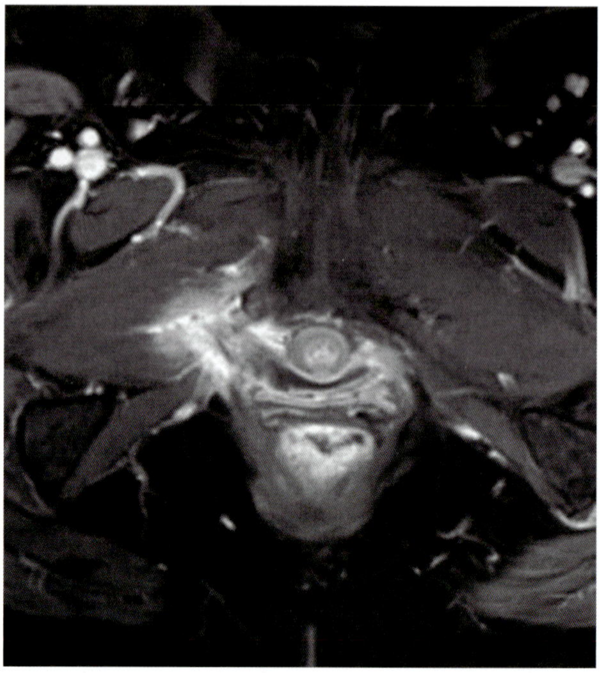

▲ 图 18–2　有经尿道中段悬吊史的女性，右腹股沟有引流窦。这张图像捕捉了尿道和阴道前壁之间的细长脓肿，脓肿导致窦道从右侧闭孔外肌和右侧股薄肌延伸到右侧腹股沟褶皱处的皮肤

二、膀胱出口梗阻

也许是最常见的并发症，尿失禁手术后膀胱出口梗阻的确切发生率尚不清楚，尽管据估计是 2%～25%[9-12]。应该注意的是，这可能被低估了，因为因尿失禁而接受手术干预的女性可能不太可能报告排尿困难，因为他们对尿失禁的解决感到满意，而那些经常寻求的医生不是她们原来的外科医生[13]。膀胱出口梗阻的症状各不相同，其中包括急性和完全性尿潴留、自发性排尿伴尿后残余尿增多、需要拉紧或进行体位排尿、增加或新的储存症状，以及尿路感染率增加。

用于治疗压力性尿失禁任何外科手术后都可能发生术后急性尿潴留。据报道，41% 的接受经阴道修补悬吊术的女性出现急性尿潴留[14]，接受耻骨后悬吊术的女性高达 27%[15]，接受耻骨阴道吊带的患者为 5%～20%[16, 17]，尿道中段吊带悬吊患者为 2.5%～25%[18-21]。对于尿道中段悬吊术术后尿潴留危险因素建议包括年龄较大、伴随手术、阴道穹窿脱垂、术前尿流低流率和逼尿肌收缩性差[22]。

急性尿潴留的诊断相对简单，最常见的诊断是在恢复室的排尿试验失败后做出的，尽管对一个成功的排尿试验的定义绝不是标准化的。然而，患者偶尔也会在恢复室进行成功的排尿试验，并以延迟的方式出现，在 Punjani 等[21]报道的 595 556 例女性中，有 3.4% 出现。这种表现相对

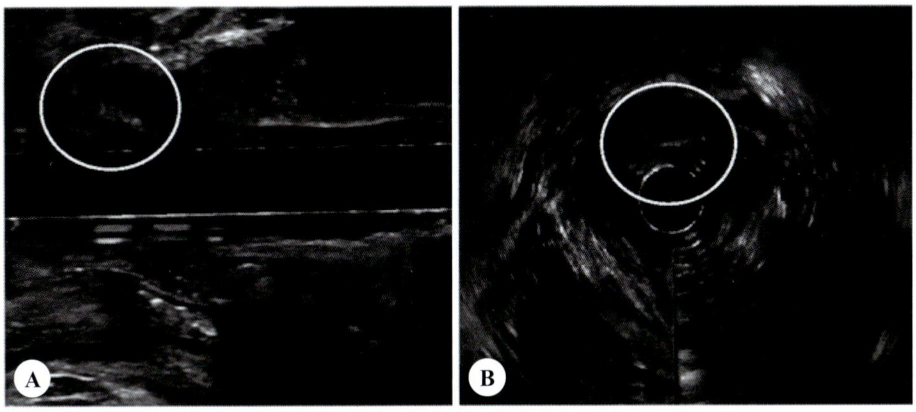

◀ 图 18-3　一名有经尿道中段吊带病史，右侧腹股沟有引流窦女性的阴道内超声图片。在矢状面（A）和冠状面（B）超声图像上的白色圆圈内可见网格

简单，如完全不能排空、弱流、紧张或体位排尿，或者可能更微妙，如新发尿急、频率或急迫性尿失禁。对于医生来说，对于术后立即出现新的排尿症状的患者，高度怀疑潴留是很重要的，因为在没有完全不能排尿的情况下可能存在潴留。

泌尿科医生和妇科医生对压力性尿失禁[23]手术干预后膀胱出口梗阻的适当治疗策略缺乏共识。急性尿潴留随着时间的推移能通过保守治疗解决，可能并不总是需要手术干预。据估计，5% 接受阴骨后和经阴道悬吊，阴骨阴道悬吊的尿潴留率高于尿道中段悬吊术[10]。最近，据报道，尿道中段悬吊术术后需要手术以缓解出口梗阻的平均发生率仅 1%～2%[24]。此外，据报道，81%～87.5% 的[25, 26]术后急性尿潴留女性需要暂时间歇导尿来恢复正常自发排尿。然而，许多梗阻的女性最终能够在没有导管的情况下排尿，在初期保留期后有明显的排尿功能障碍[23, 27]。有证据表明，尿道中段悬吊术术后 30 天内的尿潴留可能与未来需要手术干预的补片问题有关，这可能促使一些人提倡早期手术干预[21]。一些研究表明，对医源性梗阻的早期干预可能与更好的预后相关[28]。然而，对压力性尿失禁术后尿潴留的早期手术干预是否能降低后续并发症的风险尚不清楚，再手术的最佳时机也不清楚。

因此，压力性尿失禁术后膀胱出口梗阻的治疗由一系列因素决定，包括患者症状的严重和复杂程度、症状与手术相关的时间关系及手术类型。考虑到耻骨阴道悬吊术术后尿潴留的风险增加，许多手术者会选择在复杂手术时放置耻骨上导管，特别是对于既往有复杂的尿道中段悬吊术放置史或需要再次修补或移除的并发症的患者。通常需要保持在适当的位置，直到在 1～4 周内恢复正常的尿排空。另外，许多外科医生选择在经耻骨阴道吊带放置手术后常规进行间歇性清洁自我导尿（CIC），并行排空膀胱后置尿管，使残余尿下降到一定阈值以下。除了这些预防措施，在压力性尿失禁手术后急性尿潴留的情况下，当患者不能进行清洁间歇插管时，可通过清洁间歇插管或留置导尿管来完成尿路引流。在许多病例中，术后膀胱出口梗阻在导尿几天后就会消失，这使得这个保守的措施通常是首选的初始治疗选择[26, 29, 30]。

当术后膀胱出口梗阻不能通过导尿解决时，手术干预是治疗的主要手段。尿道扩张，通常伴有向下压力"松开吊带"，已被报道可改善超过 80% 的膀胱出口梗阻患者的排尿功能障碍[31, 32]。尽管有成功的报道，但该手术通常耐受性不佳，可能对尿道本身和周围组织造成相当大的损伤，与未来的网片侵蚀尿道有关，因此，不推荐用于治疗医源性膀胱出口梗阻[13]。其手术选择包括吊带移动、吊带切开术和尿道松解术。

对于在吊带手术后立即出现急性尿潴留的患者，吊带松解或移动可能是最合适的治疗选择。据报道，在 87%～100% 的病例中，这成功地解决了术后尿潴留，而不影响尿失禁（表 18-1）[25, 31, 33-38]。一般来说，最简单的和最好的是在术后 2 周内进行手术[25]，但据报道在初次手术[37]后 21 天也是可行的。虽然这可以在特定患者中进行[33]，但大多数情况下，吊带松解或移动需要在手术室麻醉下进行。在局部或全身麻醉下，打开阴道切口并识别吊带，充分显露是关键，对使用自挡牵开器（如 Lone Star 牵开器或手持式牵开器）有帮助。如果外科医生仍然难以识别吊带，可以将膀胱镜或尿道探查器放入尿道，轻轻向上牵引，以帮助显露吊带。识别吊带后，使用直角钳或止血钳放在吊带后面并向下牵引以使吊带移位约 1cm 以缓解梗阻。如果最初在吊带后面放进器械有困难，可以在吊带中点拉线帮助操作[34]。

表 18-1　吊带调整率和尿失禁改善率

作　者	病例数	尿潴留缓解率	尿失禁改善率
Moksnes 等[25]	136	89.7%	92.6%
Price 等[31]	33	87.8%	100%
Klutke 等[32]	17	100%	94.1%
Chang 等[34]	5	80%	100%
Rautenberg 等[35]	61	96.7%	95.1%
Nguyen[36]	10	100%	100%
Glavind[37]	5	100%	100%
Glavind 和 Shim[38]	17	100%	94%

据报道，吊带切开术也有类似的疗效，尤其是在初次手术后超过 3 周的患者。然而，应该注意的是，与吊带移动相比，吊带切开术有更高的压力性尿失禁复发率，一般为 14%～28%[25, 39-41]，一项研究报告了多达 60% 的接受吊带切开术的患者压力性尿失禁复发[42]。一般来说，当在最初的抗尿失禁手术后 180 天以上进行干预时，压力性尿失禁复发的可能性较小[13]。各种技术已经被记录，其中包括中线吊带切开，外侧吊带切开，双侧吊带切开及吊带骨上部分的切除。当在初次手术后不久或由初次外科医生进行吊带切开时，阴道上皮的中线切口是合适的。当吊带切开术是在延后的手术时机情况下，或者由行吊带手术以外的外科医生进行手术时，需谨慎地进行倒 U 形切口，以优化显露并减少随后网片挤压或切口破裂的风险。获得以前的手术记录可以确定放置的是什么类型的吊带，有助于识别吊带。在单纯医源性梗阻的情况下，一旦吊带分离，中线切口通常足以缓解梗阻，而耻骨阴道和尿道中段吊带均无须常规的尿道松解术[39, 40, 43]。通常，在吊带被切开后，需注意吊带材料的明显的回缩和被拉紧的尿道的松解。如果出现更复杂的表现，如伴随的疼痛或网片挤压，则谨慎的做法是切除吊带的尿道上部分，我们建议切除吊带至中线左右，以防止随后的吊带显露或侵蚀。这可以通过外侧切开吊带，避免损伤尿道，然后轻轻地将吊带从两侧的尿道周围筋膜外侧剥离，直达耻骨，此时吊带的每个臂都可以横断。当合成吊带材料被切除时，应送病检，并告知患者如何获取吊带材料和病检报告。对于单纯的医源性梗阻的患者，由于尿失禁的风险增加，不建议进行完全的吊带切除、积极的切除和反切口。

当耻骨后或经阴道悬吊后出现膀胱出口梗阻时，在吊带无法识别的情况下，或者在吊带切口失败后，可能需要进行正规的尿道松解。耻骨后或经阴道针悬吊后出现膀胱出口梗阻时，在无法识别吊带的情况下，或者在失败后吊带切口，可能需要进行正式的尿道松解术。该技术可经阴道或耻骨后方法进行，治愈率为 63%～93%，复发性压力性尿失禁为 13%～18%[3, 44-49]。尿道分离术的目的是恢复尿道、膀胱颈和阴道前壁的活动能力。

耻骨后尿道松解术已经被 Webster 和 Kreder[48] 很好地讲解过，做一个低中线或平缝切口，并进入耻骨后间隙。所有耻骨后粘连均被明显切除，并切开任何可见的悬挂缝合线或吊带。剥离可能需要向外侧延伸到坐骨结节，从而造成阴道旁缺损。在最初的手术描述中，正式的阴道旁修复通常是通过将阴道旁筋膜重新近似为骨盆腱弓腱筋膜。

现在更常见的是，尿道松解术是经阴道进行的，在文献[44, 50, 51]中被广泛描述。最常见的技术是在阴道前壁上做一个倒 U 形切口，顶点在中尿道，基部在膀胱颈。一旦阴道出现裂口，沿着尿道周围筋膜向盆腔内筋膜的内侧到外侧急剧地进行剥离。然后，盆腔内筋膜被迅速穿孔进入到耻骨后间隙。采用钝性和尖锐的剥离方法从耻骨联合的下方移动尿道。

Petrou 等也描述了尿道上松解术[52]。3 点钟到 9 点钟方位，在尿道上方 1cm 处做一个半圆的倒 U 形切口。在中线切开会阴膜，在尿道上方的平面上进行剧烈的剥离，从而从耻骨和骨盆附着处释放出尿道、膀胱颈和膀胱。使用钝性解剖分离，耻骨后间隙可进入膀胱腹侧，从而通过内侧到外侧的彻底的清扫破坏阻塞的纤维附着。当梗阻存在时，阻塞的耻骨阴道吊带或悬吊缝合线可以用这种方法加以识别和划分。这种方法的潜在好处是盆腔内外侧筋膜保留，这可以改善尿道支撑结构和减少复发性压力性尿失禁。然而，报道的尿道上尿道松解成功率低于经阴道和耻骨后尿道松解，其发生率约为 65%[52]。

人们正在争论是否应该进行组织介入来减少复发性梗阻的风险，并且通常是特殊的情况下保留的，如之前的尿道松解失败。这可以在耻骨后尿道松解[53]的情况下使用大网膜进行，或者通过经阴道尿道松解[54]后插入 Martius 唇脂肪垫移植物来进行。

三、慢性刺激症状

压力性尿失禁手术后可能会出现刺激性（储存）症状，如尿频、尿急和急迫性尿失禁，无论是持续性症状还是新发症状。应告知患者在术后初期预期刺激症状会有所恶化，并且这些症状可能会持续 4 周。当术后出现急性刺激症状时，重要的是要确认患者排空良好，并排除感染。在这些患者中，可以在急性恢复期开始使用短期的抗胆碱能药物或 β_3 受体激动药。

既往有刺激症状的患者术后可能更易出现症状。在一项大型研究中，36%～66% 的接受耻骨后悬吊手术的女性、54% 的接受经阴道悬吊手术的女性和 34%～46% 的接受悬吊手术的女性存在持续的术后急症。与术前无紧急情况的女性相比，在耻骨后悬吊的患者中有 8%～16%，经阴道悬吊患者中有 3%～10%，使用了吊带的有 3%～11%[10]。一些研究报道了混合性尿失禁（MUI）患者在尿道中段悬吊术后的刺激症状缓解。Segal 等指出，在因混合性尿失禁而接受尿道中段悬吊术治疗的女性中，术前有尿频、尿急缓解率为 57.3%，术前急迫性尿失禁缓解率为 63%，57.7% 的接受混合性尿失禁和尿道中段悬吊术治疗的女性停用抗胆碱能药物[55]。Zyczynski 等发现，大多数混合性尿失禁女性在压力性尿失禁手术治疗 1 年后膀胱过度活动症有所改善，阴骨阴道悬吊后改善率为 56.6%，耻骨后悬吊后改善率为 67.9%，尿道中段悬吊术术后改善率为 65%～70%。这种改善在 5 年时下降到 36.5%～54.1%[56]。尽管有这些发现，但大多数研究表明，混合性尿失禁中具有冲动情况的女性在手术后会出现更糟的情况[17, 57-59]，因此必须适当地诊断并在手术干预之前为患者提供咨询，以便对患者的期望进行妥善管理。令人惊讶的是，在一项比较耻骨后悬吊和耻骨阴道吊带的研究中，92% 的混合性尿失禁女性希望她们的尿频、尿急和夜尿情况得到改善，尽管咨询的结果与此相反[60]。这强调了在压力性尿失禁手术干预前，详细的混合性尿失禁咨询以适当设定期望的重要性，并强调了任何刺激症状的持续存在如何有害地影响患者对成功的感知。虽然对于压力性尿失禁手术后刺激性症状的解决没有明确的预测指标，但随着年龄的增长，首次手术时间增加[17, 56]和既往尿失禁手术次数增加，似乎与术后刺激性排尿症状的高发生率相关[55]。

当压力性尿失禁术后最初恢复期出现刺激症状持续时，第一步是排除膀胱出口梗阻和侵蚀。在持续性尿失禁患者或那些有多次抗尿失禁手术的患者中，UDS 可能在评估中有用。在没有梗阻或侵蚀的情况下，刺激性排尿症状可用膀胱过度活动的任何治疗方案进行处理，其中包括行为改变、盆底物理治疗、抗胆碱能药物、抗胆碱能药、β_3受体激动药、神经调节药或逼尿肌肌内注射肉毒杆菌毒素。

四、感染

尿路感染（UTI）是压力性尿失禁手术后常见的并发症，根据术后监测 4.5%～46.7% 的患者术后发生尿路感染，取决于术后监测时间和使用[61-68]的诊断标准。术后尿路感染的危险因素包括：复发性尿路感染史[63, 66, 69]、手术时间较[70]长、年龄＞65 岁[71]、体重指数＞40kg/m^2[71]，最显著的是术后残余尿[63, 72]升高和术后使用导管[66, 73]。多达 80% 的术后尿路感染归因于留置导尿管[74]，在接受尿道中段悬吊术和术后需要膀胱导尿的患者中，尿路感染发生率为 4.3%～32%[75]。尽管风险较高，但良好的抗生素管理对于控制超级细菌的出现至关重要。对于压力性尿失禁手术后需要导尿的女性的抗生素预防仍存在争议。虽然一些研究支持在这一人群中使用预防性抗生素[76, 77]，但其他研究没有从中受益。基于现有的最佳证据，与安慰剂相比[75]，术后口服抗生素似乎不能有效降低经尿道导尿术后女性的尿路感染率。当患者在术后几个月出现急性尿路感染症状时，评估尿潴留和获得尿培养是很重要的。如果培养呈阳性，则需要使用适当的抗生素进行治疗。在没有培养的情况下，对压力性尿失禁术后刺激性排尿症状的经验性治疗应尽可能加以限制，因为在没有感染的情况下，刺激性症状可能会在术后立即增加。在尿失禁手术后复发性尿路感染的情况下，应进行膀胱镜检查以排除缝合或补片侵蚀。

伤口感染是一种较不常见的并发症，发生率为 0.1%～16%，这取决于所进行的尿失禁手术[67, 68, 78-80]。在一项对华盛顿州 30 723 例女性在引入尿道中段悬吊术前后接受了压力性尿失禁手术的研究报告中，尿道中段悬吊术时代的伤口感染率为 0.1%，而在引入尿道中段悬吊术之前为 0.4%[80]。与侵袭性较低的尿道中段悬吊术相比，经阴道吊带后的伤口感染更常见，一项研究报告，接受经阴道吊带的患者中有 7.7% 的伤口感染[68]，而无张力性阴道悬吊术后为 0.4%[81]。手术部位感染的危险因素与任何其他手术过程相似，其中包括肥胖、糖尿病、吸烟状况和再手术。术前使用抗生素、从阴道手术场过渡到腹部手术场时更换手套、伤口冲洗等策略已被证明可以减少术后感染[82, 83]。盆腔脓肿很少见，但在尿道中段悬吊术放置后感染血肿的情况下也有报道。在尿道中段悬吊术后 2 例感染血肿的病例中，使用超声引导抽吸和静脉广谱抗生素均成功治疗。两例患者均不需要手术干预或摘除补片，并保持了下来[84]。

五、疼痛

术后疼痛和神经病变是公认的压力性尿失禁手术的风险。疼痛的机制可能与缝合或吊带轨迹中的盆腔肌肉和（或）神经的参与、吊带张力、感染或侵蚀有关。压力性尿失禁手术后术后疼痛的真实发生率难以评估，部分原因是使用了异质性术语来消除疼痛和疼痛位置。使用图表来确定疼痛的位置已被证明有助于评估尿失禁手术后的新发疼痛[85]。当患者出现与检查不成比例的疼痛，特别是伴有刺激性排尿症状或复发性尿路感染时，应考虑进行膀胱尿道镜检查以排除网片侵蚀[86]。据报道，尿道中吊带后腹股沟疼痛的发生率为 1.3%～32%[85, 87-91]。使用严格的评估患者，二次分析试验表明，尿道吊带手术后手术疼痛完全解决大约 70% 在术后 2 周，90% 在术后 6 周，疼痛解决的概率每天增加 12%，手术后第 6 周，经创伤组和耻骨后组中分别只有 5.4% 和 3.4% 的患者使用与手术相关的疼痛药物[92]。还应该注意的是患者对手术的满意度似乎在很大程度上与术后疼痛无关[85, 92]。当保守的疼痛治疗失败时，阴道尿道下尿道中段悬吊术可缓解 60%～80% 女性的疼痛[93-96]。在 52 例接受尿道下尿道中段悬吊术的女性中，只有 31% 在持续疼痛时需要二次手术摘除吊带臂，而在那些接受完全切除补片的女性中，

56% 的疼痛不变或更严重[93]。有一些争议是是否有限的阴道垫切除足以缓解疼痛或是否需要更广泛的切除，在尿道中段悬吊术后出现疼痛的个体中，没有可能受益于部分和完全补片切除的特异性决定因素[93, 97]。与完全补片切除相关的发病率并不重要，在进行手术前应彻底告知患者这些风险，包括持续疼痛的风险。我们的做法是保持保守，并支持一种分阶段的方法，除了在独特的情况下，有人担心网片感染是疼痛的来源。

闭孔神经可能会因行尿道中段悬吊术而有损伤风险，特别是通过经闭孔神经入路。尸检表明，经闭孔器尿道中段悬吊术距离闭孔神经分支约 20mm[98]。闭孔神经损伤可能是由于吊带太靠外造成的。这可以通过确保患者的腿正确定位以避免过度屈曲并提供足够的外展来预防。症状可能包括大腿内侧或腹股沟疼痛、腿部内收无力和大腿内侧感觉丧失。据报道，经闭孔尿道中段悬吊术[88]后大腿疼痛的发生率约为 5%，但在 0.7‰～0.9‰ 尿道中段悬吊术放置时[99]，真正的闭孔神经损伤要低得多。治疗闭孔神经损伤的关键是早期诊断，通常仅基于临床诊断。通过局部麻醉渗透到该区域减轻症状可用于诊断诊断和提供短期疼痛管理[100, 101]。目前还没有足够的文献来确定闭孔神经损伤的最佳治疗方法。通常采用保守治疗后会自发恢复；然而，如果患者有明显的神经症状或症状持续超过 6 周，建议进行手术干预，包括完全切除受累的补片臂[101, 102]。虽然经闭孔尿道中段悬吊术后闭孔神经损伤后的初级神经修复或移植是意外的，但在出现严重的神经症状时，神经外科咨询是必要的。

髂腹股沟神经的解剖结构使它容易在腹股沟上环出口处被卡住，在那里它几乎位于耻骨结节正上方。髂腹股沟神经的卡压或损伤可发生在耻骨上横切口、针头或套管针通过时。髂腹股沟神经卡压会导致疼痛从耻骨上区域开始，并辐射到腹股沟内侧、阴部、大阴唇和大腿内侧，并可能随着行走而加重。通过针和套管针更靠近中线和靠近耻骨，可以减少髂腹股沟神经损伤的风险。据报道，多达 8%～16% 的[103-105]患者在针悬吊及无张力阴道吊带放置[106]后出现这种并发症。该诊断可以在短期内通过髂腹股沟神经阻滞进行处理。症状可以通过保守治疗得到解决，其中包括髂腹股沟神经阻滞、物理治疗和辅助助行器，而不需要缝合或摘除补片。然而，如果疼痛持续超过 6 周或保守措施不足，可能需要手术干预缝合或补片去除[104]。

六、阴道网片显露或挤压

合成网状尿道吊带为压力性尿失禁提供可靠和有效的长期治疗尿失禁。因此，聚丙烯网片尿道吊带被泌尿流动力学、女性盆腔医学和泌尿生殖系统重建协会（SUFU），以及美国泌尿妇科学会（AUGS）[107] 支持作为“压力性尿失禁外科治疗的标准护理”。尽管使用合成网片中尿道吊带背后的证据级别为 A 级，但使用经阴道网片治疗压力性尿失禁并非没有风险。其中一个更常见和更独特的并发症是补片显露。美国食品药物管理局对 1996—2011 年所有发表的文献进行了系统回顾，报道术后 1 年阴道的显露与挤压率为 2%[108]。为了更好地帮助讨论独特的补片并发症，国际妇科泌尿外科协会和国际尿控协会发布了联合分类，以标准化手术补片相关并发症的术语[109]。术语“显露”将用于描述视觉或通过触诊识别的阴道网片，而“挤压”描述网片通过身体结构或组织，可以包括网片逐渐通过阴道壁的延迟过程（图 18–4）。

如前所述，网片显露或挤压率约发生在其中 2% 的吊带放置中，在文献中报道为 0%～8.1%[108, 110, 111]。报道的是 1 型大孔单孔聚丙烯网，这是目前合成吊带的标准。旧的吊带，如硬带和尿带有较高的显露率和挤压，因为他们是由不同的网状材料，不多孔，不允许足够的组织生长，有更高的感染率[112]。可能导致网片显露和挤压的危险因素包括糖尿病患者、活跃吸烟者、营养状况及外科医生的经验[113-116]。补片显露或挤压的可能原因是吊带放置过程中的错误、阴道切

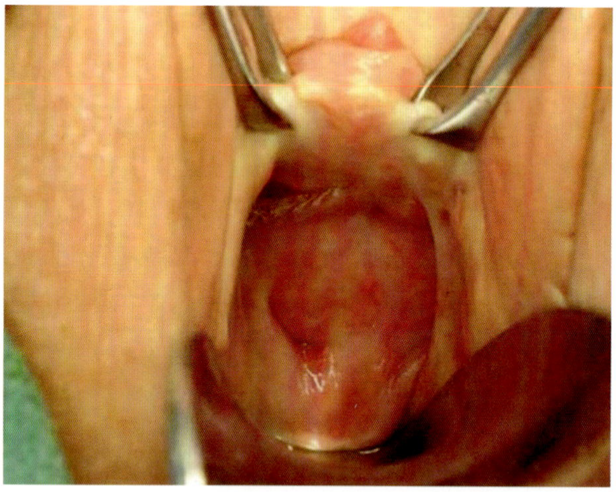

▲ 图 18—4 在手术室用半窥镜和两个全侧窥镜夹检查右侧阴道穹窿的网状挤压（图片由 Anne Cameron MD 提供）

口闭合不足、阴道切口破裂、亚临床感染、伤口愈合受损或补片收缩。

补片显露或挤压的临床表现差异是很大的。患者在表现时无症状且仅通过检查进行诊断并不罕见。性交中伴侣疼痛也可能是吊带显露的第一个迹象[117]。其他症状可能包括阴道出血或分泌物、性交困难、反复感染，或者在自检时可触及补片[112, 118]。

当怀疑网片显露或挤压时，应用半镜进行盆腔检查。显露的网可通过阴道组织呈现可见或可触及的网或肉芽组织区域。对吊带的操作过程应进行目视检查和触诊。如果由于患者不适或习惯而存在高度怀疑，无法彻底检查吊带的过程，阴道镜可作为辅助检查。如果担心伴随的网片挤压，也可以进行膀胱尿道镜检查。当患者在由其他外科医生进行了首次手术后出现补片挤压或显露时，获得手术记录以指导评估和治疗是有价值的。放置的吊带类型也可能影响延迟网片显露的位置，注意套管针的轨迹，经导管入路经常显露在穹窿处。耻骨后吊带术后网片显露率 1.3%，相比于经闭孔吊带 0.7%，耻骨后吊带更容易发生术后网片显露[119]。

在确定补片显露或挤压后，治疗将取决于许多因素，其中包括患者的症状和麻烦程度，首次手术和补片显露 / 挤压之间的时间长短、显露的大小和位置，以及患者的阴道组织的情况。对于无症状或轻微症状的小显露＜0.5cm 的女性，保守治疗 6～12 周是合理的，高达 40% 的患者可能成功[96, 120]。对于适当选择的患者，可以考虑使用显露网格的小的，容易看到的网格修剪。然而，这种治疗选择具有挑战性，因为患者不适和缺乏显露，这可能导致不同的可视化片。应告知女性补网的成功率较低，大多数患者最终需要在手术室进一步探查和切除[120]。

对于较大的网片显露，特别是那些在手术后 6 周内出现早期伤口分离的患者，可以在显露部位形成局部阴道瓣，并在显露的网片上提前闭合。这种治疗选择很吸引人，因为它能保持。评价阴道伤口闭合成功率的文献报道了 36%～100%[121-123] 的混合成功率，但需要注意的是，在这些研究中，从首次手术到显露的时间变化很大，包括阴道伤口闭合网片侵蚀和显露。根据我们的经验，对于手术切口早期补片显露，阴道假片闭合是首选的一线治疗方法。

如果保守措施失败，或者对于较大或更多延迟的补片挤压，应提供部分补片切除。决定切除多少补片部分取决于显露的位置和大小，应该注意的是，切除后的尿失禁率似乎随着补片的额外长度而增加。在最近的一项研究中评估在部分网片切除（只切除吊带显露的一部分）与完整网片切除（切除双侧分支）后的尿失禁率，复发性压力性尿失禁有 7% 的患者为部分切除，59% 的人为切除双侧分支[124]。在单纯补片显露或挤压的情况下，很少需要全补片切除，但当存在感染或严重盆腔疼痛时可以考虑。患者应了解全吊带切除的风险和好处，包括持续疼痛和复发性压力性尿失禁的风险。

七、尿道侵蚀

网片或缝合线侵蚀到泌尿道是压力性尿失禁手术治疗的罕见并发症。2001 年首次报道[125]，随着时间的推移，网状侵蚀有所增加，目前的发病率为 0.02%～5.4%[10, 126]。尿路侵蚀的危险因素包括吊置时未识别的套管针穿孔、剥离离尿道太近且组织变薄和断流、吊置后尿道扩张、过度牵拉或未识别的直接尿道损伤。患者可表现为刺激性或梗阻性排尿症状、复发性尿路感染或血尿。如前所述，在评估这些患者时需要高度怀疑，应该进行膀胱尿道镜检查。已侵蚀到尿路的缝合线或吊带可能成为结石形成的病灶（图 18–5）。

内镜治疗是对膀胱或尿道侵蚀的一个合理的一线治疗选择。内镜治疗可以进行激光或内镜切除使用电极环或内镜剪刀。在一项对 198 例网片侵蚀患者的内镜治疗的系统回顾中，激光切除的初始成功率为 67%，而环切除或剪刀切除的初始成功率为 80%。许多患者随后接受了重复的内镜下切除，只有 2%～7% 需要随后的开放手术切除，最终成功率为 92%～98%。激光和内镜下的并发症发生率分别为 24% 和 28%，分别有 21% 的患者经历了复发性压力性尿失禁。需要注意的是，在使用电极环或剪刀治疗 [127] 的组中发生了 3 例膀胱阴道瘘管。

当内镜下切除不成功时，应进行手术切除被侵蚀的补片。这可以通过经阴道入路进行尿道或膀胱颈侵蚀，或者在网状臂侵蚀膀胱时通过耻骨上膀胱切开术进行。腹腔镜或机器人入路膀胱切开术是补片侵蚀膀胱的合理替代方法，已在许多病例系列中被成功描述，没有主要并发症 [128, 129]（图 18–6）。

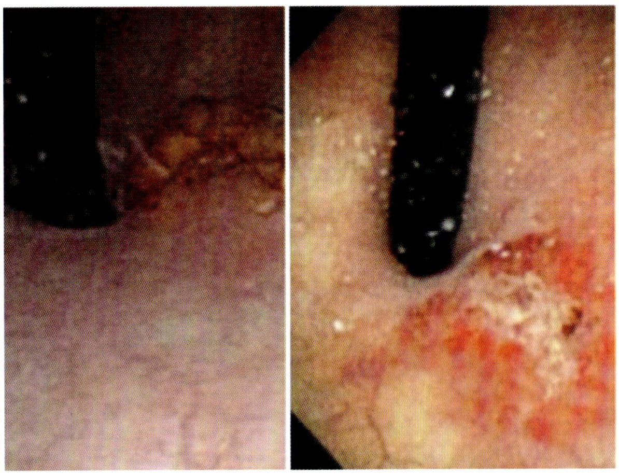

▲ 图 18–5　激光治疗前后的膀胱颈侵蚀的柔性膀胱尿道镜评估（图片由 Anne Cameron MD 提供）

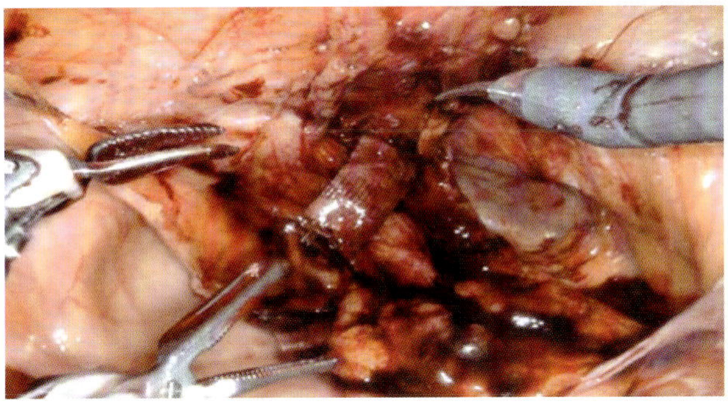

▲ 图 18–6　机器人辅助腹腔镜膀胱切开术切除被侵蚀到膀胱内的经阴道胶带网臂

八、性功能障碍

据报道，42%～56% 的尿失禁女性存在性功能障碍 [130]。阴道神经支配可能集中在阴道前，可能受压力性尿失禁手术的影响 [131, 132]。据推测，阴道前壁神经支配的破坏可能与性交困难的发展有关 [133]。Cayan 等发现，在接受压力性尿失禁手术的女性中，与阴道吊带相比，接受 Burch 膀胱阴道悬吊手术的女性性功能下降更多，尤其是在唤醒、润滑和性高潮评分方面 [134]。Mazouni 及其同事报道，25.6% 的女性在无张力性阴道悬吊术放置后性功能有所恶化 [135]。相反，一些研究报道了压力性尿失禁手术治疗后性功能的改善 [130, 136, 137]。需要进一步的前瞻性研究来识别手术治疗压力性尿失禁对性功能的影响。

总结

压力性尿失禁手术治疗后的并发症并不少见。在进行治疗前，进行一次完整的病史和体格检查是很重要的，以便能够选择最合适的个人手术方法。共享决策，即患者了解一系列治疗方案以及他们的成功率和并发症发生率，将有助于培养信任和患者满意度。当患者在接受压力性尿失禁手术治疗后出现新的排尿或储存症状、尿潴留、复发性尿路感染或疼痛时，医生应高度怀疑并发症。当怀疑有并发症时，应进行彻底的病史和体格检查，并谨慎地使用额外的诊断测试，如膀胱尿道镜检查或尿流动力学检查。每种并发症的治疗选择应包括对患者的评估，并应包括讨论关于压力性尿失禁复发或未能缓解症状的风险，特别是关于盆腔疼痛，因为这在本质上可能是多因素的，可以不同的治疗。

参考文献

[1] Milsom IAD, Lapitan MC, Nelson R, Sillen U, Thom D. Epidemiology of urinary (UI) and faecal (FI) incontinence and pelvic organ prolapse (POP). Committee 1. International Continence Society; 2009.
[2] Legendre G, Fritel X, Panjo H, Zins M, Ringa V. Incidence and remission of stress, urge, and mixed urinary incontinence in midlife and older women: a longitudinal cohort study. Neurourol Urodyn [Internet]. 2020;39(2):650–7. Available from: https://onlinelibrary.wiley. com/doi/abs/10.1002/nau.24237.
[3] Tse V, Chan L. Outlet obstruction after sling surgery. BJU Int [Internet]. 2011;108:24–8. Available from: http://doi.wiley.com/10.1111/j.1464-410X.2011.10712.x.
[4] Nitti VW, Tu LM, Gitlin J. Diagnosing bladder outlet obstruction in women. J Urol [Internet]. 1999;161(5):1535–40. Available from: http://www.ncbi.nlm.nih.gov/pubmed/10210391.
[5] Gracely A, Major N, Zheng Y, Silverii H, Lim C, Rittenberg L, et al. Do urodynamics predict urinary retention after sling placement in the complex patient: the value of reproducing symptoms on urodynamics. Int Urogynecol J [Internet]. 2021;32(1):81–6. Available from: http://link.springer.com/10.1007/s00192-020-04623-8.
[6] Rodrigues P, Hering F, Dias EC. Female obstruction after incontinence surgery may present different urodynamic patterns. Int Urogynecol J [Internet]. 2013;24(2):331–6. Available from: http://link.springer.com/10.1007/s00192-012-1869-x.
[7] Brucker BM, Shah S, Mitchell S, Fong E, Nitti MD, Kelly CE, et al. Comparison of urodynamic findings in women with anatomical versus functional bladder outlet obstruction. Female Pelvic Med Reconstr Surg [Internet]. 2013;19(1):46–50. Available from: http:// journals.lww.com/01436319-201301000-00010.
[8] Gammie A, Kirschner-Hermanns R, Rademakers K. Evaluation of obstructed voiding in the female. Curr Opin Urol [Internet]. 2015;1. Available from: http://journals.lww. com/00042307-900000000-99465.
[9] Welk B, Al-Hothi H, Winick-Ng J. Removal or revision of vaginal mesh used for the treatment of stress urinary incontinence. JAMA Surg [Internet]. 2015;150(12):1167. Available from: http://archsurg.jamanetwork.com/article.aspx?doi=10.1001/jamasurg.2015.2590.
[10] Leach GE, Dmochowski RR, Appell R, Blaivas JG, Hadley HR, Luber KM, et al. Female stress urinary incontinence clinical guidelines panel summary report on surgical management of female stress urinary incontinence. J Urol [Internet]. 1997;875–80. Available from: http://journals.lww.com/00005392-199709000-00054.
[11] Dmochowski RR, Blaivas JM, Gormley EA, Juma S, Karram MM, Lightner DJ, et al. Update of AUA guideline on the surgical management of female stress urinary incontinence. J Urol [Internet]. 2010;183(5):1906–14. Available from: http://www.jurology.com/doi/10.1016/j. juro.2010.02.2369.
[12] Plagakis S, Tse V. The autologous pubovaginal fascial sling: an update in 2019. LUTS Low Urin Tract Symptoms [Internet]. 2020;12(1):2–7. Available from: https://onlinelibrary.wiley. com/doi/abs/10.1111/luts.12281.
[13] Malacarne DR, Nitti VW. Post-sling urinary retention in women. Curr Urol Rep [Internet]. 2016 27;17(11):83. Available from: http://link.springer.com/10.1007/s11934-016-0639-6.
[14] Kelly M, Zimmern, Philippe E, Leach G. Complications of bladder neck suspension procedures. Urol Clin N Am. 1991;18(2):339.
[15] Parnell JP, Marshall VF, Vaughan ED. Management of recurrent urinary stress incontinence by the Marshall-Marchetti-Krantz vesicourethropexy. J Urol [Internet]. 1984;132(5):912–914. Available from: http://www.jurology.com/doi/10.1016/S0022-5347%2817%2949943-5.
[16] Athanasopoulos A, Gyftopoulos K, McGuire EJ. Efficacy and preoperative prognostic factors of autologous fascia rectus sling for treatment of female stress urinary incontinence. Urology [Internet]. 2011;78(5):1034–1038. Available from: https://linkinghub.elsevier.com/retrieve/ pii/S0090429511021923.
[17] Chaikin DC, Rosenthal J, Blaivas JG. Pubovaginal fascial sling for all types of stress urinary incontinence: long-term analysis. J Urol [Internet]. 1998;160(4):1312–6. Available from: http://www.ncbi.nlm.nih.gov/pubmed/9751343.
[18] Levin I, Groutz A, Gold R, Pauzner D, Lessing JB, Gordon D. Surgical complications and medium-term outcome results of tension-free vaginal tape: a prospective study of 313 consecutive patients. Neurourol Urodyn [Internet]. 2004;23(1):7–9. Available from: http://doi. wiley.com/10.1002/nau.10164.
[19] Karram M. Complications and untoward effects of the tension-free vaginal tape procedure. Obstet Gynecol [Internet]. 2003;101(5):929–932. Available from: http://linkinghub.elsevier. com/retrieve/pii/S0029784403001224.
[20] de Tayrac R, Deffieux X, Droupy S, Chauveaud-Lambling A, Calvanèse-Benamour L, Fernandez H. RETRACTED: a prospective randomized trial comparing tension-free vaginal tape and transobturator suburethral tape for surgical treatment of stress urinary incontinence. Am J Obstet Gynecol [Internet]. 2004;190(3):602–608. Available from: https://linkinghub. elsevier.com/retrieve/pii/S0002937803019380.
[21] Punjani N, Winick-Ng J, Welk B. Postoperative urinary retention and urinary tract infections predict midurethral sling mesh complications. Urology [Internet]. 2017;99:42–48. Available from: https://linkinghub.elsevier.com/retrieve/pii/S0090429516307324.
[22] Takacs P, Medina CA. Tension-free vaginal tape: poor intraoperative cough test as a predictor of postoperative urinary retention. Int Urogynecol J [Internet]. 2007;18(12):1445–1447. Available from: http://link.springer.com/10.1007/s00192-007-0364-2.
[23] Hashim H, Terry T. Management of recurrent stress urinary incontinence and urinary retention following midurethral sling insertion in women. Ann R Coll Surg Engl [Internet]. 2012;94(7):517–522. Available from: https://publishing.rcseng.ac.uk/doi/10.130 8/003588412X13373405385610.
[24] Jonsson Funk M, Siddiqui NY, Pate V, Amundsen CL, Wu JM. Sling revision/removal for mesh erosion and urinary retention: long-term risk and predictors. Am J Obstet Gynecol [Internet]. 2013;208(1):73.e1–7. Available from: https://linkinghub.elsevier.com/retrieve/pii/S0002937812010782.
[25] Moksnes LR, Svenningsen R, Schiøtz HA, Moe K, Staff AC, Kulseng-Hanssen S. Sling mobilization in the management of urinary retention after mid-urethral sling surgery. Neurourol Urodyn [Internet]. 2017;36(4):1091–6. Available from: http://www.ncbi.nlm.nih. gov/pubmed/27241330.
[26] Hong B, Park S, Kim HS, Choo M. Factors predictive of urinary retention after a tension- free vaginal tape procedure for female stress urinary incontinence. J Urol [Internet]. 2003;170(3):852–6. Available

from: http://www.ncbi.nlm.nih.gov/pubmed/12913715.

[27] Çetinel B, Tarcan T. Management of complications after tension-free midurethral slings. Korean J Urol [Internet]. 2013;54(10):651. Available from: https://icurology.org/DOIx. php?id=10.4111/kju.2013.54.10.651.

[28] Abraham N, Makovey I, King A, Goldman HB, Vasavada S. The effect of time to release of an obstructing synthetic mid-urethral sling on repeat surgery for stress urinary incontinence. Neurourol Urodyn [Internet]. 2017;36(2):349–353. Available from: http://doi.wiley.com/10.1002/nau.22927.

[29] Shukla A, Paul SK, Nishtar A, Bibby J. Factors predictive of voiding problems following insertion of tension-free vaginal tape. Int J Gynecol Obstet [Internet]. 2007;96(2):122–126. Available from: http://doi.wiley.com/10.1016/j.ijgo.2006.10.013.

[30] Bailey C, Matharu G. Conservative management as an initial approach for post-operative voiding dysfunction. Eur J Obstet Gynecol Reprod Biol [Internet]. 2012;160(1):106–109. Available from: https://linkinghub.elsevier.com/retrieve/pii/S0301211511005409.

[31] Price N, Slack A, Khong S-Y, Currie I, Jackson S. The benefit of early mobilisation of tension- free vaginal tape in the treatment of post-operative voiding dysfunction. Int Urogynecol J [Internet]. 2009;20(7):855–858. Available from: http://link.springer.com/10.1007/s00192–009–0858–1.

[32] Klutke C, Siegel S, Carlin B, Paszkiewicz E, Kirkemo A, Klutke J. Urinary retention after tension-free vaginal tape procedure: incidence and treatment. Urology [Internet]. 2001;58(5):697–701. Available from: http://www.ncbi.nlm.nih.gov/pubmed/11711343.

[33] Greiman A, Kielb S. Revisions of mid Urethral slings can be accomplished in the office. J Urol [Internet]. 2012;188(1):190–193. Available from: http://www.jurology.com/doi/10.1016/j. juro. 2012.02.2560.

[34] Chang W-C, Sheu B-C, Huang S-C, Wu M-T, Hsu W-C, Chou L-Y, et al. Postoperative transvaginal tape mobilization in preventing voiding difficulty after tension-free vaginal tape procedures. Int Urogynecol J [Internet]. 2010;21(2):229–33. Available from: http://www.ncbi. nlm. nih.gov/pubmed/19834633.

[35] Rautenberg O, Kociszewski J, Welter J, Kuszka A, Eberhard J, Viereck V. Ultrasound and early tape mobilization-a practical solution for treating postoperative voiding dysfunction. Neurourol Urodyn [Internet]. 2014;33(7):1147–51. Available from: http://www.ncbi.nlm.nih. gov/pubmed/23818418.

[36] Nguyen JN. Tape mobilization for urinary retention after tension-free vaginal tape procedures. Urology [Internet]. 2005;66(3):523–6. Available from: http://www.ncbi.nlm.nih.gov/ pubmed/16140070.

[37] Glavind K, Glavind E. Treatment of prolonged voiding dysfunction after tension-free vaginal tape procedure. Acta Obstet Gynecol Scand [Internet]. 2007;86(3):357–60. Available from: http://www.ncbi.nlm.nih.gov/pubmed/17364313.

[38] Glavind K, Shim S. Incidence and treatment of postoperative voiding dysfunction after the tension-free vaginal tape procedure. Int Urogynecol J [Internet]. 2015;26(11):1657–60. Available from: http://www.ncbi.nlm.nih.gov/pubmed/26068102.

[39] Moore CK, Goldman HB. Simple sling incision for the treatment of iatrogenic bladder outlet obstruction. Int Urogynecol J [Internet]. 2013;24(12):2145–2146. Available from: http://link. springer.com/10.1007/s00192–013–2241–5.

[40] Wu S-Y, Kuo H-C. Long-term outcomes of anti-incontinence surgery and subsequent transvaginal sling incision for urethral obstruction. Int Urogynecol J [Internet]. 2019;30(5):761–766. Available from: http://link.springer.com/10.1007/s00192–018–3733–0.

[41] Yoost T, Rames R, Lebed B, Bhavsar R, Rovner E. Predicting for postoperative incontinence following sling incision. Int Urogynecol J [Internet]. 2011;22(6):665–669. Available from: http://link.springer.com/10.1007/s00192–010–1339–2.

[42] Viereck V, Rautenberg O, Kociszewski J, Grothey S, Welter J, Eberhard J. Midurethral sling incision: indications and outcomes. Int Urogynecol J [Internet]. 2013;24(4):645–653. Available from: http://link.springer.com/10.1007/s00192–012–1895–8.

[43] Nitti VW, Carlson K V, Blaivas JG, Dmochowski RR. Early results of pubovaginal sling lysis by midline sling incision. Urology [Internet]. 2002;59(1):47–51. Available from: https://linkinghub. elsevier.com/retrieve/pii/S009042950101559X.

[44] Foster HE, McGuire EJ. Management of urethral obstruction with transvaginal urethrolysis. J Urol [Internet]. 1993;150(5 Part 1):1448–51. Available from: http://www.jurology.com/ doi/10.1016/S0022–5347%2817%2935805–6.

[45] Nitti VW, Raz S. Obstruction following anti-incontinence procedures: diagnosis and treatment with transvaginal urethrolysis. J Urol [Internet]. 1994;152(1):93–98. Available from: http://www.jurology.com/doi/10.1016/S0022–5347%2817%2932825–2.

[46] Anger JT, Amundsen CL, Webster GD. Obstruction after Burch colposuspension: a return to retropubic urethrolysis. Int Urogynecol J [Internet]. 2006;17(5):455–459. Available from: http://link.springer.com/10.1007/s00192–005–0037–y.

[47] Petrou SP, Young PR. Rate of recurrent stress urinary incontinence after retropubic urethrolysis. J Urol [Internet]. 2002;613–5. Available from: http://journals.lww. com/00005392–200202000–00035.

[48] Webster GD, Kreder KJ. Voiding dysfunction following cystourethropexy: its evaluation and management. J Urol [Internet]. 1990;144(3):670–673. Available from: http://www.jurology. com/doi/10.1016/S0022–5347%2817%2939550–2.

[49] Starkman JS, Duffy JW, Wolter CE, Kaufman MR, Scarpero HM, Dmochowski RR. The evolution of obstruction induced overactive bladder symptoms following urethrolysis for female bladder outlet obstruction. J Urol [Internet]. 2008;179(3):1018–1023. Available from: http:// www.jurology.com/doi/10.1016/j.juro.2007.10.051.

[50] Cross CA, Cespedes RD, English SF, McGuire EJ. Transvaginal urethrolysis for urethral obstruction after anti-incontinence surgery. J Urol [Internet]. 1998;159(4):1199–201. Available from: http://www.ncbi.nlm.nih.gov/pubmed/9507832.

[51] Zimmern PE, Hadley HR, Leach GE, Raz S. Female urethral obstruction after Marshall- Marchetti-Krantz operation. J Urol [Internet]. 1987;138(3):517–520. Available from: http:// www.jurology.com/doi/10.1016/S0022–5347%2817%2943244–7.

[52] Petrou SP, Brown JA, Blaivas JG. Suprameatal transvaginal urethrolysis. J Urol [Internet]. 1999;161(4):1268–71. Available from: http://www.ncbi.nlm.nih.gov/pubmed/10081883.

[53] Carr LK, Webster GD. Voiding dysfunction following incontinence surgery: diagnosis and treatment with retropubic or vaginal urethrolysis. J Urol [Internet]. 1997;157(3):821–3. Available from: http://www.ncbi.nlm.nih.gov/pubmed/9072576.

[54] Carey JM, Chon JK, Leach GE. Urethrolysis with martius labial fat pad graft for iatrogenic bladder outlet obstruction. Urology [Internet]. 2003;61(4):21–25. Available from: https:// linkinghub.elsevier.com/retrieve/pii/S0090429503001171.

[55] Segal JL, Vassallo B, Kleeman S, Silva WA, Karram MM. Prevalence of persistent and de novo overactive bladder symptoms after the tension-free vaginal tape. Obstet Gynecol [Internet]. 2004;104(6):1263–9. Available from: http://www.ncbi.nlm.nih.gov/pubmed/15572487.

[56] Zyczynski HM, Albo ME, Goldman HB, Wai CY, Sirls LT, Brubaker L, et al. Change in overactive bladder symptoms after surgery for stress urinary incontinence in women. Obstet Gynecol [Internet]. 2015;126(2):423–30. Available from: http://www.ncbi.nlm.nih.gov/pubmed/26241434.

[57] Chou EC-L, Flisser AJ, Panagopoulos G, Blaivas JG. Effective

treatment for mixed urinary incontinence with a pubovaginal sling. J Urol [Internet]. 2003;170(2 Pt 1):494–7. Available from: http://www.ncbi.nlm.nih.gov/pubmed/12853807.

[58] Stoffel JT, Smith JJ, Crivellaro S, Bresette JF. Mixed incontinence: does preoperative urodynamic detrusor overactivity affect postoperative quality of life after pubovaginal sling? Int Braz J Urol [Internet]. 2008;34(6):765–771. Available from: http://www.scielo.br/scielo. php?script=sci_arttext&pid=S1677-55382008000600012&lng=en&tlng=en.

[59] Kulseng-Hanssen S, Husby H, Schiotz HA. The tension free vaginal tape operation for women with mixed incontinence: do preoperative variables predict the outcome? Neurourol Urodyn [Internet]. 2007;26(1):115–21; discussion 122. Available from: http://www.ncbi.nlm. nih.gov/pubmed/16894616.

[60] Mallett VT, Brubaker L, Stoddard AM, Borello-France D, Tennstedt S, Hall L, et al. The expectations of patients who undergo surgery for stress incontinence. Am J Obstet Gynecol [Internet]. 2008;198(3):308.e1–6. Available from: http://www.ncbi.nlm.nih.gov/pubmed/18313452.

[61] Debodinance P, Delporte P, Engrand JB, Boulogne M. Complications of urinary incontinence surgery: 800 procedures. J Gynecol Obstet Biol Reprod (Paris) [Internet]. 2002;31(7):649–62. Available from: http://www.ncbi.nlm.nih.gov/pubmed/12457137.

[62] Anger JT, Litwin MS, Wang Q, Pashos CL, Rodríguez LV. Complications of sling surgery among female Medicare beneficiaries. Obstet Gynecol [Internet]. 2007;109(3):707–14. Available from: http://www.ncbi.nlm.nih.gov/pubmed/17329524.

[63] Nygaard I, Brubaker L, Chai TC, Markland AD, Menefee SA, Sirls L, et al. Risk factors for urinary tract infection following incontinence surgery. Int Urogynecol J [Internet]. 2011;22(10):1255–65. Available from: http://www.ncbi.nlm.nih.gov/pubmed/21560012.

[64] Brubaker L, Norton PA, Albo ME, Chai TC, Dandreo KJ, Lloyd KL, et al. Adverse events over two years after retropubic or transobturator midurethral sling surgery: findings from the Trial of Midurethral Slings (TOMUS) study. Am J Obstet Gynecol [Internet]. 2011;205(5):498.e1–6. Available from: http://www.ncbi.nlm.nih.gov/pubmed/21925636.

[65] Schimpf MO, Rahn DD, Wheeler TL, Patel M, White AB, Orejuela FJ, et al. Sling surgery for stress urinary incontinence in women: a systematic review and metaanalysis. Am J Obstet Gynecol [Internet]. 2014;211(1):71.e1–27. Available from: http://www.ncbi.nlm.nih.gov/pubmed/24487005.

[66] Varasteh Kia M, Long JB, Chen CCG. Urinary tract infection after midurethral sling. Female Pelvic Med Reconstr Surg [Internet]. 2021;27(1):e191–5. Available from: http://www.ncbi. nlm.nih.gov/pubmed/32427625.

[67] Lee RA, Symmonds RE, Goldstein RA. Surgical complications and results of modified Marshall-Marchetti-Krantz procedure for urinary incontinence. Obstet Gynecol [Internet]. 1979;53(4):447–50. Available from: http://www.ncbi.nlm.nih.gov/pubmed/440646.

[68] Chan PT, Fournier C, Corcos J. Short-term complications of pubovaginal sling procedure for genuine stress incontinence in women. Urology [Internet]. 2000;55(2):207–11. Available from: http://www.ncbi.nlm.nih.gov/pubmed/10688080.

[69] Sutkin G, Alperin M, Meyn L, Wiesenfeld HC, Ellison R, Zyczynski HM. Symptomatic urinary tract infections after surgery for prolapse and/or incontinence. Int Urogynecol J [Internet]. 2010;21(8):955–61. Available from: http://www.ncbi.nlm.nih.gov/pubmed/20354678.

[70] Gehrich AP, Lustik MB, Mehr AA, Patzwald JR. Risk of postoperative urinary tract infections following midurethral sling operations in women undergoing hysterectomy. Int Urogynecol J [Internet]. 2016;27(3):483–90. Available from: http://www.ncbi.nlm.nih.gov/pubmed/26467938.

[71] Vigil HR, Mallick R, Nitti VW, Lavallée LT, Breau RH, Hickling DR. Risk factors for urinary tract infection following mid urethral sling Surgery. J Urol [Internet]. 2017;197(5):1268–73. Available from: http://www.ncbi.nlm.nih.gov/pubmed/28034608.

[72] Doganay M, Cavkaytar S, Kokanali MK, Ozer I, Aksakal OS, Erkaya S. Risk factors for postoperative urinary tract infection following midurethral sling procedures. Eur J Obstet Gynecol Reprod Biol [Internet]. 2017;211:74–7. Available from: http://www.ncbi.nlm.nih.gov/pubmed/28192735.

[73] Dieter AA, Amundsen CL, Edenfield AL, Kawasaki A, Levin PJ, Visco AG, et al. Oral antibiotics to prevent postoperative urinary tract infection: a randomized controlled trial. Obstet Gynecol [Internet]. 2014;123(1):96–103. Available from: http://www.ncbi.nlm.nih.gov/pubmed/24463669.

[74] Sedor J, Mulholland SG. Hospital-acquired urinary tract infections associated with the indwelling catheter. Urol Clin N Am [Internet]. 1999;26(4):821–8. Available from: http://www.ncbi.nlm.nih.gov/pubmed/10584622.

[75] Sanaee MS, Hutcheon JA, Larouche M, Brown HL, Lee T, Geoffrion R. Urinary tract infection prevention after midurethral slings in pelvic floor reconstructive surgery: a systematic review and meta-analysis. Acta Obstet Gynecol Scand [Internet]. 2019;98(12):1514–22. Available from: http://www.ncbi.nlm.nih.gov/pubmed/31112286.

[76] Marschall J, Carpenter CR, Fowler S, Trautner BW, CDC Prevention Epicenters Program. Antibiotic prophylaxis for urinary tract infections after removal of urinary catheter: metaanalysis. BMJ [Internet]. 2013;346:f3147. Available from: http://www.ncbi.nlm.nih.gov/ pubmed/23757735.

[77] Sutkin G, Lowder JL, Smith KJ. Prophylactic antibiotics to prevent urinary tract infection during clean intermittent self-catheterization (CISC) for management of voiding dysfunction after prolapse and incontinence surgery: a decision analysis. Int Urogynecol J Pelvic Floor Dysfunct [Internet]. 2009;20(8):933–8. Available from: http://www.ncbi.nlm.nih.gov/ pubmed/19582384.

[78] KIRBY RS, Whiteway JE. Assessment of the results of stamey bladder neck suspension. Br J Urol [Internet]. 1989;63(1):21–23. Available from: http://doi.wiley.com/10.1111/ j.1464-410X.1989.tb05117.x.

[79] Morgan JE. The suprapubic approach to primary stress urinary incontinence. Am J Obstet Gynecol [Internet]. 1973;115(3):316–20. Available from: http://www.ncbi.nlm.nih.gov/ pubmed/4682824.

[80] Stewart LE, Eston MA, Symons RG, Fialkow MF, Kirby AC. Stress urinary incontinence surgery in Washington state before and after introduction of the mesh midurethral sling. Female Pelvic Med Reconstr Surg [Internet]. 2019;25(5):358–61. Available from: http://www.ncbi. nlm.nih.gov/pubmed/29894326.

[81] Abouassaly R, Steinberg JR, Lemieux M, Marois C, Gilchrist LI, Bourque J-L, et al. Complications of tension-free vaginal tape surgery: a multi-institutional review. BJU Int [Internet]. 2004;94(1):110–3. Available from: http://www.ncbi.nlm.nih.gov/ pubmed/15217442.

[82] Vij SC, Kartha G, Krishnamurthi V, Ponziano M, Goldman HB. Simple operating room bundle reduces superficial surgical site infections after major urologic surgery. Urology [Internet]. 2018;112:66–8. Available from: http://www.ncbi.nlm.nih.gov/pubmed/29122621.

[83] Harris JA, Sammarco AG, Swenson CW, Uppal S, Kamdar N, Campbell D, et al. Are perioperative bundles associated with reduced postoperative morbidity in women undergoing benign hysterectomy? Retrospective cohort analysis of 16,286 cases in Michigan. Am J Obstet Gynecol [Internet]. 2017;216(5):502.e1–11. Available from: http://www.ncbi.nlm. nih.gov/pubmed/28082214.

[84] Neuman M. Infected hematoma following tension-free vaginal tape implantation. J Urol. 2002;168(6):2549.

[85] Cadish LA, Hacker MR, Modest AM, Rogers KJ, Dessie S, Elkadry EA. Characterization of pain after inside-out transobturator midurethral sling. Female Pelvic Med Reconstr Surg [Internet]. 2014;20(2):99–

103. Available from: http://www.ncbi.nlm.nih.gov/ pubmed/24566214.
[86] Hilton P, Mohammed KA, Ward K. Postural perineal pain associated with perforation of the lower urinary tract due to insertion of a tension-free vaginal tape. BJOG [Internet]. 2003;110(1):79–82. Available from: http://www.ncbi.nlm.nih.gov/pubmed/12504943.
[87] Laurikainen E, Valpas A, Kivelä A, Kalliola T, Rinne K, Takala T, et al. Retropubic compared with transobturator tape placement in treatment of urinary incontinence: a randomized controlled trial. Obstet Gynecol [Internet]. 2007;109(1):4–11. Available from: http://www.ncbi. nlm.nih.gov/pubmed/17197581.
[88] Meschia M, Bertozzi R, Pifarotti P, Baccichet R, Bernasconi F, Guercio E, et al. Peri-operative morbidity and early results of a randomised trial comparing TVT and TVT-O. Int Urogynecol J Pelvic Floor Dysfunct [Internet]. 2007;18(11):1257–61. Available from: http://www.ncbi.nlm.nih.gov/pubmed/17345002.
[89] de Leval J. Novel surgical technique for the treatment of female stress urinary incontinence: transobturator vaginal tape inside-out. Eur Urol [Internet]. 2003;44(6):724–30. Available from: http://www.ncbi.nlm.nih.gov/pubmed/14644127.
[90] Neuman M, Sosnovski V, Goralnik S, Diker B, Bornstein J. Comparison of two inside-out transobturator suburethral sling techniques for stress incontinence: early postoperative thigh pain and 3-year outcomes. Int J Urol [Internet]. 2012;19(12):1103–7. Available from: http:// www.ncbi.nlm.nih.gov/pubmed/22882761.
[91] Giberti C, Gallo F, Cortese P, Schenone M. Transobturator tape for treatment of female stress urinary incontinence: objective and subjective results after a mean follow-up of two years. Urology [Internet]. 2007;69(4):703–7. Available from: http://www.ncbi.nlm.nih.gov/ pubmed/17445655.
[92] Thomas TN, Siff LN, Jelovsek JE, Barber M. Surgical pain after transobturator and retropubic midurethral sling placement. Obstet Gynecol [Internet]. 2017;130(1):118–25. Available from: http://www.ncbi.nlm.nih.gov/pubmed/28594776.
[93] Fuentes JL, Finsterbusch C, Christie AL, Zimmern PE. Mesh sling arm removal for persistent pain after an initial vaginal suburethral mesh sling removal procedure. Female Pelvic Med Reconstr Surg [Internet]. 2020. Available from: http://www.ncbi.nlm.nih.gov/pubmed/33208654.
[94] Hou JC, Alhalabi F, Lemack GE, Zimmern PE. Outcome of transvaginal mesh and tape removed for pain only. J Urol [Internet]. 2014;192(3):856–60. Available from: http://www. ncbi.nlm.nih.gov/pubmed/24735934.
[95] Ismail S, Chartier-Kastler E, Reus C, Cohen J, Seisen T, Phé V. Functional outcomes of synthetic tape and mesh revision surgeries: a monocentric experience. Int Urogynecol J [Internet]. 2019;30(5):805–13. Available from: http://www.ncbi.nlm.nih.gov/pubmed/30069725.
[96] Tijdink MM, Vierhout ME, Heesakkers JP, Withagen MIJ. Surgical management of meshrelated complications after prior pelvic floor reconstructive surgery with mesh. Int Urogynecol J [Internet]. 2011;22(11):1395–1404. Available from: http://link.springer.com/10.1007/ s00192-011-1476-2.
[97] Wolff GF, Winters JC, Krlin RM. Mesh excision: is total mesh excision necessary? Curr Urol Rep [Internet]. 2016;17(4):34. Available from: http://www.ncbi.nlm.nih.gov/ pubmed/26905696.
[98] Shah NM, Jackson LA, Phelan JN, Corton MM. Medial thigh anatomy in female cadavers: clinical applications to the transobturator midurethral sling. Female Pelvic Med Reconstr Surg [Internet]. 2020;26(9):531–5. Available from: http://www.ncbi.nlm.nih.gov/pubmed/30045054.
[99] Kuuva N, Nilsson CG. A nationwide analysis of complications associated with the tensionfree vaginal tape (TVT) procedure. Acta Obstet Gynecol Scand [Internet]. 2002;81(1):72–77. Available from: http://doi.wiley.com/10.1034/j.1600-0412.2002.810113.x.
[100] Corona R, De Cicco C, Schonman R, Verguts J, Ussia A, Koninckx PR. Tension-free vaginal tapes and pelvic nerve neuropathy. J Minim Invasive Gynecol [Internet]. 15(3):262–7. Available from: http://www.ncbi.nlm.nih.gov/pubmed/18439494.
[101] Aydogmus S, Kelekci S, Aydogmus H, Ekmekci E, Secil Y, Ture S. Obturator nerve injury: an infrequent complication of TOT procedure. Case Rep Obstet Gynecol [Internet]. 2014;2014:290382. Available from: http://www.ncbi.nlm.nih.gov/pubmed/25343052.
[102] Lee SH, Jung JH, Chung WS, Park YY, Yoon H. Obturator nerve injury complicating a tension- free vaginal tape. BJU Int [Internet]. 2003;92(Suppl 3):e12. Available from: http://www. ncbi.nlm.nih.gov/pubmed/19125469.
[103] Monga M, Ghoniem GM. Ilioinguinal nerve entrapment following needle bladder suspension procedures. Urology [Internet]. 1994;44(3):447–50. Available from: http://www.ncbi. nlm.nih.gov/pubmed/8073565.
[104] Miyazaki F, Shook G. Ilioinguinal nerve entrapment during needle suspension for stress incontinence. Obstet Gynecol [Internet]. 1992;80(2):246–8. Available from: http://www. ncbi.nlm.nih.gov/pubmed/1635738.
[105] Kelly MJ, Zimmern PE, Leach GE. Complications of bladder neck suspension procedures. Urol Clin N Am [Internet]. 1991;18(2):339–8. Available from: http://www.ncbi.nlm.nih.gov/ pubmed/2017815.
[106] Geis K, Dietl J. Ilioinguinal nerve entrapment after Tension-free Vaginal Tape (TVT) Procedure. Int Urogynecol J [Internet]. 2002;13(2):136–138. Available from: http://link. springer.com/10.1007/s001920200029.
[107] Nager C, Tulikangas P, Miller D, Rovner E, Goldman H. Position statement on mesh midurethral slings for stress urinary incontinence. Female Pelvic Med Reconstr Surg [Internet]. 2014;20(3):123–125. Available from: http://journals.lww.com/01436319-201405000-00001.
[108] Devices CF, Health R. Urogynecologic surgical mesh implants-considerations about surgical mesh for SUI. [Internet]. Available from: http://www.fda.gov/MedicalDevices/ ProductsandMedicalProcedures/ ImplantsandProsthetics/UroGynSurgicalMesh/ucm345219.htm.
[109] Haylen BT, Freeman RM, Swift SE, Cosson M, Davila GW, Deprest J, et al. An International Urogynecological Association (IUGA)/ International Continence Society (ICS) joint terminology and classification of the complications related directly to the insertion of prostheses (meshes, implants, tapes) and grafts in female pelvic flo. Neurourol Urodyn [Internet]. 2011;30(1):2–12. Available from: http://www.ncbi.nlm.nih.gov/pubmed/21181958.
[110] Clemons JL, Weinstein M, Guess MK, Alperin M, Moalli P, Gregory WT, et al. Impact of the 2011 FDA transvaginal mesh safety update on AUGS members' use of synthetic mesh and biologic grafts in pelvic reconstructive surgery. Female Pelvic Med Reconstr Surg [Internet]. 19(4):191–8. Available from: http://www.ncbi.nlm.nih.gov/pubmed/23797515.
[111] Osborn DJ, Dmochowski RR, Harris CJ, Danford JJ, Kaufman MR, Mock S, et al. Analysis of patient and technical factors associated with midurethral sling mesh exposure and perforation. Int J Urol [Internet]. 2014;21(11):1167–70. Available from: http://www.ncbi.nlm.nih. gov/pubmed/25039945.
[112] Giusto LL, Zahner PM, Goldman HB. Management of the exposed or perforated midurethral sling. Urol Clin N Am [Internet]. 2019;46(1):31–40. Available from: http://www.ncbi.nlm. nih.gov/pubmed/30466700.
[113] Linder BJ, El-Nashar SA, Carranza Leon DA, Trabuco EC. Predictors of vaginal mesh exposure after midurethral sling placement: a case-control study. Int Urogynecol J [Internet]. 2016;27(9):1321–6. Available from: http://www.ncbi.nlm.nih.gov/pubmed/26811112.
[114] Kokanalı MK, Cavkaytar S, Kokanalı D, Aksakal O, Doganay M. A

comperative study for short-term surgical outcomes of midurethral sling procedures in obese and non-obese women with stress urinary incontinence. J Obstet Gynaecol [Internet]. 2016;36(8):1080–5. Available from: http://www.ncbi.nlm.nih.gov/pubmed/27759469.

[115] Velemir L, Amblard J, Jacquetin B, Fatton B. Urethral erosion after suburethral synthetic slings: risk factors, diagnosis, and functional outcome after surgical management. Int Urogynecol J Pelvic Floor Dysfunct [Internet]. 2008;19(7):999–1006. Available from: http://www.ncbi.nlm.nih.gov/pubmed/18202812.

[116] Withagen MI, Vierhout ME, Hendriks JC, Kluivers KB, Milani AL. Risk factors for exposure, pain, and dyspareunia after tension-free vaginal mesh procedure. Obstet Gynecol [Internet]. 2011;118(3):629–36. Available from: http://www.ncbi.nlm.nih.gov/pubmed/21860293.

[117] Petri E, Ashok K. Partner dyspareunia-a report of six cases. Int Urogynecol J [Internet]. 2012;23(1):127–9. Available from: http://www.ncbi.nlm.nih.gov/pubmed/21800200.

[118] Bergersen A, Hinkel C, Funk J, Twiss CO. Management of vaginal mesh exposure: a systematic review. Arab J Urol [Internet]. 2019;17(1):40–8. Available from: http://www.ncbi.nlm. nih.gov/pubmed/31258942.

[119] Richter HE, Albo ME, Zyczynski HM, Kenton K, Norton PA, Sirls LT, et al. Retropubic versus transobturator midurethral slings for stress incontinence. N Engl J Med [Internet]. 2010;362(22):2066–76. Available from: http://www.ncbi.nlm.nih.gov/pubmed/20479459.

[120] Abbott S, Unger CA, Evans JM, Jallad K, Mishra K, Karram MM, et al. Evaluation and management of complications from synthetic mesh after pelvic reconstructive surgery: a multicenter study. Am J Obstet Gynecol [Internet]. 2014;210(2):163.e1–8. Available from: http://www.ncbi.nlm.nih.gov/pubmed/24126300.

[121] Giri SK, Sil D, Narasimhulu G, Flood HD, Skehan M, Drumm J. Management of vaginal extrusion after tension-free vaginal tape procedure for urodynamic stress incontinence. Urology [Internet]. 2007;69(6):1077–80. Available from: http://www.ncbi.nlm.nih.gov/pubmed/17572190.

[122] Kim SY, Park JY, Kim HK, Park CH, Kim SJ, Sung GT, et al. Vaginal mucosal flap as a sling preservation for the treatment of vaginal exposure of mesh. Korean J Urol [Internet]. 2010;51(6):416–9. Available from: http://www.ncbi.nlm.nih.gov/pubmed/20577609.

[123] Karmakar D, Dwyer PL, Nikpoor P. Mid-urethral sling revision for mesh exposure-long-term outcomes of two surgical techniques from a comparative clinical retrospective cohort study. BJOG [Internet]. 2020;127(8):1027–33. Available from: http://www.ncbi.nlm.nih.gov/pubmed/32107882.

[124] Jambusaria LH, Heft J, Reynolds WS, Dmochowski R, Biller DH. Incontinence rates after midurethral sling revision for vaginal exposure or pain. Am J Obstet Gynecol [Internet]. 2016;215(6):764.e1–5. Available from: http://www.ncbi.nlm.nih.gov/pubmed/27448731.

[125] Koelbl H, Stoerer S, Seliger G, Wolters M. Transurethral penetration of a tension-free vaginal tape. BJOG [Internet]. 2001;108(7):763–5. Available from: http://www.ncbi.nlm.nih.gov/ pubmed/11467707.

[126] Novara G, Galfano A, Boscolo-Berto R, Secco S, Cavalleri S, Ficarra V, et al. Complication rates of tension-free midurethral slings in the treatment of female stress urinary incontinence: a systematic review and meta-analysis of randomized controlled trials comparing tension-free midurethral tapes to other surgical procedures and d. Eur Urol [Internet]. 2008;53(2):288–308. Available from: http://www.ncbi.nlm.nih.gov/pubmed/18031923.

[127] Karim SS, Pietropaolo A, Skolarikos A, Aboumarzouk O, Kallidonis P, Tailly T, et al. Role of endoscopic management in synthetic sling/mesh erosion following previous incontinence surgery: a systematic review from European Association of Urologists Young Academic Urologists (YAU) and Uro-technology (ESUT) groups. Int Urogynecol J [Internet]. 2020;31(1):45–53. Available from: http://www.ncbi.nlm.nih.gov/pubmed/31468095.

[128] Misrai V, Rouprêt M, Xylinas E, Cour F, Vaessen C, Haertig A, et al. Surgical resection for suburethral sling complications after treatment for stress urinary incontinence. J Urol [Internet]. 2009;181(5):2198–202; discussion 2203. Available from: http://www.ncbi.nlm. nih.gov/pubmed/19296973.

[129] Macedo FIB, O'Connor J, Mittal VK, Hurley P. Robotic removal of eroded vaginal mesh into the bladder. Int J Urol [Internet]. 2013;20(11):1144–6. Available from: http://www.ncbi.nlm. nih.gov/pubmed/23600850.

[130] Thiagamoorthy G, Srikrishna S, Cardozo L. Sexual function after urinary incontinence surgery. Maturitas [Internet]. 2015;81(2):243–7. Available from: http://www.ncbi.nlm.nih.gov/ pubmed/25899565.

[131] Hilliges M, Falconer C, Ekman-Ordeberg G, Johansson O. Innervation of the human vaginal mucosa as revealed by PGP 9.5 immunohistochemistry. Acta Anat (Basel) [Internet]. 1995;153(2):119–26. Available from: http://www.ncbi.nlm.nih.gov/pubmed/8560964.

[132] Zivkovic F, Tamussino K, Ralph G, Schied G, Auer-Grumbach M. Long-term effects of vaginal dissection on the innervation of the striated urethral sphincter. Obstet Gynecol [Internet]. 1996;87(2):257–60. Available from: http://www.ncbi.nlm.nih.gov/pubmed/8559535.

[133] Lemack GE, Zimmern PE. Sexual function after vaginal surgery for stress incontinence: results of a mailed questionnaire. Urology [Internet]. 2000;56(2):223–227. Available from: https://linkinghub.elsevier.com/retrieve/pii/S0090429500006269.

[134] Cayan F, Dilek S, Akbay E, Cayan S. Sexual function after surgery for stress urinary incontinence: vaginal sling versus Burch colposuspension. Arch Gynecol Obstet [Internet]. 2008;277(1):31–6. Available from: http://www.ncbi.nlm.nih.gov/pubmed/17653739.

[135] Mazouni C, Karsenty G, Bretelle F, Bladou F, Gamerre M, Serment G. Urinary complications and sexual function after the tension-free vaginal tape procedure. Acta Obstet Gynecol Scand [Internet]. 2004;83(10):955–961. Available from: http://doi.wiley. com/10.1111/j.0001–634.2004.00524.x.

[136] Zyczynski HM, Rickey L, Dyer KY, Wilson T, Stoddard AM, Gormley EA, et al. Sexual activity and function in women more than 2 years after midurethral sling placement. Am J Obstet Gynecol [Internet]. 2012;207(5):421.e1–6. Available from: http://www.ncbi.nlm.nih. gov/pubmed/22840975.

[137] Glavind K, Tetsche MS. Sexual function in women before and after suburethral sling operation for stress urinary incontinence: a retrospective questionnaire study. Acta Obstet Gynecol Scand [Internet]. 2004;83(10):965–968. Available from: http://doi.wiley.com/10.1111/j.0001–6349.2004.00555.x.

第 19 章　压力性尿失禁治疗的失败

Failure of Treatment of Stress Urinary Incontinence

Caroline Dowling　Sandra Elmer　著

一、吊带失效的病理生理学和治疗

吊带失效，对患者和外科医生来说都是毁灭性的。人们对成功和功能正常化的期望很高，术前对预期的设定往往是不充分的[1]。

随着 2011 年美国食品药品管理局（FDA）发出的警告，以及随后围绕合成材料或网片、压力性尿失禁（SUI）管理的诉讼，在压力性尿失禁的管理中，吊带失效的分析显著也受到了影响。当地专业机构[2]继续在其算法中包括用于原发性尿失禁的尿道中段悬吊术（MUS），但临床实践和监管机构已经不再使用网状尿道中段悬吊术[3]，特别是经闭孔途径和在失败时重复合成吊带。

由于缺乏高质量的系统数据和对吊带基本工作原理的不完全了解，阻碍了对吊带治疗压力性尿失禁失败的分析。众所周知，根据尿流动力学参数，如 Q_{max}、膀胱出口梗阻指数（BOOI）、pDet 增加和残余尿量增加，压力性尿失禁手术的成功与尿道阻力增加有关，这表明吊带成功的关键在于尿道阻力的产生[4]。

尿道功能研究领域的最新进展是一个重要的提示，即对吊带机制的理解是不完整的[5]。从历史上看，人们一直关注尿道运动亢进过度矫正和内在括约肌功能障碍（ISD）的相互作用，更关注尿道的活动作为关键机制。在过度活动已经得到纠正的复发病例中，这成了一个挑战。

（一）失败的定义

失败可定义为术后主观上或客观上压力性尿失禁持续存在。复发性压力性尿失禁是指患者在干燥 6 周或以上，出现急迫性尿失禁（膀胱过度活动症），并发症包括梗阻和排尿功能障碍，以及合成材料、显露、糜烂和疼痛[6-8]。

Escobar[9]在最近对尿流动力学进行的全面回顾中评价失败，其中包括 3 个定义，即复发性压力性尿失禁、新的或恶化的膀胱过度活动症，以及新发排尿功能障碍或膀胱出口梗阻（BOO）。在本章中，我们将讨论复发性压力性尿失禁，包括持久性和新发的膀胱过度活动症。排尿功能障碍、疼痛和网片特异性并发症见第 18 章。

在查看二次手术的结果时，需要检查是失败还是复发，并且在术后 12 个月之前发生失败或在此时间之后复发时考虑失败[6]。据报道，5 年随访的失败率差异很大（8%～57%）[7]，超过 50% 的患者在压力性尿失禁手术治疗疗效试验（SISTeR）和经闭孔尿道中段悬吊术（TOMUS）试验在第一年内重新治疗[10]。约 15% 的数字似乎是有用和有效的。同样重要的是，很少有复发性尿失禁患者在就诊时有实际孤立的复发性压力性尿失禁的表现[11]。

一旦失败，患者就会对他们的外科医生失去信心，尤其是认为评估不充分的情况下。这可能会影响失败频数图表[12]。

（二）失败的病理生理学

尿失禁再发的原因尚不完全清楚，但大多数治疗尿失禁失败的因素包括持续性内在括约肌功能障碍、尿道过度活动和混合症状等。既往抗尿失禁手术本身就是失败的独立危险因素[13]。

如下是一些公认的导致吊带失败的危险因素。Stav研究[14]表明，体重指数（BMI）>25kg/m^{2}的患者、术前有混合症状的患者、之前接受过尿失禁手术的患者、糖尿病患者和术前存在压力性尿失禁的患者，吊带治疗失败的风险增加。Stav发现，盆腔器官脱垂（POP）的伴随手术与较低的失败风险相关，但大多数其他研究认为伴随手术会增加失败风险[14]。Pradhan在2013年关于尿道中段悬吊术治疗复发性尿失禁的疗效进行的系统评价表明，手术治疗后复发性或持续性尿失禁的危险因素包括年龄、肥胖、内科合并症（如糖尿病）、既往重度尿失禁、混合性尿失禁和既往手术失败[15]。

Richter在一项对600多例女性的研究中表明，既往尿失禁手术、最大Q尖偏移和衬垫重量超重都是失败的独立危险因素[16]。这项关于经闭孔尿道中段悬吊术与耻骨后尿道中段悬吊术大型随机研究（TOMUS研究）证实了Stav发现的混合症状是失败的危险因素，另外还注意到在术前评估中存在衬垫重量、年龄和严重程度评分的增加[16, 17]。

吊带相对于尿道长度的位置已被证明是会影响失败的危险因素。Bogusiewicz在一项基于经闭孔的吊带研究中表明更近端放置与更高的失败率相关[18]。与联合的关系也已经用超声检查过，联合显示无张力性阴道悬吊术越靠近联合的位置效果更好[19]。一些进一步的研究试图将吊带后的超声发现（如动态压缩）与临床结果相关联，如动态压缩（如果缺失可能意味着吊带松动），以及从吊带到尿道和吊带到耻骨的距离等，但在很大程度上尚无定论，而且技术还正在发展，其目前的应用最好在有经验的中心进行研究和使用[20]。

Ghoniem综述研究了自体筋膜吊带在视频尿质动力学治尿失禁中的机制，并表明自体筋膜吊带需要在活动期间压缩尿道[21]。因此，它沿尿道的位置和张力与过度紧张相关，也比缺乏张力更相关。

（三）失败的管理

无论材料如何，复发性压力性尿失禁的管理都应逐步进行，仔细评估病史，重点是发病，严重程度（主观尿垫使用）和当前症状的特征，以及与术前症状的区别，并确定是否在第一次对尿失禁治疗时判断的类型和治疗是正确的。麻烦的程度非常重要。应重新评估手术的类型、方法、使用的合成植入物、最好带有原始手术报道，以及术前的尿流动力学参数（如果存在）。推荐膀胱日记和标准化问卷［如国际尿失禁咨询问卷（ICIQ）］[7]。

对患者的检查应包括对尿道流动性的评估（尽管这一标准尚未建立）、是否有盆腔器官脱垂和盆腔器官脱垂的程度、咳嗽压力测试中压力性尿失禁的客观证据、是否有绝经泌尿生殖系统综合征（GSM）、注意尿道中段悬吊术的独特问题，其中包括挤压、糜烂和疼痛，以及任何神经系统症状的评估。患者应使用舒适的膀胱充盈检查，并对伴有咳嗽和Valsalva的压力性尿失禁进行客观评估。在Escobar[9]和Fontenot[22]的优秀评论中对评估患者术后失败的方法进行了全面讨论。在这些评估中使用经过验证的工具是重复性的关键。

尽管在压力性尿失禁手术中强制性术前尿流动力学检查是一个争议点，正如Clarke[23]的综述中总结的那样，但在失败的情况下，它们存在的重要性变得显而易见。术前尿流动力学检查的能力突然变得高度相关。失败与下腹部漏点压力对尿流动力学的影响有关，如几位作者所证明的，在初次手术前未能认识到这一点，从而固有地增加了不良结局的风险[24]。继续寻找成功或失败的尿流动力学预测因子，最近发表的一篇关于首次渗漏时膀胱容量作为不良结果预测因子效用的出版物证明了这一点[25]。Escobar和Brucker[9]详细介绍了尿流动力学研究的细节，但应包括一项评估压力性尿失禁本身的减法研究和对括约肌功能障碍的评估，但也包括逼尿肌过度活动的存在及对排尿的影响。手术失败后的尿流动力学是国家健康和护理卓越研究所（NICE）指南[26]所推荐的。

调查应至少包括对残余尿量的评估和中流尿（MSU）的显微镜和培养分析。增加柔性膀胱镜或带 70° 镜的膀胱镜以充分检查膀胱颈部，特别是在以前的尿道中段悬吊术[6, 27]的情况下，这取决于复杂性、对存在膀胱网孔穿孔的可能性的担忧、残余尿量的发现和患者进一步手术的动机[28]。为指导是否存在吊带错位并提高重复吊带的选择[29]，国际指南[26, 30]支持通过成像查看尿道中段悬吊术中吊带相对于中尿道的位置。然后，外科医生应该能够根据这些评估对失败的可能原因做出判断，并就最佳的前进方向与患者进行共同决策。这是在理解指导这一决策的证据不完全的情况下进行的，尤其是在合成吊带方面，当地指导方针和监管安排的快速变化。最近在 Cochrane 数据库[31]上发表的文章得出了一个发人深省的结论，即尽管有大量的尿道中段悬吊术被实施，但没有任何证据比较失败时的管理替代方案，并且“临床医生必须在很大程度上依赖专家意见和个人经验”[31]。

（四）新的膀胱过度活动症

约 9% 的患者在吊带手术后发生新生的膀胱过度活动症，并且尚未系统地证明在一种吊带入路中发生的频率比另一个更高[32]。新的膀胱过度活动症是一种令人不安的症状，与较低的术后生活质量评分紧密相关[33]。在没有阻塞、感染和网状物显露的情况下，新发的膀胱过度活动症的机制尚不清楚，但手术解剖导致自主神经支配中断已被判定。毫无疑问，放置吊带的外科医生认为，这种症状与患者的高不满率有关。有一些可识别的危险因素应考虑，如年龄、曾做过压力性尿失禁手术、增加的产次和剖宫产，以及曾做过抗胆碱能治疗增加了术后膀胱过度活动症的风险[34]。

新发膀胱过度活动症的管理应通过如前所述的仔细评估逐步进行，特别注意症状的时间，以确定它们是新发的而不是预先存在的，以及重要的因果病理，如激素状态、神经病理、尿路感染、结石和盆腔器官脱垂。病史和检查应重点关注这些情况。

所有患者都应进行尿液分析和残余尿量评估。如果在这些和临床评估后出现不复杂的图像，则有理由尝试膀胱过度活动症的一线和二线治疗，就像在先证者中一样，因为预期的自发消退率很高[34]。

膀胱镜检查和尿流动力学检查应用于怀疑膀胱出口梗阻、异物 / 网状物穿孔进入膀胱、以前未被识别的神经病学的情况。当怀疑膀胱出口梗阻时应进行尿流动力学检查，并在怀疑逼尿肌过度活动的情况下注意减慢填充。

研究表明，二线抗胆碱能药物治疗悬吊术后新发膀胱过度活动症是有效的[35]。β_3 药物尚未经过系统研究或证明同样有效，但可以安全地进行试验，但需要注意与指示病例相同的注意事项。在使用肉毒杆菌毒素 A 的情况下，由于缺乏数据也阻碍了悬吊术后新发膀胱过度活动症的三线治疗。Miotla[36]比较了 53 例特发性和 49 例尿道中段悬吊术后用 100U 肉毒杆菌毒素 A 治疗并证明了相似的结果。有 4 例患者因有症状的膀胱排空不全需要间歇性自我导尿，其中 3 例在吊带组。然而，这些例数太少，无法得出确切的结论。骶神经调节的研究较少，但研究表明，一项试验更有可能在稍微年轻患者（65 岁以下）和吊带放置 4 年内成功[37]。

二、复发性压力性尿失禁失败吊带的治疗

（一）保守治疗和药物治疗

如果发生复发性压力性尿失禁，治疗应从讨论保守措施开始，如减肥、盆底锻炼、失禁子宫托和雌激素替代。这方面的证据主要是从原发性压力性尿失禁的治疗中推断出来的，并且在失败的情况下没有得到很好的研究。加拿大妇产科协会建议保守措施作为复发性压力性尿失禁的一线管理[38]。然而，对于手术失败后物理治疗的作用尚未达成共识，该领域需要进一步研究。一些专

家表示要求女性再次这样做是不公平的，而其他专家意见则认为应该重新审视[7]，并且在轻度复发性压力性尿失禁病例中有一些证据表明它是有效的[15]。然而，保守措施不如手术有效，应主要考虑在拒绝手术或不适合手术或症状非常轻微的女性中。

度洛西汀已在欧洲被批准用于治疗压力性尿失禁，并且已被证明对女性压力性尿失禁有效[39]，但据报道其不良反应的相关危害，特别是胃肠道和精神方面的危害超过了益处[40]。NICE 指南建议不应将度洛西汀用作压力性尿失禁的一线治疗或常规作为二线治疗，因为盆底肌训练比度洛西汀更有效且成本更低，并且手术比度洛西汀更具成本效益[26, 28]。由于其心脏不良反应，不鼓励使用超说明书的丙咪嗪来增加括约肌张力[22]。

（二）复发性压力性尿失禁的手术治疗

对复发性压力性尿失禁进行重复手术的决定必须由患者和外科医生共同决定，并得到充分的咨询。重复手术的结果普遍低于初次手术[13, 41]。应仔细考虑重复手术的风险与获益之间的平衡。尽管越来越多地认识到使用合成材料的风险，特别是重复使用，以及自 FDA 警告。尿道填充术（UBA）新材料的出现使其成为更具吸引力和低风险的管理选择。自体筋膜吊带在 2015 年的回顾[42]中发现有 79.3% 的合并成功率，并且是 TOMUS 试验中失败的外科医生的首选[10]。

从 2014 年开始对复发性压力性尿失禁管理方案的研究表明，大多数泌尿妇科医生会选择第二个尿道中段悬吊术，泌尿科医生会在 27% 的病例中推荐自体筋膜吊带[28]。81.5% 和 48.6% 的受访者在尿道中段悬吊术失败后研究了有利于重复耻骨后尿道中段悬吊术和尿道填充术作为抢救的首选方案。这种实践模式已经随着围绕盆腔器官脱垂和压力性尿失禁管理使用经阴道合成网片的问题而改变，但除了已确定减少合成网片材料的使用外，这种做法尚未得到很好的记录[43, 44]。

可能影响复发性压力性尿失禁手术决策的因素包括初次手术后是否存在尿道过度活动、平均尿道闭合压力（MUCP）和原发性尿道中段悬吊术情况下原始吊带的位置[28]。在考虑重复尿道中段悬吊术时，如果尿道黏膜在剥离过程中被破坏（包括憩室或瘘管修复）或在切除侵蚀的合成吊带后尿道黏膜破裂[27]，则不应该推荐合成材料。现在确定了某些其他高风险群体，其中最好避免使用合成物，包括复杂的盆腔疼痛和（或）性交困难、慢性类固醇治疗、先前的照射或广泛的组织纤维化和瘢痕。

值得注意的是，英国的 NICE 指南[26]建议，由多学科团队在三级中心管理因抗失禁手术失败而被转介的女性，这将与最佳实践相一致。最终，这是一个共同的决定，并受到围绕接受合成材料和愿意进行主要程序的因素的影响[45]。疗效和发病率之间存在公认的权衡[46]。

吊带管理失败的手术选择按实用性的大致顺序呈现，并针对每种干预的特定情况提出警告。对所有干预方案的评估受到以病例系列、短期随访、异质人群，以及历史程序和设备为主的低质量研究的限制。

- 自体筋膜吊带（AFS）。
- 填充剂。
- 重复尿道中段合成吊带（包括可调节吊带）。
- 阴道悬吊——腹腔镜或开放式。
- 吊带折叠和操作。
- 膀胱颈悬吊技术。
- 螺旋或阻塞自体筋膜吊带。
- 可调节尿失禁疗法（ACT）。
- 干细胞治疗。
- 人工尿道括约肌。

1. 自体筋膜吊带

Welk 和 Herschorn 在 2012 年发表了第一个系列，其中 33 例患者尿道中段悬吊术失败后使用自体筋膜吊带。他们证明，使用 13cm × 2cm 吊带可显著减少垫子的使用并获得良好的患者满意度。2015 年以后的出版物承认，由于围绕使用合成材料管理压力性尿失禁和盆腔器官脱垂[29]存在争议，实践发生了转变。作为首选的抢救手术[21]已转向自体筋膜吊带。

将自体筋膜吊带作为压力性尿失禁的主要和次要治疗方法的分析受到文献中不同手术方法的限制。一项对288例接受McGuire型[47]自体筋膜吊带的女性进行的大型研究检查了该队列中59例既往进行尿道中段悬吊术的患者，其中25例患有尿道中段悬吊术并发症，需要吊带松解术或显露或阻塞。该研究显示，原发性和继发性自体筋膜吊带的主观和客观结果相当（59.9% vs. 62.4%客观治愈率和66.1% vs. 69%主观治愈率）。继发性自体筋膜吊带的情况下保留和重复手术较多[48]。

Milose[49]研究了66例继发性自体筋膜吊带患者，结果显示客观治愈率仅为37.7%，而主观治愈率为69.7%。Petrou进行的一项小型回顾性研究表明，21例吊带术后使用自体筋膜吊带的患者，52.4%是干性的，重要的是，切除之前的吊带没有统计学上的显著影响[50]。需要将更大手术（如自体筋膜吊带）导致更严重并发症的风险纳入术前咨询，静脉血栓栓塞风险为0.3%[51]。

自体筋膜吊带与耻骨后尿道中段悬吊术的比较，在224例患者中进行了回顾性系列，其中1/3采用自体筋膜吊带，2/3进行耻骨后尿道中段悬吊术，采用患者选择驱动的方法[52]。主要手术是吊带，2/3采用人工合成吊带进行尿道中段悬吊术。在中位随访29个月中，自体筋膜吊带和尿道中段悬吊术的预后相当，合成组治愈率为61.4%和自体筋膜吊带组治愈率为66.1%，无统计学差异。合成组中的6例患者需要进行第三次手术，即自体筋膜吊带手术。目前还不清楚有多少患者共使有2个合成吊带，以及这是否影响结局或后来网片特定并发症的发展的因素。

近10年前于2011年发表的一项研究观察了英国泌尿妇科医师在治疗复发性或持续性压力性尿失禁吊带术后管理方面的当前实践，结果表明51%的人会在2次失败的手术后考虑自体筋膜吊带[28]。当时，一篇评论文章指出，自体筋膜吊带“不太可能是在尿道中段悬吊术失败后复发性压力性尿失禁的常用手术”[53]。这在当代实践中不太可能发生。

在网片切除时或随后放置自体筋膜吊带的决定取决于网片切除时是否存在压力性尿失禁，如果存在广泛的尿道周围夹层或组织质量有问题，则更倾向于使用自体筋膜吊带。网片切除的原因也为选择提供了依据。患者需要参与关于伴随或分阶段方法的决策[21]，关于网片切除的原因，只有少数具有广泛变量的研究发表；因此，我们只能听取专家意见。

考虑到吊带的阻塞性和排空进一步变差的可能性，在选择自体筋膜吊带来治疗复发性压力性尿失禁时，需要考虑重要的临床和尿流动力学因素，如不完全排空或逼尿肌活动不足[54]。这与较长的手术和恢复时间以及术后需要间歇性清洁自我导尿（CIC）的风险相结合[51]使得尿道扩张成为许多患者的合理选择。

对传统McGuire[47]技术的修改正在不断发展，以使自体筋膜吊带的病态性降低，并且更类似于其合成物。在Malde的小型病例系列中，通过3cm耻骨上切口使用6cm×1cm吊带的患者中有26%用于治疗复发性压力性尿失禁[55]。10例复发性压力性尿失禁组中80%报道总体改善，这与原发组（82%）没有显著差异。在整个38例患者的队列中，3例发生了新发膀胱过度活动症，其中2例在复发性压力性尿失禁组。包括标准化张力在内的进一步修改将改善自体筋膜吊带在原发性尿失禁和复发性压力性尿失禁管理中的结果。目前，澳大利亚的数据显示当打结缝合在直肌筋膜上方时，可以通过松弛的吊带高度预测术后排尿功能障碍。该研究得出结论，松弛的吊带高度＜40mm与较高的术后尿潴留风险，以及需要间歇性自我导尿和尿道溶解术相关[56]。

2. 填充剂

由于较新的药物的出现及其FDA的批准，尿道填充术的疗效评估变得困难。所有药物的数据都有限，以小型单系列研究为主。目前最广泛使用的试剂包括碳涂层锆（Durasphere®）；羟基磷灰石钙（Coaptite®）；聚二甲基硅氧烷弹性体（Macroplastique®）和聚丙烯酰胺水凝胶（PAHG，Bulkamid®）。最新产品 PDMS-U（Urolastic®）是一种在注射时会聚合的硅胶。

最佳的尿道填充术将是生物相容的、耐用的、非迁移和低致敏性的，同时有利于愈合及形成最小的瘢痕。考虑到这一点，聚丙烯酰胺水凝胶具有最大的效用。在复发性压力性尿失禁人群中，在一项针对 60 例女性的观察性研究中，包括约 1/3 的混合症状或括约肌功能障碍，聚丙烯酰胺水凝胶治疗与 83.6% 的治愈率相关，或者在 12 个月时改善，如阴性咳嗽压力测试或尿垫重量＜2g [57]。耐用性始终是尿道填充术的问题。对初级人群中聚丙烯酰胺水凝胶最长的随访时间为 2 年，结果显示持续缓解 [58]。长期证据是可用的，并证明了持久的疗效。数据表明，当 Bulkamid® 用作压力性尿失禁的一线治疗时，80% 的患者在 7 年内治愈或改善 [59]。英国一项 3 年随访研究数据显示，3 个月时治愈率达到 82% 显著改善，最终随访结果保持不变 [60]。

较旧的药物（如基于硅树脂的 Macroplastique®）存在显露风险，导致结石形成、复发性尿路感染和难以去除的风险，这些在短期文献中很少见 [61]。Macroplastique® 作为一种补救剂，在小系列（23 例女性）的不到一年的随访中公布的治愈率约为 35%，但据说 77% 的患者对结果感到满意 [62]。在 Dray [11] 的系列中，71% 的患者对 Macroplastique® 或胶原蛋白有阳性反应，平均持续 35 个月。有趣的是，超过 50% 的研究对象的体重指数＞30kg/m^2，超过 50% 的研究对象被跟踪到 40 个月。只有 12.3% 的患者进行了进一步手术，大多数选择自体筋膜吊带。在对 Macroplastique® 的回顾性研究中取得了类似的结果，在注射前移除吊带的人群中，通常需要第二次注射才能实现 83% 的主观改善，平均随访时间为 46.4 个月，这驳斥了以下理论：吊带的存在支持注射剂并提高其功效，但这尚未得到系统研究 [63]。胶原蛋白（戊二醛处理的牛胶原蛋白）因其被重吸收并导致症状复发于 2011 年在全球范围内被淘汰 [64]。Durasphere® 已在 74 例患者吊带后进行了研究，成功率为 40% [65]。

在一项回顾性队列研究中，尿道填充术（67 例患者）与重复尿道中段悬吊术（165 例患者）的比较显示，尿道填充术组的失败率为 38.8%，而尿道中段悬吊术组的失败率为 11.2% [66]。接受研究设计的局限性，需要与患者进行讨论，讨论重复吊带的公认风险与尿道填充术组稍微降低的疗效之间的关系，再次合理化疗效 / 发病率权衡的复杂关系 [46]。

基于这些总体较差的结果，Kavanagh 在 2017 年 [66] 建议不应使用尿道填充术，除非在老年人或有进一步吊带禁忌证的情况下。与关于自体筋膜吊带消亡的评论一样，这可能不再反映当代实践，美国泌尿外科协会（AUA）指南推荐尿道填充术作为一种选择，它可以为患者提供更短的恢复时间和更少的侵入性手术，但患者应就成功率和重复治疗的风险进行咨询 [27]。

3. 重复尿道中段合成吊带，包括使用可调节吊带

随着时间的推移，曾经流行的重复尿道中段悬吊术正在减少。前几年发表了几项研究，Stav [41] 对 1100 例患者进行了具有里程碑意义的大型系列研究，其中 77 例是重复吊带，证明耻骨后（PR）路径在重复手术中优于经闭孔（TO）路径。同一组发表了耻骨后路径治疗括约肌功能障碍的改善结果，括约肌功能障碍通常是初始治疗失败的原因 [67]。一项针对 637 例括约肌功能障碍患者的回顾性研究中得到了证实，该研究表明，继发性尿道中段悬吊术患者的失败风险增加 12 倍 [6]。

如果发生第二次尿道中段悬吊术，这本身就是发生复发性压力性尿失禁的高风险情况，不能推荐经闭孔路径 [40, 68, 69]。一项对大约 10 个回顾性系列研究表明，成功率差异很大（40%～100% 有效），且疗效远低于初次治疗，在重复治疗中推荐耻骨后路径 [7]。2017 年 Cochrane 评价发现耻骨后尿道中段悬吊术降低了原发病例（括约肌功能障碍）再手术的风险 [70]。

与此相反，Abdel-Fattah 在一项大型经闭孔吊带研究的亚组分析中进行了为期 9 年的随访，观察了 46 例将经闭孔吊带作为二次手术的患者，并发现在 PGI-I 上的结果与主要队列相比更有利。然而，该研究表明，在小队列中腹股沟疼痛和糜烂的发生率很高，并且受到人数的限制，只有 63% 的组有完整的 9 年随访[71]。

未管理的尿道过度活动的存在对于预测那些可能从第二次吊带手术中受益的人是有意义的，无论是合成的还是自体筋膜吊带。这表明员带失败后更严重的群体是用自体筋膜吊带管理的，但这可能会涉及排尿功能、较高的并发症发生率和较长的恢复时间的平衡，因此需要明确的咨询[7]。重复尿道中段悬吊术失败后的随访 11 年的女性，Burch 或尿道中段悬吊术的主观治愈率为 67%，客观治愈率为 65%，生活质量评分令人满意，PGI-I 的成功率为 78%[72]。

由于吊带过度拉紧和压力性尿失禁治疗不足之间的细微差别，可调节吊带的概念一直受到呼吁。然而，这些吊带在原发性或复发性尿失禁中尚未得到广泛使用。然而，这种吊带在 102 例女性的回顾性系列研究中被报道在复发病例中有使用，平均随访时间超过 2 年[73]。使用经验化的尿失禁严重程度指数来评估结果，87.2% 的患者感到满意。与不可调节吊带的文献相比，这似乎很高，但由于数量少、回顾性设计和需要延迟吊带调整的比例接近 14%，该技术需要进一步评估才能被主流采用。2018 年欧洲指南建议这些吊带仅用于试验[30]。

应根据具体情况考虑在二次尿道中段悬吊术之前去除网片的作用。如果没有与合成网状材料相关的并发症，则在复发性压力性尿失禁手术时没有将其移除的指征，也没有这方面的文献指导[68]。在第二次吊带之前进行移除的 2 个系列显示了第二次吊带的可比结果，但没有足够的文献来确定是否需要这样做，并且应该根据具体情况和任何并发症（如网眼显露）的背景进行考虑[46, 74]。鉴于与未移除的重复尿道中段悬吊术相比，发生率相似，因此很难证明在没有特定网片并发症的情况下移除主要吊带的合理性。

在这一点上，有名誉暂停并考虑复发性压力性尿失禁手术治疗的 3 种主要选择，即自体筋膜吊带（AFS）、尿道填充术（DBA）和尿道中段悬吊术，它们是最有可能提供的手术[22, 27]。很明显，手术各不相同，患者和临床医生都很难做出决策。在临床实践中使用科学信息图形（图 19–1）进行决策可能有助于这一过程，并允许患者直观地了解他们的恢复时间、其他合并症、括约肌功能障碍的存在、最初进行的手术以及他们是否愿意再次或首次进行网片手术，是否存在诸如辐射、瘘管或过度瘢痕等并发症问题、以前的腹部手术和膀胱过度活动症，以及是否需要考虑使用紧吊带和永久性间歇性清洁自我导尿（CIC）。重复合成尿道中段悬吊术后的自体筋膜吊带的明确适应证包括疼痛、网片糜烂或瘘管[13]。外科医生更有可能建议重复尿道中段悬吊术，但女性更有可能将已经失败的手术排除在选择列表之外，仅从数字来看，这更有可能是尿道中段悬吊术[75]。

4. 阴道悬吊术：腹腔镜或开腹

使用阴道悬吊术进行检索的文献非常少以至于该方法没有写入主要指南[27]。一项对 16 例复发性压力性尿失禁女性的研究表明，开腹阴道悬吊术后初次手术失败的定义不清，客观治愈率为 55%，主观治愈率 93%[76]。2011 年 Giarenis 研究结果表明尿道中段悬吊术失败后行开腹阴道悬吊术的客观治愈率为 77%，主观治愈率为 85%[40]。Nikolopoulos 系统综述的汇总分析显示客观治愈率为 76%[42]。开腹 Burch 膀胱尿道悬吊术损伤大，增加盆腔器官脱垂风险，并且不能完全解决括约肌功能障碍问题。腹腔镜和机器人 Burch 膀胱尿道悬吊术因是微创方法而一直极具吸引力，并在术中可同时进行盆腔器官脱垂手术。

5. 吊带折叠法

个案报道了有关吊带折叠的结果[77]、使用聚丙烯[78]可调技术或吊带缩短[79]，但样本量均较少。5 项回顾性研究汇总后分析，总体成功率为

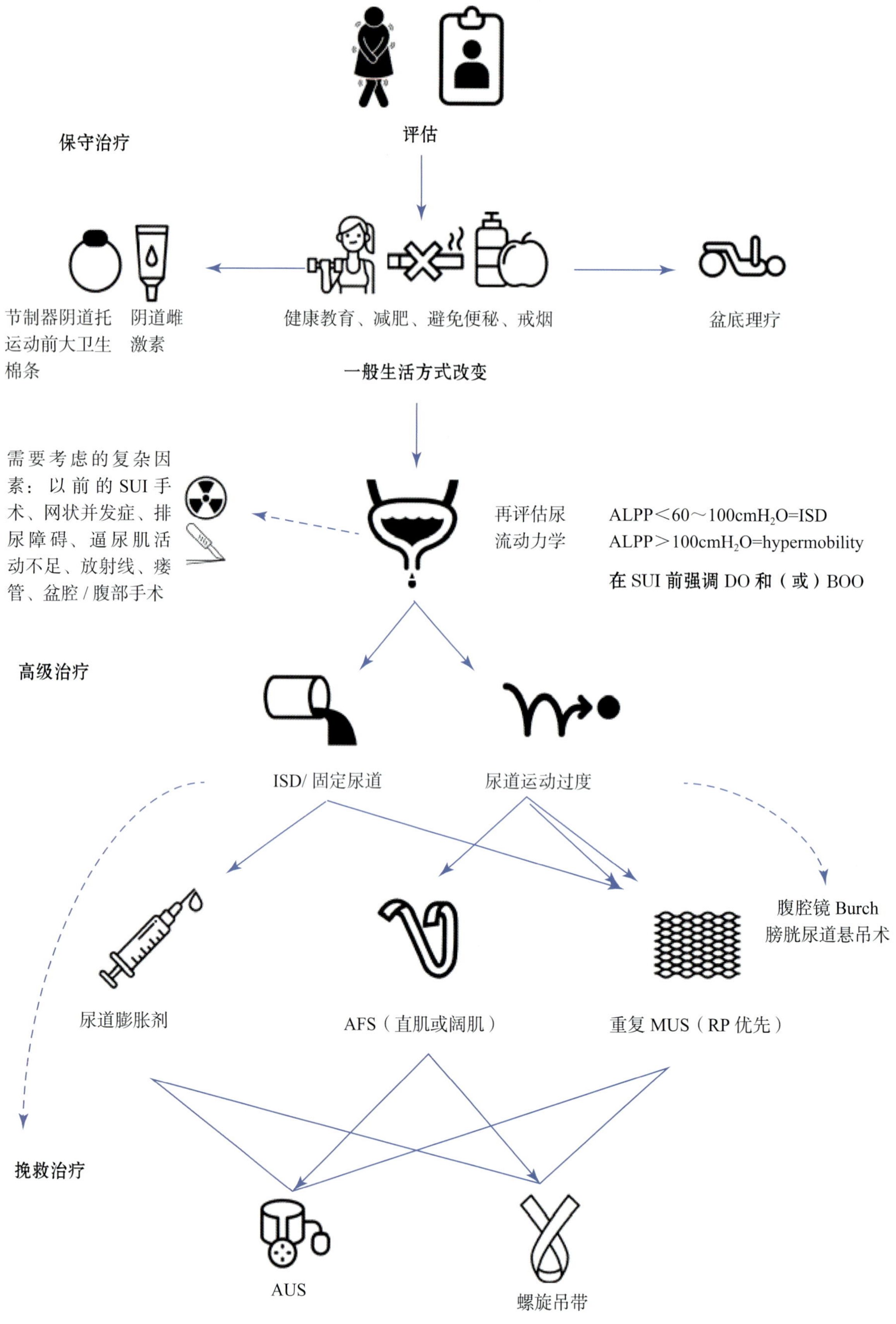

▲ 图 19-1　吊带失败和复发性压力性尿失禁

SUI. 压力性尿失禁；ALPP. 腹部漏尿点压力；ISD. 括约肌功能障碍；AFS. 自体筋膜吊带；MUS. 人工尿道括约肌；AUS. 尿道中段悬吊术；BOO. 膀胱出口梗阻

61%[80]，耻骨后路径组成功率高于经闭孔路径组。由于缺乏该领域的数据和持续发表的文章，导致这些作者得出了与 Kavanagh[7] 相同的结论，即不建议治疗失败后使用吊带折叠法。

尽管如此，在临床中该技术仍继续应用，并在 2019 年的一篇病例报告中报道了 36 例患者[81]，其中约有 3/4 的患者行耻骨后路径悬吊术，1/4 的患者行经闭孔路径悬吊术，折叠前的持续时间仅 6.8 周。成功率为 76%，在耻骨后路径组中成功率更高（$P= 0.034$），并且随访时间短于 2 年。对于这种治疗方案，建议采取谨慎的个体化治疗方法。

6. 膀胱颈悬吊术

通过阴道、耻骨后入路的膀胱颈悬吊术（BNS）有长期实践史，但并未得到广泛应用。然而，在人工合成材料日益受到关注的时代，一种无须设备的技术通过悬挂膀胱颈并改善活动时的排尿功能。曾经应用的传统的阴道前壁折叠术已被证明在治疗压力性尿失禁时失败率很高，因而已摒弃使用[82]。Rashid 等[29] 得出结论，膀胱颈悬吊术在阴道前壁脱垂修复中可能发挥作用，在这种修复中，若存在持续性过度活动或复发性压力性尿失禁，尿道中段悬吊术是禁忌的，但该技术已被尿道中段悬吊术取代，并且作为一种基于全球实践的补救技术，不如自体筋膜吊带或尿道填充术。

7. 螺旋吊带或阻塞吊带

多年来，螺旋吊带和阻塞吊带一直用于挽救性手术。初次吊带手术治疗失败的患者由于尿道纤维化、去神经支配和尿道周围筋膜断裂，使得尿道难以被压迫，出现不活动或管状尿道，使得手术难度大。患有神经系统疾病的女性患者中，尽管膀胱压力正常，但间歇性清洁自我导尿仍存在并且漏尿，以故意阻塞的方式压迫尿道有治疗作用。用自体组织或合成材料制成的螺旋或阻塞吊带为人工括约肌或膀胱颈闭合以及可控尿流改道提供了一种恰当的选择。

在治疗神经系统功能正常的病例时，对于腹部漏尿点压力（ALPP）<60cmH$_2$O 且愿意并能够进行清洁间歇导尿的患者，应考虑使用螺旋吊带。如果担心在不加压的情况下无法实现节制，则可以考虑具有较高腹部漏尿点压力的患者。

围术期应阴道局部使用雌激素。对患者的术前评估应根据之前的建议，特别注意相关的尿流动力学检查结果、神经病变情况下的腹部漏尿点压力和膀胱压力，复杂病例中还应评估 EMG 和影像学检查[83]。对于较高腹部漏尿点压力患者，如果膀胱压力不受控制，再加上吊带产生的出口阻塞，会造成上尿路损伤，也会加重由逼尿肌过度活动引起的尿失禁。

该手术操作时要在放置吊带之前，仔细进行尿道分离，以达到最大限度地压缩，吊带可交叉放置于相对于尿道的背侧或腹侧。吊带尺寸是不同的，也取决于使用的是合成材料还是自体材料。在一项研究中使用了 16cm × 1cm 的合成材料[84]。在手术中，尿道被移动，吊带从尿道背侧穿过并从尿道腹侧交叉，然后用一个 Allis 夹固定以防止在随后跨过耻骨后吊带臂时尿道周围过度牵拉。靠近骨膜有助于安全通过尿道背侧，以避免损伤尿道或背侧静脉复合体，建议使用小型弯曲 Satinsky 钳仔细解剖以实现该步骤。实际上，许多这样的病例已经进行了多次手术，类似于膀胱颈人工尿道括约肌，可能需要改良的开放式或腹腔镜或机器人辅助，以确保其他结构不会穿孔并允许吊带准确放置。在所有文献中，解剖过程中出现尿道和膀胱颈医源性损伤的比例较高。

Rodriguez 进行了一项研究，21 例患者使用合成吊带，5 例使用自体吊带，3 例在交叉后将吊带置于外侧（双侧肢体在一侧）。患者在就诊时平均接受 3.5 次手术，每天 7 个垫子，90% 的患者腹部漏尿点压力<60cmH$_2$O。其中 1 例一侧合成吊带失败，5 例双侧合成吊带失败。失败组各有两侧需要填充。自体吊带手术均成功。平均垫子使用量降至每天 0.9 个，平均随访期为 15 个月。除了 3 例需要间歇性清洁自我导尿（全部来自合成吊带组）之外，该组在改善括约肌功能障碍的同时能维持自发排尿。新发膀胱过度活动症的发生率较

低[75]。从技术上讲，作者认为吊带臂中的张力对于保持低张力至关重要，然后依靠包裹来达到效果，因为低张力可以维持排尿能力。一项平均随访26个月的28例女性的研究得出了类似的结论，并且在71.4%的患者中使用带有背侧交叉的聚丙烯网状包裹物，"治愈"了压力性尿失禁[85]。

Raz等[86]最初的螺旋吊带研究用于治疗神经系统疾病或先天性疾病导致的尿道功能不全、多次尿失禁手术失败导致的医源性损伤，螺旋吊带使用的15cm×1cm聚丙烯网，两端用柔软的聚乳酸共聚物零缝合。在随访12个月的47例患者中，40例的结果相似，7例失访也被认为失败，则成功率为68%。45%的患者没有使用垫子。在研究的40例患者中，仅3例需要进行膀胱颈闭合和尿道分流。总体而言，没有其他患者需要清洁间歇导尿。

如此高的成功率和维持自发排尿的机制尚不清楚，但推测可能与支持中段尿道并周向应对腹压增加有关[39]。了解这些患者在排尿功能、新发膀胱过度活动症和12个月后的网片特异性并发症等方面的长期结果，以及在放置网片之前对原位网片的操作，是很有价值的。该研究中神经系统疾病的数量和性质也没有明确说明。我们目前对此类病例的处理方法是常规放置自体筋膜吊带，在放置22F膀胱镜鞘时收紧，该鞘与尿道在一个水平面。在膀胱阴道瘘修复术后尿失禁的患者中，采用类似技术通常导致明显的阴道纤维化，被描述为使用填充染料的膀胱收紧Valsalva[87]。40例患者接受了这种手术并进行了阔筋膜移植。只有一例患者术后需要持续清洁间歇导尿。这项研究受到随访和设计的限制。螺旋吊带在受辐射人群中的应用尚未得到系统评估。

8. 可调节性控制（ACT）

这种器械的功能类似于可调节的置入式膨胀剂，作为一种治疗选择从未引起重视，在原发性或继发性压力性尿失禁治疗中使用的研究也很少。以垫重<2gm为临界值，58%的患者吊带失败（垫重≥2g），52%的患者垫重<2g。80%的患者随着尿失禁严重程度的增加，改善效果越差[88]。

Kocjancic[89]研究了57例既往括约肌功能障碍手术失败的女性，其中22例是前次吊带失败的女性。随访5年，垫子的使用量从每天5.6个减少到1.6个。28%的并发症较轻，5%的并发症较严重，器械导致的并发症为18%。Freton比较了ACT®装置与人工尿道括约肌AMS 800治疗女性括约肌功能障碍所致压力性尿失禁的结果。研究表明人工尿道括约肌可以降低USP压力性尿失禁评分（–7.6 vs. –3.2），每24小时垫数（–4.6 vs. –2.3），PGII评分（PGII=1分，61.1% vs. 12%）和治愈率（71.4% vs. 21.7%）。该研究得出结论：与ACT®相比，人工尿道括约肌置入具有更好的功能效果，但术中并发症发生率更高、手术时间更长以及住院时间更长（Freton，2018 #147）。

2013年发表的一篇关于可调节性控制的系统综述[90]，报道了8项异质性研究中的各种结果，结论是该技术与括约肌功能障碍治疗失败的患者相关，对于这些患者不适合使用人工尿道括约肌。由于先前的手术，这些患者也可能有使用螺旋吊带的禁忌证。

9. 干细胞疗法

已有文献报道使用脂肪和肌肉来源干细胞治疗的相关研究[91-93]。Mitterberger在20例患有括约肌功能障碍的女性中使用了干细胞治疗，2年后治愈率为89%。很少有文献报道干细胞在继发性括约肌功能障碍或失败病例中的应用，最近的指南建议它们只在试验中使用[27]。

10. 人工尿道括约肌（适应证和方法）

(1) 介绍：既往压力性尿失禁手术后复发或持续压力性尿失禁的治疗方案包括保守治疗和（或）手术治疗。自体筋膜吊带、尿道填充术和重复尿道中段悬吊术是大多数国家的主要选择方案。人工尿道括约肌AMS 800（Boston Scientifc™; Inc. USA）是一种可替代手术的选择；然而在美国，这种方法并不常用，因为它未经FDA批准[94]，并且被大多数国际指南视为"最后的方案"。与此相反，法国指南推荐人工尿道括约肌作为括约肌功能障碍所致压力性尿失禁女性患者的治疗标准[95]。

在目前的临床实践中，人工尿道括约肌主要用于前列腺切除术后尿失禁的男性患者，尽管其最初是为女性设计的。支持在女性患者中使用人工尿道括约肌的证据缺乏且质量差，仅有回顾性病例研究。人工尿道括约肌袖带通常采用腹部入路置入膀胱颈水平，尽管曾有阴道入路的研究，但由于效果不佳，很快就被摒弃。人工尿道括约肌置入具有挑战性和矛盾性。在 20 世纪 90 年代中期，人工尿道括约肌未获得 FDA 批准时，人工尿道括约肌治疗女性压力性尿失禁的应用大多在欧洲，尤其是法国，采用开腹方法植入人工尿道括约肌。近年来，微创手术的兴起，以及技术设备的改进，帮助解决了人工尿道括约肌在置入时的技术复杂性，提高了置入成功率，未来人工尿道括约肌的作用可能会越来越大[96]。未来需要高质量的研究作为证据，更好地阐明人工尿道括约肌在治疗括约肌功能障碍所致压力性尿失禁女性患者中的疗效。

(2) 女性人工尿道括约肌的适应证：尽管尿道中段悬吊术是治疗女性尿道过度活动所致压力性尿失禁的金标准手术方法，但对于括约肌功能障碍相关压力性尿失禁的治疗方法尚不明确[97]。括约肌功能障碍被认为是由于出口阻力降低导致的尿道管腔不完全覆盖，通常见于既往治疗尿失禁手术失败的患者或神经源性压力性尿失禁患者[96]。然而，括约肌功能障碍引起的压力性尿失禁还没有普遍认可的定义。Cour 等描述的临床标准包括咳嗽压力试验中的明显压力性尿失禁且伴尿道活动障碍、Marshall/Bonney 试验阴性（尿道固定后渗漏）、尿流动力学检查中的最大尿道闭合压较低或检查时的“固定尿道”[95]，结合临床怀疑括约肌功能障碍的其他标准［首次抗失禁手术失败、高压力性尿失禁评分、日常活动持续渗漏和（或）腹部用力导致渗漏］[97]。

AMS 800 具有 3 个相互连接的主要组件：充气袖带（环绕膀胱颈）、液压泵（放置在大阴唇）和压力调节球囊（PRB）（放置在膀胱前间隙）。在膀胱周期的有储阶段期间，储存期的正常静息模式下，袖带充满水，周向挤压膀胱颈，增加出口阻力。在排尿阶段，袖带减压，膀胱颈打开，出口阻力降低。理论上人工尿道括约肌可以恢复膀胱正常储存和排尿功能。当怀疑存在括约肌功能障碍时，可考虑人工尿道括约肌治疗女性压力性尿失禁，如既往抗尿失禁手术后出现复发性压力性尿失禁或持续性压力性尿失禁[97]、神经源性压力性尿失禁（通常由于脊髓损伤、脊柱裂、马尾综合征或骨盆外伤）[98]，考虑到人工尿道括约肌几乎不可能发生阻塞，它可能是严重逼尿肌活动不足女性患者的有用选择[97]。

人工尿道括约肌置入的最佳时机存在争议。虽然括约肌功能障碍是人工尿道括约肌置入的主要适应证，但并非所有具有此适应证的女性都会立即行此手术，并且很少将人工尿道括约肌作为女性压力性尿失禁的主要手术方案，除了一些神经源性患者[99]。Chartier-Kastler 等提出了人工尿道括约肌置入成功率随着术前手术干预次数的增加而降低的难题，因此，他们建议在术前至少 1 次但最多 2 次干预失败后考虑人工尿道括约肌置入，而不是在所有术前手术均失败后作为最后补救措施[99]。

(3) 结果：支持人工尿道括约肌在女性患者中使用的证据水平低且质量差。已有许多系统评价，评估人工尿道括约肌治疗女性压力性尿失禁的效果。Rue 评估了人工尿道括约肌治疗非神经源性严重女性压力性尿失禁的短期至长期疗效和安全性。这项综述收录的 12 篇文章没有随机研究或前瞻性研究，他们发现报道的零垫率为 42%～86%，修正率为 6%～44%，机械故障率为 2%～41%。他们发现，手术严重不良事件发生率为 2%～54%，设备严重不良反应的发生率为 2%～27%[100]。

按照 PRISMA 声明和 Cochrane 手册建议，在国际尿控协会主持下进行的另一项系统评价中，Peyronnet 发现手术方法、手术量和经验最有可能影响围术期发病率和设备存活率。手术达到完全自制的概率为 61.1%～100%。术后并发症发生率差异很大，在机器人手术中发生率为 16.7%～33.3%，在开腹手术中发生率为 4.1%～75%。在腹腔镜和机器人手术中，侵蚀率和解释率分别为 0%～8.1% 和 0%～22.2%，中位随访时间为 37.5 个月和 18.9 个月。两个最多样本量的研究报告了开腹人工尿道括约肌置入手术的最低设备解释率（7% 和 12.8%）和机械故障率（13.6% 和 15.5%）[97, 101, 102]。最近，机器人辅助手术的研究显示出了进一步改善的结果，侵蚀和术后并发症的发生率分别低至 2.1% 和 4.1%，在最后的随访中，81.6% 患者达到完全自制，12.2% 患者尿失禁得到改善，6.1% 患者尿失禁没有改善[103]。

未来需要高水平的研究作为证据，帮助更好地阐明人工尿道括约肌在女性括约肌功能障碍所致压力性尿失禁中的治疗作用。

(4) 手术技术：自美国医疗系统公司（Boston Scientifc, Minnetonka, MN, USA）在 30 多年前推出第一款人工尿道括约肌（AMS 721）以来，该设备经历多次修改，成为目前的 AMS 800 型号，该型号在世界范围内仅在少数医疗机构置入女性体内[99]。AMS 800 的置入可采用以下 2 种方法：耻骨后入路[104]或经阴道入路[105]。经阴道入路因其较高的复发率和感染率而很快被摒弃[99]。充气袖带的放置位置可因尿失禁的病因而异；然而，大多数患者接受膀胱颈放置。人工尿道括约肌置入最初是采用开腹方法进行，近几年微创技术的应用有助于克服技术复杂性，降低复发率[97]。

(5) 术前注意事项：在决定人工尿道括约肌置入时，患者需要权衡长期成功率和生活质量(QoL）改善与不可忽视并发症和未来复发的利弊。由于 AMS 800 置入后由患者自己在每次排空膀胱时自行操作，因此必须患者自愿行人工尿道括约肌置入，并且在术前准确告知患者有关装置的重要信息[99]。人工尿道括约肌放置之前需要评估患者的手部灵活性和精神状态，以确定患者有能力操作装置。术前进行全面的病史询问、辅助检查和尿流动力学检查，术后患者要进行排尿记录、尿垫测试和填写问卷表对病情评估都有意义。应行膀胱镜检查评估尿道组织的状况并排除狭窄或网片侵蚀（需要在人工尿道括约肌置入前进行干预和处理）。术前必须进行尿培养，围术期使用的抗生素能预防皮肤和泌尿道病原体感染，以避免置入物感染。适当给予预防深静脉血栓形成（DVT）的治疗措施。

(6) 机器人辅助 AMS 800 膀胱颈置入术：在有或没有机器人辅助的情况下通过腹腔镜置入人工尿道括约肌具有以下优点：保留腹壁、视野清楚、显露于设备的时间短，可以降低感染风险[106]。备皮包括脐下腹部、生殖器和会阴部，根据制造商的说明，建议在手术前用聚维酮碘肥皂擦洗皮肤 10min（对于碘过敏者可以使用洗必泰擦洗）。

(7) 膀胱颈解剖：在 Peyronnet 等描述的技术中[103]，患者位于 23° 头低足高卧位，双臂沿身体放置并保持在扶手上，下肢取低位截石位。插入 14Fr Foley 导管并引流膀胱。放置了 4 个 8mm 机器人端口（脐部的摄像头端口，右侧腹中 1 个，左右腹直肌外侧边缘 2 个）和左侧腹中附加的 12mm 辅助端口。四臂 Da Vince Si/Xi 机器人放置在右侧对接位置。使用了 3 种机器人仪器：双极 Prograsp 镊子（左臂）、剪刀（右臂内）和基本 Prograsp 镊子（右臂外）。AMS 800 的 3 个组件是根据制造商的指导准备的。

膀胱充满 100～300ml 的生理盐水以确定其边界，然后使膀胱从前腹壁下降。找到 Retzius 间隙，然后显露膀胱颈和盆腔内筋膜，一定要准确识别膀胱颈。助手将一个手指放在阴道外侧穹窿中，向上和横向推膀胱颈。用助手的手指钝性剥离膀胱颈，进入膀胱周围筋膜，当阴道出现闪亮的白色平面（“秃顶平面”），在该位置必须进行膀胱颈剥离。一旦解剖达到中线，解剖膀胱颈的另一侧，直到两侧被解剖的间隙接合。助手确认阴道壁完好无损，膀胱内充满亚甲蓝以验证膀胱颈部的完整性[103]。

Gondran-Tellier 等也描述了膀胱颈和膀胱阴道间隙的后入路[59]。借助阴道瓣膜将膀胱和阴道之间的平面从膀胱颈后部切开，然后横向到盆腔内筋膜。后壁剥离完成后，外科医生将剥离物前移，打开 Retzius 间隙，然后显露左右盆腔内筋膜，确定膀胱颈。用马里兰双极钳小心地从后平面进入到前平面。

(8) AMS 800 放置：沿圆周切开膀胱颈后，使用通过 12mm 端口引入的卷尺测量周长。然后将充气袖带穿过相同的 12mm 端口并放置在膀胱颈部周围，小心轻拿袖带避免损坏。经耻骨上 3cm 切口将 61～70cmH_2O 压力调节球囊置入膀胱前间隙并注满水。通过相同的耻骨上切口抓住并从袖带取出管子。腹膜用带刺缝线封闭，封闭端口部位用局部麻醉剂浸润。通过从耻骨上切口开始形成皮下通道，将液压泵置入其中一个大阴唇。来自袖带、压力调节球囊和泵的管道通过耻骨上切口连接，然后关闭该切口，设备停用[103]。患者用 Foley 导管进行夜间监测，第二天早上进行排尿试验。许多外科专家在患者出院后使用短疗程广谱口服抗生素，尽管 AUA 指南不推荐这样做。

总结

总体而言，在复发性或持续性压力性尿失禁的管理中，很少有系统的数据来指导决策。吊带操作和网状吊带的使用正在减少，现在大多数患者可能会接受尿道填充术或自体筋膜吊带，这取决于其合并症和漏尿程度。存在括约肌功能障碍时，AUA 指南建议考虑重复尿道中段悬吊术、自体筋膜吊带或尿道填充术[27]。可能有在女性人工尿道括约肌植入或螺旋或阻塞吊带的独特情况。显然要在失败的领域进行持续的随访和研究，以更好地为这些患者提供治疗。

致谢：感谢莫纳什大学的 Tina Lam 和奥克兰理工大学的 Cassandra Khoo 在准备图 19-1 的平面设计元素方面提供的宝贵帮助。感谢我们家人的耐心，并感谢他们在完成这篇重要出版物的工作时给予的支持。

参考文献

[1] Wai CY, Curto TM, Zyczynski HM, Stoddard AM, Burgio KL, Brubaker L, et al. Patient satisfaction after midurethral sling surgery for stress urinary incontinence. Obstet Gynecol. 2013;121(5):1009–16.
[2] Treatment options for stress urinary incontinence. Information for consumers. Patient resource. https://www.safetyandqualitygovau/sites/default/files/2020-11/treatment_options_for_stress_urinary_incontinence_sui_-transvaginal_tv_mesh_-information_for_consumers_patient_resourcepdf.
[3] TGA information for medical practitioners on pending up-classification of surgical mesh devices. https://www.tgagovau/information-medical-practitioners- pending- classification- surgical- mesh- devices.
[4] Liu HH, Kuo HC. Durability of retropubic suburethral sling procedure and predictors for successful treatment outcome in women with stress urinary incontinence. Urology. 2019;131:83–8.
[5] Khayyami Y, Klarskov N, Lose G. The promise of urethral pressure reflectometry: an update. Int Urogynecol J. 2016;27(10):1449–58.
[6] Smith AR, Artibani W, Drake MJ. Managing unsatisfactory outcome after mid-urethral tape insertion. Neurourol Urodyn. 2011;30(5):771–4.
[7] Kavanagh A, Sanaee M, Carlson KV, Bailly GG. Management of patients with stress urinary incontinence after failed midurethral sling. Can Urol Assoc J. 2017;11(6Suppl2):S143–S6.
[8] Gormley EA. Evaluation and management of the patient with a failed midurethral synthetic sling. Can Urol Assoc J. 2012;6(5 Suppl 2):S123–S4.
[9] Escobar C, Brucker B. Urodynamics for the "failed" midurethral sling. Curr Bladder Dysfunct Rep. 2020;15(4):245–58.
[10] Zimmern PE, Gormley EA, Stoddard AM, Lukacz ES, Sirls L, Brubaker L, et al. Management of recurrent stress urinary incontinence after burch and sling procedures. Neurourol Urodyn. 2016;35(3):344–8.
[11] Dray EV, Hall M, Covalschi D, Cameron AP. Can urethral bulking agents salvage failed slings? Urology. 2019;124:78–82.
[12] Rodrigues P, Hering F, D'Imperio M, Campagnari JC. One hundred cases of SUI treatment that failed: a prospective observational study on the behavior of patients after surgical failure. Int Braz J Urol. 2014;40(6):790–801.
[13] MacLachlan LS, Rovner ES. Management of failed stress urinary incontinence surgery. Curr Urol Rep. 2014;15(8):429.
[14] Stav K, Dwyer PL, Rosamilia A, Schierlitz L, Lim YN, Lee J. Risk factors of treatment failure of midurethral sling procedures for women with urinary stress incontinence. Int Urogynecol J. 2010;21(2):149–55.
[15] Pradhan A, Jain P, Latthe PM. Effectiveness of midurethral slings in recurrent stress urinary incontinence: a systematic review and meta-analysis. Int Urogynecol J. 2012;23(7):831–41.
[16] Richter HE, Litman HJ, Lukacz ES, Sirls LT, Rickey L, Norton P, et al. Demographic and clinical predictors of treatment failure one year after midurethral sling surgery. Obstet Gynecol. 2011;117(4):913–21.
[17] Richter HE, Albo ME, Zyczynski HM, Kenton K, Norton PA, Sirls LT, et al. Retropubic versus transobturator midurethral slings for stress incontinence. N Engl J Med. 2010;362(22):2066–76.
[18] Bogusiewicz M, Monist M, Galczynski K, Wozniak M, Wieczorek AP, Rechberger T. Both the middle and distal sections of the urethra may be regarded as optimal targets for 'outside- in' transobturator tape placement. World J Urol. 2014;32(6):1605–11.
[19] Pedraszewski P, Wlazlak E, Wlazlak W, Krzycka M, Pajak P, Surkont G. The role of TVT position in relation to the pubic symphysis in eliminating the symptoms of stress urinary incontinence and urethral funneling. J Ultrason. 2019;19(78):207–11.
[20] Chan L, Tse V. Pelvic floor ultrasound in the diagnosis of sling complications. World J Urol. 2018;36(5):753–9.
[21] Mahdy A, Ghoniem GM. Autologous rectus fascia sling for treatment of stress urinary incontinence in women: a review of the literature. Neurourol Urodyn. 2019;38(Suppl 4):S51–S8.

[22] Fontenot PA, Padmanabhan P. Management of recurrent stress urinary incontinence after failed mid-urethral sling placement. Curr Bladder Dysfunct Rep. 2018;13(3):93–100.
[23] Clarke A Do urodynamic findings influence the approach to mid-urethral sling surgery for stress urinary incontinence? Br J Nurs. 2018;27(11):600–5.
[24] Nager CW, Sirls L, Litman HJ, Richter H, Nygaard I, Chai T, et al. Baseline urodynamic predictors of treatment failure 1 year after mid urethral sling surgery. J Urol. 2011;186(2):597–603.
[25] Hill B, Fletcher S, Blume J, Adam R, Ward R. Volume at first leak is associated with sling failure among women with stress urinary incontinence. Female Pelvic Med Reconstr Surg. 2019;25(4):294–7.
[26] NICE guidelines urinary-incontinence-and-pelvic-organ-prolapse-in-women-management-pdf- 66141657205189.pdf.
[27] Kobashi KC, Albo ME, Dmochowski RR, Ginsberg DA, Goldman HB, Gomelsky A, et al. Surgical treatment of female stress urinary incontinence: AUA/SUFU guideline. J Urol. 2017;198(4):875–83.
[28] Giarenis I, Thiagamoorthy G, Zacche M, Robinson D, Cardozo L. Management of recurrent stress urinary incontinence after failed midurethral sling: a survey of members of the International Urogynecological Association (IUGA). Int Urogynecol J. 2015;26(9):1285–91.
[29] Rashid TG, De Ridder D, Van der Aa F. The role of bladder neck suspension in the era of mid-urethral sling surgery. World J Urol. 2015;33(9):1235–41.
[30] Lucas MG, Bosch RJ, Burkhard FC, Cruz F, Madden TB, Nambiar AK, et al. EAU guidelines on surgical treatment of urinary incontinence. Eur Urol. 2012;62(6):1118–29.
[31] Bakali E, Johnson E, Buckley BS, Hilton P, Walker B, Tincello DG. Interventions for treating recurrent stress urinary incontinence after failed minimally invasive synthetic midurethral tape surgery in women. Cochrane Database Syst Rev. 2019;9:CD009407.
[32] Pergialiotis V, Mudiaga Z, Perrea DN, Doumouchtsis SK. De novo overactive bladder following midurethral sling procedures: a systematic review of the literature and meta-analysis. Int Urogynecol J. 2017;28(11):1631–8.
[33] Sajadi KP, Vasavada SP. Overactive bladder after sling surgery. Curr Urol Rep. 2010;11(6):366–71.
[34] Marcelissen T, Van Kerrebroeck P. Overactive bladder symptoms after midurethral sling surgery in women: risk factors and management. Neurourol Urodyn. 2018;37(1):83–8.
[35] Serati M, Braga A, Sorice P, Siesto G, Salvatore S, Ghezzi F. Solifenacin in women with de novo overactive bladder after tension-free obturator vaginal tape-is it effective? J Urol. 2014;191(5):1322–6.
[36] Miotla P, Futyma K, Cartwright R, Bogusiewicz M, Skorupska K, Markut-Miotla E, et al. Effectiveness of botulinum toxin injection in the treatment of de novo OAB symptoms following midurethral sling surgery. Int Urogynecol J. 2016;27(3):393–8.
[37] Sherman ND, Jamison MG, Webster GD, Amundsen CL. Sacral neuromodulation for the treatment of refractory urinary urge incontinence after stress incontinence surgery. Am J Obstet Gynecol. 2005;193(6):2083–7.
[38] Lovatsis D, Easton W, Wilkie D. No. 248–guidelines for the evaluation and treatment of recurrent urinary incontinence following pelvic floor surgery. J Obstet Gynaecol Can. 2017;39(9):e309–e14.
[39] Nadeau G, Herschorn S. Management of recurrent stress incontinence following a sling. Curr Urol Rep. 2014;15(8):427.
[40] Giarenis I, Cardozo L. Management of stress urinary incontinence following a failed midurethral tape. Curr Bladder Dysfunct Rep. 2011;6(2):67–9.
[41] Stav K, Dwyer PL, Rosamilia A, Schierlitz L, Lim YN, Chao F, et al. Repeat synthetic mid urethral sling procedure for women with recurrent stress urinary incontinence. J Urol. 2010;183(1):241–6.
[42] Nikolopoulos KI, Betschart C, Doumouchtsis SK. The surgical management of recurrent stress urinary incontinence: a systematic review. Acta Obstet Gynecol Scand. 2015;94(6):568–76.
[43] Rac G, Younger A, Clemens JQ, Kobashi K, Khan A, Nitti V, et al. Stress urinary incontinence surgery trends in academic female pelvic medicine and reconstructive surgery urology practice in the setting of the food and drug administration public health notifications. Neurourol Urodyn. 2017;36(4):1155–60.
[44] Hansen MF, Lose G, Kesmodel US, Gradel KO. Repeat surgery after failed midurethral slings: a nationwide cohort study, 1998–2007. Int Urogynecol J. 2016;27(7):1013–9.
[45] Plagakis S, Tse V. The autologous pubovaginal fascial sling: an update in 2019. Low Urin Tract Symptoms. 2020;12(1):2–7.
[46] Giarenis I, Malde S, Harding C, Robinson D, Gajewski J, Rahnamai M, et al. Do we need better information to advise women with stress incontinence on their choice of surgery? Report from the ICI-RS 2018. Neurourol Urodyn. 2019;38(Suppl 5):S98–S103.
[47] McGuire EJ, Lytton B. Pubovaginal sling procedure for stress incontinence. J Urol. 1978;119:82–4.
[48] Parker WP, Gomelsky A, Padmanabhan P. Autologous fascia pubovaginal slings after prior synthetic anti-incontinence procedures for recurrent incontinence: a multi-institutional prospective comparative analysis to de novo autologous slings assessing objective and subjective cure. Neurourol Urodyn. 2016;35(5):604–8.
[49] Milose JC, Sharp KM, He C, Stoffel J, Clemens JQ, Cameron AP. Success of autologous pubovaginal sling after failed synthetic mid urethral sling. J Urol. 2015;193(3):916–20.
[50] Petrou SP, Davidiuk AJ, Rawal B, Arnold M, Thiel DD. Salvage autologous fascial sling after failed synthetic midurethral sling: greater than 3–year outcomes. Int J Urol. 2016;23(2):178–81.
[51] Albo ME, Richter HE, Brubaker L, Norton P, Kraus SR, Zimmern PE, et al. Burch colposuspension versus fascial sling to reduce urinary stress incontinence. N Engl J Med. 2007;356:2143–55.
[52] Aberger M, Gomelsky A, Padmanabhan P. Comparison of retropubic synthetic mid-urethral slings to fascia pubovaginal slings following failed sling surgery. Neurourol Urodyn. 2016;35(7):851–4.
[53] Walsh CA. Recurrent stress urinary incontinence after synthetic mid-urethral sling procedures. Curr Opin Obstet Gynecol. 2011;23(5):355–61.
[54] Sanses TV, Brubaker L, Xu Y, Kraus SR, Lowder JL, Lemack GE, et al. Preoperative hesitating urinary stream is associated with postoperative voiding dysfunction and surgical failure following Burch colposuspension or pubovaginal rectus fascial sling surgery. Int Urogynecol J. 2011;22(6):713–9.
[55] Malde S, Moore JA. Autologous mid-urethral sling for stress urinary incontinence: preliminary results and description of a contemporary technique. J Clin Urol. 2015;9(1):40–7.
[56] Preece PD, Chan G, O'Connell HE, Gani J. Optimising the tension of an autologous fascia pubovaginal sling to minimize retentive complications. Neurourol Urodyn. 2019;38(5):1409–16.
[57] Zivanovic I, Rautenberg O, Lobodasch K, von Bunau G, Walser C, Viereck V. Urethral bulking for recurrent stress urinary incontinence after midurethral sling failure. Neurourol Urodyn. 2017;36(3):722–6.
[58] Toozs-Hobson P, Al-Singary W, Fynes M, Tegerstedt G, Lose G. Two-year follow-up of an open-label multicenter study of polyacrylamide hydrogel [Bulkamid(®)] for female stress and stress-predominant mixed incontinence. Int Urogynecol J. 2012;23(10):1373–8.
[59] Brosche T, Kuhn A, Lobodasch K, Sokol ER. Seven-year efficacy and safety outcomes of Bulkamid for the treatment of stress urinary incontinence. Neurourol Urodyn. 2021;40(1):502–8.
[60] Pai A, Al-Singary W. Durability, safety and efficacy of polyacrylamide hydrogel [Bulkamid(®)] in the management of stress and mixed urinary incontinence: three year follow up outcomes. Cent Eur J Urol. 2015;68(4):428–33.

[61] Rodriguez D, Jaffer A, Hilmy M, Zimmern P. Bladder neck and urethral erosions after Macroplastique injections. Low Urin Tract Symptoms. 2021;13(1):93–7.
[62] Lee HN, Lee YS, Han JY, Jeong JY, Choo MS, Lee KS. Transurethral injection of bulking agent for treatment of failed mid-urethral sling procedures. Int Urogynecol J. 2010; 21(12):1479–83.
[63] Rodriguez D, Carroll T, Alhalabi F, Carmel M, Zimmern PE. Outcomes of Macroplastique injections for stress urinary incontinence after suburethral sling removal. Neurourol Urodyn. 2020;39(3):994–1001.
[64] Siddiqui ZA, Abboudi H, Crawford R, Shah S. Intraurethral bulking agents for the management of female stress urinary incontinence: a systematic review. Int Urogynecol J. 2017;28(9):1275–84.
[65] Kim J, Lee W, Lucioni A, Govier F, Kobashi K. 1360 long-term efficacy and durability of Durashpere. urethral bulking after failed urethral sling for stress urinary incontinence. The J Urol. 2012;187:552.
[66] Gaddi A, Guaderrama N, Bassiouni N, Bebchuk J, Whitcomb EL. Repeat midurethral sling compared with urethral bulking for recurrent stress urinary incontinence. Obstet Gynecol. 2014;123(6):1207–12.
[67] Schierlitz L, Dwyer PL, Rosamilia A, Murray C, Thomas E, De Souza A, et al. Three-year follow-up of tension-free vaginal tape compared with transobturator tape in women with stress urinary incontinence and intrinsic sphincter deficiency. Obstet Gynecol. 2012;119(2 Pt 1):321–7.
[68] Speed JM, Mishra K. What to do after a mid-urethral sling fails. Curr Opin Obstet Gynecol. 2020;32(6):449–55.
[69] Kim A, Kim MS, Park YJ, Choi WS, Park HK, Paick SH, et al. Retropubic versus transobturator mid urethral slings in patients at high risk for recurrent stress incontinence: a systematic review and meta-analysis. J Urol. 2019;202(1):132–42.
[70] Ford AA, Rogerson L, Cody JD, Aluko P, Ogah JA. Mid-urethral sling operations for stress urinary incontinence in women. Cochrane Database Syst Rev. 2017;7:CD006375.
[71] Abdel-Fattah M, Cao G, Mostafa A. Long-term outcomes of transobturator tension-free vaginal tapes as secondary continence procedures. World J Urol. 2017;35(7):1141–8.
[72] Ulrich D, Bjelic-Radisic V, Grabner K, Avian A, Trutnovsky G, Tamussino K, et al. Objective outcome and quality-of-life assessment in women with repeat incontinence surgery. Neurourol Urodyn. 2017;36(6):1543–9.
[73] Park BH, Kim JC, Kim HW, Kim YH, Choi JB, Lee DH. Midterm efficacy and complications of readjustable midurethral sling (Remeex system) in female stress urinary incontinence with recurrence or intrinsic sphincter deficiency. Urology. 2015;85(1):79–84.
[74] Kociszewski J, Majkusiak W, Pomian A, Tomasik P, Horosz E, Kuszka A, et al. The outcome of repeated mid urethral sling in SUI treatment after vaginal excisions of primary failed sling: preliminary study. Biomed Res Int. 2016;2016:1242061.
[75] Tincello DG, Armstrong N, Hilton P, Buckley B, Mayne C. Surgery for recurrent stress urinary incontinence: the views of surgeons and women. Int Urogynecol J. 2018;29(1):45–54.
[76] De Cuyper EM, Ismail R, Maher CF. Laparoscopic Burch colposuspension after failed sub-urethral tape procedures: a retrospective audit. Int Urogynecol J Pelvic Floor Dysfunct. 2008;19(5):681–5.
[77] Kim S, Son JH, Kim HS, Ko JS, Kim JC. Tape shortening for recurrent stress urinary incontinence after transobturator tape sling: 3-year follow-up results. Int Neurourol J. 2010;14(3):164–9.
[78] Schmid C, Bloch E, Amann E, Mueller MD, Kuhn A. An adjustable sling in the management of recurrent urodynamic stress incontinence after previous failed midurethral tape. Neurourol Urodyn. 2010;29(4):573–7.
[79] de Landsheere L, Lucot JP, Foidart JM, Cosson M. Management of recurrent or persistent stress urinary incontinence after TVT-O by mesh readjustment. Int Urogynecol J. 2010;21(11):1347–51.
[80] Patterson D, Rajan S, Kohli N. Sling plication for recurrent stress urinary incontinence. Female Pelvic Med Reconstr Surg. 2010;16(5):307–9.
[81] Maheshwari D, Jones K, Solomon E, Harmanli O. Sling plication for failed midurethral sling procedures: a case series. Female Pelvic Med Reconstr Surg. 2019;25(1):e4–6.
[82] Glazener CM, Cooper K, Mashayekhi A. Anterior vaginal repair for urinary incontinence in women. Cochrane Database Syst Rev. 2017;7:CD001755.
[83] Dray EV, Cameron AP, Bergman R. Stress urinary incontinence in women with neurogenic lower urinary tract dysfunction. Curr Bladder Dysfunct Rep. 2018;13(2):75–83.
[84] Rodriguez AR, Hakky T, Hoffman M, Ordorica R, Lockhart J. Salvage spiral sling techniques: alternatives to manage disabling recurrent urinary incontinence in females. J Urol. 2010;184(6):2429–33.
[85] Onol SY, Sevket O, Onol FF, Erdem R, Tepeler A. Minimum 1-year results of mesh spiral-sling procedure in managing refractory and primary disabling stress urinary incontinence. Int Urogynecol J. 2014;25(10):1399–404.
[86] Rutman MP, Deng DY, Shah SM, Raz S, Rodríguez LV. Spiral sling salvage anti-incontinence surgery in female patients with a nonfunctional urethra: technique and initial results. J Urol. 2006;175(5):1794–9.
[87] Lengmang S, Shephard S, Datta A, Lozo S, Kirschner CV. Pubovesical sling for residual incontinence after successful vesicovaginal fistula closure: a new approach to an old procedure. Int Urogynecol J. 2018;29(10):1551–6.
[88] Aboseif SR, Sassani P, Frankc EI, Nash SD, Slutsky JN, Baum NH, et al. Treatment of moderate to severe female stress urinary incontinence with the adjustable continence therapy (ACT) device after failed surgical repair. World J Urol. 2011;29(2):249–53.
[89] Kocjancic E, Crivellaro S, Ranzoni S, Bonvini D, Grosseti B, Frea B. Adjustable continence therapy for severe intrinsic sphincter deficiency and recurrent female stress urinary incontinence: long-term experience. J Urol. 2010;184(3):1017–21.
[90] Phe V, Nguyen K, Roupret M, Cardot V, Parra J, Chartier-Kastler E. A systematic review of the treatment for female stress urinary incontinence by ACT(R) balloon placement (Uromedica, Irvine, CA, USA). World J Urol. 2014;32(2):495–505.
[91] Staack A, Rodriguez LV. Stem cells for the treatment of urinary incontinence. Curr Urol Rep. 2011;12(1):41–6.
[92] Mitterberger M, Pinggera G-M, Marksteiner R, Margreiter E, Fussenegger M, Frauscher F, et al. Adult stem cell therapy of female stress urinary incontinence. Eur Urol. 2008;53(1):169–75.
[93] Tran C, Damaser MS. The potential role of stem cells in the treatment of urinary incontinence. Ther Adv Urol. 2015;7(1):22–40.
[94] Gomelsky A, Athanasiou S, Choo MS, Cosson M, Dmochowski RR, Gomes CM, et al. Surgery for urinary incontinence in women: report from the 6th international consultation on incontinence. Neurourol Urodyn. 2019;38(2):825–37.
[95] Cour F, Le Normand L, Lapray JF, Hermieu JF, Peyrat L, Yiou R, et al. Intrinsic sphincter deficiency and female urinary incontinence. Prog Urol. 2015;25(8):437–54.
[96] Peyronnet B, Greenwell T, Gray G, Khavari R, Thiruchelvam N, Capon G, et al. Current use of the artificial urinary sphincter in adult females. Curr Urol Rep. 2020;21(12):53.
[97] Peyronnet B, O'Connor E, Khavari R, Capon G, Manunta A, Allue M, et al. AMS-800 artificial urinary sphincter in female patients with stress urinary incontinence: a systematic review. Neurourol Urodyn. 2019;38(Suppl 4):S28–s41.
[98] Phé V, Léon P, Granger B, Denys P, Bitker MO, Mozer P, et al. Stress urinary incontinence in female neurological patients: long-term

functional outcomes after artificial urinary sphincter [AMS 800(TM)] implantation. Neurourol Urodyn. 2017;36(3):764–9.
[99] Chartier-Kastler E, Van Kerrebroeck P, Olianas R, Cosson M, Mandron E, Delorme E, et al. Artificial urinary sphincter (AMS 800) implantation for women with intrinsic sphincter deficiency: a technique for insiders? BJU Int. 2011;107(10):1618–26.
[100] Reus CR, Phe V, Dechartres A, Grilo NR, Chartier-Kastler EJ, Mozer PC. Performance and safety of the artificial urinary sphincter (AMS 800) for non-neurogenic women with urinary incontinence secondary to intrinsic sphincter deficiency: a systematic review. Eur Urol Focus. 2020;6(2):327–38.
[101] Vayleux B, Rigaud J, Luyckx F, Karam G, Glémain P, Bouchot O, et al. Female urinary incontinence and artificial urinary sphincter: study of efficacy and risk factors for failure and complications. Eur Urol. 2011;59(6):1048–53.
[102] Costa P, Poinas G, Ben Naoum K, Bouzoubaa K, Wagner L, Soustelle L, et al. Long-term results of artificial urinary sphincter for women with type III stress urinary incontinence. Eur Urol. 2013;63(4):753–8.
[103] Peyronnet B, Capon G, Belas O, Manunta A, Allenet C, Hascoet J, et al. Robot-assisted AMS-800 artificial urinary sphincter bladder neck implantation in female patients with stress urinary incontinence. Eur Urol. 2019;75(1):169–75.
[104] Costa P, Mottet N, Rabut B, Thuret R, Ben Naoum K, Wagner L. The use of an artificial urinary sphincter in women with type III incontinence and a negative Marshall test. J Urol. 2001;165(4):1172–6.
[105] Abbassian A. A new operation for insertion of the artificial urinary sphincter. J Urol. 1988;140(3):512–3.
[106] Gondran-Tellier B, Boissier R, Baboudjian M, Rouy M, Gaillet S, Lechevallier E, et al. Robot-assisted implantation of an artificial urinary sphincter, the AMS-800, via a posterior approach to the bladder neck in women with intrinsic sphincter deficiency. BJU Int. 2019;124(6):1077–80.

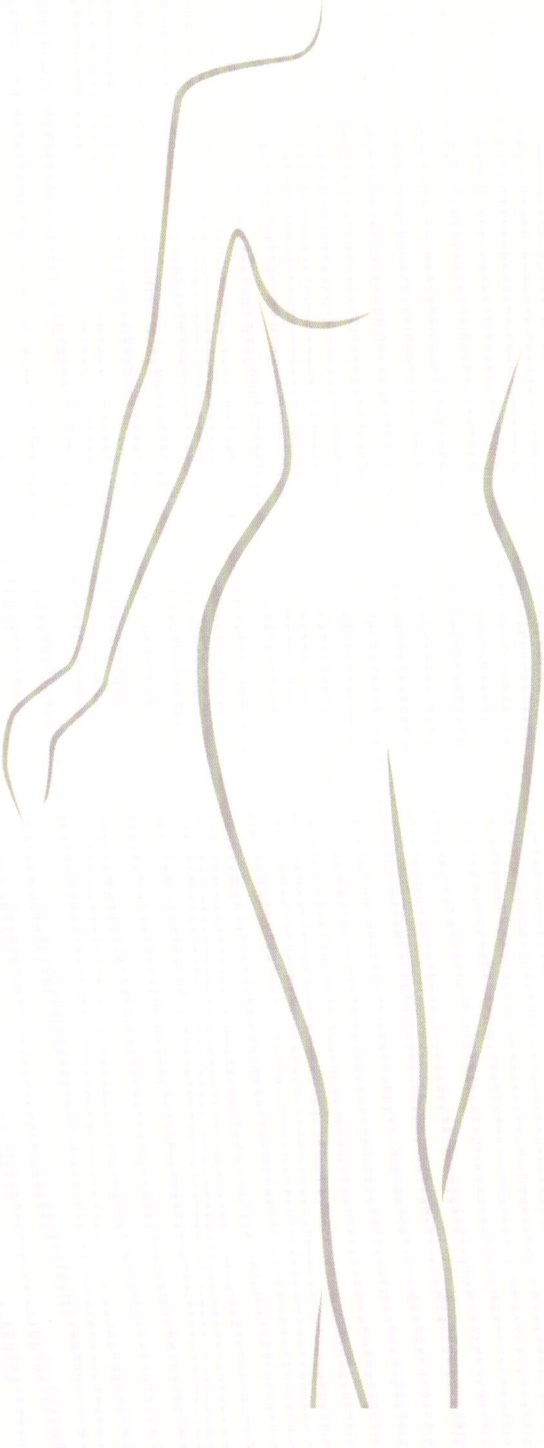

第五篇 尿失禁的其他因素和原因

Other Contributors and Causes of Incontinence

第20章 盆腔脏器脱垂是压力性尿失禁和急迫性尿失禁的一个危险因素

Prolapse as a Contributing Factor to Stress and Urgency Urinary Incontinence

Whitney Horner Carolyn W. Swenson 著

一、脱垂的流行病学

（一）定义

盆腔器官脱垂是盆腔器官向下移位，伴有症状[1]。盆腔器官包括阴道前壁和后壁、子宫、阴道顶端和邻近的器官，如膀胱、肠道。常见脱垂症状为阴道膨出或受压，排尿不全需要夹板或指状，出血、分泌物或腰痛[1, 2]。脱垂在超出阴道口时最具症状。通过临床检查进行诊断，脱垂的定量可以使用盆腔器官脱垂定量（POP-Q）[3]或Baden-Walker分级系统[4]。根据受影响的腔室进行分类：阴道前壁脱垂（膀胱膨出）、阴道后壁脱垂（直肠膨出）、子宫/宫颈脱垂、阴道穹窿脱垂（如果是子宫切除术后的情况）和肠膨出（膀胱切除术后小肠疝）。

（二）患病率

据报道，脱垂的患病率为3%～50%，这取决于脱垂的定义。在一项针对近2000例美国女性的人群的研究中，2.9%的受访者自我报道有症状性阴道隆起[5]。在其他类似的人群的研究中报道症状脱垂的患病率为6%～8%[6]。当通过体检确定脱垂时，脱垂的患病率要高得多。Swift等的一项研究发现，在常规妇科护理中无脱垂症状的女性中，50.3%的人在检查中出现POP-Q2期（脱垂距离处女膜1cm以内）或3期（脱垂距离处女膜1cm外）[7]。

在不同类型的脱垂中，阴道前壁脱垂最常见，影响超过1/3的50岁女性，其次是阴道后壁脱垂（约1/5）和子宫脱垂（1/7）[8]。对于美国女性来说，脱垂手术的终生风险估计为12.6%[9]。

（三）危险因素

脱垂是一种多因素疾病，由解剖因素、分娩相关结构变化、合并症和遗传风险共同导致[10]。年龄可能是脱垂的最大危险因素，在≥80岁的女性中，脱垂和脱垂手术的比例最高[11]。在女性健康倡议对16 616例女性的横断面分析中，与50—59岁的女性相比，70—79岁的女性子宫脱垂的概率增加36%，阴道后壁脱垂的概率增加18%，阴道前壁脱垂的概率增加35%[9]。衰老和脱垂之间的关系还不完全清楚。然而，与年龄相关的骨骼肌变化、神经肌肉和结缔组织损伤以及随着时间的推移反复的盆底负荷都可能起作用。

阴道分娩是脱垂的另一个重要危险因素，每多一次分娩就有累积风险[12-16]。肛提肌是构成盆底“底板”的骨骼肌，在阴道分娩时经历了显著的拉伸和变形。产钳辅助阴道分娩是肛提肌损伤风险最高的分娩方式，与自然分娩相比，其概率增加了11～26倍[17]。MRI和超声检测显示，34%～55%的脱垂女性存在肛提肌缺损[18, 19]。严重的肛提肌缺损会使脱垂的概率增加7倍[20]。即使在没有明显损伤的情况下，盆底肌肉也会因阴道分娩而遭受神经损伤。一项对初产妇在分娩前和产后 6 周和 6 个月进行肛门括约肌电图检查的研究发现，24.1% 的女性患有提肛神经病变，只有 64% 的女性在 6 个月后恢复[21]。在三维计算机模拟阴道分娩过程中，DeLancey 等发现直肠下神经和会阴神经分支分别被拉伸到原来长度的 35% 和 33%，超过了已知造成永久性神经损伤的 15% 应变阈值[22]。盆底肌肉去神经会损害提肌维持正常骨盆支撑的功能，增加脱垂发展的风险。在一项使用特殊设计的器械窥镜评估肛提肌强度的研究中，DeLancey 等发现脱垂的女性阴道闭合力（盆底肌肉最大收缩时产生的力）比不脱垂的女性低 40%[18]。

虽然剖宫产能显著降低盆底疾病的风险，但并不能完全保护胎儿。在一项对 1528 例首次分娩后 5～10 年的女性的纵向研究中，发现采用手术阴道分娩（产钳或真空）的女性盆底障碍的发生率最高，而采用剖宫产分娩并以自发阴道分娩为参照组的女性盆底障碍发生率最低。然而，剖宫产组仍报告有盆底症状，脱垂占 5%，压力性尿失禁占 13%，膀胱过度活动占 10.4%[23]。Lukacz 等进行了一项需要治疗的数字分析，并确定有 7 例女性必须通过剖宫产来分娩，以防止女性患盆底疾病[15]。因此，单独的妊娠压力，独立于分娩路线，可能会带来盆底紊乱的风险，包括脱垂。

一些研究表明，脱垂的遗传易感性与双胞胎的脱垂高度一致，并且患有结缔组织疾病的女性脱垂风险增加[20, 24-26]。一级家庭成员（如姐妹或母亲）患有脱垂的女性，其自身脱垂的风险显著增加[13]。最近的一项 Meta 分析和系统综述发现了支持胶原蛋白基因（COL1A1）与脱垂[27]之间关联的证据。HOXa11 是一种参与泌尿生殖道胚胎发育的同源异型盒基因，据报道，与对照组相比，脱垂女性的子宫骶韧带（USL）（子宫和阴道上部的主要支撑结构）中 HOXa11 显著减少。尽管有这些研究，“脱垂基因”尚未被确定，脱垂的遗传风险仍然未知。

最后，对盆底结构的长期重复负荷会增加脱垂的风险。重复负荷是指导致腹内和盆腔压力重复增加的活动或状况。这包括肥胖[8, 16]、慢性紧张便秘[28]，以及重体力劳动（如农场和工厂工人）[13]。

二、脱垂如何导致尿失禁

（一）常见危险因素

虽然并非所有脱垂女性都有尿失禁的经历，但由于共同的疾病机制，这两种疾病经常共存。上一节讨论的脱垂的许多危险因素，如年龄和阴道分娩，也是尿失禁的危险因素。

在不同类型的脱垂中，考虑到膀胱、尿道和阴道前壁之间的解剖关系，阴道前壁（AVW）脱垂最有可能伴有尿失禁。因此，本节将重点讨论阴道前壁脱垂与尿失禁之间的因果关系。

（二）脱垂和压力性尿失禁

高达 80% 的脱垂女性还伴有压力性尿失禁[29, 30]。阴道前壁脱垂（图 20-1）通常被称为“膀胱囊肿”，这错误地暗示了这种情况是由膀胱病理引起的。事实上，膀胱和尿道脱垂是一个结果，而不是原因，阴道前壁脱垂是由于在三层骨盆支持的任何一层结缔组织支持受损所致[31]。

正如 DeLancey 所描述的，阴道前壁结缔组织和骨盆内筋膜形成了一个吊床状的支撑，支撑着尿道和膀胱，锚定在外侧的腱弓筋膜骨盆[32]。随着腹腔内和囊泡内压力的增加，出现尿道压迫这个吊床，导致腔内尿道压力增加从而维持平衡。阴道前壁脱垂被认为是导致压力性尿失禁的原因，因为当支持性吊床失效时，尿道和尿道膀胱连接无法抵消腹内压力的增加，导致“尿道高流动性”和尿道腔的闭合受损。

对阴道前壁脱垂和压力性尿失禁的研究表明，这种相关性在较低的脱垂阶段最强，一旦脱垂大到足以“扭结”尿道并导致出口梗阻，压力性尿失禁的发生率实际上会降低（图 20-2）。Burrows 等对 330 例女性进行了回顾性研究，以确定脱垂与膀胱症状之间的关系，发现无压力性尿失禁的女性最大阴道前壁脱垂更低（即 POP-Q 强阳性）（+1.0 vs. 0.0cm，$P<0.001$），无压力性尿失禁的女性顶端位置也更明显（0.0 vs. –5.0cm，$P<0.001$）[33]。

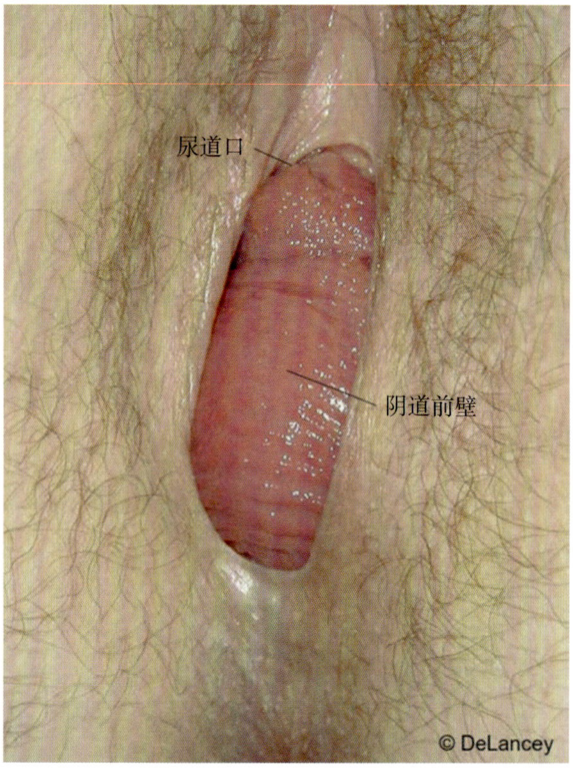

▲ 图 20-1 膀胱囊肿的临床图片显示尿道口向上倾斜，阴道前壁支撑受损

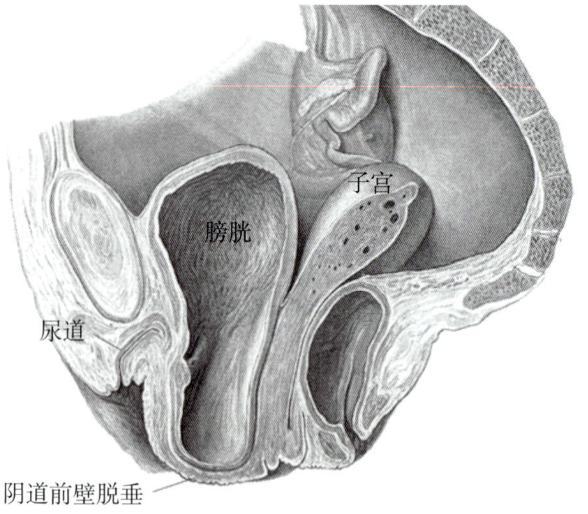

▲ 图 20-2 解剖图显示膀胱、尿道和阴道前壁之间的正中矢状关系，伴阴道前壁大面积脱垂。可见尿道“扭结”

相反，在需要人工辅助排空膀胱的女性中，阴道前壁和根尖脱垂明显更大（+3.0 vs. 0.0cm，$P<0.001$；+1.5 vs. −5.0cm，$P<0.001$）。这些结果表明膀胱出口梗阻对压力性尿失禁具有保护作用。

与压力性尿失禁最密切相关的因素是最大尿道闭合压力（MUCP），有压力性尿失禁的女性比没有压力性尿失禁的女性低 42%[34]。如前所述，增大阴道前壁脱垂尺寸与压力性尿失禁症状减少相关，因此，人们可以假设与尿道梗阻相关的最大尿道闭合压力增加是其潜在机制。然而，观察最大尿道闭合压力与阴道前壁脱垂大小之间关系的研究显示了相互矛盾的结果。在 Bai 等的一项研究中，最大尿道闭合压力在 4 期阴道前壁脱垂女性中最高［68.7 ± 20.3mmHg（2 期）vs. 67.0 ± 20.2mmHg（3 期）vs. 79.0 ± 30.9mmHg（4 期）］；但三组间差异无统计学意义（P=0.07）[35]。相反，Chang 等的一项研究报告，压力尿道闭合压力随着脱垂阶段的增加而降低，对于 1、2 和 3 期阴道前壁脱垂，压力尿道闭合压力分别为 69.3cmH_2O、62.3cmH_2O 和 52.2cmH_2O（均 $P<0.05$）[36]。然而，在控制了其他临床因素如年龄、更年期状况和阴道胎次后，这些关联的意义减弱了。年龄是最大尿道闭合压力的主要决定因素，每 10 年减少 15mmHg[37]，也是脱垂的主要危险因素；因此，压力性尿失禁和脱垂之间的另一种解释可能仅仅是衰老的共同风险因素。这些研究看似相互矛盾的结果表明，阴道前壁脱垂与尿道功能之间存在复杂的关系。尿道过度运动和尿道闭合压力对压力性尿失禁发病机制的相对贡献可能取决于每个女性独特的危险因素和阴道前壁脱垂的程度。因此，未来研究的一个潜在领域可以集中于量化每个危险因素对阴道前壁脱垂女性压力性尿失禁发展的患者特异性贡献。

最后，在晚期阴道前壁脱垂的女性中，由于没有事先的紧急情况和盆底肌肉收缩而手动压迫膀胱而引起的活动或某些位置的变化可发生意外压力性尿失禁。

（三）脱垂和急迫性尿失禁

22%～88% 的脱垂女性有急迫性尿失禁[38]。据报道，急迫性尿失禁合并脱垂的相对风险为 1.1～5.8[39-41]。虽然脱垂的治疗与急迫性尿失禁的改善相关，但急迫性尿失禁的治疗并不能改善脱垂，这表明共同的疾病机制主要与膀胱和尿道支持功能受损有关[42]。

脱垂和急迫性尿失禁之间的关联机制已经被提出，但没有一个在人体研究中得到明确证明。晚期阴道前壁脱垂可引起膀胱出口梗阻和膀胱排空不全，以及移位膀胱的机械压迫。随着时间的推移，这些因素会导致逼尿肌的刺激和重塑以及尿路上皮的机械创伤。一些动物研究表明，尿路上皮细胞会在化学或机械刺激下释放乙酰胆碱和 ATP，从而引发逼尿肌收缩和过度活动[40, 43-45]。

三、脱垂治疗如何改善压力性尿失禁和急迫性尿失禁

如上文所讨论的，脱垂和尿失禁通常同时存在，这是由于密切相关的疾病机制。因此，通过子宫托或手术矫正脱垂，可以通过解决膀胱出口梗阻和（或）改进阴道前壁支架来改善尿路症状[38, 46]。

（一）使用子宫托

子宫托可有效治疗脱垂症状，改善脱垂程度[47]。也有数据显示使用子宫托可改善泌尿系统症状（包括急迫性尿失禁和压力性尿失禁）。在一项对 73 例脱垂女性的前瞻性研究中，使用子宫托 2 个月后，45% 的女性压力性大小便失禁得到改善，46% 的女性强烈性大小便失禁得到改善，53% 的女性排尿困难得到改善[48]。另一项研究报告称，在 97 例成功安装阴道子宫托的女性中，使用 4 个月后，37% 的人的急迫性下降，28% 的人的急迫性尿失禁下降，但压力性尿失禁没有明显改善[49]。相反，Hanson 等报道使用子宫托的女性急迫性尿失禁治愈率为 58%。

除了主观改善尿失禁症状，客观改善尿流动力学研究尿流量测量使用子宫托已被证明。Romanzi 等发现 72% 脱垂女性尿流动力学检查提示有尿道梗阻，其中 94% 的女性在子宫托插入后得到缓解[50]。同样，另一项研究表明，子宫托使用 3 个月后，最大流量、平均流量、排出量和排出后剩余容积显著改善。在同一项研究中，76.9% 的女性报告急迫性尿失禁改善，58.1% 的压力性尿失禁改善。然而，20% 的女性在子宫托使用后发生了新的压力性尿失禁[51]。

（二）手术

手术修复脱垂与重建和清除程序也可以改善恼人的泌尿症状。需要注意的是，虽然脱垂矫正可以改善压力性尿失禁或急迫性尿失禁症状，但脱垂手术的主要目标是治疗脱垂症状，而不是泌尿系统症状。此外，脱垂矫正实际上可能导致新的急迫性尿失禁或压力性尿失禁症状，在脱垂手术前对病情严重的患者进行适当的评估和咨询[52]。

Baessler 等在第六届国际尿失禁会议中回顾了脱垂手术对膀胱功能的影响。他们报道说，在接受脱垂手术的女性中，高达 40% 的术前膀胱过度活动症（OAB）症状可能会得到缓解[53]。Chang 等在膀胱日记和尿流动力学上主客观均显示脱垂修复后下尿路症状（LUTS）明显改善[32]。在这项研究中，尽管液体摄入量、总排尿量和每次排尿的最大排尿量没有变化，但除了多项排尿日记参数（夜尿发作、日间频率、急症发作和失禁发作）外，关于下尿路症状和生活质量的验证问卷也得到了显著改善。在 De Boer 等的一篇综述中，研究了脱垂修复术前后未伴随失禁手术的膀胱过度活动症症状。7 项研究的术后随访时间为 12～30 个月。在所有研究中，逼尿肌过度活动在术后均有所下降，其下降比例为 25%～80%[42]。在对脱垂进行重建手术与闭锁手术比较时，可以观察到类似的紧急症状和症状频率的改善[54]。

虽然一些研究显示膀胱过度活动症有显著改善，但脱垂修复后仍有出现新的膀胱过度活动症的风险。在 Cochrane 对脱垂手术治疗的回顾中，12% 的女性在接受脱垂手术后出现了新的膀胱过度活动症[55]。

在脱垂手术前患有压力性尿失禁的女性中，压力性尿失禁仅通过脱垂手术而不伴随失禁手术解决的可能性很低。仅脱垂手术术后压力性尿失禁的风险为 39%，而伴有中尿道吊带的风险为 8%～19%[55]。在患有隐匿性压力性尿失禁的女

性中，仅脱垂手术后发生压力性尿失禁的风险为34%，而伴有中尿道吊带的风险为10%～22%[55]。Colombo等比较了前阴道切开术和Burch膀胱尿道悬吊术治疗阴道前壁脱垂和压力性尿失禁。在本研究中，52%仅行前路修复的女性压力性尿失禁主观治愈[56]。Baessler等在第六届尿失禁国际会议中分析发现，与脱垂修复时伴有失禁手术的女性相比，未伴有失禁手术的女性发生持续性压力性尿失禁的概率增加了11倍[53]。同样，术前隐匿性压力性尿失禁检查呈阳性且在脱垂修复时未进行伴随性尿失禁手术的女性，术后发生新的或"重新发生"压力性尿失禁的概率比同时进行尿失禁手术的女性高10倍。Borstad等的研究表明，仅29%的女性通过自体组织脱垂手术治愈压力性尿失禁，且不需要禁尿手术[57]。

阴道补片在脱垂修补术中的使用也会影响复发压力性尿失禁的风险。在Cochrane关于脱垂手术处理的综述中，发现阴道前网修复与前路原位组织修复相比，术后新生压力性尿失禁略有增加（RR=1.58）[55]。Baessler等报道称，前路修复术后新生压力性尿失禁率为8%，而前路臂网修复术后新生压力性尿失禁率为14%[53]。

四、盆腔器官脱垂修复术何时应进行失禁手术

所有计划接受脱垂手术的女性都应筛查泌尿系统症状并评估隐匿性压力性尿失禁，以最大限度地降低脱垂手术后重新发生压力性尿失禁的风险，其风险为15%～51%[55, 58-61]。隐匿性压力性尿失禁患者中，接受脱垂手术而无尿失禁的患者术后压力性尿失禁发生率明显高于伴有尿失禁手术的患者（OR=9.8，95%CI 7.1%～13.6%）[57, 59, 60, 62]。Liang等的研究表明，术前隐匿性压力性尿失禁合并子宫托的患者在术后18～21个月未接受中尿道吊带的患者中，与术后18～21个月接受吊带的患者相比，出现新生压力性尿失禁的患者明显更多（53% vs. 0%，P＜0.001）[59]。

由于术前隐匿性压力性尿失禁显著增加脱垂手术后重新发生压力性尿失禁的风险，计划脱垂手术的女性应在术前进行常规评估。隐匿性压力性尿失禁可通过减压试验或尿流动力学试验进行评估。减压压力测试评估脱垂"减少"的控制力，模拟脱垂的解决方案，就像子宫托或手术一样。减压试验技术的标准方案尚未达成共识；然而，典型的程序是手动减少脱垂，然后让患者咳嗽或做Valsalva动作多达3次，膀胱舒适地充满或回填到300ml。脱垂减少可以使用大尖端棉镜，检查者的手或子宫托。Visco等通过减压测试发现，在27%计划施行骶直肠固定术治疗脱垂的压力较大的女性中，有隐匿性压力性尿失禁[60]。对于选择手术前子宫托试验的女性，这也是一个评估隐匿性尿失禁的机会。

不幸的是，减压测试的预测价值是有限的，因为39%的阴性测试的女性仍然会出现新的压力性尿失禁[60]。由于没有办法完美地预测谁会发生新生压力性尿失禁，所有患者都应该被告知发生新生压力性尿失禁的可能性，尽管减压测试呈阴性。

尿流动力学研究通常在女性失禁手术前进行，以确认诊断或指导治疗决定。然而，Nager等表明，对于无并发症、可证实的压力性尿失禁的女性，与单独的办公室评估（包括刺激性压力测试、尿空后剩余容量、尿道活动能力评估和膀胱无感染）相比，尿流动力学测试并不能提高治疗成功率（77.2% vs. 76.9%）[63]。当对脱垂的女性患者进行尿流动力学治疗时，应在脱垂减轻的情况下进行压力操作，特别是对晚期脱垂患者。

五、脱垂手术何时应同时进行尿失禁手术

所有接受脱垂手术的女性都应该被告知伴随性尿失禁手术的选择。下面，我们将讨论有助于指导咨询和决策的注意事项。

（一）明显的压力性尿失禁

对于同时存在压力性尿失禁和脱垂的患者，通常建议在脱垂手术时同时进行尿失禁手

术。与同时进行失禁手术的患者相比，接受脱垂手术而不进行失禁手术的患者发生持续性压力性尿失禁的风险明显更高（OR=10.9，95%CI 7.9～15.0）[55, 53]。然而，在一小部分女性中，仅在脱垂修复后压力性尿失禁可得到改善或解决[55, 57]。因此，可能首选分阶段方法。

（二）隐匿性压力性尿失禁

减压试验中隐匿的压力性尿失禁和脱垂发生或进展前的压力性尿失禁史是咨询患者术后压力性尿失禁风险时考虑的重要因素。与可证明性压力性尿失禁相似，隐秘性压力性尿失禁的女性在脱垂修复后有复发性压力性尿失禁的风险（OR=9.8，95%CI 7.1～13.6）[53]。

（三）尿失禁女性的预防性手术

在接受脱垂修复术的尿失禁女性中，应该讨论重新压力性尿失禁的风险和伴随失禁手术的风险和益处。预测谁将从预防性失禁手术中受益在临床上具有挑战性。对于有过禁药史的女性，降低复发压力性尿失禁风险的一种选择包括在脱垂修复时实施失禁手术。Brubaker 等的研究表明，与单纯的骶直肠固定术相比，在腹部骶直肠固定术时同时进行 Burch 膀胱尿道悬吊术可显著降低两年后复发压力性尿失禁症状的风险（41.8% vs. 57.9%；P=0.020）[58]。而为预防 1 例尿失禁而行伯氏阴道悬吊术的患者为 6.2 例。Wei 等在 12 个月后证实，阴道脱垂手术时接受无张力性阴道悬吊术也比单纯脱垂手术显著降低尿失禁的风险（27.3% vs. 43.0%，P=0.002）[61]。与 Brubaker 的研究相似，为预防 1 例尿失禁，需要无张力性阴道悬吊术治疗的人数为 6.3 人。因此，如果所有接受脱垂修复术的女性同时接受失禁手术，57% 的女性将接受不必要的手术并面临相关风险。

（四）危险因素的存在和以患者为中心的结果

提供者和患者之间的共同决策对于确定脱垂手术时伴随的失禁程序是否合适是很重要的。脱垂发生前的压力性尿失禁症状、目前的症状和生活质量、全膀胱减压压力测试和（或）尿流动力学的结果应有助于指导咨询。然而，术前讨论患者的偏好和目标是必要的，因为未达到的目标与治疗后患者的不满有关[64]。例如，如果患者对补片有强烈的厌恶感，尽管有新生压力性尿失禁的风险因素，但可能会拒绝使用吊带。相反，如果患者有强烈的愿望避免新生压力性尿失禁的风险，尽管没有隐匿性压力性尿失禁或危险因素，也可以进行伴随性尿失禁手术。此外，决定是否增加一个伴随失禁程序也可能取决于计划手术。在使用阴道补片进行修复的大陆女性中，与原生组织修复相比，发生新生压力性尿失禁的风险更高；然而，这些产品已不再上市（RR=1.58，95%CI 1.05～2.37）（9% vs. 14%）[55]。

（五）新发压力性尿失禁的风险评估

风险分层模型通常是共享决策的有用工具。Jelovsek 等建立了一个模型来预测女性新生压力性尿失禁的个体风险[65]。列线图量表使用危险因素包括手术年龄、阴道分娩次数、体重指数、术前压力测试、是否进行失禁手术、与紧迫感相关的尿漏、糖尿病诊断来预测脱垂修复的女性发生新生压力性尿失禁的风险。这些信息可以用来指导决定在脱垂修复时进行尿失禁手术。

（六）策划过程

对于那些选择分期手术的患者，脱垂修复术单独进行，术后监测泌尿系统症状。如果麻烦的从头开始压力性尿失禁发展，失禁程序可以作为第二次手术进行。在同时放置和延迟放置中尿道吊带的比较中，主观结果似乎没有差异（压力性尿失禁风险 1%～16% vs. 11%）[57]。

如果仅靠脱垂手术不能治疗尿失禁，需要进行干预，则尿失禁的治疗应与没有脱垂修复史的人相似。

总结

盆腔器官脱垂和尿失禁是女性常见的疾病，由于共同的疾病机制和共同的危险因素，往往同时存在。虽然脱垂矫正后尿路症状可以改善，但脱垂修复后仍有持续或重新出现尿失禁的风险。伴随性尿失禁的程序可以提供脱垂修复或治疗既有的或防止新的压力性尿失禁。

风险分层和患者偏好对于确定脱垂修复时伴随失禁的手术是否合适很重要。

参考文献

[1] Haylen BT, Maher CF, Barber MD, Camargo S, Dandolu V, Digesu A, et al. An International Urogynecological Association (IUGA)/International Continence Society (ICS) joint report on the terminology for female pelvic organ prolapse (POP). Int Urogynecol J. 2016;27(4):655–84. https://doi.org/10.1007/s00192-016-3003-y.

[2] Rogers RG. Female pelvic medicine and reconstructive surgery: clinical practice and surgical atlas. 1st ed. New York: McGraw-Hill; 2013.

[3] Bump RC, Mattiasson A, Bo K, Brubaker LP, DeLancey JO, Klarskov P, et al. The standardization of terminology of female pelvic organ prolapse and pelvic floor dysfunction. Am J Obstet Gynecol. 1996;175(1):10–7.

[4] Baden WF, Walker T. Surgical repair of vaginal defects. Philadelphia: Lippincott; 1992.

[5] Nygaard I, Barber MD, Burgio KL, Kenton K, Meikle S, Schaffer J, et al. Prevalence of symptomatic pelvic floor disorders in US women. JAMA. 2008;300(11):1311–6. https://doi. org/10.1001/jama.300.11.1311.

[6] Barber MD, Maher C. Epidemiology and outcome assessment of pelvic organ prolapse. Int Urogynecol J. 2013;24(11):1783–90. https://doi.org/10.1007/s00192-013-2169-9.

[7] Swift SE. The distribution of pelvic organ support in a population of female subjects seen for routine gynecologic health care. Am J Obstet Gynecol. 2000;183(2):277–85. https://doi. org/10.1067/mob.2000.107583.

[8] Hendrix SL, Clark A, Nygaard I, Aragaki A, Barnabei V, McTiernan A. Pelvic organ prolapse in the Women's Health Initiative: gravity and gravidity. Am J Obstet Gynecol. 2002;186(6):1160–6.

[9] Dieter AA, Wilkins MF, Wu JM. Epidemiological trends and future care needs for pelvic floor disorders. Curr Opin Obstet Gynecol. 2015;27(5):380–4. https://doi.org/10.1097/GCO.0000000000000200.

[10] Delancey JO, Kane Low L, Miller JM, Patel DA, Tumbarello JA. Graphic integration of causal factors of pelvic floor disorders: an integrated life span model. Am J Obstet Gynecol. 2008;199(6):610, e1–5. https://doi.org/10.1016/j.ajog.2008.04.001.

[11] Wu JM, Vaughan CP, Goode PS, Redden DT, Burgio KL, Richter HE, et al. Prevalence and trends of symptomatic pelvic floor disorders in U.S. women. Obstet Gynecol. 2014;123(1):141–8. https://doi.org/10.1097/AOG.0000000000000057.

[12] Akervall S, Al-Mukhtar Othman J, Molin M, Gyhagen M. Symptomatic pelvic organ prolapse in middle-aged women: a national matched cohort study on the influence of childbirth. Am J Obstet Gynecol. 2020;222(4):356, e1–e14. https://doi.org/10.1016/j.ajog.2019.10.007.

[13] Chiaffarino F, Chatenoud L, Dindelli M, Meschia M, Buonaguidi A, Amicarelli F, et al. Reproductive factors, family history, occupation and risk of urogenital prolapse. Eur J Obstet Gynecol Reprod Biol. 1999;82(1):63–7. https://doi.org/10.1016/s0301-2115(98)00175-4.

[14] Handa VL, Blomquist JL, Roem J, Munoz A. Longitudinal study of quantitative changes in pelvic organ support among parous women. Am J Obstet Gynecol. 2018;218(3):320, e1–e7. https://doi.org/10.1016/j.ajog.2017.12.214.

[15] Lukacz ES, Lawrence JM, Contreras R, Nager CW, Luber KM. Parity, mode of delivery, and pelvic floor disorders. Obstet Gynecol. 2006;107(6):1253–60. https://doi.org/10.1097/01.AOG.0000218096.54169.34.

[16] Moalli PA, Jones Ivy S, Meyn LA, Zyczynski HM. Risk factors associated with pelvic floor disorders in women undergoing surgical repair. Obstet Gynecol. 2003;101(5 Pt 1):869–74. https://doi.org/10.1016/s0029-7844(03)00078-4.

[17] Kearney R, Fitzpatrick M, Brennan S, Behan M, Miller J, Keane D, et al. Levator ani injury in primiparous women with forceps delivery for fetal distress, forceps for second stage arrest, and spontaneous delivery. Int J Gynaecol Obstet. 2010;111(1):19–22. https://doi.org/10.1016/j.ijgo.2010.05.019.

[18] DeLancey JO, Morgan DM, Fenner DE, Kearney R, Guire K, Miller JM, et al. Comparison of levator ani muscle defects and function in women with and without pelvic organ prolapse. Obstet Gynecol. 2007;109(2 Pt 1):295–302. https://doi.org/10.1097/01.AOG.0000250901.57095.ba.

[19] Dietz HP, Simpson JM. Levator trauma is associated with pelvic organ prolapse. BJOG. 2008;115(8):979–84. https://doi.org/10.1111/j.1471-0528.2008.01751.x.

[20] Lammers K, Lince SL, Spath MA, van Kempen LC, Hendriks JC, Vierhout ME, et al. Pelvic organ prolapse and collagen-associated disorders. Int Urogynecol J. 2012;23(3):313–9. https://doi.org/10.1007/s00192-011-1532-y.

[21] Weidner AC, Jamison MG, Branham V, South MM, Borawski KM, Romero AA. Neuropathic injury to the levator ani occurs in 1 in 4 primiparous women. Am J Obstet Gynecol. 2006;195(6):1851–6. https://doi.org/10.1016/j.ajog.2006.06.062.

[22] Lien KC, Morgan DM, Delancey JO, Ashton-Miller JA. Pudendal nerve stretch during vaginal birth: a 3D computer simulation. Am J Obstet Gynecol. 2005;192(5):1669–76. https://doi. org/10.1016/j.ajog.2005.01.032.

[23] Blomquist JL, Munoz A, Carroll M, Handa VL. Association of delivery mode with pelvic floor disorders after childbirth. JAMA. 2018;320(23):2438–47. https://doi.org/10.1001/ jama.2018.18315.

[24] Allen-Brady K, Cannon-Albright L, Farnham JM, Teerlink C, Vierhout ME, van Kempen LCL, et al. Identification of six loci associated with pelvic organ prolapse using genome-wide association analysis. Obstet Gynecol. 2011;118(6):1345–53. https://doi.org/10.1097/AOG.0b013e318236f4b5.

[25] Carley ME, Schaffer J. Urinary incontinence and pelvic organ prolapse in women with Marfan or Ehlers Danlos syndrome. Am J Obstet Gynecol. 2000;182(5):1021–3. https://doi. org/10.1067/mob.2000.105410.

[26] Ward RM, Velez Edwards DR, Edwards T, Giri A, Jerome RN, Wu JM. Genetic epidemiology of pelvic organ prolapse: a systematic review. Am J Obstet Gynecol. 2014;211(4):326–35. https://doi.org/10.1016/j.ajog.2014.04.006.

[27] Cartwright R, Kirby AC, Tikkinen KA, Mangera A, Thiagamoorthy G, Rajan P, et al. Systematic review and metaanalysis of genetic association studies of urinary symptoms and prolapse in women. Am J Obstet Gynecol. 2015;212(2):199, e1–24. https://doi.org/10.1016/j.ajog.2014.08.005.

[28] Snooks SJ, Barnes PR, Swash M, Henry MM. Damage to the innervation of the pelvic floor musculature in chronic constipation.

Gastroenterology. 1985;89(5):977–81. https://doi. org/10.1016/0016–5085(85)90196–9.

[29] Bai SW, Jeon MJ, Kim JY, Chung KA, Kim SK, Park KH. Relationship between stress urinary incontinence and pelvic organ prolapse. Int Urogynecol J Pelvic Floor Dysfunct. 2002;13(4):256–60.; discussion 60. https://doi.org/10.1007/s001920200053.

[30] Muniz KS, Pilkinton M, Winkler HA, Shalom DF. Prevalence of stress urinary incontinence and intrinsic sphincter deficiency in patients with stage IV pelvic organ prolapse. J Obstet Gynaecol Res. 2020;47(2):640–4. https://doi.org/10.1111/jog.14574.

[31] Hoyte LPJ, Damaser M. Biomechanics of the female pelvic floor. London/San Diego: Academic Press is an imprint of Elsevier; 2016.

[32] DeLancey JO. Structural support of the urethra as it relates to stress urinary incontinence: the hammock hypothesis. Am J Obstet Gynecol. 1994;170(6):1713–20.; discussion 20–3. https://doi.org/10.1016/s0002–9378(94)70346–9.

[33] Burrows LJ, Meyn LA, Walters MD, Weber AM. Pelvic symptoms in women with pelvic organ prolapse. Obstet Gynecol. 2004;104(5 Pt 1):982–8. https://doi.org/10.1097/01. AOG.0000142708.61298.be.

[34] DeLancey JO, Trowbridge ER, Miller JM, Morgan DM, Guire K, Fenner DE, et al. Stress urinary incontinence: relative importance of urethral support and urethral closure pressure. J Urol. 2008;179(6):2286–90.; discussion 90. https://doi.org/10.1016/j.juro.2008.01.098.

[35] Bai SW, Cho JM, Kwon HS, Park JH, Shin JS, Kim SK, et al. The relationship between maximal urethral closure pressure and functional urethral length in anterior vaginal wall prolapse patients according to stage and age. Yonsei Med J. 2005;46(3):408–13. https://doi.org/10.3349/ ymj.2005.46.3.408.

[36] Chang HW, Ng SC, Chen GD. Correlations between severity of anterior vaginal wall prolapse and parameters of urethral pressure profile. Low Urin Tract Symptoms. 2020;13(2):238–43. https://doi.org/10.1111/luts.12357.

[37] Trowbridge ER, Wei JT, Fenner DE, Ashton-Miller JA, Delancey JO. Effects of aging on lower urinary tract and pelvic floor function in nulliparous women. Obstet Gynecol. 2007;109(3):715–20. https://doi.org/10.1097/01.AOG.0000257074.98122.69.

[38] Cameron AP. Systematic review of lower urinary tract symptoms occurring with pelvic organ prolapse. Arab J Urol. 2019;17(1):23–9. https://doi.org/10.1080/2090598X.2019.1589929.

[39] Bradley CS, Nygaard IE. Vaginal wall descensus and pelvic floor symptoms in older women. Obstet Gynecol. 2005;106(4):759–66. https://doi.org/10.1097/01.AOG.0000180183.03897.72.

[40] Fritel X, Varnoux N, Zins M, Breart G, Ringa V. Symptomatic pelvic organ prolapse at midlife, quality of life, and risk factors. Obstet Gynecol. 2009;113(3):609–16. https://doi.org/10.1097/AOG.0b013e3181985312.

[41] Tegerstedt G, Maehle-Schmidt M, Nyren O, Hammarstrom M. Prevalence of symptomatic pelvic organ prolapse in a Swedish population. Int Urogynecol J Pelvic Floor Dysfunct. 2005;16(6):497–503. https://doi.org/10.1007/s00192–005–1326–1.

[42] de Boer TA, Salvatore S, Cardozo L, Chapple C, Kelleher C, van Kerrebroeck P, et al. Pelvic organ prolapse and overactive bladder. Neurourol Urodyn. 2010;29(1):30–9. https://doi. org/10.1002/nau.20858.

[43] Birder LA, de Groat WC. Mechanisms of disease: involvement of the urothelium in bladder dysfunction. Nat Clin Pract Urol. 2007;4(1):46–54. https://doi.org/10.1038/ncpuro0672.

[44] Ferguson DR, Kennedy I, Burton TJ. ATP is released from rabbit urinary bladder epithelial cells by hydrostatic pressure changes-a possible sensory mechanism? J Physiol. 1997;505(Pt 2):503–11. https://doi.org/10.1111/j.1469–7793.1997.503bb.x.

[45] Keay SK, Birder LA, Chai TC. Evidence for bladder urothelial pathophysiology in functional bladder disorders. Biomed Res Int. 2014;2014:865463. https://doi.org/10.1155/2014/865463.

[46] Glazener CM, Cooper K, Mashayekhi A. Anterior vaginal repair for urinary incontinence in women. Cochrane Database Syst Rev. 2017;7:CD001755. https://doi.org/10.1002/14651858. CD001755. pub2.

[47] Handa VL, Jones M. Do pessaries prevent the progression of pelvic organ prolapse? Int Urogynecol J Pelvic Floor Dysfunct. 2002;13(6):349–51.; discussion 52. https://doi. org/10.1007/s001920200078.

[48] Clemons JL, Aguilar VC, Tillinghast TA, Jackson ND, Myers DL. Patient satisfaction and changes in prolapse and urinary symptoms in women who were fitted successfully with a pessary for pelvic organ prolapse. Am J Obstet Gynecol. 2004;190(4):1025–9. https://doi.org/10.1016/j.ajog.2003.10.711.

[49] Fernando RJ, Thakar R, Sultan AH, Shah SM, Jones PW. Effect of vaginal pessaries on symptoms associated with pelvic organ prolapse. Obstet Gynecol. 2006;108(1):93–9. https://doi. org/10.1097/01. AOG.0000222903.38684.cc.

[50] Romanzi LJ, Chaikin DC, Blaivas JG. The effect of genital prolapse on voiding. J Urol. 1999;161(2):581–6.

[51] Ding J, Chen C, Song XC, Zhang L, Deng M, Zhu L. Changes in prolapse and urinary symptoms after successful fitting of a ring pessary with support in women with advanced pelvic organ prolapse: a prospective study. Urology. 2016;87:70–5. https://doi.org/10.1016/j.urology.2015.07.025.

[52] American Urogynecologic Society Guidelines Statements Committee, Carberry CL, Tulikangas PK, Ridgeway BM, Collins SA, Adam RA. American urogynecologic society best practice statement: evaluation and counseling of patients with pelvic organ prolapse. Female Pelvic Med Reconstr Surg. 2017;23(5):281–7. https://doi.org/10.1097/SPV.0000000000000424.

[53] Abrams P, Cardozo L, Wagg A, Wein A, editors. Incontinence. 6th ed. Bristol: International Continence Society; 2017.

[54] Foster RT Sr, Barber MD, Parasio MF, Walters MD, Weidner AC, Amundsen CL. A prospective assessment of overactive bladder symptoms in a cohort of elderly women who underwent transvaginal surgery for advanced pelvic organ prolapse. Am J Obstet Gynecol. 2007;197(1):82, e1–4. https://doi.org/10.1016/j.ajog.2007.02.049.

[55] Maher C, Feiner B, Baessler K, Schmid C. Surgical management of pelvic organ prolapse in women. Cochrane Database Syst Rev. 2013;(4):CD004014. https://doi.org/10.1002/14651858. CD004014. pub5.

[56] Colombo M, Vitobello D, Proietti F, Milani R. Randomised comparison of Burch colposuspension versus anterior colporrhaphy in women with stress urinary incontinence and anterior vaginal wall prolapse. BJOG. 2000;107(4):544–51. https://doi.org/10.1111/j.1471–0528.2000. tb13276.x.

[57] Borstad E, Abdelnoor M, Staff AC, Kulseng-Hanssen S. Surgical strategies for women with pelvic organ prolapse and urinary stress incontinence. Int Urogynecol J. 2010;21(2):179–86. https://doi.org/10.1007/s00192–009–1007–6.

[58] Brubaker L, Cundiff GW, Fine P, Nygaard I, Richter HE, Visco AG, et al. Abdominal sacrocolpopexy with Burch colposuspension to reduce urinary stress incontinence. N Engl J Med. 2006;354(15):1557–66. https://doi.org/10.1056/NEJMoa054208.

[59] Liang CC, Chang YL, Chang SD, Lo TS, Soong YK. Pessary test to predict postoperative urinary incontinence in women undergoing hysterectomy for prolapse. Obstet Gynecol. 2004;104(4):795–800. https://doi.org/10.1097/01.AOG.0000140689.90131.01.

[60] Visco AG, Brubaker L, Nygaard I, Richter HE, Cundiff G, Fine P, et al. The role of preoperative urodynamic testing in stress-continent women undergoing sacrocolpopexy: the Colpopexy and Urinary Reduction

Efforts (CARE) randomized surgical trial. Int Urogynecol J Pelvic Floor Dysfunct. 2008;19(5):607–14. https://doi.org/10.1007/s00192–007– 0498–2.

[61] Wei JT, Nygaard I, Richter HE, Nager CW, Barber MD, Kenton K, et al. A midurethral sling to reduce incontinence after vaginal prolapse repair. N Engl J Med. 2012;366(25):2358–67. https://doi.org/10.1056/NEJMoa1111967.

[62] Ellstrom Engh AM, Ekeryd A, Magnusson A, Olsson I, Otterlind L, Tobiasson G. Can *de novo* stress incontinence after anterior wall repair be predicted? Acta Obstet Gynecol Scand. 2011;90(5):488–93. https://doi.org/10.1111/j.1600–0412.2011.01087.x.

[63] Nager CW, Brubaker L, Litman HJ, Zyczynski HM, Varner RE, Amundsen C, et al. A randomized trial of urodynamic testing before stress-incontinence surgery. N Engl J Med. 2012;366(21):1987–97. https://doi.org/10.1056/NEJMoa1113595.

[64] Hullfish KL, Bovbjerg VE, Steers WD. Patient-centered goals for pelvic floor dysfunction surgery: long-term follow-up. Am J Obstet Gynecol. 2004;191(1):201–5. https://doi. org/10.1016/j.ajog.2004.03.086.

[65] Jelovsek JE. Predicting urinary incontinence after surgery for pelvic organ prolapse. Curr Opin Obstet Gynecol. 2016;28(5):399–406. https://doi.org/10.1097/GCO.0000000000000308.

第21章 复杂泌尿系统重建后尿失禁：原位新膀胱及性别确定手术

Incontinence After Complex Urinary Reconstruction: Orthotopic Neobladder and Gender-Affirming Surgery

Amanda C. Chi　Nancy Ye　Virginia Li　Krystal DePorto　Polina Reyblat　著

尿失禁是各种泌尿重建手术严重的并发症。在本章中，我们关注原位新膀胱重建和性别确定手术后各种类型的尿失禁。虽然这些患者有详细的病史和体格检查，但在治疗时还要考虑细微差别和重要因素。

一、原位尿流改道术后女性尿失禁

治疗肌层浸润性膀胱癌和高危非浸润性膀胱癌的金标准是根治性膀胱切除术和尿流改道术[1]。在女性患者中，根治性膀胱切除术和尿流改道指的是盆腔前全切除术，包括膀胱切除术、子宫切除术、双侧输卵管－卵巢切除术、阴道前壁切除术和尿道切除术，并采用回肠储尿囊或输尿管皮肤造瘘[2]。当原位移植新膀胱首次应用时，考虑到女性尿道长度较短，最初对女性的肿瘤学和功能结果表示担忧，此后的研究解决了这些问题，提示女性膀胱癌患者中尿道受累的比例相对较小，从而更详细地了解了女性的控尿机制，并且在保留尿道用于原位新膀胱的特定女性患者中显示了可接受的肿瘤学和功能结局[3-10]。

二、原位尿流改道术的原则

虽然原位尿流改道术有多种不同的手术方式，但成功的关键原则是：①非梗阻尿道，保留足够的外括约肌机制；②顺应性储尿囊，允许低压储尿；③储尿囊容量足够（300～500ml）[11]。各种肠段均可以用来构造一个储尿囊，然而，回肠新膀胱已被证明比结肠新膀胱[12]更具顺应性。无论使用何种肠段，重要的是进行充分的去管化和创建一个球形。一般认为，去管化肠段会破坏蠕动收缩，从而允许降低管腔内压力和便于低压储存。球面几何允许对给定的表面积[13]进行最大体积的存储。

三、控尿机制

为了了解女性原位尿道改道与尿失禁相关的功能结果，我们必须了解女性尿道失禁机制。女性尿道括约肌由横纹肌和平滑肌组成。在过去，人们认为女性膀胱颈控尿，这解释了最初对女性创建原位尿流改道术的怀疑。然而，研究表明括约肌中横纹肌对尿失禁至关重要。通过尸体解剖对女性横纹肌进行了仔细的评估，发现横纹肌在尿道前侧至盆内筋膜[3]处最坚固。阴部神经分支深入骨盆内筋膜，并向外侧进入尿道尾部，支配横纹肌[3, 14]。尿流动力学研究也表明，膀胱切除术和原位尿流改道术后女性的主要控尿区是尿道的中1/3[15]。术中应谨慎操作，将尿道剥离范围限制在盆内浅筋膜，避免损伤横纹肌及其神经支配，导致术后尿失禁。

尿道括约肌的平滑肌部分主要由阴道外侧的自主神经支配，保留这些自主神经的必要性存在争议。虽然一些人认为保留自主神经对排尿至关重要[6, 9, 16-18]，但另一些人则认为依赖于横纹肌括约肌的阴部神经支配[19, 20]即可。鉴于缺乏回答这个问题的随机对照试验，当病情允许时，尽可能保留自主神经丛[21]。

四、原位尿流改道术后的尿失禁

由于缺乏标准化结果报告，评估原位改道术后尿失禁的真实发生率和患病率非常具有挑战性。术后6～12个月，储液囊逐渐成熟并获得稳定的最大容量[22]。一些人建议，进一步的评估和治疗应该推迟到术后12～18个月，以便使控尿状态达到平台期[10, 15, 23]。但尿失禁的定义、尿失禁的严重程度、收集和报告数据的方法、随访的时间，以及很少使用有效的调查问卷，使得研究结果之间难以进行有意义的比较。此外，报道原位新膀胱失禁的研究倾向于根据尿失禁时间（日间与夜间），而不是症状（压力、急迫性、过度）来分类。

据报道，日间尿失禁率为77%～90%，夜间尿失禁率为57%～86%[5, 23-25]。在最初的6～12个月期间，日间的尿失禁似乎逐渐改善，而夜间的尿失禁通常改善较慢，并可延长至[11]第二年。研究表明，糖尿病和子宫切除术是尿失禁的危险因素[26-28]。1996—2011年，Anderson等对49例接受根治性膀胱切除术和原位新膀胱术的女性进行了回顾性研究，确定了日间尿失禁的唯一预测因素是既往或同时行子宫切除术。在这些尿失禁患者中，子宫切除术后尿失禁发生率（51.2%）高于保留子宫尿失禁发生率（13.3%）（$P<0.01$）。在国内患者中，62.8%的患者尝试保留双侧神经，34.9%的患者尝试保留单侧神经；在尿失禁患者中，保留双侧神经的占36.7%，保留单侧神经的占53.3%（$P=0.02$）[17]。2017年，一项回顾性研究评估了保留盆腔器官的根治性膀胱切除术与标准根治性膀胱切除术在尿道改流术患者中的肿瘤学和功能结局。保留盆腔器官的根治性膀胱切除术包括神经保留、阴道切除或生殖器保留。在接受保留盆腔器官的根治性膀胱切除术[29]治疗的患者中，日间尿失禁率为57.1%～100%，夜间失禁率为42.9%～100%，差异很大。本研究存在一些局限性，其中包括研究间的异质性、叙述综合方法和缺乏术前尿功能状态。然而，这是关于保留盆腔器官的根治性膀胱切除术的首次系统评价，并指出需要进行前瞻性多中心研究，以进一步评估接受保留盆腔器官根治性膀胱切除术女性的功能结局。

病例的选择也可能改善结局。术前静息时尿道闭合压力较高、功能性尿道长度较长的女性与术后尿失禁[17]相关。术前压力性尿失禁与日间尿失禁严重程度相关。年龄也被认为是一个影响因素；在一项对41例患者平均随访5.7年的研究中，手术时年龄＞65岁是与日间尿失禁[30]相关的唯一因素。在另一项研究中，年龄较大与夜间尿失禁的存在和严重程度有关[27]。其中一个原因可能是继发于与年龄增加相关的生理性夜间多尿[31]。

夜间尿失禁被认为是由于横纹括约肌松弛、生理性利尿和感觉下降导致新膀胱过度膨胀，过大的容量抑制尿道关闭机制[28]。最初的治疗可能包括晚间减少液体量，睡觉前排空尿液，夜间增加醒来次数以排空新膀胱，以及根据需要定时排尿[28, 32]。

五、评估和检查

尿失禁的初步评估应包括回顾相关病史和体格检查。需要进行重点体检，其中包括腹部、尿道、阴道、会阴、直肠、肛门和下肢的感觉和适当的反射测试。阴道检查应包括使用内镜来确定潜在的新膀胱阴道瘘[33]。评估肾功能和排除感染性尿失禁的病因包括基础代谢检查和尿培养在内的实验室检查。门诊诊断性检查包括尿流率测定、排尿后残余尿测定、评估多饮或夜间多尿的排尿记录，以及尿流动力学检查[28]。残余尿量高的患者可能需要做脱垂检查，因为这类人群中约6%发生脱垂。在开始任何治疗之前，必须排除新膀胱阴道瘘的存在（图21–1）。

六、治疗

（一）物理治疗

1948年，盆底物理治疗由Arnold Kegel博士

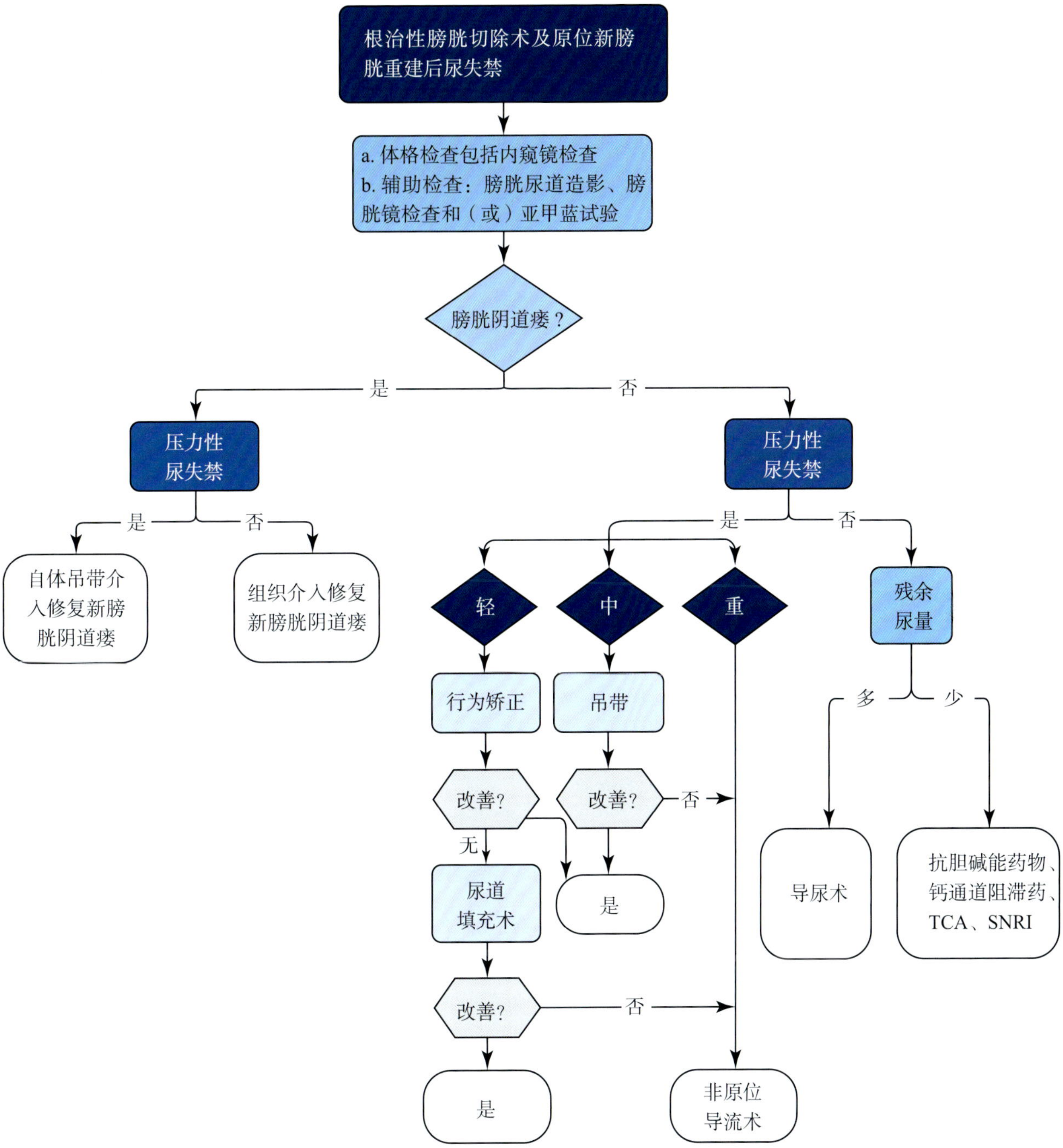

▲ 图 21-1　新膀胱尿失禁患者详细检查流程

提出，是治疗压力性尿失禁[35]的首选无创治疗方案。针对性的治疗锻炼有助于加强盆底肌组织，增加尿道稳定性，最终改善排尿控制。对于接受根治性膀胱切除术 + 原位新膀胱重建术的患者，建议在手术干预前开始盆底物理治疗[36, 37]。该建议是根据 Centemero 等公布的数据推断得出。他们研究了术前和术后均接受盆底物理治疗、术后接受单纯盆底物理治疗的患者在前列腺切除术后的控尿恢复情况。那些完成术前和术后盆底物理治疗的患者在术后 1 个月的控尿率比对照组高 24%。通过术前盆底肌物理治疗，患者可以在神经肌肉再兴奋的关键阶段更快速地兴奋盆底肌。虽然对于膀胱切除术和新膀胱重建术后出现尿失禁的女性，目前还没有金标准治疗方案，但 Johnson 等提出了一种治疗方案（表 21-1）。通过内镜、摄像机、肌电图描记或抽象图形表示的视觉生物反馈是帮助患者神经肌肉连接重建的重要辅助手段[36]。术后 8～12 个月可考虑进行盆底物理治疗[37]。

（二）药物治疗

抗胆碱能药物适用于治疗逼尿肌过度活动。常见的不良反应包括眼干、口干和肠道蠕动降低，这可能有助于改善新膀胱患者的尿失禁。单独使用羟丁尼或维拉帕米（一种钙通道阻滞药）已被证明可增加首次排尿意愿时的容量，并降低无抑制的新膀胱收缩的频率和幅度。在最初的研究中，奥昔布宁有较好的主观反应，70% 的患者报告夜间遗尿有所改善，而使用维拉帕米[38]的患者则有 55% 的患者得到改善。这 2 种药物都可以考虑用于那些以肠道代替膀胱作为容量的过度活动。然而，考虑到接受根治性膀胱切除术的女性平均年龄，建议避免使用抗胆碱能药物，因为它会增加不良反应和痴呆的风险。目前还没有对膀胱切除术后患者使用更新的抗胆碱能药物或新型 β 肾上

表 21-1　盆底物理治疗指南[36]

1. 术前盆底训练（术前 4～6 周开始）	盆底肌肉协调训练和有意识的正确控制
	提升盆底肌 10 次 ×4 组 / 天
	收缩盆底肌时间 5～10s，10 次 ×2 组 / 天
2. 术后	早期活动：改变下床活动策略，用腹部支撑从坐到站，避免负重和紧张
	改善日常活动：每天至少 3 次 10min 的短时间步行，以提高耐力并协助胃肠道活动
	充分补水
3. 尿管拔除后术后约 3 周	开始盆底肌意识训练：学习运用盆底肌肉，减少臀肌、腹部和臀部的辅助使用，以提高括约肌控制
	避免 Valsalva 动作
	新膀胱再训练：定时排尿（将排尿间隔提高到至少每 1.5 小时），同时使用警报器、液体起搏和盆底肌肉练习
	夜间排尿唤醒：每 2 小时 1 次
4. 盆底物理治疗神经肌肉再训练（4～6 周）	生物反馈训练（视觉或手动反馈），用于盆底肌的意识训练
	提升盆底肌 10 次 ×4 组，收缩盆底肌（根据客观发现）5s 保持 10 次 ×3 组 / 天
	盆腔收缩反射训练配合咳嗽以改善协调性
	在仰卧位进行臀肌 / 核心肌群的强化
	活动能力（从坐到站）的增强和运动前使用腹横肌协同对盆底肌功能的加强
	患者再教育：健康恢复和饮食自如，如厕技巧，以及排尿 / 排便的盆底肌协调
5. 恢复期（8～12 周）	盆底肌在直立姿势加强收缩，并与腹横肌共同收缩
	持续时间为 10s，15s，20s
	在直立状态下，将运动控制与提升、收缩盆底肌训练相结合
	运动控制的生物反馈：金字塔、阶梯式盆底肌视觉训练
	认知干扰下的盆底肌肉锻炼对不自主运动的影响
	功能性运动训练：举重、弯腰、步态、恢复到以前的活动水平（运动、徒步旅行、健身房锻炼）
	实现日间和夜间每 4 小时排尿间隔，漏尿量最小

腺素受体激动药的评估，但由于这些患者缺失逼尿肌，对肠道没有影响的药物可能是无效的。去氨加压素是一种抗利尿激素的合成类似物，在多项试验中已显示出改善尿失禁和夜尿症的临床疗效[39-41]。Goldberg 等研究了原位新膀胱重建术后夜间遗尿症患者使用小剂量去氨加压素的情况。通过减少排尿量，50% 的患者排尿间隔时间延长，生活质量得到改善。去氨加压素的常见不良反应包括头痛、头晕、失眠、口干和恶心。考虑到低钠血症风险[42]，应在使用去氨加压素时监测患者电解质的改变。

虽然目前还没有公开的数据表明，在原位新膀胱患者中，尚无丙咪胺或度洛西汀是否可改善膀胱功能的数据，但许多研究人员已经建议使用这些药物[37, 43]。丙咪嗪是一种三环胺抗抑郁药，已被证明能引起逼尿肌松弛和膀胱颈及尿道收缩，是治疗混合性尿失禁的有效选择[44, 45]。度洛西汀对压力性尿失禁的疗效源于 Onuf 细胞核选择性抑制 5- 羟色胺和去甲肾上腺素的突触前再摄取。在膀胱充盈过程中，Onuf 细胞核受体的刺激通过保护反射导致尿道张力的增加[46]。

对于那些特发性和神经性逼尿肌过度活动的患者，膀胱内注射肉毒杆菌毒素是很有效的。也有报道将其注射到直肠黏膜下层[47]用于治疗便秘。Michel 等研究了肉毒杆菌毒素 A 注射在神经源性逼尿肌过度活动的肠囊成形术患者中的应用。在膀胱和肠补片注射肉毒杆菌毒素 A 均无严重并发症[48]。Hoag 等将 100～200U 的肉毒杆菌毒素 A 注射到患者的肠道储尿囊以治疗新膀胱过度活动。平均随访 8.3 个月，患者主观上均有不同程度的改善。可能的括约肌功能不全和依赖通过 Valsalva 排尿的这些患者在膀胱内注射肉毒杆菌毒素 A 后发生尿潴留的风险较低。因此，推荐注射 200U，但有关其使用情况的数据有限[49]。

（三）尿道填充注射术

在经过严格筛选的患者中，经尿道注射填充剂可以为原位膀胱重建后持续性压力性尿失禁提供一种微创治疗选择。小型研究表明，缓解情况多变且不持久。在一项研究中，12 例患者共注射了 25 次胶原蛋白或不可吸收的碳涂层珠，在平均 22.5 个月的随访中，17% 的患者尿漏完全消失，33% 的患者有一定的改善，50% 的患者症状没有改变。根据疾病严重程度分层时，66% 的轻至中度疾病患者（定义为每日使用≤4 片尿垫）有改善或治愈，而只有 33% 的重度疾病患者[50]获益。Tchetgen 等报道了 3 例经尿道注射胶原蛋白的女性患者，最初的结果是希望所有女性无漏尿。然而，为了持续控制症状，需要进行维持注射，仅 1 例患者恢复到术前尿失禁[51]的基线水平。

目前，胶原蛋白不再用于经尿道注射。Bailey 等描述了 6 例女性运用 Defux、Macroplastique、Coaptite、Contingen 或 Dursphere 的经验。75% 的患者症状只是暂时改善，其中 1 例出现继发性新膀胱阴道瘘[33]。上述研究未确定经尿道注射填充剂的确切位置，但 Pruthi 等先前的研究建议在远离新膀胱颈[52]的位置前注射填充剂。综上所述，经尿道注射膨胀剂对于原位膀胱重建术后轻度压力性尿失禁的患者是一种值得谨慎考虑的治疗选择。应告知患者需要多次手术的可能性高、疗效不确定、新膀胱阴道瘘形成的风险，以及未经证实的长期获益。

（四）吊带

使用耻骨阴道自体吊带和合成经闭孔吊带治疗保守治疗失败的患者的压力性尿失禁。与支持其他治疗方式的数据相似，压力性尿失禁保守治疗失效的患者使用耻骨阴道自体吊带和合成经闭孔吊带，评估吊带放置结果的研究是有限的，长期结果显示具有显著发病率和死亡率的可能性。

在原位新膀胱重建术后接受耻骨阴道悬吊术的 4 例患者中（2 例自体直肌悬吊术和 2 例真皮悬吊术），50% 的患者出现了与耻骨后剥离相关的严重并发症[53]。不幸的是，套管针穿过耻骨后间隙导致一名患者出现肠 – 新膀胱瘘，另一名患者随后死于败血症。接受真皮移植悬吊术的患者术后过度失禁，需要清洁的间歇导尿。考虑到新膀胱和肠道损伤的风险，一些人提倡使用耻骨下骨锚来避免在放置吊带时进入骨盆[21, 33, 54]。

利用骨膜下途径放置的4个耻骨阴道吊带和4个经闭孔吊带的研究显示效果不佳；没有一个女性是仅次于悬吊术的。经闭孔悬吊术在该人群中是有利的，因为它避免了骨盆入口，降低了新膀胱和（或）肠道损伤的风险[33]。更有希望的结果见于一系列接受经闭孔阴道吊带（内翻）放置的6例患者；66%显示完全的日间和夜间干燥，17%显示相对改善，17%报道无变化。平均随访18个月，结果是持久的。报道漏尿无改善的患者术前患有严重的压力性尿失禁[54]。

虽然尿道中段合成吊带的放置是治疗索引患者压力性尿失禁的金标准，但它在原位新膀胱重建术后压力性尿失禁患者中仅显示出适度的成功。根治性膀胱切除术中需要进行广泛的骨盆解剖，这导致瘢痕形成和相对缺血的环境，两者都使吊带放置变得复杂。尿道中段悬吊传统上是无张力放置的。然而，在这一人群中，目标是相对尿道梗阻，以恢复尿失禁。对于部分性尿道梗阻，反过来有很高的尿潴留风险并且随后需要长期间歇性导尿。患者术前必须被告知，并愿意和能够进行清洁的间歇导尿。此外，在缺血环境下张力放置吊带会增加侵蚀的风险[55]。

在膀胱重建术后患有严重压力性尿失禁的患者中，微创治疗方案可能成功有限并且具有风险。患者经常面临将新膀胱转换为回肠导管或考虑可插入导管的储尿袋的决定[43]。在这种情况下，由于压力性尿失禁的治疗选择有限，在选择尿流改道类型之前，需要仔细评估尿失禁状态。关于尿流改道选择的咨询和共同决策应该受到患者术前尿失禁状态的强烈影响。

七、膀胱重建后阴道瘘

原位新膀胱重建术的一个不常见但极具破坏性的并发症是发生新膀胱阴道瘘，发生率为0%～10%[33, 55-57]。发生新膀胱阴道瘘的已知风险因素包括解剖过程中对阴道前壁的损伤，特别是在尿道水平处[58]，缝合线重叠，由于先前的手术或放疗导致的血管化组织不良，癌症复发，以及尿道填充剂的使用[55, 57]。此外，相对较薄的新膀胱壁使其更容易凝固[58]。新膀胱阴道瘘可在膀胱切除术后立即或数月出现，大多数在3～6个月内出现[33, 56]。间歇性与持续性尿失禁的存在不能可靠地将新膀胱阴道瘘与术后尿失禁的其他原因区分开来[56]。在鉴别新膀胱阴道瘘形成和其他类型的尿失禁时必须保持警惕，因为它们可能相似或同时出现，并需要不同的处理。大多数新膀胱阴道瘘可以通过检查确定。其他诊断选项包括排尿性膀胱尿道造影、膀胱镜检查和（或）染色试验[28, 56, 59]。当发现新膀胱阴道瘘时，最可能的位置是尿道新膀胱吻合处，其次是阴道残端。

精确的手术是预防新膀胱阴道瘘形成的最重要因素[56]。需要仔细解剖膀胱阴道平面，以防止对阴道的意外损伤[58, 60]。防止新膀胱阴道瘘形成的其他操作包括闭合阴道残端并将其从后面远离新膀胱尿道吻合术，将直肠前壁的腹膜边缘缝合固定到阴道残端，并将带蒂网膜瓣固定在阴道残端和新膀胱尿道吻合术之间[23, 60]。

用全胃肠外营养和膀胱减压保守治疗新膀胱阴道瘘已被证明是无效的；大多数患者需要手术修复[13]。如果临床检查怀疑有癌症复发，需要在手术修复前进行活检。建议在手术前使用经阴道雌激素以优化阴道组织质量。与经腹手术相比，经阴道手术通常被推荐用于输卵管修补，或者改为可控性或尿失禁手术。如果可行，经阴道途径可提供良好的功能结果，且不会损害外尿道括约肌[57, 61]。

修复新膀胱阴道瘘的关键是多层非重叠层的闭合。插入层的组织选项包括Martius瓣、网膜瓣、股薄肌瓣、腹膜瓣、自体筋膜移植物，在极少数情况下，还包括生物胶[55-57]。插入层提供了额外的血管分布、淋巴引流和上皮形成的表面积，并防止缝合线重叠。如果怀疑初次出现压力性尿失禁，可以考虑在手术中使用自体筋膜吊带作为中间层。建议使用耻骨下骨锚以防止切开耻骨后间隙。合成吊带不应与股骨假体修复同时使用[33]。

新膀胱阴道瘘修补的成功率差异很大（25%～100%）[33, 55, 57, 61]。那些在尿道－新膀胱吻合处有尿道瘘的患者往往比那些近端有更多尿道瘘患者的情况更差，并且有更高的转化为非正位新膀胱分流术的比率[55]。在那些保留原位新膀胱的患者中，许多人继发内在括约肌功能不全的尿失禁，并最终需要治疗[56]。

八、超连续性

虽然原位尿流改道后尿失禁在女性中很常见，但高达 69% 的女性也报道了某种程度的尿失禁[27, 62]。原位新膀胱后尿失禁在文献中被定义为超过 150ml 的排空后残留或无法排空[63]。已知的防止原位新膀胱重建术后尿失禁的因素也有助于增加尿失禁的风险。这些包括保留子宫、保留双侧神经和延长功能性尿道长度[17]。在高达 80% 的患者中，保留阴道和子宫颈固定术与尿失禁有关[64]。患者也可能因储尿池过大、新膀胱和括约肌复合体协同失调或形成膀胱膨出导致尿道扭结而无法排空[18, 63, 65]。Finley 等发现，原位新膀胱术后尿道平均扭结 18° 的患者伴有尿潴留，这些通常是由于膀胱膨出引起的。滞留的患者最初可以用清洁的间歇导尿来处理。对于患有膀胱膨出的患者，他们可以将手指放入阴道内，以减少新膀胱脱垂，从而排尿。术后初期持续性尿失禁的患者可以通过矫正脱垂来矫正尿道，从而改善排空[66, 67]。

九、性别确定手术后尿失禁

（一）女性化手术

在跨性别女性的泌尿生殖系统性别确定手术中，近 50% 的患者会有排尿不适，据报道尿失禁的发生率为 5%～19%[68-70]。尽管患者在外部表现为女性泌尿生殖系统综合征，但在内部，前列腺仍然存在。简言之，全深度阴道成形术包括双侧睾丸切除术、切除体部、形成新阴道管、用皮肤或腹膜移植物衬管、缩短尿道的尿道成形术、阴蒂成形术和阴唇成形术。患者也可以接受零深度阴道成形术（与外阴成形术或浅深度阴道成形术同义），在这种手术中不会产生新的阴道管。目前实践中有多种技术和方法，但没有明确的证据支持一种特定的技术。新阴道管的发育依赖于沿着 Denonvilliers 筋膜仔细解剖前列腺后部和直肠前部之间的潜在空间。Hugh Hampton Young 在描述会阴前列腺切除术的技术时为理解这一解剖结构奠定了基础[71]。

患者在阴道成形术或外阴成形术后的短期内经常有各种各样的排尿主诉。大多数主诉集中在尿流变化、喷溅、尿后滴沥和会阴区总体湿度增加。随着切口愈合和术后水肿的改善，这些症状在恢复期的早期是常见的。此外，在缩短尿道的坐姿下，新的排泄动力学将不可避免地导致尿液偶尔喷到阴唇或大腿内侧。一旦证实完全排空，患者应该放心，大多数尿流异常将随着恢复进展而消失。

当排尿症状持续超过至术后急性期时，应对患者进行全面的评估，包括一次彻底的尿道检查和一次内镜检查。彻底的检查可以确定尿道狭窄、尿道阴道或膀胱阴道瘘以及尿道异常扭曲 / 成角。1%～6% 的阴道成形术后患者出现尿道狭窄，而 0.9%～3.9% 的患者出现尿道阴道瘘[72-74]。尿道狭窄的患者可能出现溢流性尿失禁和与梗阻相关的刺激症状。根据尿道阴道瘘的位置，尿道阴道瘘患者可能会经历分流、阴道积液和持续湿润。此外，在没有尿道瘘的情况下，单独的阴道积液症状也可以被认为是尿失禁。在大多数情况下，阴道积液可以解释为尿道的非生理性成角、尿道口的回缩位置或由于尿道口附近多余组织引起的血流改道。在某些情况下，我们观察到患者在排尿时没有张开双腿跨在马桶上，这可能导致尿液滞留在阴道中，并且在站立时滞留的尿液会泄漏。尿道过度向上倾斜或尿道不对称也会导致喷溅或向上流；这可以通过手术修正尿道口的位置来纠正。

检查应该从全面的病史和体格检查、排尿后残余物的评估和无创性血流测定开始（如果需要的话）。重要的是要认识到，尽管大多数性别确定手术患者已经进行了长期雌激素补充，并伴有或不伴有雄激素阻断，但他们仍有发展为良性前列腺增生并伴有下尿路症状的风险。关于去势对前列腺增生发展的影响，证据仍不清楚，尽管文献确实显示了几例跨性别女性患者尽管去势仍发展为前列腺癌，表明雄激素合成的替代来源仍影响前列腺生长[75-78]。一方面，根据患者开始激素阻断的年龄，患者可能在移植前已经出现前列腺增生相关的膀胱出口梗阻症状。另一方面，研究认为激素治疗导致前列腺变小可能会使排尿更容易并导致压力性尿失禁[79]。

详细的病史有助于分析患者是否有急迫性、压力性、溢流性、持续性或混合性尿失禁。性别确定手术前的基线泌尿症状也有助于识别尿失禁的来源。除了术前有压力性尿失禁风险的患者外，下尿路症状在术后可能保持稳定。在接受阴道成形术之前，必须评估患者的排尿症状。至少，我们建议在初次咨询时采用美国泌尿协会症状评分（AUASS）。随后应对已确定的症状进行检查。此外，在手术重建早期进行骨盆底物理治疗，可以改善许多患者的排尿功能，并将排尿功能障碍降到最低。与仅接受术后治疗的患者相比，至少进行过1次术前骨盆底物理治疗的患者发生骨盆底功能障碍的可能性较低（27% vs. 86%）。然而，即使术前没有诊断，患者仍将受益于术后盆底理疗[80]。

既往有根治性前列腺切除术史的患者面临着特殊的挑战。传统的治疗术后尿失禁的方法，如放置人工尿道括约肌或男性吊带，变得困难且有潜在的风险。在阴道成形术中，海绵体通常在隆起的尿道处逐渐变细，在尿道和覆盖的吊带或括约肌袖带之间留下非常少的组织。此外，因为球海绵体肌通常被切除，所以植入的装置可能缺乏足够的覆盖。已经考虑了几种方法，包括在阴道成形术时同时放置人工尿道括约肌或男性吊带，分阶段手术，或者机器人方法将括约肌袖带定位在膀胱颈部。迄今为止，还没有数据可以得出有意义的结论。对于在评估时没有出现尿失禁的术后患者，咨询需要包括在提肌复合体附近的会阴切开术中出现新的压力性尿失禁的可能性。强烈建议有根治性前列腺切除术病史的患者行零深度阴道成形术。这主要是由于直肠损伤的风险增加，并且有很大的可能重新发展或现有尿失禁的恶化。在某种程度上，这也适用于有经尿道前列腺切除术病史的患者，其中功能性内括约肌已作为手术的一部分被切除[81]。

（二）男性化手术

在跨性别男性患者中，可以通过阴茎成形术和阴蒂阴茎化手术来达到性别确认的目的。阴蒂阴茎化手术包括利用现有的生殖器组织创造一个新生殖器。对于那些希望从他们的新阴茎顶端排尿的人来说，完成了尿道延长术，由此将阴道口前庭的黏膜内层重新排列和装管，以构建从原尿道延伸到新阴茎顶端的新尿道。这部分尿道被称为固定部（图21-2）。通常，阴道切除术也在尿道延长的同时进行。阴茎成形术包括使用组织瓣来创造新阴茎。常见的供体部位包括前臂桡侧、大腿前外侧、背阔肌和腹部组织瓣。根据组织瓣供体部位的不同，阴茎干内的新尿道可以在阴茎成形术时通过将筋膜皮组织瓣置于阴茎干内而形成，也可以在不同的阶段形成。可以预料，潜在尿道并发症的区域主要集中在分水岭区域，通常在原尿道和固定部之间的吻合处以固定部和阴茎尿道（下垂部）之间的吻合处[82]。

阴道切除术和新尿道重建是男性化手术的组成部分，通常导致排尿功能障碍。最显著的尿道并发症是狭窄和尿道成形。尿道狭窄的发生率很高，超过50%，而尿道狭窄发生在10%～64%的患者中[83-89]。狭窄可能导致尿潴留和溢流性尿失禁的症状，而尿道狭窄最初可能表现为尿失禁。固定部和远端的狭窄可能导致阴道残端的重新开放和假性憩室的形成。这些患者可以表现为弱流

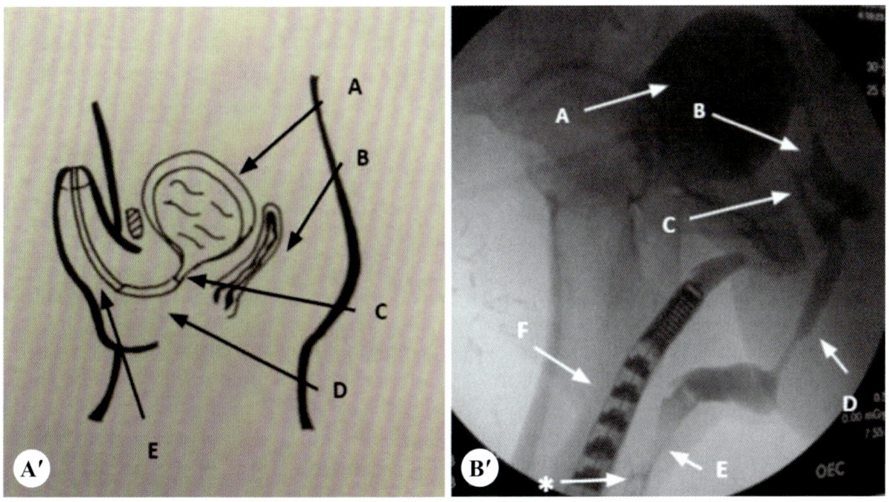

◀ **图 21-2 A′. 跨性别男性新阴茎解剖学矢状面图；B′. 新阴茎逆行尿道造影（RUG）**

A. 膀胱；B. 阴道残体；C. 原生尿道；D. 固定部；E. 摆部；F. 阴茎植入物；*. 尿道充盈缺损

和尿后滴沥，通常有恶臭的尿液和（或）复发性尿路感染。对这些患者的评估需要膀胱镜检查，伴或不伴逆行尿道造影，以确定重建的解剖结构。在尿道狭窄修复时，需切除任何阴道残余物并重新阻塞阴道腔。在某些情况下，股薄肌组织瓣用于为修复提供额外的支持。对于患有瘘管的患者，高达 66% 的瘘管将通过保守治疗解决，如使用导尿管进行尿流改道[84]。对于那些患有持续性尿道皮肤瘘的患者，首先评估整个尿道以排除任何可能导致尿道瘘形成的远端狭窄区域是很重要的。一旦这一问题得到解决，重建修复与尿道皮肤瘘患者相似，根据需要切除尿道瘘管并在组织瓣覆盖下多层缝合。阴茎成形术后患者的尿道狭窄通常需要手术修复。根据我们的经验，尿道扩张后尿道狭窄通常会复发。由于尿道缺乏灵活性和组织冗余，切除和一期吻合术很少是可行的选择。采用颊部移植或全层皮肤移植替代尿道成形术。短狭窄和固定部狭窄通常可以用颊黏膜移植一期尿道成形术修复，而长狭窄和下垂部狭窄通常需要用皮肤移植分期尿道成形术。

阴茎成形术患者可能会经历尿后滴沥，通常是由于尿道中的尿液滞留[90]。因为新尿道没有支持结构，如球海绵体肌，所以与原尿道相比，新尿道更可能含有残余尿。这些患者需学会用手从阴茎底部按压到其尖端部来排液[91]。

总结

原位新膀胱和性别确定手术后的尿失禁在表现和结构病因学上有所不同。最初，接受膀胱切除术的女性只有尿失禁改道术或可插入导管的膀胱术两种选择。外科技术的进步和对女性骨盆底解剖的更好理解使得膀胱切除术后女性能够经尿道排尿。这一进步存在各种类型尿失禁的挑战。有许多方法可以改善原位新膀胱女性的尿失禁状况；然而，如果所有的努力都失败了，可能需要转化为回肠导管或可插入导管的管道结构，以达到理想的期望值。在性别确定手术中，彻底了解重建和保留的原生解剖结构在尿失禁的检查中至关重要。详尽的病史和体格检查结合泌尿医疗设备的各种诊断性检查是确定尿失禁原因的关键。这些病例在识别和治疗上都提出了技术和智力上的挑战。

参考文献

[1] Stein JP, Lieskovsky G, Cote R, Groshen S, Feng AC, Boyd S, Skinner E, Bochner B, Thangathurai D, Mikhail M, Raghavan D, Skinner DG. Radical cystectomy in the treatment of invasive bladder cancer: long-term results in 1,054 patients. J Clin Oncol. 2001;19:666–75.
[2] Marshall FF, Treiger BFG. Radical cystectomy (anterior exenteration) in the female patient. Urol Clin North Am. 1991;18:765–75.

[3] Colleselli K, Stenzl A, Eder R, Strasser H, Poisel S, Bartsch G. The female urethral sphincter: a morphological and topographical study. J Urol. 1998;160:49–54.
[4] Stein JP, Penson DF, Wu SD, Skinner DG. Pathological guidelines for orthotopic urinary diversion in women with bladder cancer: a review of the literature. J Urol. 2007;178:756–60.
[5] Stein JP, Penson DF, Lee C, Cai J, Miranda G, Skinner DG. Long-term oncological outcomes in women undergoing radical cystectomy and orthotopic diversion for bladder cancer. J Urol. 2009;181:2052–8. discussion 2058–9.
[6] Stenzl A, Colleselli K, Poisel S, Feichtinger H, Pontasch H, Bartsch G. Rationale and technique of nerve sparing radical cystectomy before an orthotopic neobladder procedure in women. J Urol. 1995;154:2044–9.
[7] Stenzl A, Colleselli K, Poisel S, Feichtinger H, Bartsch G. The use of neobladders in women undergoing cystectomy for transitional-cell cancer. World J Urol. 1996;14:15–21.
[8] Nesrallah LJ, Almeida FG, Dall'Oglio MF, Nesrallah AJ, Srougi M. Experience with the orthotopic ileal neobladder in women: a mid-term follow-up. J Urol. 2006;175:987–8.
[9] Turner WH, Danuser H, Moehrle K, Studer UE. The effect of nerve sparing cystectomy technique on postoperative continence after orthotopic bladder substitution. J Urol. 1997;158:2118–22.
[10] Studer UE, Burkhard FC, Schumacher M, Kessler TM, Thoeny H, Fleischmann A, Thalmann GN. Twenty years experience with an ileal orthotopic low pressure bladder substitute- lessons to be learned. J Urol. 2006;176:161–6.
[11] Skinner EC, Daneshmand DS. Orthotopic urinary diversion. In: Partin AW, Peters CA, Kavoussi LR, Dmochowski RR, Wein AJ, editors. Campbell-Walsh-Wein urology. 12th ed. Philadelphia: Elsevier; 2020. p. 3233–57.
[12] Hinman F. Selection of intestinal segments for bladder substitution: physical and physiological characteristics. J Urol. 1998;139:519–23.
[13] Amini E, Djaladat H. Long-term complications of urinary diversion. Curr Opin Urol. 2015;25:50–7.
[14] Hinata N, Murakami G, Abe S-I, Honda M, Isoyama T, Sejima T, Takenaka A. Detailed histological investigation of the female urethra: application to radical cystectomy. J Urol. 2012;187:451–6.
[15] Grossfeld GD, Stein JP, Bennett CJ, Ginsberg DA, Boyd SD, Lieskovsky G, Skinner DG. Lower urinary tract reconstruction in the female using the kock ileal reservoir with bilat- eral ureteroileal urethrostomy: update of continence results and fluorourodynamic findings. Urology. 1996;48:383–8.
[16] Dhar NB, Kessler TM, Mills RD, Burkhard F, Studer UE. Nerve-sparing radical cystectomy and orthotopic bladder replacement in female patients. Eur Urol. 2007;52:1006–14.
[17] Gross T, Meierhans Ruf SD, Meissner C, Ochsner K, Studer UE. Orthotopic ileal bladder substitution in women: factors influencing urinary incontinence and hypercontinence. Eur Urol. 2015;68:664–71.
[18] Hautmann RE. The ileal neobladder to the female urethra. Urol Clin North Am. 1997;24:827–35.
[19] Ali-El-Dein B. Oncological outcome after radical cystectomy and orthotopic bladder substitution in women. Eur J Surg Oncol. 2009;35:320–5.
[20] Stein JP, Dunn MD, Quek ML, Miranda G, Skinner DG. The orthotopic T pouch ileal neobladder: experience with 209 patients. J Urol. 2004;172:584–7.
[21] Zlatev DV, Skinner EC. Orthotopic urinary diversion for women. Urol Clin North Am. 2018;45:49–54.
[22] Hautmann RE. Urinary diversion: ileal conduit to neobladder. J Urol. 2003;169:834–42.
[23] Granberg CF, Boorjian SA, Crispen PL, Tollefson MK, Farmer SA, Frank I, Blute ML. Functional and oncological outcomes after orthotopic neobladder reconstruction in women. BJU Int. 2008;102:1551–5.
[24] Stenzl A, Jarolim L, Coloby P, Golia S, Bartsch G, Babjuk M, Kakizoe T, Robertson C. Urethra-sparing cystectomy and orthotopic urinary diversion in women with malignant pelvic tumors. Cancer. 2001;92:1864–71.
[25] Lee CT, Hafez KS, Sheffield JH, Joshi DP, Montie JE. Orthotopic bladder substitution in women: nontraditional applications. J Urol. 2004;171:1585–8.
[26] Ahmadi H, Skinner EC, Simma-Chiang V, Miranda G, Cai J, Penson DF, Daneshmand S. Urinary functional outcome following radical cystoprostatectomy and ileal neobladder reconstruction in male patients. J Urol. 2013;189:1782–8.
[27] Anderson CB, Cookson MS, Chang SS, Clark PE, Smith JA, Kaufman MR. Voiding function in women with orthotopic neobladder urinary diversion. J Urol. 2012;188:200–4.
[28] Steers WD. Voiding dysfunction in the orthotopic neobladder. World J Urol. 2000;18:330–7.
[29] Veskimäe E, Neuzillet Y, Rouanne M, MacLennan S, Lam TB, Yuan Y, Comperat E, Cowan NC, Gakis G, van der Heijden AG, Ribal MJ, Witjes JA, Lebret T. Systematic review of the oncological and functional outcomes of pelvic organ-preserving radical cystectomy (RC) compared with standard RC in women who undergo curative surgery and orthotopic neobladder substitution for bladder cancer. BJU Int. 2017;120:12–24.
[30] Rouanne M, Legrand G, Neuzillet Y, Ghoneim T, Cour F, Letang N, Yonneau L, Hervé J-M, Botto H, Lebret T. Long-term women-reported quality of life after radical cystectomy and orthotopic ileal neobladder reconstruction. Ann Surg Oncol. 2014;21:1398–404.
[31] Kim S-O, Kim JS, Kim HS, Hwang EC, Oh KJ, Kwon D, Park K, Ryu SB. Age related change of nocturia in women. Int Neurourol J. 2010;14:245–9.
[32] Hoy NY, Cohn JA, Kowalik CG, Kaufman MR, Stuart Reynolds W, Dmochowski RR. Management of voiding dysfunction after female neobladder creation. Curr Urol Rep. 2017;18:33.
[33] Bailey GC, Blackburne A, Ziegelmann MJ, Lightner DJ. Outcomes of surgical management in patients with stress urinary incontinence and/ or neovesicovaginal fistula after orthotopic neobladder diversion. J Urol. 2016;196:1478–83.
[34] Badawy AA, Abolyosr A, Mohamed ER, Abuzeid AM. Orthotopic diversion after cystectomy in women: a single-centre experience with a 10–year follow-up. Arab J Urol. 2011;9:267–71.
[35] Marques A, Stothers L, Macnab A. The status of pelvic floor muscle training for women. Can Urol Assoc J. 2010;4:419–24.
[36] Johnson EV, Kirages DJ. Pelvic floor rehabilitation for orthotopic diversion. In: Daneshmand S, editor. Urinary diversion. Los Angeles: Springer; 2017. p. 143–52.
[37] Zhang Y-G, Song Q-X, Song B, Zhang D-L, Zhang W, Wang J-Y. Diagnosis and treatment of urinary incontinence after orthotopic ileal neobladder in China. Chin Med J. 2017;130:231–5.
[38] El-Bahnasawy MS, Shaaban H, Gomha MA, Nabeeh A. Clinical and urodynamic efficacy of oxybutynin and verapamil in the treatment of nocturnal enuresis after formation of orthotopic ileal neobladders. A prospective, randomized, crossover study. Scand J Urol Nephrol. 2008;42:344–51.
[39] Hjalmas K, Hanson E, Hellstrom AL, Kruse S, Sillen U. Long-term treatment with desmopressin in children with primary monosymptomatic nocturnal enuresis: an open multicentre study. Swedish enuresis trial (SWEET) group. Br J Urol. 1998;82:704–9.
[40] Naghizadeh S, Kefi A, Serkan Dogan H, Burgu B, Akdogan B, Tekgul S. Effectiveness of oral desmopressin therapy in posterior urethral valve patients with polyuria and detection of factors affecting the therapy. Eur Urol. 2005;48:819–25.
[41] Eckford SD, Carter PG, Jackson SR, Penney MD, Abrams P. An open,

in-patient incremental safety and efficacy study of desmopressin in women with multiple sclerosis and nocturia. Br J Urol. 1995;76:459–63.
[42] Goldberg H, Baniel J, Mano R, Gillon G, Kedar D, Yossepowitch O. Low-dose oral desmopressin for treatment of nocturia and nocturnal enuresis in patients after radical cystectomy and orthotopic urinary diversion. BJU Int. 2014;114:727–32.
[43] Schneider MP, Burkhard FC. Management of incontinence after orthotopic bladder substitution post-radical cystectomy. Curr Bladder Dysfunct Rep. 2019;14:125–9.
[44] Dave S, Grover VP, Agarwala S, Mitra DK, Bhatnagar V. The role of imipramine therapy in bladder exstrophy after bladder neck reconstruction. BJU Int. 2002;89:557–60.
[45] Mahony DT, Laferte RO, Mahoney JE. Studies of enuresis. VI. Observations on sphincter-augmenting effect of imipramine in children with urinary incontinence. Urology. 1973;1:317–23.
[46] Jost W, Marsalek P. Duloxetine: mechanism of action at the lower urinary tract and Onuf's nucleus. Clin Auton Res. 2004;14:220–7.
[47] Bridoux V, Gourcerol G, Kianifard B, Touchais J-Y, Ducrotte P, Leroi A-M, Michot F, Tuech J-J. Botulinum A toxin as a treatment for overactive rectum with associated faecal incontinence. Color Dis. 2012;14:342–8.
[48] Michel F, Ciceron C, Bernuz B, Boissier R, Gaillet S, Even A, Chartier-Kastler E, Denys P, Game X, Ruffion A, Le Normand L, Perrouin-Verbe B, Saussine C, Manuta A, Forin V, De Seze M, Grise P, Tournebise H, Schurch B, Karsenty G. Botulinum toxin type A injection after failure of augmentation enterocystoplasty performed for neurogenic detrusor overactivity: preliminary results of a salvage strategy. The ENTEROTOX study. Urology. 2019;129:43–7.
[49] Hoag N, Tse V, Wang A, Chung E, Gani J. Intravesical onabotulinumtoxinA injection for overactive orthotopic ileal neobladder: feasibility and efficacy. Int Neurourol J. 2016;20:81–5.
[50] Wilson S, Quek ML, Ginsberg DA. Transurethral injection of bulking agents for stress urinary incontinence following orthotopic neobladder reconstruction in women. J Urol. 2004;172:244–6.
[51] Tchetgen MB, Sanda MG, Montie JE, Faerber GJ. Collagen injection for the treatment of incontinence after cystectomy and orthotopic neobladder reconstruction in women. J Urol. 2000;163:212–4.
[52] Pruthi RS, Petrus CD, Bundrick WS. New onset vesicovaginal fistula after transurethral collagen injection in women who underwent cystectomy and orthotopic neobladder creation: presentation and definitive treatment. J Urol. 2000;164:1638–9.
[53] Quek ML, Ginsberg DA, Wilson S, Skinner EC, Stein JP, Skinner DG. Pubovaginal slings for stress urinary incontinence following radical cystectomy and orthotopic neobladder reconstruction in women. J Urol. 2004;172:219–21.
[54] Badawy AA, Saleem MD, Abolyosr A, Abuzeid AM. Transobturator vaginal tape (inside-out) for stress urinary incontinence after radical cystectomy and orthotopic reconstruction in women. Arab J Urol. 2012;10:182–5.
[55] Rosenberg S, Miranda G, Ginsberg DA. Neobladder-vaginal fistula: the University of Southern California experience. Neurourol Urodyn. 2018;37:1380–5.
[56] Kaufman MR. Neobladder-vaginal fistula: surgical management techniques. Curr Urol Rep. 2019;20:67.
[57] Carmel ME, Goldman HB, Moore CK, Rackley RR, Vasavada SP. Transvaginal neobladder vaginal fistula repair after radical cystectomy with orthotopic urinary diversion in women. Neurourol Urodyn. 2016;35:90–4.
[58] Rapp DE, Corey O'Connor R, Katz EE, Steinberg GD. Neobladder-vaginal fistula after cystectomy and orthotopic neobladder construction. BJU Int. 2004;94:1092–5.
[59] Ali-El-Dein B, Shaaban AA, Abu-Eideh RH, El-Azab M, Ashamallah A, Ghoneim MA. Surgical complications following radical cystectomy and orthotopic neobladders in women. J Urol. 2008;180:206–10.
[60] Tunuguntla HSGR, Tunuguntla HSG, Manoharan M, Gousse AE. Management of neobladder-vaginal fistula and stress incontinence following radical cystectomy in women: a review. World J Urol. 2005;23:231–5.
[61] Ali-El-Dein B, Ashamallah A. Vaginal repair of pouch-vaginal fistula after orthotopic bladder substitution in women. Urology. 2013;81:198–203.
[62] Hautmann RE, Paiss T, de Petriconi R. The ileal neobladder in women: 9 years of experience with 18 patients. J Urol. 1996;155:76–81.
[63] Ismail MAA, Wishahi MM, Elsherbeeny M, Sewallam TA, Lockhart J. Hypercontinence in women after orthotopic neobladder diversion. UroToday Int J. 2009;2:1.
[64] Neymeyer J, Abdul-Wahab W, Beer M. Prevention of hypercontinence and preservation of womanhood in patients undergoing cystectomy and ileum neobladder creation for invasive bladder cancer by preserving the vagina and performing a colposacropexy with titanium coated polypropeleium mesh all in a single session; the berliner neobladder. Eur Urol Suppl. 2008;7:220.
[65] Arai Y, Okubo K, Konami T, Kin S, Kanba T, Okabe T, Hamaguchi A, Okada Y. Voiding function of orthotopic ileal neobladder in women. Urology. 1999;54:44–9.
[66] Finley DS, Lee U, McDonough D, Raz S, de Kernion J. Urinary retention after orthotopic neobladder substitution in females. J Urol. 2011;186:1364–9.
[67] Stearns G, Donahue T, Fathollahi A, Dalbagni G, Sandhu J. Formal sacrocolpopexy reduces hypercontinence rates in female neobladder formation. Neurourol Urodyn. 2018;37:2281–5.
[68] Hoebeke P, Selvaggi G, Ceulemans P, De Cuypere G, T'Sjoen G, Weyers S, Decaestecker K, Monstrey S. Impact of sex reassignment surgery on lower urinary tract function. Eur Urol. 2005;47:398–402.
[69] Ferrando CA. Vaginoplasty complications. Clin Plast Surg. 2018;45:361–8.
[70] Shoureshi P, Dy GW, Dugi D. Neovaginal canal dissection in gender-affirming vaginoplasty. J Urol. 2021;205:1110–8.
[71] Jewett HJ. The case for radical perineal prostatectomy. J Urol. 1970;103:195–9.
[72] Krege S, Bex A, Lümmen G, Rübben H. Male-to-female transsexualism: a technique, results and long-term follow-up in 66 patients. BJU Int. 2001;88:396–402.
[73] Reed HM. Aesthetic and functional male to female genital and perineal surgery: feminizing vaginoplasty. Semin Plast Surg. 2011;25:163–74.
[74] Rossi Neto R, Hintz F, Krege S, Rübben H, Vom Dorp F. Gender reassignment surgery – a 13 year review of surgical outcomes. Int Braz J Urol. 2012;38:97–107.
[75] van Kesteren P, Meinhardt W, van der Valk P, Geldof A, Megens J, Gooren L. Effects of estrogens only on the prostates of aging men. J Urol. 1996;156(4):1349–53.
[76] Roy AK, Lavrovsky Y, Song CS, Chen S, Jung MH, Velu NK, Bi BY, Chatterjee B. Regulation of androgen action. Vitam Horm. 1999;55:309–52.
[77] Deebel NA, Morin JP, Autorino R, Vince R, Grob B, Hampton LJ. Prostate cancer in transgender women: incidence, etiopathogenesis, and management challenges. Urology. 2017;110:166–71.
[78] Turo R, Jallad S, Prescott S, Cross WR. Metastatic prostate cancer in transsexual diagnosed after three decades of estrogen therapy. Can Urol Assoc J. 2013;7:544–6.
[79] Kuhn A, Hiltebrand R, Birkhäuser M. Do transsexuals have micturition disorders? Eur J Obstet Gynecol Reprod Biol. 2007;131:226–30.
[80] Jiang DD, Gallagher S, Burchill L, Berli J, Dugi D. Implementation of a pelvic floor physical therapy program for transgender women undergoing gender-affirming vaginoplasty. Obstet Gynecol.

2019;133:1003–11.
[81] Chen ML, Reyblat P, Poh MM, Chi AC. Overview of surgical techniques in gender-affirming genital surgery. Transl Androl Urol. 2019;8:191–208.
[82] Jun MS, Santucci RA. Urethral stricture after phalloplasty. Transl Androl Urol. 2019;8:266–72.
[83] Santucci RA. Urethral complications after transgender phalloplasty: strategies to treat them and minimize their occurrence. Clin Anat. 2018;31:187–90.
[84] Ascha M, Massie JP, Morrison SD, Crane CN, Chen ML. Outcomes of single stage phalloplasty by pedicled anterolateral thigh flap versus radial forearm free flap in gender confirming surgery. J Urol. 2018;199:206–14.
[85] Matti BA, Matthews RN, Davies DM. Phalloplasty using the free radial forearm flap. Br J Plast Surg. 1988;41:160–4.
[86] Fang RH, Kao YS, Ma S, Lin JT. Phalloplasty in female-to-male transsexuals using free radial osteocutaneous flap: a series of 22 cases. Br J Plast Surg. 1999;52:217–22.
[87] Leriche A, Timsit M-O, Morel-Journel N, Bouillot A, Dembele D, Ruffion A. Long-term outcome of forearm free-flap phalloplasty in the treatment of transsexualism. BJU Int. 2008;101:1297–300.
[88] Kim S-K, Moon J-B, Heo J, Kwon Y-S, Lee K-C. A new method of urethroplasty for prevention of fistula in female-to-male gender reassignment surgery. Ann Plast Surg. 2010;64:759–64.
[89] Doornaert M, Hoebeke P, Ceulemans P, T'Sjoen G, Heylens G, Monstrey S. Penile reconstruction with the radial forearm flap: an update. Handchir Mikrochir Plast Chir. 2011;43:208–14.
[90] Nassiri N, Maas M, Basin M, Cacciamani GE, Doumanian LR. Urethral complications after gender reassignment surgery: a systematic review. Int J Impot Res. 2020; https://doi. org/10.1038/s41443-020-0304- y.
[91] Heston AL, Esmonde NO, Dugi DD III, Berli JU. Phalloplasty: techniques and outcomes. Transl Androl Urol. 2019;8:254–65.

第 22 章 尿失禁的罕见病因及其治疗

Rare Conditions Causing Incontinence and Their Treatment

Ariana L. Smith Andrea C. Yeguez 著

一、膀胱阴道瘘

良性子宫切除术后约 1 周的持续漏尿是膀胱阴道瘘（VVF）的必要条件。瘘管是指两个或多个上皮或间皮内衬的体腔或皮肤表面之间的解剖结构外交通。尿路的任何部分（肾脏、输尿管、膀胱和尿道）和几乎任何其他体腔之间都有可能形成瘘管，包括生殖器官、胃肠道、胸部（胸膜腔）、淋巴管、血管系统、生殖器和皮肤。瘘管是基于相通的两个器官命名的（表 22-1）。虽然工业化国家的大多数瘘管是先天性的，但也可能由于分娩（全世界最常见的病因）、先天性畸形、恶性肿瘤、炎症和感染、放射治疗、手术伤害、外部组织创伤。异物、缺血，以及其他各种原因而发生（表 22-2）[1-3]。膀胱阴道瘘是最常见的后天性尿道瘘。顾名思义，膀胱阴道瘘是膀胱和阴道之间的通路。

（一）病因学

在发展中国家中，常规产科护理发展有限，膀胱阴道瘘最常发生的原因是长时间的难产导致盆腔组织缺血、坏死[4, 5]。在撒哈拉沙漠以南的非洲地区，据估计，产科膀胱阴道瘘的发生率为 10.3/10 万[6]。阴道前壁、三叉神经和尿道通常承受着胎儿最大的直接压力[3]。在某些情况下，膀胱阴道瘘是由于在分娩过程中使用了产钳或其他器械导致的。产科瘘管往往较大，位于阴道远端，并可能涉及尿道近端。由难产引起的一系列问题并不局限于膀胱阴道瘘，被称为“难产损伤综合征”，包括不同程度的以下问题：尿道脱落、压力性尿失禁、肾盂积水、肾功能衰竭、直肠阴道瘘、直肠闭锁、肛门括约肌功能不全、宫颈损伤、闭经、盆腔炎、继发性不孕症、阴道狭窄、耻骨骨炎和足下垂[7]。

在美国，妇科手术时对膀胱的损伤的最常见原因——通常是良性疾病的子宫切除术（80%）[8]。

表 22-1 泌尿道瘘管：与泌尿道相邻脏器出现交通

	类 型	涉及的器官	
泌尿生殖道瘘	膀胱阴道瘘	膀胱	阴道
	输尿管阴道瘘	输尿管	阴道
	膀胱子宫瘘	膀胱	子宫
	尿道阴道瘘	尿道	阴道
泌尿肠道瘘	膀胱肠道瘘	膀胱	肠道
	输尿管肠道瘘	输尿管	肠道
	肾盂肠道瘘	肾盂	肠道
	尿道肠道瘘	肠道	尿道
泌尿血管瘘	肾脏血管瘘	肾脏	脉管系统
	肾盂血管瘘	肾盂	脉管系统
	输尿管血管瘘	输尿管	脉管系统
其他类型	肾章胸膜瘘	肾脏	肺胸膜
	肾小球支气管瘘	肾脏	支气管
	膀胱皮肤瘘	膀胱	皮肤
	输尿管皮肤瘘	输尿管	皮肤
	尿道皮肤瘘	尿道	皮肤
	肾脏皮肤瘘	肾盂	皮肤

表 22-2　泌尿系统瘘管的病因

病　因	举　例
分娩	• 长时间难产 • 产科创伤 / 产钳撕裂伤 • 子宫破裂
手术 / 医源性	• 妇科、泌尿科或盆腔手术 • 剖宫产 • 使用合成网的手术
先天性异常	泌尿生殖腔畸形
恶性肿瘤	妇科、泌尿科或其他盆腔恶性肿瘤
炎症	• 子宫内膜异位症 • 盆腔炎 • 尿道憩室
感染	• 盆腔脓肿 • 直肠周围脓肿
缺血	膀胱颈 / 三角区受压导致缺血
放疗	• 外照射疗法 • 近距离放射治疗
异物	• 子宫托 • 宫内节育器 • 残留的手术材料
创伤	• 骨盆骨折 • 性暴力

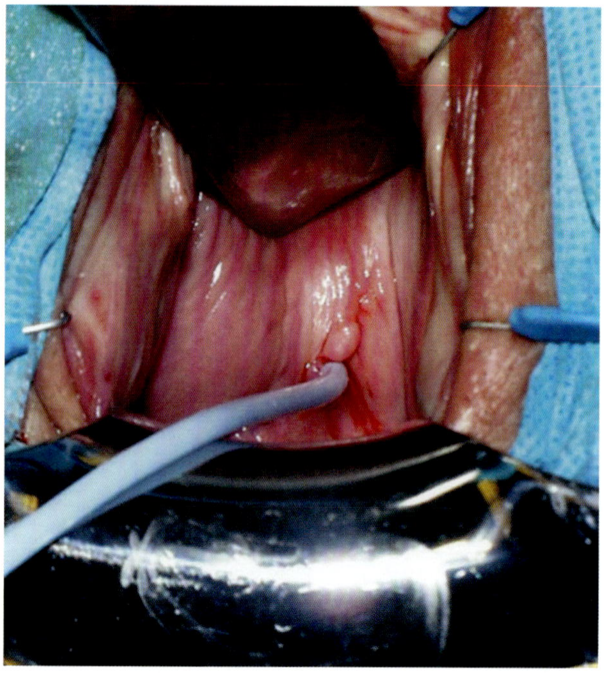

▲ 图 22-1　子宫切除术后膀胱阴道瘘，在阴道前壁与膀胱后壁处可见一个小的膀胱阴道瘘（蓝色导管穿过瘘管）

产科事件（10%）、妇科恶性肿瘤的手术干预（5%）和盆腔放疗（5%）是膀胱阴道瘘不太常见的病因[8, 9]。此外，与恶性肿瘤和既往放疗相关的瘘管一般比较复杂。

子宫切除术后的膀胱阴道瘘最常见的原因是阴道前壁附近的膀胱切开（图 22-1）。其他潜在的原因包括缝合线缝入膀胱内导致压力坏死和组织损失，电器械放置不当，以及阴道或周围组织感染。子宫切除术的手术方式是一个重要因素。与经腹子宫切除术相比，腹腔镜子宫切除术中的膀胱损伤至少高出两倍，而机器人子宫切除术中的膀胱损伤率也可能更高[2, 10]。经腹全子宫切除术和阴式子宫切除术发生瘘管的风险较低[11]。发生膀胱阴道瘘的患者更有可能膀胱损伤大，电器械使用多，子宫体积大，手术时间长，手术失血多[12, 13]。瘘管在年龄超过 50 岁的女性切除子宫时更为常见，这可能和雌激素缺乏导致的阴道组织质量变化相关[11]。

（二）影响

膀胱阴道瘘对于患者造成了相当大的身体和心理影响，而对医疗机构来说，医疗法律方面的影响也是令人生畏的。迅速的处理以尽量减少患者的不适感是至关重要的，这也是一种诚实、积极的医患关系。通过加强教育、认真做盆腔手术和精确放射治疗来预防泌尿系的医源性损伤可以减少瘘管的形成。

（三）诊断

泌尿道瘘的症状和体征是多种多样的，在很大程度上取决于所涉及的器官、潜在的尿路梗阻或感染、瘘管的大小以及相关的疾病如恶性肿瘤。膀胱阴道瘘最常见的主诉是持续的尿液排出。尽管小的瘘管可能表现为间歇性的漏尿，但由于位置，常被误认为是压力性尿失禁。膀胱阴道瘘必须与其他原因造成的尿失禁区分开来，其中包括压力性尿失禁、急迫性尿失禁和充盈性尿失禁。患者可能会表现为反复性膀胱炎、会阴部皮肤因持续潮湿而过敏、真菌性阴道炎，少数也会出现盆腔疼痛。当出现大的膀胱阴道瘘时。患者可能完全不排尿，表现为阴道持续性漏尿。子宫切除术或其他手术后的膀胱阴道瘘可能出现在尿管移除后，也可以发生在术后 1～3 周后出现阴道漏尿。子宫切除术后的膀胱阴道瘘通常位于阴道顶端或阴道前壁。放射治疗导致的阴道瘘可能在完成放射治疗后数月至数年内不会出现。这些阴道瘘因为其大小程度、复杂程度，以及膀胱放射导致的相关排尿功能障碍成为泌尿外科中最具挑战性的重建病例。放射治疗导致的组织缺血可能涉及周围的组织，也限制了重建的选择。

应该应用窥阴器进行盆腔检查找到瘘管的位置并评估瘘管的大小和数量。应进行触诊评估是否有肿块或其他在修复瘘管时处理的盆腔病变，此外，要评估瘘管周围的炎症，因为它可能影响修复的时机。将亚甲蓝注入膀胱观察阴道漏液是否变色可以确定是否存在阴道瘘。双重染料试验可以确认尿道瘘的诊断，并提示可能存在相关的输尿管阴道瘘或尿道阴道瘘。进行这种检查时，将棉条放在阴道内，口服酚苄明，并将亚甲蓝灌入膀胱内。如果棉条顶部变色为黄橙色，则提示有输尿管阴道瘘。棉条中间部分的蓝色变色表明是膀胱阴道瘘，而棉条底部的蓝染表明是尿道阴道瘘。尿路瘘的诊断和定位以及对尿路瘘损伤的评估，无论是否进行内镜评估，一般都采用包括使用膀胱尿道造影术、尿路造影术（静脉注射、CT 或逆行肾盂造影术）或其他横断面成像等方法。

膀胱尿道造影术（VCUG）可用于评估膀胱阴道瘘或尿道阴道瘘的大小和位置。除非膀胱充盈到一定程度并引起逼尿肌收缩，在 X 线片上可能无法看到一些较小的瘘管。膀胱阴道瘘也可以评估膀胱输尿管反流的情况。静脉尿路造影、计算机断层尿路造影（CTU）和（或）逆行肾盂输尿管造影（RPG）可以评估合并的输尿管损伤、狭窄和（或）输尿管阴道瘘，据报道有 12% 的患者会出现这种情况[14]。阴道内的对比剂、膀胱内的空气和膀胱壁增厚是提示存在瘘管的征兆。如果怀疑有恶性肿瘤，建议进行盆腔横断面成像［磁共振成像（MRI）/ 计算机断层扫描（CT）］，CT 膀胱造影可以在当膀胱阴道瘘因患者体型较大或瘘管道非常小等原因而无法诊断时发挥作用。

盆腔恶性肿瘤病史或怀疑有恶性肿瘤的情况可以做膀胱镜检查和可疑瘘管道活检。膀胱镜检查可以显示瘘管相对于输尿管的位置，如果瘘管涉及输尿管，修复瘘管可能需要输尿管再植入。此外，还要评估是否可以从阴道到达瘘管。是否包括缝合材料、网片和（或）膀胱结石等的异物。

（四）治疗

尿瘘管的治疗取决于以下因素：瘘管的位置、大小、病因（恶性或良性）和周围组织质量。

1. 非手术治疗膀胱阴道瘘

通过最大限度地引流和分流尿液（粪便，如果涉及）的保守治疗可以避免手术干预。当膀胱阴道瘘在临床早期被发现并且瘘管尚未有机会形成时，导尿管引流是大多数病例的初始治疗。抗生素、抗胆碱能药物和外用雌激素药膏是预防感染、促进膀胱松弛的辅助性措施。帮助膀胱放松，并促进伤口愈合。在小的（＜5mm）不复杂的瘘管中，用电灼法灌注瘘管，然后用导管引流已被证明有一定疗效。据一些小系列报道，纤维蛋白胶等辅助措施与栓塞和导管引流相结合，作为瘘管的“塞子”和“支架”帮助健康组织的生长。

2. 手术治疗膀胱阴道瘘

泌尿道瘘管的手术治疗包括多层、无张力的闭合，并插入血管良好的组织。遵循基本的手术原则是成功修复所有尿道瘘的关键。所有尿道瘘的修复在手术开始时对膀胱和输尿管进行膀胱镜评估有助于确定瘘管的准确位置并对其进行导管插管。无论采用何种方法，都必须充分显露瘘管道，以便完全解剖并分离膀胱壁和阴道壁。充分止血对于防止持续出血或术后血肿是很有必要的，不要过度使用单极烧灼，因为单极烧灼会导致组织延迟坏死和分解。应对破坏的和缺血的组织进行清创来防止坏死和破坏的瘘管闭合，但健康的瘘管道组织不需要切除。对任何残留的手术材料或其他异物应予以清除以保证瘘管内的膀胱壁的清洁、无障碍和水密闭。膀胱壁的第二层闭合通常是在第一层缝合线的基础上进行的。把蓝色染料灌注到膀胱内可以测试膀胱闭合是否充分，并检查是否需要进行缝合。在进行水密缝合之前，建议在阴道壁闭合前插入健康组织，以达到不漏水的目的。

修复的时机应考虑目前的炎症程度、是否存在感染、患者的一般健康和营养状况及患者的舒适度[15]。在发达国家，绝大多数情况下都主张早期干预。在有明显炎症、感染或辐射损伤的情况下，建议有3～6个月的等待期。无论采用何种手术方法，成功率都接近90%～98%。

对膀胱阴道瘘最佳手术方式的选择（经腹或经阴道）是有争议的，一般取决于外科医生的技能[16, 17]。没有一种方法适用于所有的膀胱阴道瘘，但是所有的膀胱阴道瘘都应该由一个训练有素的有足够的瘘管管理专业知识的外科医生来处理。经腹部（包括腹腔镜或机器人）入路非常适合位于输尿管附近的瘘管，当需要输尿管再植时，须通过阴道难以到达区域。当病因手术在腹部进行时，经阴道的方法是最理想的。

3. 经腹方法

通过脐下中线切口、横切口、腹腔镜或机器人方法，显露膀胱。在膀胱镜下通过瘘管轨道放置导管或导线，可以帮助确定所涉及的区域。可以采用膀胱外或经膀胱的方法来确定瘘管连接处。采用膀胱外侧入路时，通常在阴道内的一个筛子或海绵棒的协助下，调动膀胱并将其反映在阴道底层顶端上。在经膀胱的方法中，膀胱在矢状面被打开。在矢状面打开，直到瘘管的水平。如果担心有恶性肿瘤，则对瘘管进行活检；如果有坏死，则对组织进行清创。膀胱壁和阴道壁分别进行多层封闭，并将膀胱壁和阴道壁合并（而不是切除）。通常，一些血管发达的组织如网膜被放置在阴道和膀胱之间作为一个额外的层以促进愈合和防止复发。当网膜无法调动时，可使用腹膜作为穿插层。

4. 经阴道方法

许多阴道路径方法包括Sims、Latzko和Raz的方法都已被记录[18-23]。使用钩子和环形牵开器的固定牵开以及加权窥阴器可以是比较成功的设置。用导管或金属丝穿过瘘管的轨道可以很容易地确定阴道口的位置。一般来说，在阴道壁上做一个倒U形切口，并在瘘管道周围延伸。小心地将阴道壁从瘘管道周围移开，并将阴道壁与底层膀胱分开。这需要精细的剥离，以避免撕裂膀胱和阴道壁，通常需要使用自持式和手持式牵引器。瘘管道被切除（如果缺血或坏死），切除后的瘘管道边缘形成第一层闭合，或者瘘管道被留在原位，瘘管道边缘被卷起形成第一层闭合。然后将第一层闭合处两侧的肛周筋膜覆盖在主缝合线上形成第二层。来自唇部脂肪垫（Martius瓣）、腹膜瓣或股薄肌瓣的健康组织可以放在缝合线上，作为类似于经腹方法中网膜瓣的椭圆血管化瓣[24]。另外，或在某些情况下，可以利用修改后的拉兹科法来提供额外的覆盖。这包括扩大阴道壁切口，以便在阴道顶的水平上显露直肠前壁。然后使用直肠周围组织来覆盖封闭的膀胱壁，类似于部分结肠切除术的技术。虽然阴道切除术可以使阴道缩短几厘米，但不是所有的性行为都适合做这种手术。并非所有性行为活跃的女性都需要这种技术，但它通常可以在阴道深度没有明显变化的情况下使用。最后，阴道壁的皮瓣被推进到修复处形成最后一层闭合层。

在研究的患者中，通过经腹或经阴道入路的成功率相似。辅助组织瓣可用于任何一种入路并且可以帮助治疗复杂或复发性瘘管、盆腔放疗史或周围有广泛组织丢失的患者的手术。不管方法是什么，都要进行最大限度的尿液引流［使用尿道和（或）耻骨上导管］，通常在修复后2～3周进行膀胱造影以保证成功闭合。抗心律失常药或

β_3 受体激动药可以帮助促进膀胱放松，并帮助患者耐受导管。在适当的时候，局部阴道雌激素可以改善阴道组织质量方面。

二、输尿管阴道瘘

良性子宫切除术或盆腔手术后 1～4 周后持续漏尿并保留自主排尿是输尿管阴道瘘（UVF）最常见的表现。

（一）病因学

输尿管阴道瘘在输尿管和阴道之间形成。大多数输尿管阴道瘘是由于在妇科手术过程中未被发现的输尿管远端损伤引起的。输尿管阴道瘘是继发于妇科手术中未被确认的输尿管远端损伤，包括腹腔镜、腹部或阴道子宫切除术。剖腹产、脱垂手术和抗失禁手术[25]。这些损伤可能包括输尿管的撕裂、输尿管的完全横断、继发于血液供应丧失或烧灼伤的延迟坏死、缝合结扎或钝性撕脱。在妇科手术中，输尿管人为损伤的发生率估计为 0.03%～1.5%[10]。尿液会从受伤的输尿管溢出进入腹膜或腹膜外空间，一般会导致尿瘤的形成。尿瘤的大小和张力不断增加，导致尿液从阴道顶端排出[18]。少数时候，输尿管阴道瘘可能继发于内镜下的器械治疗、放射治疗、盆腔恶性肿瘤、穿透性盆腔创伤或其他盆腔手术（血管、肠道等）。输尿管损伤的风险因素包括既往有盆腔手术史、盆腔恶性肿瘤、肥胖、子宫内膜异位症、放射治疗和盆腔炎症（PID）。然而，许多输尿管损伤的发生没有可识别的风险因素[9, 18, 26]。高达 12% 的膀胱阴道瘘可能伴有输尿管阴道瘘[14, 27]。

（二）诊断

输尿管阴道瘘一般在术后 1～4 周出现尿漏或单侧输尿管肾积水，以及继发于部分输尿管梗阻的腹部疼痛。腹痛、恶心和发热随着盆腔手术后尿液渗漏的开始而改善提示输尿管损伤，与膀胱阴道瘘不同的是，只要对侧肾脏不受影响，输尿管阴道瘘的患者将继续保持正常的排尿模式。漏出液肌酐过高可以证实阴道漏出的是尿液，而双份染料测试（如上所述）可以区分膀胱阴道瘘和输尿管阴道瘘。

输尿管阴道瘘一般用静脉尿路造影或 CT 尿路造影来评估。尿路造影可显示部分梗阻、输尿管肾积水和阴道引流。膀胱镜检查和逆行肾盂造影可以用来评估是否有合并的膀胱损伤，并观察输尿管远端。如果肾盂输尿管出现问题，尝试进行逆行支架植入是合理的。长期的内引流（6～8 周）并进行输尿管支架手术可能会治愈输尿管瘘。CT 或 MRI 的横断面成像可能有助于评估盆腔恶性肿瘤或在持续发热的患者中评估是否有尿瘤。在长段输尿管受累的情况下，考虑采用 Boari 膀胱造影或膀胱造影可能有助于评估膀胱容量。

特别是在输尿管完全闭塞的情况下，经皮肾脏造影术和前向肾脏造影术会有帮助。对受累的肾脏进行引流然后进行前向灌注对比剂。可以为部分阻塞肾脏减压并且解剖定位和显示肾盂的位置。

（三）治疗

如上所述，输尿管阴道瘘可以通过输尿管支架手术进行保守治疗[28]。如果在败血症的情况下存在严重的部分梗阻，在进行修复之前需要经皮引流和一个疗程的抗生素治疗。如果逆行支架术不成功，但输尿管造影显示输尿管管腔通畅，那么可以尝试进行逆行支架术。支架术的目的是为输尿管减压，支架术的目的是为上尿路减压，并防止进一步的尿液外渗和尿毒症。

当支架治疗不成功且瘘管位于远端时，可进行输尿管膀胱造口术（输尿管再植术，带或不带腰肌搭桥和板瓣）。这可以通过腹腔镜或机器人的方式进行。腰肌搭接可保持膀胱的解剖位置，并在膀胱充盈和排空时保持稳定。除非膀胱输尿管反流。否则没有必要切除远端输尿管段，甚至不需要关闭输尿管。位于输尿管中 1/3 处的瘘管可能适合于输尿管膀胱造口术，并结合从膀胱推进的板瓣手术。近端瘘管需要在支架上进行近端和远端动员和初级输尿管造口术，对于较长的输尿管损伤需要进行回肠插管，甚至是自体移植。

（四）尿道阴道瘘

尿瘘情况的加重常发生于抗尿失禁手术、尿道周围网片移除术、尿道憩室切除术、阴道前壁脱垂修复术或生殖器重建术等术后，尿瘘情况加重表明可能发生尿道阴道瘘。尿漏的程度取决于瘘管沿尿道腔的大小和位置。在尿道阴道瘘患者中，有时会发现排尿困难或复发性尿路感染（UTI），通过优化术后护理可极大改善上述情况的发生。

（五）病因

尿道阴道瘘形成于尿道和阴道之间。在工业化国家，虽然尿道阴道瘘发生偶见于外伤、长时间放置尿管、放疗、骨盆骨折、阴道肿瘤或分娩等因素，但尿道阴道瘘发生通常是医源性的，常发生于抗尿失禁手术、尿道周围网片移除术、尿道憩室切除术、阴道前壁脱垂修复术、生殖器重建术等术后（图 22-2）[29, 30]。在发展中国家，尿道阴道瘘的发生率极低，大多数是由于难产造成的。在工业化国家，吊带手术时继发医源性尿道损伤的频率似乎在增加[31, 32]。值得关注的是约 20% 的尿道阴道瘘合并膀胱阴道瘘[33]。

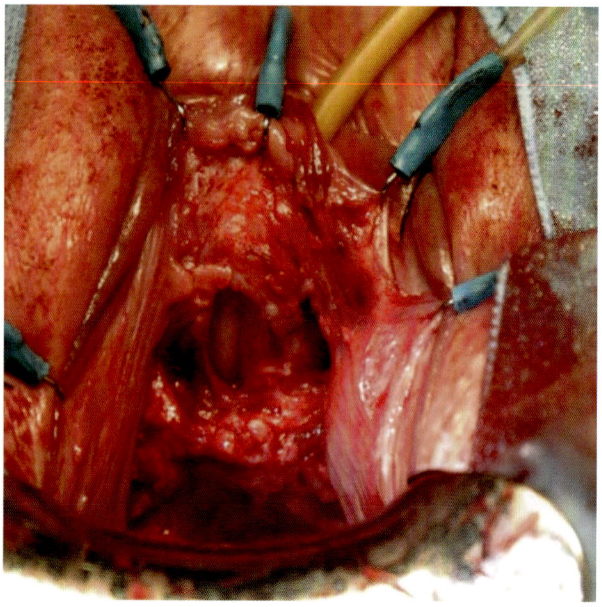

▲ 图 22-2　移除破损的网状吊带后的尿道阴道瘘（黄色导管位于尿道内）

（六）诊断

尿道阴道瘘若位于尿道远端 1/3 处（即超出控尿机制）可无相关症状出现；若尿道阴道瘘没有位于尿道远端 1/3 处，其症状表现与膀胱阴道瘘相似。尿道阴道瘘可通过对阴道远端仔细体格检查诊断出来。膀胱尿道镜也可用于观察尿道腔。然而，为了更好观察尿道腔，可能需要技术方面的考量，如使用女性膀胱镜、软膀胱镜，或者充分扩张尿道、仔细操作膀胱镜。膀胱镜检查也有助于评估膀胱和尿道并发异常，特别是用于下述方面：评估是否存在尿道和膀胱异物、评估膀胱和尿道是否出现先前吊带手术的网片材料、评估是否有残留的尿道憩室或尿道狭窄，以及评估现存尿道组织是否完整。有时尿道阴道瘘的患者可能出现压力性尿失禁或急迫性尿失禁的症状，但通过体格检查和膀胱镜检查不能确诊。在这种情况下，排泄性膀胱尿道造影（VCUG）对阴道尿道瘘的诊断非常有用。对于膀胱颈和近端尿道括约肌功能正常的患者必须获得排尿影像资料，否则将无法显示瘘管所在位置。

（七）治疗

若在尿道阴道瘘发生后及时发现尿道阴道瘘，尿管引流在少数情况下可能是有用的。经阴道修复尿道阴道瘘是最常用的方法，其原理与膀胱阴道瘘手术类似，可以对尿道腔、尿道周组织和阴道进行解剖性修复。手术修复第一步包括：分辨尿道阴道瘘管位置、仔细解剖阴道和尿道之间的平面。可使用带有挂钩的环形拉钩更好显露并观察病变部位，也有利于保留尿道周围筋膜作为一个特殊层次置入尿道和阴道之间。经阴道手术切除所有异物材料是尿道成功重建的必要条件，其中异物材料包括之前手术的材料或网片。尿道重建通常主要通过导尿管进行，但在尿道组织严重丧失的情况下，可能需要口腔颊黏膜或阴道壁组织。使用尿道周围筋膜、大阴唇球海绵体脂肪垫（板瓣）和阴道壁皮瓣进行多层闭合是最佳选择。

这种多层闭合技术允许同时或后续对压力性尿失禁进行治疗。需要注意的是，根据美国泌尿学会/泌尿动力学、女性盆腔医学与泌尿生殖系统重建学会（AUA/SUFU）最新发布的压力性尿失禁指南，不建议在尿道阴道瘘修复时同时行压力性尿失禁治疗，即放置人工合成网片材料行尿道中段悬吊[34]。然而，使用自体阴部吊带被认为是安全和有效的。对压力性尿失禁的最佳治疗时机尚存争议，一些作者认为压力性尿失禁的治疗应推迟到尿道阴道瘘后，并重新评估患者是否存在持续性压力性尿失禁[35]。

三、膀胱子宫瘘

在宫颈功能正常的情况下，漏尿症状可能不是膀胱子宫瘘的一部分原因；相反，周期性血尿和阴道水样分泌物症状可提示膀胱子宫瘘的存在。膀胱子宫瘘可出现在宫颈机能不全、先前经阴道分娩等情况下，症状可能会与膀胱阴道瘘相似。

（一）病因学

膀胱子宫瘘形成于膀胱和子宫之间。膀胱子宫瘘是罕见的瘘管，最常见发生于低位剖宫产术后[36, 37]。膀胱子宫瘘的其他潜在诱发因素包括：难产时子宫破裂、阴道手术产、既往剖宫产后经阴道分娩（VABC）和胎盘植入等[38]。据报道：宫内节育器（IUD）引起的异物反应、子宫动脉栓塞术、子宫内膜消融术、人工流产术、外伤后膀胱留置尿管和近距离放射治疗是导致膀胱子宫瘘的原因。通常情况下，若子宫和膀胱同时受损，若损伤未被及时发现或修复不充分，子宫和膀胱之间可能会形成瘘管。据推测，有些膀胱子宫瘘在产后未被发现，其症状可能被分娩后的正常产后恶露所掩盖。尿液性恶露（即尿液与恶露混合）出现时膀胱子宫瘘可被发现，但该症状仍可在其产后自行消失，消失原因可能与母乳喂养引起的激素抑制和闭经有关[39]。口服避孕药和使用促黄体生成素释放激素激动药（LHRH）抑制机体激素水平后，目前也有膀胱子宫瘘自愈的相关报道。

（二）诊断

膀胱子宫瘘所表现的临床症状基于子宫颈功能情况，因此，在评估膀胱子宫瘘的时候一般要保持高度怀疑的态度。膀胱子宫瘘的症状可表现为 Youssef 综合征（即月经不调、周期性血尿伴明显闭经、不孕和尿失禁）或出现类似于膀胱阴道瘘的尿失禁的症状。膀胱子宫瘘的诊断通常依靠膀胱镜检查和影像学检查相结合。在膀胱子宫瘘存在情况下，排泄性膀胱尿道造影（VCUG）可显示对比剂从膀胱外渗并充满子宫腔。相反，子宫输卵管造影可显示对比剂从子宫外渗并充满膀胱。使用增强 CT 或 MRI 对尿液横断面进行造影可显示尿瘘的瘘管位置，并且可能同时排除输尿管受累情况。

（三）治疗

膀胱子宫瘘的非手术治疗是有可能的，正如膀胱阴道瘘治疗方案中描述：延长尿管置入时间可能使瘘管较小患者或尿瘘未形成患者成功治愈。另外，除了延长尿管置入时间外，通过连续口服避孕药或使用激素诱导子宫复旧（即闭经）来防止月经通过瘘管也有成功报道[39]。

通常来说，膀胱子宫瘘是可通过手术治疗的。其手术方式是由患者的生育意愿决定的，并且手术方式应与患者充分讨论。若患者需要保留生育功能，则可按照膀胱阴道瘘的治疗方法，初步闭合子宫和膀胱后切除膀胱子宫瘘的瘘管并置入大网膜。若患者已完成生育，则可行子宫切除术和大网膜间置膀胱闭合术以防膀胱阴道瘘发生。现已有膀胱子宫瘘管修复后有成功分娩的报道[40]。

四、放射性膀胱炎与放射性尿瘘

膀胱刺激症状（如尿频、尿急和急迫性尿失禁）是放射性膀胱炎最常见的症状，然而，严重血尿、逼尿肌收缩性下降、膀胱排空不畅、瘘管与阴道连接、膀胱/尿道疼痛等均可是晚期放射性膀胱炎的症状。

（一）病因学

放射性膀胱炎可由局部盆腔照射（如近距离治疗）或外部辐射盆腔邻近组织引起。尽管放疗向靶区器官投放射线的技术已取得巨大进展，但射线对周围器官仍能产生极大影响。大鼠约在放疗开始约4周后出现早期放疗反应，其放疗反应显示膀胱形态（如纤维化和缺血）和膀胱功能（如顺应性和储存能力）发生改变[41]。膀胱相关症状在放疗早期很常见，尿流动力学试验常显示出膀胱早期感觉功能减退、膀胱测压能力下降和膀胱顺应性降低，这些症状有望在6个月内得到改善。晚期放疗反应不常见，但晚期放疗反应发生可能是逐步发展的且难以治疗。文献中报道放疗对尿路有害影响率为1%～12%，其中尿瘘发生率为1%～5%[38]。放射性瘘发生的风险取决于放疗所投放的辐射剂量和潜在肿瘤的类型。

（二）诊断

放射性膀胱炎的诊断可以根据患者临床病史和膀胱镜检查评估膀胱状态。放射性尿瘘的诊断可能会变得更加困难，因为放射性尿瘘起病症状缓慢、发病隐匿或缺乏引起考虑放射性尿瘘的病史。但重要的是需谨记既往远期放疗病史也可是放射性瘘发生的病因。诊断既往有放疗病史的尿瘘患者所需的评估与上述膀胱阴道瘘的评估相同（详见第22章）。对肿瘤复发的评估必须进行组织采样。

（三）治疗

通常采用以症状为导向的药物治疗来治疗尿路刺激症状，如尿频、尿急和急迫性尿失禁。戊聚糖多硫酸钠已被用于修复膀胱中有缺陷的糖胺聚糖层，而且其修复效果已取得了一定的成功；然而，对继发于色素性黄斑病变的视力变化限制了戊聚糖多硫酸钠的应用。单独使用膀胱冲洗或膀胱内联合使用药物（如透明质酸、福尔马林、氨基己酸或前列腺素）收效甚微[42]。用膀胱电灼法进行膀胱镜检查有效阻止大多数膀胱活动性出血。在膀胱严重出血的情况下，可能需要进行选择性行髂内动脉栓塞术。高压氧治疗可极大改善肉眼血尿和膀胱刺激症状，因为高压氧治疗增加了氧传递，从而恢复了组织的正常细胞组成并且促进了正常尿路上皮的再生[43]。超过80%的患者高压氧治疗后出现肉眼血尿症状消失。

放射性尿瘘的治疗通常被比非放射性尿瘘治疗更困难。放射性尿瘘患者术前在癌症史允许的情况下可在阴道局部应用雌激素治疗和高压氧治疗，上述治疗方案可以使机体组织的健康状态和完整性的得到优化。放射性尿瘘的手术修复方式与膀胱阴道瘘相同（见第22章）。放射性尿瘘患者的治疗有一定难度，当务之急是利用组织介入方式，以最大限度地提高手术治疗成功率。若不能对病灶处进行初次手术闭合，则可能需要进行尿路改道。在决定使用回肠还是横结肠进行尿路改道时，考虑放疗辐射场是很重要的。若患者无法耐受手术治疗，则可考虑使用带（或不带）输尿管线圈的双侧肾造瘘管来容纳尿液。

五、尿道憩室

尿道憩室的经典症状可概括为3个“D”，即排尿困难（dysuria）、性交困难（dyspareunia）和漏尿（dribbling）。然而，同一患者同时出现上述所有症状的情况并不多见。患者可能会出现反复的尿路感染，经常是同一病原体持续存在。鉴于尿道憩室让人难以捉摸的性质，通常需要高度怀疑来识别这种病变。

（一）病因学

尿道憩室、阴道囊肿是在尿道和阴道壁之间形成的突起或囊袋。尿道憩室的出现是由于尿道壁组织薄弱引起的，尿道壁组织薄弱可能是由于反复尿路感染、尿道周围腺体堵塞或阴道分娩时对尿道壁创伤所致。曾接受过阴道或尿道手术的女性患者可发展为尿道憩室或阴道囊肿。尿道憩室或阴道囊肿可能不会引起任何症状，但对一些患者来说，尿道憩室或阴道囊肿可能会引起疼痛、反复尿路感染、排尿不适或性交不适。当尿道憩室或阴道囊肿引起患者不适时，可通过阴道手术去除。

（二）诊断

警觉的临床医师可能会注意到尿培养中持续存在相同的致病微生物，医师对其尿路来源敏感性增加考虑。所有复发性尿路感染的女性患者都应进行仔细的盆腔检查，寻找包括尿道憩室在内的潜在病因；尽管只有一小部分病例可被发现。行阴道检查可发现尿道中段充盈或尿道中段波动感，也可在阴道检查时触及阴道前壁时发现有无尿道口排尿。磁共振成像（MRI）、排泄性膀胱尿道造影（VCUG）或膀胱镜检查可帮助诊断。T_2 加权 MRI 矢状位、轴位和冠状位图像通常对于诊断是最有帮助的，因磁共振检查下机体内充满液体的结构显示为亮白色，故尿道解剖结构可以很好地确定，若尿道存在开口则可进行识别。通常需要排泄性膀胱尿道造影（VCUG）上的侧位排尿图像来了解憩室，侧位排尿的图像可能会受到下列相关因素限制，如患者身体习惯、患者目前正留置导尿管、患者在当前位置或在他人面前排尿受限等因素。膀胱镜检查可发现尿道憩室的开口。在检查女性尿道时，操作技术要求是很重要的，可使用女性膀胱镜或软膀胱镜进行检查，或者使用冲洗液体使尿道扩张以便观察。彻底观察尿道的 5 点钟和 7 点钟方位很重要（该位置通常位于尿道皱襞中），因为尿道憩室开口可隐藏在尿道皱襞皱褶的深处。

（三）治疗

对无症状患者的尿道憩室行定期检查是合适的，患者可放心的是尿道憩室中发生癌症的风险非常低。最常见的尿道憩室手术是切除有症状的尿道憩室。尿道憩室切除术手术入路是通过阴道切口进行的，从尿道周围筋膜剥离全层阴道壁瓣。在可行的情况下，从尿道憩室上方水平切开尿道周围筋膜，并仔细地将下尿道憩室剥离。若尿道憩室呈马蹄形或延伸至前尿道，则需进行尿道切口或移位。一旦整个尿道憩室显露在手术野中，就从尿道开口处取出憩室。

很多时候，尿道开口不能被识别，并且经常在尿道没有清晰开口时就进行切除。尿道憩室若被广泛炎症所包围，则使得局部组织平面难以保存，炎症的存在也限制了尿道周围筋膜和尿道平面的保存。如果在剥离组织过程中不慎进入憩室，应进行组织拭子培养和大量冲洗。切除憩室后，应使用可吸收缝合线在 Foley 导管上重建尿道。用蓝色染料冲洗尿道可以证明尿道的水密性闭合。若尿道周围组织可用，则在尿道初步闭合的基础上进行第二层闭合，尿道闭合一般采用不重叠的缝合线。若手术医师对组织完整性有担忧，若术中没有保留筋膜层，或者预计该患者会进行后续的压力性尿失禁手术，则可以使用大阴唇球海绵体脂肪垫（Martius）置入皮瓣。手术步骤中最后行阴道壁切口闭合。整个手术是通过阴道完成的，因此在患者恢复期间可将术后不适感降至最低。

六、术后护理

鉴于尿瘘和尿道憩室患者临床症状和手术入路不同，目前尚无可普遍适用的术后临床路径。然而，有一些原则是术后通常需遵循的。膀胱尿管置入和（或）输尿管支架通常在手术修复后延长使用数天至数周，以帮助组织愈合。目前尿管持续置入的最佳时间尚不清楚，但目前已对更短时间的尿管置入是否有利于组织充分愈合进行了相关研究[44, 45]。在尿管和（或）输尿管支架去除前，许多外科医生会对瘘管和憩室重新进行评估，瘘管和憩室的评估要么使用影像学检查（如排泄性膀胱尿道造影和 CT 膀胱造影）、要么借助染料（如亚甲蓝）进行体格检查。目前，尚未出现公认的方法评估尿瘘和憩室的方法。在药物治疗方面，除术后使用镇痛药外，还可使用其他多种药物。抗胆碱能药物和（或）β_3 受体激动药可能有助于预防 Foley 导管引起的膀胱痉挛和刺激症状。

阴道雌激素治疗可能有助于改善和维持阴道组织功能、促进组织愈合。在移除 Foley 导尿管后，可以使用抗生素或尿道口清洁消毒剂（如乌洛托品）来帮助预防菌尿发生，但不推荐术后持续性药物治疗。

（一）复发 / 再治疗

术后瘘管造影可显示瘘口持续渗漏的情况。在许多情况下，延长尿管置入引流时间至术后 3 周可使瘘管有足够的时间愈合。在患者愈合期间，尽一切努力最大限度地激发患者机体愈合潜能，如鼓励患者术后健康饮食、定期走动、预防感染、阴道适当适应雌激素和（或）持续性使用抗胆碱能药物和（或）β_3 受体激动药治疗等。若延长尿管置入引流后患者瘘管仍然存在，可考虑行二次修复。二次修复通常会采取不同的修复路径，若患者初次经阴道修复，则二次修复需用经腹部进行，若患者初次修复经腹部，则二次修复需经阴道进行。对于尿瘘手术量较少、经验不足的外科医生，可参考优秀治疗中心进行重复模仿手术。同样，若在尿道憩室切除术后进行成像，可能会看到少量残留憩室或尿液渗液情况。延长尿管置入引流至术后一周可使上述病情好转。在初次手术成功进行的情况下，极少进行后续附加手术。有报道称：若尿道憩室复发，则可能需要后续手术治疗。

（二）持续尿瘘的症状管理

瘘管修复手术或尿道憩室手术的患者术后出现尿频、尿急、夜尿或急性尿失禁等刺激性膀胱症状并不少见。上述膀胱刺激症状出现时间远超出留置导尿的时间，并且这些症状的出现可使患者感觉其手术失败或手术复杂有难度。一旦患者完成术后评估，让患者放心其瘘管或憩室已消失是至关重要的。药物治疗、患者行为矫正和盆底肌肉锻炼可以大大改善膀胱相关症状和尿失禁症状。随着时间推移，许多患者可停止药物治疗。其中一小部分患者可持续存在难治性膀胱过动症的相关症状，该患者可能需要额外的膀胱过动症三线治疗方案来有效解决其相关症状。

总结

尿瘘、放射性膀胱炎和尿道憩室等均是尿失禁的病因，这些病因均可临床治疗。及时诊断和治疗可极大改善患者漏尿情况和患者生活质量。详细的病史采集、全面的盆腔体格检查是具有诊断意义的，并且能够促进临床医生对尿失禁的诊断研究。一旦发现上述导致尿失禁的病因，这些可逆性尿失禁均可通过手术治愈，从而减轻患者尿失禁症状、提高患者生活质量。

参考文献

[1] De Ridder DAP, De Vries C, Elneil S, Emasu A, Esegbono G, Gueye S, Mohammad R, Muleta M, Hilton P, Mourad S, Pickard R, Stanford E, Fistula RE. International Consultation on I. In: Abrams P, Cardozo L, Khoury S, Wein AJ, International Continence S, editors. Incontinence: 5th International Consultation on Incontinence, Paris, February 2012. Paris: ICUD-EAU; 2013. p. 1527–80.

[2] Aarts JWM, Nieboer TE, Johnson N, Tavender E, Garry R, Mol BWJ, et al. Surgical approach to hysterectomy for benign gynaecological disease. Cochrane Database Syst Rev. 2015; https:// doi.org/10.1002/14651858. CD003677.pub5.

[3] Netsch C, Bach T, Gross E, Gross AJ. Rectourethral fistula after high-intensity focused ultrasound therapy for prostate cancer and its surgical management. Urology. 2011;77(4):999–1004. https://doi.org/10.1016/ j.urology.2010.10.028.

[4] Wall L, Karshima JA, Kirschner C, Arrowsmith SD. The obstetric vesicovaginal fistula: characteristics of 899 patients from Jos, Nigeria. Am J Obstet Gynecol. 2004;190(4):1011–6. https://doi.org/10.1016/ j.ajog.2004.02.007.

[5] Hillary CJ, Osman NI, Hilton P, Chapple CR. The aetiology, treatment, and outcome of urogenital fistulae managed in well- and low-resourced countries: a systematic review. Eur Urol. 2016;70(3):478–92. https://doi. org/10.1016/j.eururo.2016.02.015.

[6] Vangeenderhuysen C, Prual A, et al. Obstetric fistulae: incidence estimates for sub-Saharan Africa. Int J Gynecol Obstet. 2001;73(1):65–6. https://doi.org/10.1016/ S0020–7292(00)00374–X.

[7] Arrowsmith S, Hamlin EC, Wall LL. Obstructed labor injury complex: obstetric fistula formation and the multifaceted morbidity of maternal birth trauma in the developing world. Obstet Gynecol Surv. 1996;51(9):568–74. https://doi.org/10.1097/00006254–199609000–00024.

[8] Chen CW, Mark D, Karram MM. Lower urinary tract fistulas. Urogynecology and reconstructive pelvic surgery. 4th ed. Elselvier Health Sciences; 2015. p. 602–21.

[9] Moss RL. Management of enterovesical fistulas. Am J Surg.

1990;159(5):514–7. https://doi. org/10.1016/s0002–9610(05)81259–0.

[10] Teeluckdharry B, Gilmour D, Flowerdew G. Urinary tract injury at benign gynecologic surgery and the role of cystoscopy: a systematic review and meta-analysis. Obstet Gynecol. 2015;126(6):1161–9. https://doi.org/10.1097/AOG.0000000000001096.

[11] Forsgren C, Lundholm C, Johansson ALV, Cnattingius S, Altman D. Hysterectomy for benign indications and risk of pelvic organ fistula disease. Obstet Gynecol. 2009;114(3):594–9. https://doi.org/10.1097/AOG.0b013e3181b2a1df.

[12] Duong TH, Gellasch TL, Adam RA. Risk factors for the development of vesicovaginal fistula after incidental cystotomy at the time of a benign hysterectomy. Am J Obstet Gynecol. 2009;201(5):512, e1–e4. https://doi.org/10.1016/j.ajog.2009.06.046.

[13] Duong TH, Taylor DP, Meeks GR. A multicenter study of vesicovaginal fistula following incidental cystotomy during benign hysterectomies. Int Urogynecol J. 2011;22(8):975–9. https:// doi.org/10.1007/s00192–011– 1375– 6.

[14] Goodwin WE, Scardino PT. Vesicovaginal and ureterovaginal fistulas: a summary of 25 years of experience. J Urol. 1980;123(3):370–4. https://doi.org/10.1016/S0022–5347(17)55941–8.

[15] Ehlert M, Haraway AM, Atiemo HO. Lesson 7: contemporary evaluation and management of vesicovaginal fistula. AUA Update Series. 2013;32:66–75.

[16] Lee D, Zimmern P. Vaginal Approach to Vesicovaginal Fistula. Urol Clin North Am. 2019;46(1):123–33. https://doi.org/10.1016/j.ucl.2018.08.010.

[17] McKay E, Watts K, Abraham N. Abdominal approach to vesicovaginal fistula. Urol Clin North Am. 2019;46(1):135–46. https://doi.org/10.1016/j.ucl.2018.08.011.

[18] Bai SW, Huh EH, Jung DJ, Park JH, Rha KH, Kim SK, et al. Urinary tract injuries during pelvic surgery: incidence rates and predisposing factors. Int Urogynecol J. 2006;17(4):360–4. https://doi.org/10.1007/s00192–005– 0015– 4.

[19] Sims J. On the treatment of vesico-vaginal fistula. Am J Med Sci. 1852;45:59–82. https://doi. org/10.1007/BF01901610.

[20] Eilber KS, Kavaler E, Rodrìguez LV, Rosenblum N, Raz S. Ten-year experience with transvaginal vesicovaginal fistula repair using tissue interposition. J Urol. 2003;169(3):1033–6. https://doi.org/10.1097/01.ju.0000049723.57485.e7.

[21] Latzko W. Postoperative vesicovaginal fistulas. Am J Surg. 1942;58(2):211–28. https://doi. org/10.1016/S0002–9610(42)90009–6.

[22] Raz S, Bregg KJ, Nitti VW, Sussman E. Transvaginal repair of vesicovaginal fistula using a peritoneal flap. J Urol. 1993;150(1):56–9. https://doi.org/10.1016/S0022–5347(17)35396–X.

[23] Luo D-Y, Shen H. Transvaginal repair of apical vesicovaginal fistula: a modified latzko techniqueóoutcomes at a high-volume referral center. Eur Urol. 2019;76(1):84–8. https://doi. org/10.1016/j.eururo.2019.04.010.

[24] Margules AC, Rovner ES. The use of tissue flaps in the management of urinary tract fistulas. Curr Urol Rep. 2019;20(6):32. https://doi.org/10.1007/s11934–019– 0892– 6.

[25] Shaw J, Tunitsky-Bitton E, Barber MD, Jelovsek JE. Ureterovaginal fistula: a case series. Int Urogynecol J. 2014;25(5):615–21. https://doi.org/10.1007/s00192–013– 2272– y.

[26] Vakili B, Chesson RR, Kyle BL, Shobeiri SA, Echols KT, Gist R, et al. The incidence of urinary tract injury during hysterectomy: a prospective analysis based on universal cystoscopy. Am J Obstet Gynecol. 2005;192(5):1599–604. https://doi.org/10.1016/j.ajog.2004.11.016.

[27] Seth J, Kiosoglous A, Pakzad M, Hamid R, Shah J, Ockrim J, et al. Incidence, type and management of ureteric injury associated with vesicovaginal fistulas: report of a series from a specialized center. Int J Urol. 2019;26(7):717–23. https://doi.org/10.1111/iju.13965.

[28] Chen YB, Wolff BJ, Kenton KS, Mueller ER. Approach to ureterovaginal fistula: examining 13 years of experience. Female Pelvic Med Reconstr Surg. 2019;25(2):e7–e11. https://doi. org/10.1097/SPV.0000000000000690.

[29] Badlani GDR, Mettu JR, Rovner ES, Wein AJ, Kavoussi LR, Partin AW. Urinary tract fistulae. Campbell-Walsh urology. 11th ed. Elsevier Saunders; 2016. p. 2103–39.

[30] Thompson IM, Marx AC. Conservative the of rectourethralfistula: five-year follow-up. Urology. 1990;35(6):533–6. https://doi.org/10.1016/0090–4295(90)80111–Y.

[31] Reisenauer C, Wallwiener D, Stenzl A, Solomayer F-E, Sievert K-D. Urethrovaginal fistulaóa rare complication after the placement of a suburethral sling (IVS). Int Urogynecol J. 2007;18(3):343–6. https://doi.org/10.1007/s00192–006– 0139– 1.

[32] Blaivas JG, Mekel G. Management of urinary fistulas due to midurethral sling surgery. J Urol. 2014;192(4):1137–42. https://doi.org/10.1016/j.juro.2014.04.009.

[33] Lee RA, Symmonds RE, Williams TJ. Current status of genitourinary fistula. Obstet Gynecol. 1988;72(3 Pt 1):313–9.

[34] Kobashi K, Albo M, et al. Surgical treatment of female stress urinary incontinence: AUA/ SUFU guideline. J Urol. 2017;198:875.

[35] Webster GD, Sihelnik SA, Stone AR. Urethrovaginal fistula: a review of the surgical management. J Urol. 1984;132(3):460–2. https://doi.org/10.1016/s0022–5347(17)49691–1.

[36] Porcaro AB, Zicari M, Antoniolli SZ, Pianon R, Monaco C, Migliorini F, et al. Vesicouterine fistulas following cesarean section: report on a case, review and update of the literature. Int Urol Nephrol. 2002;34(3):335–44. https://doi.org/10.1023/A:1024443822378.

[37] Rajamaheswari N, Chhikara AB. Vesicouterine fistulae: our experience of 17 cases and literature review. Int Urogynecol J. 2013;24(2):275–9. https://doi.org/10.1007/s00192–012– 1798– 8.

[38] De Ridder DJMK. Urinary tract fistula. In: Partin AW, Kavoussi LR, Dmochowski RR, AJW W, editors. Campbell-Walsh-Wein urology. 12th ed; 2021.

[39] Jozwik M. Spontaneous closure of vesicouterine fistula. Account for effective hormonal treatment. Urol Int. 1999;62(3):183–7. https://doi.org/10.1159/000030388.

[40] Lotocki WJ, Jozwick M. Prognosis of fertility after surgical closure of vesicouterine fistula. Eur J Obstet Gynecol Reprod Biol. 1996;64(1):87–90. https://doi. org/10.1016/0301–2115(95)02251–1.

[41] Vale JA, Bowsher WG, Liu K, Tomlinson A, Whitfield HN, Trott KR. Post-irradiation bladder dysfunction: development of a rat model. Urol Res. 1993;21(6):383–8. https://doi.org/10.1007/ BF00300073.

[42] Smit SG, Heyns CF. Management of radiation cystitis. Nat Rev Urol. 2010;7(4):206–14. https://doi.org/10.1038/nrurol.2010.23.

[43] Degener S, Pohle A, Strelow H, Mathers MJ, Zumbé JR, Roth S, et al. Long-term experience of hyperbaric oxygen therapy for refractory radio- or chemotherapy-induced haemorrhagic cystitis. BMC Urol. 2015;15:38. https://doi.org/10.1186/s12894–015– 0035– 4.

[44] Barone MA, Widmer M, Arrowsmith S, Ruminjo J, Seuc A, Landry E, et al. Breakdown of simple female genital fistula repair after 7 day versus 14 day postoperative bladder catheterisation: a randomised, controlled, open-label, non-inferiority trial. Lancet. 2015;386(9988):56–62. https://doi.org/10.1016/S0140–6736(14)62337–0.

[45] Nardos R, Menber B, Browning A. Outcome of obstetric fistula repair after 10–day versus 14–day Foley catheterization. Int J Gynecol Obstet. 2012;118(1):21–3. https://doi. org/10.1016/j.ijgo.2012.01.024.

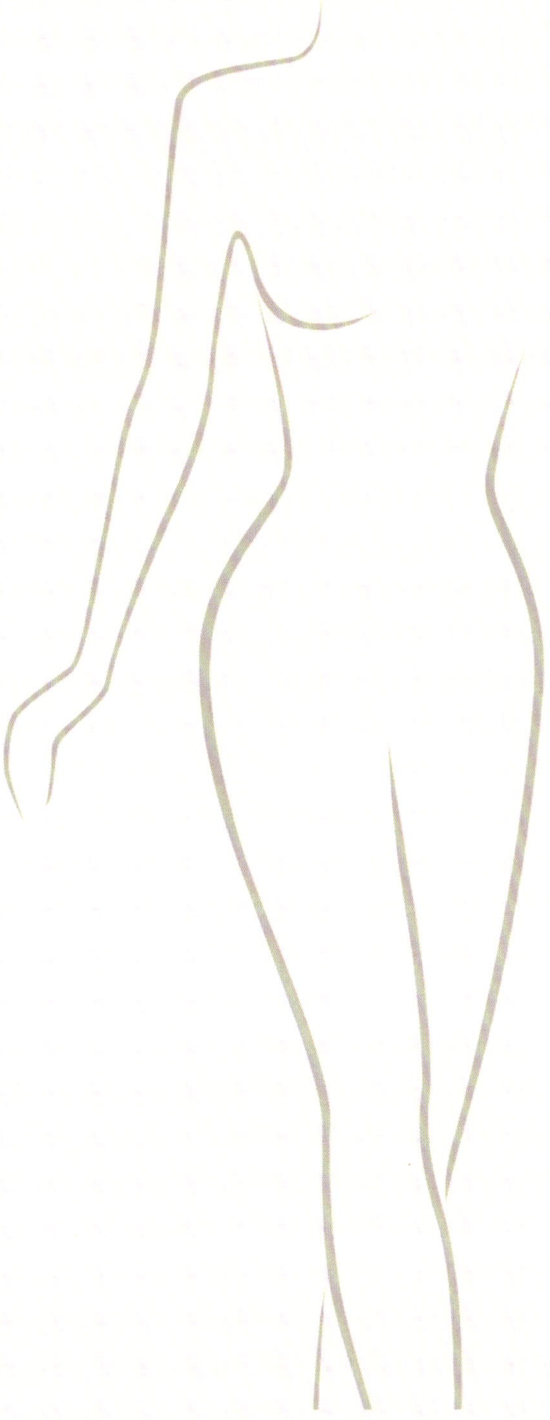

第六篇
特殊人群的尿失禁

Incontinence in Special Populations

第 23 章　大龄女孩和青少年尿失禁

Incontinence in Older Girls and Adolescents

Esther K. Liu　Kristina D. Suson　著

女性尿失禁被广泛认为是一种疾病过程，主要影响多胎或绝经期或绝经后的成年女性。大龄女孩或青春期女性的尿失禁（UI）是一个未被充分认识的群体。尿失禁会对生活质量产生负面影响：更换内衣、担心气味、避免液体摄入、避免性活动、避免体育活动，或者在性格形成期（成长期）与社会隔离[1-3]。同样重要的是要注意，它可能预示着成年期持续存在下尿路症状（LUTS）[4]。本章讨论本组压力性尿失禁（SUI）和急迫性尿失禁（UUI）的流行病学，以及先天性原因、评估和治疗。

一、背景和流行病学

（一）年龄较大的女孩和青少年中尿失禁的患病率

有限的研究集中在青少年女性尿失禁上。可以与年长女性进行比较的一个因素是胎次。排除生育的混杂因素将年轻人群的尿失禁与更常见的成年女性尿失禁区分开来，后者通常与生育创伤、更年期和合并症有关。因此，我们还可以将“年轻、健康、未生育”的女性群体（通常包括 30 岁以下的群体）的一些经验外推至青春期后的女孩。

据报道，青春期女性压力性尿失禁的患病率为 6.2%～79%[1, 5-10]。大多数研究发现压力性尿失禁比急迫性尿失禁更常见，这与成年女性不同，研究引用的急迫性尿失禁发生率为 3.4%～41.6%[1, 5, 7, 8]。Almousa 等对 18 项年轻未生育女性的研究进行了系统回顾，引用的压力性尿失禁率从 12.5% 到 79%（中位数 49.4%），急迫性尿失禁率从 15.6% 到 41.6%（中位数 31.3%）[10]。

一项包括 15 055 例来自中国的参与者的大型社区研究发现，14—21 岁人群中尿失禁的患病率为 6.6%。尿失禁在女性中更常见（7.2% vs. 6.0%），且随着年龄的增长更常见，在 19—20 岁的人群中最高达 12.3%。身体和心理健康疾病以及慢性便秘也会增加患病风险。性活动增加也是一个危险因素。然而在本研究中，急迫性尿失禁的发生率高于压力性尿失禁[11]。荷兰一项包括 8—17 岁患者的研究表明，女性也会增加尿失禁的风险。30% 的女孩报告有日间或晚上的尿失禁，只有 14.2% 的男孩注意到尿失禁（P=0.003）。他们在比较 8—12 岁和 13—17 岁的孩子时没有发现任何差异（21.5% vs. 21.8%，P=0.962）[12]。

美国一项针对 216 例 14—21 岁的青少年妇科患者的研究发现，31.5% 的患者有尿失禁。本研究还发现急迫性尿失禁发生率较高（15.7%），其次是混合性尿失禁（8.8%）和压力性尿失禁（6.9%），而夜间遗尿症（NE）发生率为 4.2%。重要的是，这些患者大多有其他主诉，通常是寻求避孕或担心月经异常。尽管报道尿失禁的人数很多，但只有 8% 的人在 1 个月内发作 1 次或更多，少于 1% 的人报道每日 / 每晚发作。一般来说，他们的尿失禁不会对他们的生活产生负面影响；4.6% 的患者将其报道为“非常小问题”，0.9% 为小问题，0.5% 为中度问题，没有患者将其视为大问题[13]。

在妊娠的青少年中，下尿路症状的发病率很高，近 80% 的人抱怨至少有 1 种症状。在 206 例妊娠少女中，27.2% 的人出现了失禁。研究中超过 50% 的患者处于妊娠晚期。更严重的症状与每天喝咖啡、吸烟、慢性咳嗽 / 便秘和尿路感染（UTI）[14] 相关。与成年女性一样，青春期女性可能会在分娩后失禁。会阴切开术会增加风险，生下一个大于胎龄且产前检查频率较低的婴儿也会增加风险 [15]。

泌尿科医生早就认识到大脑和膀胱之间的联系。行为和精神障碍与 18 岁以下儿童的尿失禁有关，尽管这些障碍在女性中发生的频率低于男性 [16]。一项包括青春期男孩和女孩的研究发现，原发性夜间遗尿症患者中社交焦虑的发生率更高。此外，社交焦虑可能延误遗尿症的治疗 [17]。在 10 岁时表现出内化（抑郁、焦虑、社交退缩和躯体不适）和外化（攻击性）行为和注意力不集中的儿童更有可能在青少年时期患有夜间遗尿症 [18]。虽然患有任何下尿路症状的儿童和青少年更可能出现情绪和行为问题，但更明显的是他们伴有肠功能障碍 [19]。很难确定女性患者的具体心理发现，因为研究通常包括两种性别 [17-19]。发育和身体发育迟缓以及睡眠障碍也与夜间遗尿症相关 [20]。

（二）青春期女性压力性尿失禁

压力性尿失禁在青春期女性中较急迫性尿失禁 [10] 更为常见。在这一年轻人群中，与压力性尿失禁相关的风险因素包括肥胖、剧烈活动或高强度训练，以及肺疾病 [如囊性纤维化（CF）][8]。经产妇压力性尿失禁背后的病理生理学归因于从分娩到盆底的创伤。很少有研究探讨未生育或青春期女性的病理生理。基于先前的研究显示盆腔器官脱垂女性胶原蛋白含量存在差异，Keane 等推测未产压力性尿失禁女性胶原蛋白含量存在类似差异，认为这是先天危险因素所致。在将经尿流动力学证实为压力性尿失禁的未产女性与大陆年轻女性对照组进行比较时，他们发现尿道周围活检的胶原蛋白含量显著降低，Ⅰ型和Ⅲ型胶原蛋白比例降低。Ⅰ型胶原蛋白更坚硬，常见于骨骼、肌腱和牙本质，而Ⅲ型胶原蛋白常见于弹性更强的组织，如血管系统和肠道。这些作者认为，由于固有的胶原蛋白薄弱，盆底训练，往往是一线治疗，可能是徒劳的，手术干预可能更有益的 [21]。

1. 肥胖症

体重指数（BMI）升高与腹内压升高呈正相关，随着时间的推移，腹压对骨盆底肌肉和神经支配施加压力。Subak 等证实，在成年女性中，体重指数每增加 5 个单位，尿失禁的风险就会增加 20%～70%。在 15—19 岁的女孩中，通过问卷接受压力性尿失禁的女孩体重明显高于大陆青少年（61kg vs. 56kg，P=0.0188）[8]。

在一组 40 例 12—17 岁的肥胖女孩（定义为＞95%BMI）中，12.5% 报告的尿失禁频率为每周 1 次，而 20 例非肥胖女孩中没有。肥胖组中还有 18 例女孩报道称，她们每月发生尿失禁的次数少于 1 次。在尿失禁严重程度评分中发现差异，泄漏频率乘以泄漏体积。肥胖组的平均得分为 1.3 分，而非肥胖组为 0.3 分（P=0.009）[23]。最后，意大利的一项研究包括了来自 10 所大学的 1936 例平均年龄为 21 岁的女性，报道称体重指数＞30kg/m^2 与尿失禁（AOR 3.0，95%CI 1.4～6.2）[1] 的风险增加相关。仍有一些争论，因为在澳大利亚的失禁诊所就诊的 862 例 5—18 岁的男孩和女孩中发现体重与尿失禁之间没有关联 [24]。

2. 高强度训练

关于女性运动员的压力性尿失禁已经有了很好的记录。腹腔内压力的增加导致膀胱颈和尿道的过度活动，这可能导致尿失禁，而不是尿道内括约肌缺乏。Carls 证实，在 86 例平均年龄为 17 岁（14—21 岁）、每周训练 3～25h 或参加多种运动的女性运动员中，28% 报告在体育活动中发生压力性尿失禁。在报道压力性尿失禁的 28% 患者中，26% 报道了相关的急迫性症状。这些运动员的压力性尿失禁也发生在赛场外，11.6% 发生在上厕所时，11.6% 发生在咳嗽时，6.9% 发生在打喷嚏时。在那些尿失禁患者中，92% 的人在问卷调查之前从未告诉过任何人他们的症状，研究中不幸的发现凸显了耻辱感 [2]。

Eliasson 等研究了一个非常特殊的群体：精英蹦床运动员的尿失禁[25, 26]。在一项研究中，35 例女性蹦床运动员完成了尿失禁问卷调查；80% 的患者承认在开始训练后平均 2.5 年开始出现不自主的尿漏。所有超过 15 岁的患者都有尿漏。值得注意的是，没有女性承认蹦床练习之外的泄漏[25]。在第二项研究中，前蹦床运动员比非蹦床运动员更有可能报道失禁。此外，训练的频率和持续时间，以及月经初潮后的训练年限，均与尿失禁[26]有关。

尽管蹦床运动员在他们的运动之外并没有注意到尿失禁，但一组女性高中运动员（其中超过 34% 的人在运动过程中出现尿失禁）也抱怨在大笑或其他日常活动时漏水。女孩参加比赛的赛季数越多，发生尿失禁的可能性就越大。尽管大多数失禁女孩报道的尿量较小，但 21% 的女孩有中度的尿漏，尿液会在外套上留下斑点，7% 的女孩会打湿短裤或裤子[27]。压力性尿失禁对女运动员的生活质量有负面影响。那些报道尿失禁的患者在生活质量总分、回避和限制性行为得分、社会心理影响得分和社交尴尬得分[28]上有统计学意义上的显著降低。

3. 饮食失调

神经性厌食症被认为是尿失禁的危险因素。348 例患者中 96.3% 为女性，平均年龄为 15.2 ± 1.8 岁，其中 1.8% 有夜间遗尿症，1.8% 有日间尿失禁，因此得出结论，他们没有增加风险[29]。然而，一项对平均年龄为 21 ± 5.3 岁的优秀女运动员的研究发现，根据饮食紊乱检查问卷（Eating Disorders Examination Questionnaire）筛选的那些饮食紊乱的人发生尿失禁的可能性是没有饮食紊乱的人的 3 倍[30]。

4. 肺部疾病（肺病）

慢性肺部疾病导致尿失禁，可能继发于咳嗽引起的腹部压力和盆底压力的反复增加。White 等首次在成人囊性纤维化患者中描述了这两者之间的联系。他们报道称，患有囊性纤维化成年女性的尿失禁发生率为 38%[31]。鉴于囊性纤维化是一个终生的疾病过程，Blackwell 等研究了儿童囊性纤维化患者尿失禁的患病率。在南安普敦的小儿囊性纤维化服务中心，共有 72 例 5—18 岁的受试者回答了一份关于非自愿尿液流失严重程度和频率的问卷。26 例女孩中有 8 例（31%）接受压力性尿失禁治疗。压力性尿失禁的严重程度随着囊性纤维化的恶化而增加，通过用力呼气量测量[32]。Nixon 等调查了青少年女性囊性纤维化患者，发现患者发生尿失禁的中位年龄为 13 岁。尿失禁最常见的诱因是咳嗽和大笑。在回应的 55 例患者中，47% 报道曾有过尿失禁发作，22% 报道每月至少发生 2 次。值得关注的是，42% 的患者认为它干扰了他们的囊性纤维化物理治疗，只有 2 例尿失禁患者曾向他们的医生提到过[33]。

（三）女性青少年尿急性尿失禁

一项针对 18—30 岁“假定健康”的年轻女医科学生的研究显示，下尿路症状包括夜尿症、日间频率、犹豫、紧张和间歇性，在这个年龄段比之前假设的更普遍。在 159 例女性中，94.3% 承认存在下尿路症状，20% 承认尿失禁。尽管该组的烦扰总分较低，但最高的烦扰得分与紧急程度有关。这些受试者之前都没有寻求过医疗建议，这说明年轻女性尿失禁比临床[7]更普遍。有人建议，膀胱过度活动症（OAB）在成年女性可能与儿童和青少年膀胱症状有关。与其把膀胱过度活动症和急迫性尿失禁仅仅发生在成年期，还不如把它们看作一个连续统一体，它可能起源于童年时期的[34]。

（四）儿童与成人尿失禁的关系

成年女性的急迫性尿失禁可能不是一个新问题，而是一个新被承认的问题。童年时期未解决或未解决的尿路问题可能会持续到青春期和成年期。2006 年，2109 例平均年龄为 56 岁的女性参与者被要求回忆她们从一年级到高中期间的泌尿系统症状。儿童日间尿失禁和夜间遗尿症与成人急迫性尿失禁的 2 倍增加相关（OR=2.6，95%CI 1.1～5.9 和 OR=2.7，95%CI 1.3～5.5）[35]。在夜间遗尿症诊所接受治疗的平均年龄<20 岁的男女青少年和成年人完成了一份关于他们童年排尿习惯和当前排尿症状的问卷。报道儿童期急症、尿频率、急迫性尿失禁、不频繁排尿或排空不完全感的患者与目前成年期急症、急迫性尿失禁和压力性尿失禁的患者之间存在显著相关性[36]。

意大利的一个小组通过邮寄调查问卷的方式，将国际尿失禁调查问卷邮寄给了患有尿失禁和尿失禁的成年女性。问卷由 47 例前患者和 111 例健康对照者提交。在 47 例患者中，28 例患者在 5—20 岁接受了尿失禁治疗（中位年龄 11 岁），而 19 例患者在 5—15 岁接受了夜间遗尿症治疗（中位年龄 10 岁）。患者组中的女性目前更有可能出现尿失禁（34% vs. 7%）[4]。

我们必须记住，当儿童进入青春期时，夜间遗尿症会以每年 14% 的速度自发消退[37]。16 岁以后的患病率保持在 2.3%，这表明如果夜间遗尿症仍然存在，自发消退的可能性很低[38]。在一项针对 107 例患有夜间遗尿症的意大利男性和女性青少年的研究中，74% 的人患有原发性夜间遗尿症，而其余 26% 的人承认有超过 6 个月的夜间干燥[39]。

（五）笑性尿失禁

被称为“笑尿”或“遗尿”，是一种罕见的情况，在笑的过程中或笑后立即发生尿漏或排空。笑尿失禁的一个关键区别是，在没有笑的情况下，膀胱功能是正常的[40]。对于咯咯笑失禁背后的病因有一点共识。Logan 等回顾了 1959 年首次描述的笑性尿失禁的历史讨论，强调了关于病理生理学的不同观点：它是神经学还是泌尿学现象[41]？虽然有些人强调笑性尿失禁的核心因素，但它可能是神经因素、腹部收缩、逼尿肌和盆底功能的组合，甚至可能带有家族因素。笑尿失禁似乎与猝倒有相似的病理生理学，笑后肌肉张力的丧失，或在强烈的感觉后，如惊讶或恐惧，并与嗜睡症相关[42]。嗜睡症和猝倒症可以用刺激性药物治疗；类似地，哌甲酯已被证明对治疗笑性尿失禁有效[42, 43]。

二、尿失禁的先天性原因

与重大出生缺陷相关的尿失禁，其大多数先天性原因，如膀胱外翻或脊髓脊膜膨出，将在出生时或出生后不久被发现。然而，还有其他更微妙的解剖原因（表 23-1）。女性异位输尿管可插入尿道括约肌外，持续尿失禁者应考虑异位输尿管。评估从肾超声开始，但通常需要磁共振尿路造影来确认诊断（图 23-1）。不是所有的患者都表现出相同的症状；因此，重点是要保持高度的怀疑。Viers 等报道了 1 例 12 岁女性，在多次治疗失败后出现终身夜间遗尿症和新发尿失禁，计算机断层扫描显示上极部分与外括约肌附近的异位输尿管插入相关，作者推测夜间遗尿症和新发尿失禁发生在括约肌张力下降时[44]。

完全性女性尿道上裂（CFE）是另一种先天性失禁原因。在外翻谱系中，完全性女性尿道上裂极为罕见，发生率约为 1/50 万。从表面上看，与女性患者的膀胱外翻相比，其临床意义似乎较小，因为腹壁和膀胱是闭合的。然而，继发于膀胱颈开放，失禁的结果是相似的[45]。完全性女性尿道上裂的体检结果可能是微妙的。虽然通常是在儿童早期发现的，但也有报道称，直到青春期才发现，然后出现持续性尿失禁[46, 47]。

青少年女性失禁的其他先天性原因包括脊柱裂。有时，甚至成人也可能出现原发性脊髓拴系综合征。超过 90% 的成人患者会主诉泌尿系统症状，其中 18.6% 没有神经系统症状。夜间遗尿症可能是唯一的抱怨[48]。一项对前往儿科和青少年妇科诊所就诊的女孩和青少年的回顾性研究确定了 32 例临床怀疑患有脊髓拴系综合征的患者。最终诊断为脊髓拴系的 18 例患者的平均年龄为 11 ± 4.6 岁。18 例患者中有 10 例出现尿失禁。重要的是，18 例患者中有 17 例接受了“松绑”。术后随访的 14 例患者中，13 例在 6 周时症状得到缓解[49]。

表 23-1 尿失禁的先天性原因

先天性病因	发病过程	评估标准	临床治疗
异位输尿管	持续尿失禁，如果反流进入下极系统，可能有发热性尿路感染史	肾脏超声、磁共振尿路造影，可能还有排尿膀胱尿道造影和膀胱镜检查	上极至下极输尿管输尿管吻合术，上极肾切除术，输尿管膀胱吻合术
完全性女性尿道上裂	连续尿失禁	肾脏超声、骨盆 X 线片、膀胱镜 / 膀胱容量测量和膀胱造影术、尿流动力学	上尿道的修复，很可能需要膀胱颈重建，也可能需要输尿管膀胱造瘘
脊髓拴系	下尿路症状包括尿路感染、日间尿失禁、夜间遗尿症、尿急、尿频。其他症状可能包括背痛、便秘和增重异常	肾超声、腰椎 MRI、尿流动力学	转诊到神经外科。根据尿流动力学的结果，可能需要抗胆碱能药物、间歇性清洁自我导尿，或者其他膀胱治疗

MRI. 磁共振成像

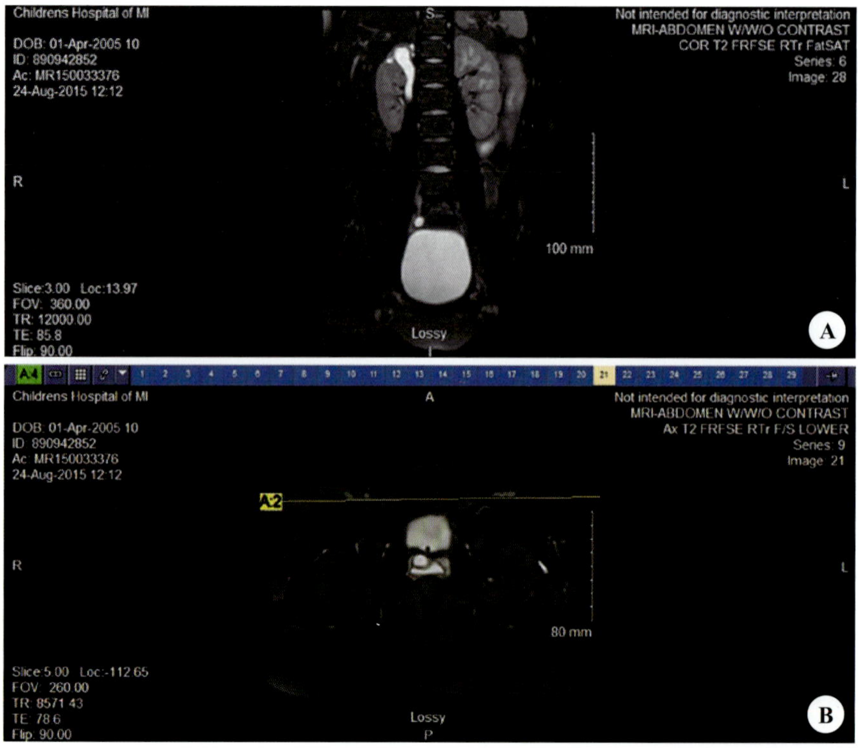

◀ **图 23-1 1 例 14 岁患儿自出生后出现持续尿失禁**

肾脏超声显示右侧重复收集系统，上极轻度扩张，因此获得磁共振成像。冠状位 T_2 加权 MRI（A）显示扩张的右上极收集系统和远端输尿管插入阴道，轴位成像（B）也显示。患者尿失禁在输尿管输尿管吻合术后得到解决

三、青少年尿失禁的评估

（一）发病过程

对失禁青少年的咨询不同于年幼的儿童或成人（表 23-2）。青少年正处于获得独立的过渡期。快速成长和身体变化往往伴随着不安全感。这就要求医生能够以一种不加评判的方式直接与青少年进行互动。虽然性史一般是受保护的，但应该对青少年设定保密限制[50]。

仔细的病史是评估尿失禁的基础。评估患者是否曾经干燥过，或者这是否是一个终生的问题。尿失禁与什么特定的活动有关吗？它发生的频率是多少，体积是多少？渗漏发生在日间还是晚上？患者排便的习惯是什么？彻底的排便习惯史也至关重要。重要的是要注意是否有儿科泌尿系统干

表 23-2 大龄女孩和青春期女性尿失禁的评估

病史

- 渗漏发生在日间、晚上，还是两者都发生？
- 泄漏的体积是多少？
- 你曾经完全干燥过吗？
- 你有尿路感染史吗？
- 是否在活动、咳嗽、大笑或紧急情况下发生渗漏？
- 你有尿后滴沥症状吗？
- 你一天排尿几次？
- 你有呼吸道问题或打鼾的病史吗？
- 是否有夜间遗尿症或肠膀胱功能障碍的家族史？
- 检查症状时，患者是否有便秘、步态异常、背部 / 颈部疼痛或肥胖？

查体

- 患者希望他们的父母在场吗（如果没有的话，找一个陪护。即使家长在场，也可以考虑带一个监护人）？
- 腹部：腹部膨胀吗？凳子上明显吗？
- 泌尿生殖系统：肋椎角有压痛吗？膀胱是否可触及 / 或触痛？生殖器附近有皮肤变化吗？阴道内有尿液淤积吗？是否可见异位输尿管口？阴蒂是否分叉？尿道出现扩张吗？
- 神经学：步态正常吗？有肛交吗？
- 背部：骶骨部位是否有异常，如毛斑或酒窝？

评定标准

- 残余尿量
- 尿液分析
- 讨论
- 若持续症状或空洞后残留升高，可采用肌电图进行尿流
- 如果反复感染或连续失禁超声检查
- 反复发热感染或超音波异常的排尿膀胱尿道造影
- 如涉及输尿管异位，行尿路磁共振造影
- 与脊髓拴系综合征有关的腰椎磁共振成像
- 尿流动力学（如持续症状，与神经系统表现有关，或与超声、排尿膀胱尿道造影或脊柱 MRI 表现有关）

预的历史。在这一年龄组应调查性史和性传播感染的潜在危险因素。此外，重要的是要对性虐待的可能性保持敏感，因为可能存在关联[51]。还要询问患者是否妊娠。

更客观的数据可以帮助进行咨询。包括体积和频率的膀胱日记可以识别尿失禁触发因素并可能证明具有治疗作用。国际尿失禁问题咨询小儿下尿路症状（ICIQ-CLUTS）是一项经过验证的调查问卷，用于筛查其他相关的下尿路症状。这份 12 项问卷在 5—18 岁时表现出敏感性和特异性[52]。对于患有尿失禁的 11—17 岁的尿失禁患者，密歇根大学的作者开发并执行了尿失禁症状指数 – 儿科（ISI-P）的初步验证。这份由患者报告的 11 项问卷将尿失禁严重程度和其他评分客观化[53]。

对症状的全面检查也可以为诊断提供线索。在到儿科和青少年妇科就诊的女孩和青少年中，除了压力性尿失禁外，患者还表现为便秘和背部疼痛[49]。特别是在夜间遗尿症患者中，确定他们是否打鼾或有其他睡眠障碍是很重要的。考虑使用行为问卷，因为这些可以识别隐匿性行为或精神疾病[16, 54]。同样，有原发性夜间遗尿症的患者也可以从社交焦虑[17]筛查中获益。

（二）体格检查

应询问患者是否希望父母 / 监护人在体检期间待在房间里[50]。腹部检查可显示大便负荷大，脏器肿大或膀胱膨胀。仔细检查生殖器，寻找异位输尿管口。注意皮肤的变化。发现阴蒂分叉和尿道扩张符合完全性女性尿道上裂[46]。对下背部的检查可以发现隐蔽性脊柱闭合障碍的迹象。神经学检查可显示步态异常。肛门反射缺失可能是感觉减退，可能是脐带系留[49]。

（三）附加试验

应进行尿液分析，以排除感染、高或特别低的比重以及葡萄糖的存在。当不确定青春期女孩是否有漏尿或生理性阴道分泌物时，尿垫试验有价值当尿漏与生理性阴道分泌物存在不确定性时，尿垫测试是有价值的。排尿后残留引起了对排尿功能障碍、神经源性病因或盆底功能障碍的担忧。肾膀胱超声可显示结构异常、上尿路扩张或膀胱壁增厚。尿流率检查可显示异常的尿流率曲线或 Q_{max} 下降，提示梗阻或排尿功能障碍。肾脏 – 输尿管 – 膀胱（KUB）平片有助于评估尿量负荷，也可能显示隐匿性脊柱侧弯。尿流动力学评估虽

然是有创检查，但可用于诊断逼尿肌过度活动、排尿功能障碍、膀胱容量增加、感觉减退和内在括约肌缺乏。如果担心神经源性膀胱，应进行该检查，但也可能提示进一步的神经系统检查。

四、临床治疗

（一）行为矫正和泌尿疗法

尿路治疗通常是下尿路症状的一线治疗，是指非药物、非手术的干预措施。尿路治疗包括教育患者规律排尿习惯和正确的排尿姿势，以鼓励患者完全排空。我们向患者提供了关于每日液体摄入量、避免可能刺激膀胱的饮料、预防便秘，以及其他排尿的建议。表 23-3 列出了改善膀胱控制的常见步骤，以及逐步增加的治疗。

表 23-3　大龄女孩和青春期女性尿失禁治疗方案的升级

尿疗法
- 定时排尿
- 双空洞
- 正确的个人卫生状况
- 增加水的摄入量
- 减少含咖啡因、碳酸、人工色素和糖的饮料摄入
- 增加纤维和粪便软化剂
- 适当时转诊到体重管理诊所
- 生物反馈
- 盆底物理治疗

药物治疗
- 抗胆碱能药物，包括奥昔布宁、托特罗定、索利那新和非索特罗定
- Mirabegron 米拉贝隆（用于治疗膀胱过度活动症）
- 去氨加压素（用于夜间遗尿症）
- 三环类抗抑郁药，包括丙咪嗪（用于夜间遗尿症）
- 哌甲酯（用于咯咯笑尿失禁）

经皮电神经刺激
- 骶骨
- 骶旁
- 胫后肌

手术的选择
- 骶神经调节
- 膀胱内注射肉毒杆菌毒素 A

国际儿童失禁学会（International Children's Continence Society）在其标准化文件中概述了 6 种具体的尿路疗法：定时排尿、膀胱训练、盆底肌训练、中枢抑制训练、神经刺激和清洁间歇导尿。每种尿路疗法都有其最适合的特定泌尿系统主诉。他们建议对各种形式的尿失禁进行膀胱训练。急迫性尿失禁也可通过定时排尿、中枢抑制训练和神经刺激进行治疗。有效的肠道管理（可能包括泻药）是关键。从教育和自我监测到条件反射和反应预防，认知行为疗法也是泌尿治疗的核心[55]。

欧洲膀胱功能障碍研究（European Bladder Dysfunction Study）纳入了 7—12 岁的女孩和男孩（171 例女孩和 46 例男孩），在被随机分配接受标准治疗和 6～12 次膀胱训练的膀胱过度活动症继发失禁儿童中，44% 实现了完全控尿。相比之下，只有 15% 的患者通过标准治疗或与尿路治疗师进行 3 次咨询，达到了控尿[56]。

对于单症状和非单症状的夜间遗尿症患儿，尿床警报已被证明是最成功的治疗方法。与其他下尿路症状患者相比，只有夜间遗尿症的患者需要更少的门诊就诊并且更快地达到干燥。仅对膀胱容量小于预期的患者开具警报，而对多尿症患者开具去氨加压素，对小膀胱和多尿症患者开具两者。他们报道了 39.9% 的单症状夜间遗尿症和 36.4% 的非单症状夜间遗尿症患者的节制率。去氨加压素对 27.8% 的单症状夜间遗尿症和 14.9% 的非单症状夜间遗尿症有效。联合治疗对 13.2% 的单症状夜间遗尿症和 18.2% 的非单症状夜间遗尿症[57]有效。

尿路疗法可以成功治疗笑尿失禁患者，特别是生物反馈。一项回顾性研究包括 10 例 6—15 岁的女孩和 2 例男孩，他们在抗胆碱能药和（或）伪麻黄碱失败后接受了生物反馈。接受至少 4 次治疗的女孩在 6 个月时达到了持久的完全缓解，但有些女孩仍在接受药物治疗。他们认为，这种治疗是成功的，因为它具有新的能力，可以募集外括约肌来防止失禁。此外，40% 的患者在尿流动力学检查中发现排尿功能障碍，尽管只有笑尿

失禁的症状；生物反馈也帮助他们学习如何放松括约肌[58]。

对于压力性尿失禁患者，盆底治疗是一种有效的辅助治疗。在 Eliasson 对 35 例优秀蹦床运动员的研究中，其中 80% 报道了压力性尿失禁，其中 21 例运动员报告"在运动结束时"出现漏尿，这表明盆底肌肉疲劳[25]。类似地，Ree 等发现年轻女性（平均年龄 24 ± 1.7 岁）[59] 在剧烈运动 90min 后，最大自主收缩压力降低 17%。在 Da Roza 等的一项研究中，16 例女性有高强度的体力活动，根据国际体力活动问卷 – 简式（IPAQ-SF）分类，每周 3000min 的代谢当量或每周 4h 的剧烈体力活动，其中 7 例女性患有尿失禁。他们每个人都接受了为期 8 周的盆底康复计划。完成后，与基线相比，阴道静息压力和最大自主收缩压力均显著增加。尿失禁频率和体积显著改善，其中 6 例患者完全消退[60]。

在欧洲膀胱功能障碍研究（European Bladder Dysfunction Study）中，49% 的继发于功能失调性排尿的失禁儿童随机接受标准治疗加盆底训练，达到了尿控；25% 的患者通过标准治疗或与尿路治疗师进行 3 次咨询获得了尿控。作为盆底训练的对照，患者还被随机分配到认知治疗组，其中 52% 的患者达到了尿控。研究人员假设社会压力可能是症状的重要因素[56]。因此，有必要对这些复杂的患者采取多学科方法。

鉴于减肥是超重和肥胖尿失禁[22] 女性的有效治疗方法，因此在青少年中研究了同样的建议。一项前瞻性研究纳入了 242 例肥胖青少年，其中 33 例女性（18%），平均年龄 17.1 岁，体重指数为 50.5kg/m^2，报道减肥手术前有尿失禁。术后随访 6 个月及 3 年，尿失禁下降至 7%[61]。

（二）药物疗法

在儿童患者中，口服奥昔布宁等抗胆碱能药物被认为是膀胱过度活动症的"金标准"。然而，与成人一样，每日多次给药的不良反应和潜在需求是有问题的[62]。对于去氨加压素和尿床警报失败的患者，抗胆碱能药物也是推荐治疗夜间遗尿症的选择。重要的是监测这些患者的残余尿量，以避免发生或加重便秘[54]。

Gleason 等在 4—16 岁的患者中研究了奥昔布宁贴剂的疗效和不良反应。由于每 3～4 天更换 1 次剂量，因此无须每日多次给药。他们发现唯一显著的不良反应是 35% 的患者在贴片部位的皮肤刺激。在研究组中，69% 的患者因口干、便秘或行为改变而停止了口服奥昔布宁治疗，而使用贴剂时未出现上述情况。该贴片非常有效，97% 的患者报告症状改善；57% 报告完全解决[62]。

在奥昔布汀和托特罗定治疗失败后，索利那新被提议用于治疗难治性膀胱过度活动症[63, 64]。一项研究包括 138 例患有某种程度的日间或夜间尿失禁的男孩和女孩，他们中的大多数人曾服用过其他抗胆碱能药物。治疗 3 个月后，99 例患者完成评估，其中 45 例完全控尿，另外 39 例患者达到部分缓解，其中 17 例在日间干燥。6.5% 的患者出现了不良反应，其中包括多动、嗜睡、便秘、腹痛和粪便嵌塞[63]。另一项研究报道索利那新治疗膀胱过度活动症继发尿失禁的成功率为 94%。虽然有效，但 38% 的患者出现了不良反应，最常见的是口干和便秘。当考虑尿流动力学数据时，膀胱容量从 128ml 增加到 340ml，并且不受抑制的逼尿肌收缩幅度从 70cmH_2O 减少到 18cmH_2O。每天的失禁次数显著减少，患者和父母对失禁的看法也得到改善[64]。

非索特罗定也被用于治疗儿童和青少年膀胱过度活动症患者的尿失禁。一项比较 4～8mg 非索特罗定与缓释奥昔布宁的研究表明，两者的疗效相同。两组在便秘、口干等不良反应方面差异无统计学意义。然而，那些被随机分配到非索特罗定组的人的心率增加了。两种药物均改善了中位排尿量和失禁发作次数，生活质量也有所改善。作者将 23 例患儿的治疗延长了 12 个月。在未纳入扩展研究的 34 例儿童中，68% 在平均 18 个月随访时获得了控尿。在扩展的参与者中，78% 获得了控尿[65]。

米拉贝隆是一种用于治疗成人膀胱过度活动症的 β_3 肾上腺素受体激动药，虽然尚未被批准用于儿童的治疗，但有研究报告其结局良好。在中位年龄为 10.1 岁的 58 例膀胱过度活动症患者中，抗胆碱能治疗失败或出现不可接受的不良反应，其中 52 例报告控尿改善。没有发现严重的不良反应[66]。

三环类抗抑郁药历来用于治疗儿童夜间遗尿症。Cochran 的一篇综述发现，与安慰剂相比，三环类药物减少了夜间遗尿的次数。此外，有更大比例的患者能够达到 14 天的甚至更长时间的控尿。他们发现与安慰剂相比有益处的药物包括丙咪嗪、阿米替林和地昔帕明。他们注意到治疗停止后夜间遗尿症复发。这些研究没有包含足够的数据来比较三环化合物。他们确实将其疗效与去氨加压素进行了比较，发现其与单药治疗相似，但一项研究发现去氨加压素 / 奥昔布宁联合治疗优于丙咪嗪单药治疗。虽然三环药物比行为矫正更有效，但尿床警报在短期内和停止治疗时更有效[67]。国际儿童尿失禁学会仅在患者使用去氨加压素、尿床报警器和抗胆碱能药物（因为存在心脏毒性[54]风险）失败的情况下推荐三环药物。

当患者持续尿失禁且对一种耐受性良好的药物有部分反应时，双重抗胆碱能治疗可能是一种选择。在一项包括 6 例平均年龄为 10.5 ± 2 岁的非神经源性膀胱功能障碍女性的研究中，提供了第二种抗胆碱能药物，其组合包括奥昔布宁和托特罗定、奥昔布宁和索利那新，以及托特罗定和索利那新。最常见的不良反应是口干，但没有患者因此而停止治疗。所有患者的控尿能力均得到改善[68]。

Morin 等报道了他们加用米拉贝隆的经验，而不是加用第二种抗胆碱能药物。他们的前瞻性研究包括 35 例患者（中位年龄 10.3 岁），大多数为男性，有持续性尿失禁，对缓释型抗胆碱能药有部分应答。最终 29 例患者接受了索利那新联合米拉贝隆治疗，3 例患者接受了奥昔布宁缓释联合米拉贝隆治疗，3 例患者接受了非索特罗定联合米拉贝隆治疗。所有患者均报告症状改善，34% 报道完全控尿，66% 报告失禁发作减少 50%～99%。尿量随治疗而增加。20% 的患者报道了不良反应，3% 报道了中度不良反应[69]。

类似地，去氨加压素和奥昔布宁二联疗法可提高夜间遗尿症患者的缓解率。一项对 61 例夜间遗尿症患者（平均年龄 11.6 ± 2.6 岁）的回顾性研究发现，最大剂量 0.6mg 去氨加压素的应答率为 69%，这些患者有单症状或日间症状得到控制。然后，对于去氨加压素单药治疗失败的患者，他们将每晚加用 5mg 奥昔布宁，并将剂量增加 2.5mg 至最多 10mg。在开始联合治疗的 25 例患者中，68% 在接受 5mg 奥昔布宁治疗后转为干性。在继续接受大剂量奥昔布宁治疗的 8 例患者中，75% 变得干燥，去氨加压素单药治疗或联合治疗的最终成功率为 97%。男性和女性患者对单药治疗的应答相似，但女性患者对联合治疗的应答似乎优于男性，100% 达到干燥。在患者中，没有去氨加压素单药治疗的不良反应报告，也没有任何接受联合治疗的儿童因口干或便秘接受治疗[70]。

笑性尿失禁是尿失禁的一个子集，因此有一个独特的医学疗法。一组 20 例平均年龄 12.4 岁的纯笑性尿失禁患者首先接受了标准的行为矫正治疗，并在可能增加笑声的活动前进行预期性排尿。其中 13 例患者报道症状无改善。我们向所有患者提供了哌甲酯试验，15 例接受。15 例患者中有 12 例在上学时间尿失禁缓解。2 个月时停止用药，12 例既往干燥的患者中有 9 例[43]症状复发。

（三）更强化的治疗

尿失禁可对生活质量产生显著影响。加拿大的一个研究小组对患者和照护者进行了调查，发现 71% 的患者和 89% 的照护者意识到其生活质量受到中度至重度影响。此外，他们愿意尝试经皮神经刺激（54%）或植入骶神经调节（42%）[3]。对骶神经调节技术的改进可能使其更具微创性，减少了辐射显露并改善了美容效果[71]。

（四）经皮神经调节

与置入设备相比，经皮神经电刺激疗法（TENS）的侵入性更小，已被提议作为儿科患者的更好选择。已经描述了不同的电极位置，包括骶骨、骶旁和胫骨后。一项纳入 14 岁以下儿童的骶神经经皮神经电刺激疗法对照试验发现，主动治疗组 61% 的患者日间尿失禁严重程度降低，而假治疗组为 17%（$P<0.01$）。他们日间发生的尿失禁也较少。研究人员还评估了尿流动力学参数，试图阐明该方法有效的原因，但他们无法确定膀胱容量的差异[72]。

一项前瞻性研究纳入了 83 例接受骶旁经皮神经电刺激疗法治疗的患者，其中大多数为女性，但只有 25% 的患者年龄>10 岁，研究发现使用夜间遗尿症时成功率较低。96.4% 的患者报道有显著改善，56.6% 的患者完全缓解。当比较有或无夜间遗尿症的患者时，只有 45.5% 的有夜间遗尿症的患者达到完全缓解，而无夜间遗尿症的患者为 78.6%。10 岁及以上患者与 9 岁及以下患者相比，无统计学显著性差异（66.7% vs. 55.9%，$P=0.97$）[73]。骶旁经皮神经电刺激疗法也能改善便秘，但其效果似乎与治疗尿失禁无关[74]。

胫后经皮神经电刺激疗法也被证明能有效治疗患有膀胱过度活动症和排尿功能障碍的男孩和女孩的日间失禁和夜间遗尿症。排尿功能障碍患者的反应甚至优于膀胱过度活动症患者，85% 的患者实现了日间控尿。大多数排尿功能障碍的儿童在 2 岁时仍保持其反应。许多未治愈的患者对慢性每月刺激有很好的反应[75]。

一项前瞻性研究比较了生物反馈和骶旁经皮神经电刺激疗法作为膀胱过度活动症、排尿功能障碍或膀胱过度活动症和排尿功能障碍的治疗模式。他们发现，这两种方法都能改善日间尿失禁，且成功率无差异。然而，他们确实注意到，生物反馈在较少的疗程后是成功的[76]。另一项研究比较了骶旁经皮神经电刺激疗法和奥昔布宁。他们将患者随机分组，一组接受骶旁经皮神经电刺激疗法联合安慰剂治疗，另一组接受假肩胛电治疗联合奥昔布宁治疗。他们发现，骶旁经皮神经电刺激疗法组的所有患者便秘均得到改善，并且没有患者出现奥昔布宁组观察到的抗胆碱能不良反应。"在评估排尿功能障碍严重程度评分的改善时，他们发现治疗成功率没有差异。"两组患者每天的最大排尿量和平均排尿量以及排尿次数均有改善[77]。

（五）手术疗法

骶神经调控术可成功治疗青少年尿失禁患者。大多数研究需要保守治疗和（或）药物治疗失败。在一项包括 3 例男孩和 15 例女孩的研究中，他们平均年龄 15 岁，有不同程度的下尿路功能障碍，15 例在测试阶段后，他们的症状至少有 50% 的改善，并置入了脉冲发生器。在使用器械的患者中，50% 在短期内达到完全缓解，28% 达到部分缓解。平均随访 28.8 ± 43.8 个月时，报道完全或部分缓解的患者比例略有下降至 73%。在主要指征为尿失禁的 10 例患者中，6 例完全缓解，3 例部分缓解[78]。经过中等长度的随访（中位数为 3.9 年），在保守治疗失败后接受骶神经调节治疗的儿童中，74% 的儿童认为其症状改善，其中部分儿童在移除装置后仍有改善[79]。

与经皮神经电刺激疗法一样，置入式骶神经调节似乎对日间尿失禁更有效。在一项对日间或夜间尿失禁患者的研究中，16 例日间尿失禁患者中，75% 的症状消失，另外 13% 的症状得到改善；而 16 例夜间遗尿症患者中，38% 的症状消失，另外 25% 的症状得到改善[80]。

除了改善控尿，骶神经调节还对社会心理生活质量评分产生积极影响，而对身体生活质量评分没有影响[81]。随着随访时间的延长，患者的泌尿系统症状和生活质量评分均有持续改善。特别是无抑制收缩的患者可能对骶神经调节反应更好[82]。

然而，在大多数研究中，很难确定患者的年龄，一项研究确实分层了顽固性功能失调性排泄综合征 / 肠和膀胱功能障碍儿童对骶神经调节的反应。他们发现，在 52 例年龄≥9 岁的患者中，87% 的患者日间尿失禁得到改善，44% 的患者尿失禁得到缓解。在该年龄组的 44 例夜间遗尿症患者中，73% 好转，23% 报道治愈[83]。

置入性骶神经调节的一个缺点是需要额外的手术。即使手术成功，器械最终也会被取出。在 61 例患者中，32.4% 的患者在放置装置后 4 年内拆除了装置以达到治愈，关闭装置至少 6 个月，且症状未复发[84]。患者也可能因为并发症而需要翻修 / 更换或切除。由于感染或治疗失败等原因，并发症的清除率为 8%～25%[79, 84, 85]。再手术率为 19.7%～54%[79, 83-85]，最常见的原因是导线移位、断裂或装置故障。低体重指数的患者即使创伤很小，也可能增加导线断裂的风险[82]，尽管其他人没有发现年龄、性别或体重指数可以预测并发症[85]。

膀胱内注射肉毒杆菌毒素 A 也用于年龄较大的尿失禁儿童和青少年。与骶神经调节术一样，患者应首先用尽保守疗法。成功率各不相同，完全缓解率为 32%～55%，另有患者报道部分缓解[86-88]。除改善尿失禁外，患者的尿频、尿急、夜尿症状也可能减轻[87]。生活质量评分也有所提高[89]。在一项包括注射前和注射后尿流动力学的研究中，75% 的患者无抑制的收缩消退，而其余 25% 的收缩幅度减小[90]。并发症发生率不一，从无并发症[86, 90]到术后尿潴留和尿路感染[87, 88, 90]。患者和家长的满意度很高，在 43 例接受了膀胱内注射肉毒杆菌毒素 A 的患者中，只有 1 例发现注射效果不佳[91]。

Burch 膀胱尿道悬吊术，无论是开腹还是腹腔镜，已经在顽固性尿失禁和影像尿流动力学检查证实膀胱颈功能不全的女孩中有报道。“对 18 例连续的腹腔镜和 18 例连续的开放阴道悬吊术的研究包括了首先失败的日间尿路治疗的女孩，然后进行了为期 10 天的强化住院培训的女孩。”最终，所有女孩都对治疗产生抗药性至少 2 年。接受腹腔镜手术的女孩平均年龄为 13.5 岁，接受开腹手术的女孩平均年龄为 11.5 岁。腹腔镜组 44% 的患者和开腹组 38% 的患者达到了完全控尿，而腹腔镜组 28% 的患者和开腹组 17% 的患者达到了部分控尿，即患者报道的压力性尿失禁发作较少。他们没有报道并发症[92]。PubMed 检索显示，在无其他先天性畸形（如膀胱外翻或尿道上裂）的情况下，没有关于吊带手术或人工尿路括约肌治疗儿童或青少年非神经源性膀胱功能障碍的报道。

总结

总之，在年龄较大的女孩和青春期女性中，尿失禁是一种认识不足，但可能影响生活的疾病，运动员和患有肥胖或肺部疾病等慢性疾病的患者尤其危险。虽然罕见，但可能是解剖学原因，因此，评估时应排除先天性原因。治疗从行为矫正和尿路治疗开始，但可升级为经皮或植入神经调节或膀胱内注射肉毒杆菌毒素 A。不幸的是，那些在青年时期遭受下尿路症状的患者在成年后有继续患下尿路症状的风险，但他们的生活质量可以通过干预措施得到改善。

参考文献

[1] Bardino M, Di Martino M, Ricci E, Parazzini F. Frequency and determinants of urinary incontinence in adolescent and young nulliparous women. J Pediatr Adolesc Gynecol. 2015;28(6):462–70.
[2] Carls C. The prevalence of stress urinary incontinence in high school and college-age female athletes in the Midwest: implications for education and prevention. Urol Nurs. 2007;27(1):21–4, 39.
[3] Dos Santos J, Marcon E, Pokarowski M, Vali R, Raveendran L, O'Kelly F, Amirabadi A, Elterman D, Foty R, Lorenzo A, Koyle M. Assessment of needs in children suffering from refractory non-neurogenic urinary and fecal incontinence and their caregivers' needs and attitudes toward alternative therapies (SNM, TENS). Front Pediatr. 2020;8:558.
[4] Petrangeli F, Capitanucci ML, Marciano A, Mosiello G, Alvaro R, Zaccara A, Finazzi-Agro E, De Gennaro M. A 20-year study of persistence of lower urinary tract symptoms and urinary incontinence in young women treated in childhood. J Pediatr Urol. 2014;10(3):441–5.
[5] O'Halloran T, Bell RJ, Robinson PJ, Davis SR. Urinary incontinence in young nulligravid women: a cross-sectional analysis. Ann Intern Med. 2012;157(2):87–93.
[6] Hägglund D, Olsson H, Leppert J. Urinary incontinence: an unexpected large problem among young females. Results from a population-based study. Fam Pract. 1999;16(5):506–9.
[7] van Breda HM, Bosch JL, de Kort LM. Hidden prevalence of lower

urinary tract symptoms in healthy nulligravid young women. Int Urogynecol J. 2015 ov;26(11):1637–43.
[8] Alnaif B, Drutz HP. The prevalence of urinary and fecal incontinence in Canadian secondary school teenage girls: questionnaire study and review of the literature. Int Urogynecol J Pelvic Floor Dysfunct. 2001;12(2):134–7.
[9] Parden AM, Griffin RL, Hoover K, Ellington DR, Gleason JL, Burgio KL, Richter HE. Prevalence, awareness, and understanding of pelvic floor disorders in adolescent and young women. Female Pelvic Med Reconstr Surg. 2016;22(5):346–54.
[10] Almousa S, Bandin van Loon A. The prevalence of urinary incontinence in nulliparous adolescent and middle-aged women and the associated risk factors: a systematic review. Maturitas. 2018;107:78–83.
[11] Luo Y, Zou P, Wang K, Cui Z, Li X, Wang J. Prevalence and associated factors of urinary incontinence among Chinese Adolescents in Henan Province: a cross-sectional survey. Int J Environ Res Public Health. 2020;17(17):6106.
[12] Linde JM, Nijman RJM, Trzpis M, Broens PMA. Prevalence of urinary incontinence and other lower urinary tract symptoms in children in the Netherlands. J Pediatr Urol. 2019;15(2):164.e1–7.
[13] Arbuckle JL, Parden AM, Hoover K, Griffin RL, Richter HE. Prevalence and awareness of pelvic floor disorders in female adolescents seeking gynecologic care. J Pediatr Adolesc Gynecol. 2019;32(3):288–92.
[14] Aydın A, Kocaöz S, Kara P. Prevalence of lower urinary tract symptoms in pregnant adolescents and the influencing factors. J Pediatr Adolesc Gynecol. 2020;33(2):160–6.
[15] Babini D, Lemos A. Risk factors for urinary incontinence in primiparous adolescents after vaginal delivery: a cohort study. J Pediatr Adolesc Gynecol. 2020;33(5):500–5.
[16] von Gontard A, Mattheus H, Anagnostakou A, Sambach H, Breuer M, Kiefer K, Holländer T, Hussong J. Behavioral comorbidity, overweight, and obesity in children with incontinence: an analysis of 1638 cases. Neurourol Urodyn. 2020;39(7):1985–93.
[17] Eray Ş, Tekcan D, Baran Y. More anxious or more shy? Examining the social anxiety levels of adolescents with primary enuresis nocturna: a controlled study. J Pediatr Urol. 2019;15(4):343.e1–5.
[18] Vasconcelos MMA, East P, Blanco E, Lukacz ES, Caballero G, Lozoff B, Gahagan S. Early behavioral risks of childhood and adolescent daytime urinary incontinence and nocturnal enuresis. J Dev Behav Pediatr. 2017;38(9):736–42.
[19] Dourado ER, de Abreu GE, Santana JC, Macedo RR, da Silva CM, Rapozo PMB, Netto JMB, Barroso U. Emotional and behavioral problems in children and adolescents with lower urinary tract dysfunction: a population-based study. J Pediatr Urol. 2019;15(4):376.e1–7.
[20] Shah S, Jafri RZ, Mobin K, Mirza R, Nanji K, Jahangir F, Patel SJ, Ejaz MS, Qaiser I, Iftikhar H, Aziz K, Khan W, Maqbool HS, Ahmed H. Frequency and features of nocturnal enuresis in Pakistani children aged 5 to 16 years based on ICCS criteria: a multi-center cross-sectional study from Karachi, Pakistan. BMC Fam Pract. 2018;19(1):198.
[21] Keane DP, Sims TJ, Abrams P, Bailey AJ. Analysis of collagen status in premenopausal nulliparous women with genuine stress incontinence. Br J Obstet Gynaecol. 1997;104(9):994–8.
[22] Subak LL, Whitcomb E, Shen H, Saxton J, Vittinghoff E, Brown JS. Weight loss: a novel and effective treatment for urinary incontinence. J Urol. 2005;174(1):190–5.
[23] Schwartz B, Wyman JF, Thomas W, Schwarzenberg SJ. Urinary incontinence in obese adolescent girls. J Pediatr Urol. 2009;5(6):445–50.
[24] Monkhouse K, Caldwell PH, Barnes EH. The relationship between urinary incontinence and obesity in childhood. J Paediatr Child Health. 2019;55(6):625–31.
[25] Eliasson K, Larsson T, Mattsson E. Prevalence of stress incontinence in nulliparous elite trampolinists. Scand J Med Sci Sports. 2002;12(2):106–10.
[26] Eliasson K, Edner A, Mattsson E. Urinary incontinence in very young and mostly nulliparous women with a history of regular organised high-impact trampoline training: occurrence and risk factors. Int Urogynecol J Pelvic Floor Dysfunct. 2008;19(5):687–96.
[27] Logan BL, Foster-Johnson L, Zotos E. Urinary incontinence among adolescent female athletes. J Pediatr Urol. 2018;14(3):241.e1–9.
[28] Hagovska M, Svihra J, Bukova A, Horbacz A, Svihrova V. The impact of physical activity measured by the International Physical Activity questionnaire on the prevalence of stress urinary incontinence in young women. Eur J Obstet Gynecol Reprod Biol. 2018;228:308–12.
[29] Mattheus HK, Wagner C, Becker K, Bühren K, Correll CU, Egberts KM, Ehrlich S, Fleischhaker C, Föcker M, Hahn F, Hebebrand J, Herpertz-Dahlmann B, Jaite C, Jenetzky E, Kaess M, Legenbauer T, Pfeiffer JP, Renner TJ, Roessner V, Schulze U, Sinzig J, Wessing I, von Gontard A. Incontinence and constipation in adolescent patients with anorexia nervosa-Results of a multicenter study from a German web-based registry for children and adolescents with anorexia nervosa. Int J Eat Disord. 2020;53(2):219–28.
[30] Carvalhais A, Araújo J, Natal Jorge R, Bø K. Urinary incontinence and disordered eating in female elite athletes. J Sci Med Sport. 2019;22(2):140–4.
[31] White D, Stiller K, Roney F. The prevalence and severity of symptoms of incontinence in adult cystic fibrosis patients. Physiother Theory Pract. 2000;16:35–42.
[32] Blackwell K, Malone PS, Denny A, Connett G, Maddison J. The prevalence of stress urinary incontinence in patients with cystic fibrosis: an under-recognized problem. J Pediatr Urol. 2005;1(1):5–9.
[33] Nixon GM, Glazner JA, Martin JM, Sawyer SM. Urinary incontinence in female adolescents with cystic fibrosis. Pediatrics. 2002;110(2 Pt 1):e22.
[34] Salvatore S, Serati M, Origoni M, Candiani M. Is overactive bladder in children and adults the same condition? ICI-RS 2011. Neurourol Urodyn. 2012;31(3):349–51.
[35] Fitzgerald MP, Thom DH, Wassel-Fyr C, Subak L, Brubaker L, Van Den Eeden SK, Brown JS, Reproductive Risks for Incontinence Study at Kaiser Research Group. Childhood urinary symptoms predict adult overactive bladder symptoms. J Urol. 2006;175(3 Pt 1):989–93.
[36] Bower WF, Sit FK, Yeung CK. Nocturnal enuresis in adolescents and adults is associated with childhood elimination symptoms. J Urol. 2006;176(4 Pt 2):1771–5.
[37] Forsythe WI, Redmond A. Enuresis and spontaneous cure rate. Study of 1129 enuretis. Arch Dis Child. 1974;49(4):259–63.
[38] Yeung CK, Sihoe JD, Sit FK, Bower W, Sreedhar B, Lau J. Characteristics of primary nocturnal enuresis in adults: an epidemiological study. BJU Int. 2004;93(3):341–5.
[39] Nappo S, Del Gado R, Chiozza ML, Biraghi M, Ferrara P, Caione P. Nocturnal enuresis in the adolescent: a neglected problem. BJU Int. 2002;90(9):912–7.
[40] Austin PF, Bauer SB, Bower W, Chase J, Franco I, Hoebeke P, Rittig S, Vande Walle J, von Gontard A, Wright A, Yang SS, Nevéus T. The standardization of terminology of lower urinary tract function in children and adolescents: update report from the Standardization Committee of the International Children's Continence Society. J Urol. 2014;191(6):1863–1865.e13.
[41] Logan BL, Blais S. Giggle incontinence: evolution of concept and treatment. J Pediatr Urol. 2017;13(5):430–5. https://doi.org/10.1016/j.jpurol.2017.04.021.
[42] Sher PK, Reinberg Y. Successful treatment of giggle incontinence with

methylphenidate. J Urol. 1996;156(2 Pt 2):656–8.
[43] Berry AK, Zderic S, Carr M. Methylphenidate for giggle incontinence. J Urol. 2009;182(4 Suppl):2028–32.
[44] Viers BR, Trost LW, Kramer SA. Ectopic ureter in an adolescent female presenting with primary nocturnal enuresis and new onset urinary incontinence. J Urol. 2011;185(2):689.
[45] Suson KD, Preece J, Baradaran N, Di Carlo HN, Gearhart JP. The fate of the complete female epispadias and exstrophy bladder-is there a difference? J Urol. 2013;190(4 Suppl):1583–8.
[46] Tantibhedhyangkul J, Copland SD, Haqq AM, Price TM. A case of female epispadias. Fertil Steril. 2008;90(5):2017.e1–3.
[47] Atilgan D, Uluocak N, Erdemir F, Parlaktas BS. Female epispadias: a case report and review of the literature. Kaohsiung J Med Sci. 2009;25(11):613–6.
[48] Son HS, Kim JH. Urological presentations of adult primary tethered cord syndrome. Neurourol Urodyn. 2020;39(2):633–41.
[49] Granada C, Loveless M, Justice T, Moriarty T, Mutchnick I, Dietrich JE, LaJoie AS, Hertweck P. Tethered cord syndrome in the pediatric-adolescent gynecologic patient. J Pediatr Adolesc Gynecol. 2015;28(5):309–12.
[50] Barnes HV. The adolescent patient. In: Walker HK, Hall WD, Hurst JW, editors. Clinical methods: the history, physical, and laboratory examinations. 3rd ed. Boston: Butterworths; 1990. Chapter 223.
[51] Yildirim A, Uluocak N, Atilgan D, Ozcetin M, Erdemir F, Boztepe O. Evaluation of lower urinary tract symptoms in children exposed to sexual abuse. Urol J. 2011;8(1):38–42.
[52] De Gennaro M, Niero M, Capitanucci ML, von Gontard A, Woodward M, Tubaro A, Abrams P. Validity of the international consultation on incontinence questionnaire-pediatric lower urinary tract symptoms: a screening questionnaire for children. J Urol. 2010;184(4 Suppl):1662–7.
[53] Nelson CP, Park JM, Bloom DA, Wan J, Dunn RL, Wei JT. Incontinence Symptom Index-Pediatric: development and initial validation of a urinary incontinence instrument for the older pediatric population. J Urol. 2007;178(4 Pt 2):1763–7.
[54] Nevéus T, Fonseca E, Franco I, Kawauchi A, Kovacevic L, Nieuwhof-Leppink A, Raes A, Tekgül S, Yang SS, Rittig S. Management and treatment of nocturnal enuresis-an updated standardization document from the international Children's continence society. J Pediatr Urol. 2020 Feb;16(1):10–9.
[55] Nieuwhof-Leppink AJ, Hussong J, Chase J, Larsson J, Renson C, Hoebeke P, Yang S, von Gontard A. Definitions, indications and practice of urotherapy in children and adolescents: – A standardization document of the International Children's Continence Society (ICCS). J Pediatr Urol. 2020:S1477–5131(20)30630–6.
[56] van Gool JD, de Jong TP, Winkler-Seinstra P, Tamminen-Möbius T, Lax H, Hirche H, Nijman RJ, Hjälmås K, Jodal U, Bachmann H, Hoebeke P, Walle JV, Misselwitz J, John U, Bael A, European Bladder Dysfunction Study (EU BMH1–CT94–1006). Multi-center randomized controlled trial of cognitive treatment, placebo, oxybutynin, bladder training, and pelvic floor training in children with functional urinary incontinence. Neurourol Urodyn. 2014;33(5):482–7.
[57] Rittig N, Hagstroem S, Mahler B, Kamperis K, Siggaard C, Mikkelsen MM, Bower WF, Djurhuus JC, Rittig S. Outcome of a standardized approach to childhood urinary symptoms-long- term follow-up of 720 patients. Neurourol Urodyn. 2014;33(5):475–81.
[58] Richardson I, Palmer LS. Successful treatment for giggle incontinence with biofeedback. J Urol. 2009;182(4 Suppl):2062–6.
[59] Ree ML, Nygaard I, Bø K. Muscular fatigue in the pelvic floor muscles after strenuous physical activity. Acta Obstet Gynecol Scand. 2007;86(7):870–6.
[60] Da Roza T, Poli de Araujo M, Viana R, Viana S, Jorge RN, Bo K, Mascarenhas T. Pelvic floor muscle training to improve urinary incontinence in young, nulliparous sport students: a pilot study. Int Urogynecol J. 2012;23:1069–73.
[61] DeFoor WR Jr, Inge TH, Jenkins TM, Jackson E, Courcoulas A, Michalsky M, Brandt M, Kollar L, Xie C. Prospective evaluation of urinary incontinence in severely obese adolescents presenting for weight loss surgery. Surg Obes Relat Dis. 2018;14(2):214–8.
[62] Gleason JM, Daniels C, Williams K, Varghese A, Koyle MA, Bägli DJ, Pippi Salle JL, Lorenzo AJ. Single center experience with oxybutynin transdermal system (patch) for management of symptoms related to non-neuropathic overactive bladder in children: an attractive, well tolerated alternative form of administration. J Pediatr Urol. 2014;10(4):753–7.
[63] Hoebeke P, De Pooter J, De Caestecker K, Raes A, Dehoorne J, Van Laecke E, Vande WJ. Solifenacin for therapy resistant overactive bladder. J Urol. 2009;182(4 Suppl):2040–4.
[64] Nadeau G, Schröder A, Moore K, Genois L, Lamontagne P, Hamel M, Pellerin E, Bolduc S. Long-term use of solifenacin in pediatric patients with overactive bladder: extension of a prospective open-label study. Can Urol Assoc J. 2014;8(3–4):118–23.
[65] Ramsay S, Naud É, Simonyan D, Moore K, Bolduc S. A randomized, crossover trial comparing the efficacy and safety of fesoterodine and extended-release oxybutynin in children with overactive bladder with 12–month extension on fesoterodine: the FOXY study. Can Urol Assoc J. 2020;14(6):192–8.
[66] Blais AS, Nadeau G, Moore K, Genois L, Bolduc S. Prospective pilot study of mirabegron in pediatric patients with overactive bladder. Eur Urol. 2016;70(1):9–13.
[67] Caldwell PH, Sureshkumar P, Wong WC. Tricyclic and related drugs for nocturnal enuresis in children. Cochrane Database Syst Rev. 2016;1:CD002117.
[68] Bolduc S, Moore K, Lebel S, Lamontagne P, Hamel M. Double anticholinergic therapy for refractory overactive bladder. J Urol. 2009;182(4 Suppl):2033–8.
[69] Morin F, Blais AS, Nadeau G, Moore K, Genois L, Bolduc S. Dual therapy for refractory overactive bladder in children: a prospective open-label study. J Urol. 2017;197(4):1158–63.
[70] Berkenwald A, Pires J, Ellsworth P. Evaluating use of higher dose oxybutynin in combination with desmopressin for refractory nocturnal enuresis. J Pediatr Urol. 2016;12(4):220.e1–6.
[71] McGee SM, Routh JC, Granberg CF, Roth TJ, Hollatz P, Vandersteen DR, Reinberg Y. Sacral neuromodulation in children with dysfunctional elimination syndrome: description of incisionless first stage and second stage without fluoroscopy. Urology. 2009;73(3):641–4.
[72] Hagstroem S, Mahler B, Madsen B, Djurhuus JC, Rittig S. Transcutaneous electrical nerve stimulation for refractory daytime urinary urge incontinence. J Urol. 2009;182(4 Suppl):2072–8.
[73] Hoffmann A, Sampaio C, Nascimento AA, Veiga ML, Barroso U. Predictors of outcome in children and adolescents with overactive bladder treated with parasacral transcutaneous electrical nerve stimulation. J Pediatr Urol. 2018;14(1):54.e1–6.
[74] Veiga ML, Costa EV, Portella I, Nacif A, Martinelli Braga AA, Barroso U Jr. Parasacral transcutaneous electrical nerve stimulation for overactive bladder in constipated children: The role of constipation. J Pediatr Urol. 2016;12(6):396.e1–6.
[75] Capitanucci ML, Camanni D, Demelas F, Mosiello G, Zaccara A, De Gennaro M. Long-term efficacy of percutaneous tibial nerve stimulation for different types of lower urinary tract dysfunction in children. J Urol. 2009;182(4 Suppl):2056–61.
[76] Dos Reis JN, Mello MF, Cabral BH, Mello LF, Saiovici S, Rocha FET. EMG biofeedback or parasacral transcutaneous electrical nerve stimulation in children with lower urinary tract dysfunction: a prospective and randomized trial. Neurourol Urodyn. 2019;38(6):1588–94.

[77] Quintiliano F, Veiga ML, Moraes M, Cunha C, de Oliveira LF, Lordelo P, Bastos Netto JM, Barroso JU. Transcutaneous parasacral electrical stimulation vs oxybutynin for the treatment of overactive bladder in children: a randomized clinical trial. J Urol. 2015;193(5 Suppl):1749–53.
[78] Groen LA, Hoebeke P, Loret N, Van Praet C, Van Laecke E, Ann R, Vande Walle J, Everaert K. Sacral neuromodulation with an implantable pulse generator in children with lower urinary tract symptoms: 15-year experience. J Urol. 2012;188(4):1313–7.
[79] Boswell TC, Hollatz P, Hutcheson JC, Vandersteen DR, Reinberg YE. Device outcomes in pediatric sacral neuromodulation: a single center series of 187 patients. J Pediatr Urol. 2020:S1477-5131(20)30568-4.
[80] Roth TJ, Vandersteen DR, Hollatz P, Inman BA, Reinberg YE. Sacral neuromodulation for the dysfunctional elimination syndrome: a single center experience with 20 children. J Urol. 2008;180(1):306–11.
[81] Stephany HA, Juliano TM, Clayton DB, Tanaka ST, Thomas JC, Adams MC, Brock JW 3rd, Pope JC 4th. Prospective evaluation of sacral nerve modulation in children with validated questionnaires. J Urol. 2013;190(4 Suppl):1516–22.
[82] Mason MD, Stephany HA, Casella DP, Clayton DB, Tanaka ST, Thomas JC, Adams MC, Brock JW 3rd, Pope JC 4th. Prospective evaluation of sacral neuromodulation in children: outcomes and urodynamic predictors of success. J Urol. 2016;195(4 Pt 2):1239–44.
[83] Dwyer ME, Vandersteen DR, Hollatz P, Reinberg YE. Sacral neuromodulation for the dysfunctional elimination syndrome: a 10-year single-center experience with 105 consecutive children. Urology. 2014;84(4):911–7.
[84] Rensing AJ, Szymanski KM, Dunn S, King S, Cain MP, Whittam BM. Pediatric sacral nerve stimulator explanation due to complications or cure: a survival analysis. J Pediatr Urol. 2019;15(1):39.e1–6.
[85] Fuchs ME, Lu PL, Vyrostek SJ, Teich S, Alpert SA. Factors predicting complications after sacral neuromodulation in children. Urology. 2017;107:214–7.
[86] McDowell DT, Noone D, Tareen F, Waldron M, Quinn F. Urinary incontinence in children: botulinum toxin is a safe and effective treatment option. Pediatr Surg Int. 2012;28(3):315–20.
[87] Blackburn SC, Jones C, Bedoya S, Steinbrecher HA, Malone PS, Griffin SJ. Intravesical botulinum type-A toxin (Dysport®) in the treatment of idiopathic detrusor overactivity in children. J Pediatr Urol. 2013;9(6 Pt A):750–3.
[88] Uçar M, Akgül AK, Parlak A, Yücel C, Kılıç N, Balkan E. Non-invasive evaluation of botulinum- A toxin treatment efficacy in children with refractory overactive bladder. Int Urol Nephrol. 2018;50(8):1367–73.
[89] Al Edwan GM, Mansi HH, Atta ONM, Shaath MM, Al Adwan R, Mahafza W, Afram KM, Ababneh O, Al Adwan D, Muheilan MM. Objective and subjective improvement in children with idiopathic detrusor overactivity after intravesical botulinum toxin injection: a preliminary report. J Pediatr Surg. 2019;54(3):595–9.
[90] Léon P, Jolly C, Binet A, Fiquet C, Vilette C, Lefebvre F, Bouché-Pillon-Persyn MA, Poli-Mérol ML. Botulinum toxin injections in the management of non-neurogenic overactive bladders in children. J Pediatr Surg. 2014;49(9):1424–8.
[91] El-Dakhakhny AS, El-Karamany TM, El-Atrebi M, Gharib T. Efficacy and safety of intradetrusor onabotulinumtoxinA injection for managing paediatric non-neurogenic overactive bladder: a prospective case-series study. Arab J Urol. 2019;17(2):143–9.
[92] Dobrowolska-Glazar BA, Groen LA, Nieuwhof-Leppink AJ, Klijn AJ, de Jong TPVM, Chrzan R. Open and laparoscopic colposuspension in girls with refractory urinary incontinence. Front Pediatr. 2017;5:284.

第 24 章 女性神经源性尿失禁
Female Neurogenic Incontinence

Jenny N. Nguyen Doreen E. Chung 著

众所周知，尿失禁会对生活质量产生严重的负面影响。然而，在神经源性下尿路功能障碍（NLUTD）女性中，她们通常活动受限，尿失禁可能对她们的生活质量产生更大的负面影响[1-4]。患有神经源性下尿路功能障碍的女性可能会遭受与无神经源性下尿路功能障碍女性相同类型的尿失禁。然而，一些额外的疾病过程可能会叠加。取决于神经损伤，由此产生的膀胱表现可能有所不同。女性神经源性尿失禁有时可以预防上尿路功能障碍，并可作为下尿路对上尿路构成危险的警告。此外，在这些女性中，尿失禁也可能是皮肤破裂、褥疮和伤口等并发症的危险因素。本章描述了女性神经源性尿失禁的原因、不同表现，其中包括尿流动力学研究、检查和治疗。

一、神经源性尿失禁的病因

女性神经源性尿失禁的病因可根据神经病变的位置进行分类。正常排尿反射涉及整个中枢神经系统的多个部位。这些包括脑桥排尿中心（脑干）、副交感神经和躯体骶排尿中心和胸腰椎交感神经的组成部分[5, 6]。

脑干上方的损伤影响大脑对排尿反射的抑制作用。这会导致逼尿肌过度活动，随后出现尿急、尿频和夜尿症[7]。此外，一些患者可能因非自愿排尿而出现尿失禁，因为他们能够感觉到逼尿肌的非自愿收缩并自愿收缩其横纹肌括约肌，但无法实际停止逼尿肌收缩[8]。

脑桥下方和骶脊髓上方的损伤中断了先前允许同时进行逼尿肌收缩和尿道括约肌松弛的路径。因此，这种中断导致逼尿肌括约肌协同失调，以及逼尿肌收缩和松弛与尿道括约肌收缩之间的不协调关系[9, 10]。换句话说，神经源性逼尿肌过度活动和未受抑制的膀胱收缩伴随着外括约肌的不协调收缩。非自愿逼尿肌收缩导致尿失禁，而不协调的括约肌收缩导致膀胱出口梗阻、尿潴留和潜在的高储存压力[11]。

骶神经损伤的表现形式可能不同，取决于神经束副交感神经、交感神经或躯体部分的损伤。对于导致副交感神经完全中断的损伤，这会导致逼尿肌无反射和尿潴留。尿潴留也可能导致溢流性尿失禁。导致交感神经损伤的损伤可表现为近端尿道功能不全引起的括约肌尿失禁。最后，影响阴部神经的躯体神经损伤导致会阴和肛周感觉丧失，以及球海绵体反射丧失，从而改变尿道和肛门括约肌的自愿收缩。后者可能表现为尿失禁和大便失禁，并导致固有括约肌缺陷。

躯体神经损伤的常见原因包括椎间盘突出、糖尿病、多发性硬化和骶骨肿瘤。此外，广泛的骨盆手术，如腹会阴直肠切除术和根治性子宫切除术，都是骶骨和体神经损伤的常见外科原因[8]。例如，对 ⅠB_1～ⅡB 期宫颈癌根治性子宫切除术后尿潴留需要泌尿外科干预的患者进行的一项研究显示，近 54% 的患者出现＞100ml 的空隙后残余[12]。

重要的是不要忘记，神经源性女性患者中遇到的慢性留置尿道导管可能会导致无功能性括约肌机制的侵蚀和扩张尿道，导致明显的尿失禁（图 24-1）[13]。此外，对于有盆腔辐射史、盆腔手术史或近期创伤性阴道分娩史的患者，还必须记住，即使在神经源性女性患者的情况下，尿瘘也可能发展并成为尿失禁的原因。

二、不同的临床表现

当神经源性下尿路功能障碍患者发生尿失禁时，可单独或联合归因于 3 种功能障碍之一。这些是逼尿肌过度活动、膀胱顺应性差和尿道括约肌 / 膀胱颈功能不全[11]。

- 逼尿肌过度活动引起的尿失禁，膀胱完全排空（平衡排尿），骶脊髓以上神经系统疾病的患者将出现逼尿肌过度活动，并导致急迫性尿失禁。流动性有限往往会加剧这种情况。尽管这些患者能够完全排空，但偶尔这些患者仅通过非自愿逼尿肌收缩排空，而不能通过意志排空，在这种情况下，可能需要使用间歇性清洁自我导尿（CIC）进行治疗，以使患者自制。这是治疗膀胱储能的附加疗法。
- 逼尿肌过度活动（DO）和（或）膀胱排空不完全顺应性差导致的尿失禁，脑桥排尿中心以下病变的患者通常有 DESD 逼尿肌过度活动。除了逼尿肌过度活动引起的尿失禁外，这些患者还经常出现排空不良（由于 DESD 引起的膀胱出口梗阻）。由于低容量或高膀胱存储压力下因顺应性差而发生的反射逼尿肌过度活动，它们的功能能力也低得多。
- 无张力膀胱伴括约肌功能不全或罕见膀胱排空伴清洁间歇性导尿引起的溢流性尿失禁。骶神经或周围神经损伤的患者通常有无张力膀胱，导致尿潴留，这是一种低存储压力；然而，如果这些女性括约肌功能不全或达到极限容量，她们仍可能出现渗漏。让他们更频繁地导尿通常是一个好的解决方案。
- 压力性尿失禁，一些患者的一个或多个尿括约肌有神经损伤。这些患者会出现不同程度的压力性尿失禁，有时会出现完全性尿失失禁，或者由于体位改变或腹内压增加而出现压力性尿失禁。一些患者也会因妊娠和分娩前尿道过度活动而出现压力性尿失禁。这些女性可能有较轻的压力性尿失禁，仅在腹内压增加时发生，类似于非神经源性女性的压力性尿失禁。

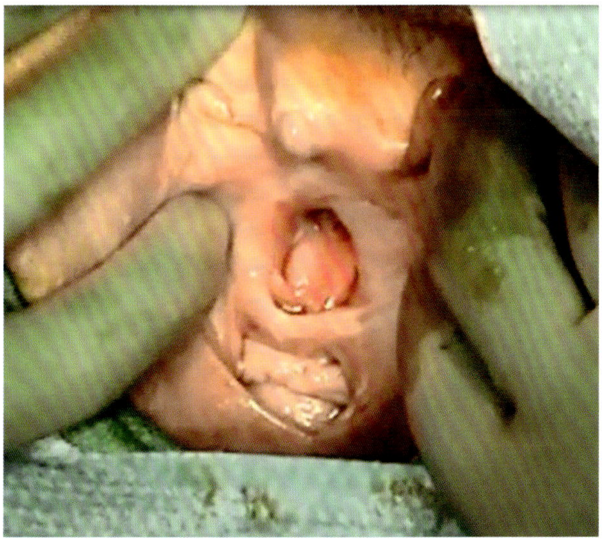

▲ **图 24-1　在 T_6 脊髓损伤（SCI）患者中，随着时间的推移，Foley 导管从 14F 逐渐增大至 24F，保留气囊从 10ml 增大至 30ml，尿道侵蚀逐渐发生。侵蚀是如此深刻；骨盆检查可见三角区。患者在尿道闭合时阴道入路失败，最终需要进行尿流改道**

图片由 Anne Cameron MD 提供

三、尿流动力学研究

由于肾损伤和最终肾功能衰竭的潜在无症状风险，尿流动力学是评估神经源性下尿路功能障碍患者的关键。这种类型的肾衰竭通常是由于膀胱内高压、膀胱顺应性差、膀胱输尿管反流、感染和（或）肾积水[11, 14]。除了评估潜在的上尿路损害外，尿流动力学还可用于评估症状的病因和直接治疗（有关尿流动力学的详细说明见第 4 章）。

（一）存储问题

填充过程中的低膀胱压力是防止上呼吸道损伤的关键。已发现逼尿肌泄漏点压力和> 40cmH_2O 的储存压力会使上段处于危险中[15]。此外，在充盈期间，还可以看到未受抑制的逼尿肌收缩，并可导致尿失禁。

在骶神经或周围神经损伤的患者中，可以看到固定的开放性尿括约肌，这可能导致尿失禁。慢性留置导管插入术也可能导致括约肌损伤，导致出口不畅和压力性尿失禁。在无逼尿肌收缩的情况下，Valsalva 泄漏点压力＜60cmH_2O 也可在神经源性患者中发现，并可识别固有括约肌缺陷[16]。

最后，膀胱顺应性可计算为膀胱顺应性异常时体积随逼尿肌压力变化的变化，一般认为小于 20ml/cmH_2O[16]。膀胱顺应性是一个重要的尿流动力学参数，因为顺应性异常是泌尿系统并发症的危险因素。

（二）排空问题

尿流动力学评估显示逼尿肌收缩力差、逼尿肌无力或括约肌协同失调，也可提供神经源性患者的信息，并帮助指导治疗。根据这些发现，通常会发现不完全排空和尿潴留。此外，对于女性而言，评估骨盆器官脱垂是否是尿道扭结导致排空不全的原因非常重要，即使是神经源性患者[16]。

（三）尿流动力学时间

在脊柱休克期结束后，约 90 天或检查时可诱发脊柱反射时，必须对所有新诊断的神经源性下尿路功能障碍患者进行基线尿流动力学研究[17]。通常，周期性尿流动力学与上尿路成像一起进行。然而，这是根据患者的症状和（或）上尿路或肾功能的变化而定制的[14, 18]。

四、安全检查

在对神经源性下尿路功能障碍患者进行常规泌尿外科护理之前，肾衰竭是最常见的死亡原因[19]。女性神经源性尿失禁的安全检查完全依赖于神经源性下尿路功能障碍管理原则。虽然在随访和监测的确切时间框架上没有共识，但公布的数据建议至少每 2 年，最多每 3～6 个月对非淋病患者进行常规泌尿外科护理[14, 18, 20]。随访应包括病史、体检和血清肌酐。然而，在肌肉质量较小的神经源性下尿路功能障碍患者中，血清肌酐可能不准确，并且在血清肌酐显著升高之前可能发生实质性肾功能丧失。在怀疑肾功能不全的情况下，可以进行功能性肾扫描，因为这是肾功能降低或梗阻的最敏感测试。胱抑素 C 虽然昂贵，但也可作为肾功能和 GFR 的替代和更准确的代表，因为它不受质量、年龄或性别的影响[21]。

就常规上尿路成像而言，大多数泌尿科医生认为肾脏超声是排除肾积水和评估肾结石疾病的充分成像。用于检测结石疾病的其他测试包括静脉肾盂造影或非对比 CT 检查，但这些测试会使患者显露于电离辐射[14, 20]。

如前所述，应在初始评估时（在任何此类脊柱休克期结束后）进行尿流动力学评估，随后的间隔由临床医生决定。神经源性患者的重要尿流动力学参数包括评估膀胱顺应性和逼尿肌泄漏点压力。较低的膀胱充盈压力对上尿路保护至关重要，＞40cmH_2O 的膀胱储存压力使患者有上尿路损伤的风险。此外，逼尿肌泄漏点压力＞40mmHg 也被证明是上尿路恶化的危险因素[15]。

由于缺乏显示实用性的质量数据，通常不推荐常规尿细胞学检查。虽然无症状菌尿在神经源性下尿路功能障碍患者中很常见，但除非在泌尿外科手术中，否则不应治疗[22]。

虽然历史数据显示，慢性留置导管脊髓损伤（SCI）患者膀胱癌的发病率较高[22]，但更新的研究表明，脊髓损伤患者膀胱癌风险显著降低，特别是随着间歇性导管插入术的出现。由于膀胱结石的高风险和导尿时间的延长是膀胱癌的危险因素，一些泌尿科医生将筛查膀胱镜作为常规泌尿科监测的一部分。然而，没有足够的证据支持无症状脊髓损伤患者的膀胱镜筛查膀胱癌。这些相同的原则可适用于所有神经源性下尿路功能障碍患者[14, 20]。

如果出现尿失禁、复发性尿路感染（UTI）、肉眼血尿或新的体征或症状，应尽早进行随访和进一步的尿路成像、膀胱镜检查或尿流动力学评估[14]。

五、膀胱治疗

逼尿肌过度活动（有或无尿失禁）和（或）膀胱顺应性差的患者可首先接受抗美沙林药物试验。常见的抗毒蕈碱药物，如氧丁宁、索利非那星和托特罗定，通过阻断位于膀胱平滑肌的毒蕈碱 M3 受体发挥作用。然而，鉴于与这些抗胆碱能药物相关的认知损害数据，针对膀胱 β_3 肾上腺素受体的新型抗胆碱能药更受青睐，但尚未获得 FDA 批准或在神经源性下尿路功能障碍患者中正式试验[24]，其中包括米拉贝格隆和 FDA 批准的最新药物维贝格隆[25, 26]。特别是在可能同时存在认知障碍问题的非淋病患者中，如多发性硬化症或帕金森病，较新的 β_3 肾上腺素受体靶向药物越来越多地被用作该人群的一线口服药物，而不是抗胆碱药。例如，在一项多发性硬化症患者的研究中，米拉贝格隆和去氨加压素的组合已被证明比单独使用索利非那星更能改善逼尿肌过度活动[27]。

对口服药物难治的神经源性下尿路功能障碍患者可以通过逼尿肌内注射肉毒杆菌毒素进行试验。最常用的是血清型肉毒杆菌毒素 A。肉毒杆菌毒素 A 通过抑制神经末梢突触前乙酰胆碱的释放，从而降低毒蕈碱受体活化[28]。这导致膀胱容量改善和逼尿肌过度活动减少，临床上改善了尿失禁发作。在美国市场上可买到肉毒杆菌毒素 A，研究使用了 200U 注射和 300U 注射治疗神经源性下尿路功能障碍患者[28]。自愿排尿的患者必须告知尿潴留的风险。对于导管插入术的患者，200U 是最佳起始剂量，因为不考虑滞留，而对于排尿患者，100U 更合适，不太可能导致滞留。在断奶有效后，增加膀胱成形术或增加剂量的情况下，可以增加注射频率，最多每 3 个月 1 次（图 24–2）

特别是对于多发性硬化症患者和其他保留排尿的神经源性下尿路功能障碍患者，还研究了骶神经调节对尿潴留和逼尿肌过度活动的影响[23, 29]。新一代骶神经刺激器现在与 MRI 兼容，因为 MRI 对于许多此类疾病的神经随访至关重要。

神经源性下尿路功能障碍患者低膀胱容量 / 顺应性的膀胱扩大成形术，需要将一小部分去管小肠或结肠缝合到广泛开放的膀胱中，以增加总尿量。这反过来减轻了任何高逼尿肌填充压力，并有助于防止泄漏和增加总膀胱容量。在经过适当治疗的神经源性下尿路功能障碍患者中，这可能是另一种有助于控制尿失禁和整个膀胱的选择，也可能是年轻患者的早期选择，因为预计会有无数次肉毒杆菌毒素注射，他们可能希望有更明确的选择，或在导尿方面有困难，需要构建导尿通道[23]。本程序的完整描述见第 12 章。

六、出口的处理

对于患有尿失禁的女性神经源性下尿路功能障碍患者，通常需要对出口进行治疗，并且存在多种选择。选择包括耻骨阴道吊带、膀胱颈重建、尿道填塞剂、人工尿道括约肌（AUS）和尿流改道。

对于尿道扩张或固有括约肌缺陷的女性神经源性下尿路功能障碍患者，自体筋膜耻骨阴道吊带是具有高疗效和低发病率的最佳手术选择之一。患者可以通过耻骨阴道吊带轻松进行间歇性清洁自我导尿（CIC），无须担心中尿道吊带存在的网状腐蚀。患有括约肌功能障碍的神经源性女性似乎与非神经源性女性具有相似的结果[30]。一项对 33 例患有脊髓脊膜膨出或脊髓损伤和括约肌功能障碍的女性患者的研究显示，放置耻骨阴道吊带后，25 例患者完全干燥，5 例患者明显改善[31]。虽然存在合成网的选择，但自体筋膜耻骨阴道吊带可能更适合需要每日间断导尿的神经源性下尿路功能障碍患者。

膀胱颈重建是患有括约肌功能障碍的女性神经源性下尿路功能障碍患者的另一种选择。有几种技术的主要目的是增加膀胱出口阻力[30]。在女性神经源性下尿路功能障碍患者中，由于长期留置尿道导管导致尿道破坏性扩张，由于残余尿道组织不足以重建或允许使用耻骨阴道吊带，可能需要膀胱颈闭合。如果患者需要节制并具有良好的手动灵活性，则同时创建使用阑尾或回肠的大陆导管造口，以允许膀胱引流。否则，同时放置耻骨上管[32, 33]。膀胱颈闭合的方法可以是经阴道或耻骨后。一项对 64 例接受膀胱颈闭合术和耻骨上导管置入术的女性的研究表明，两种方法在实现尿道自控方面没有显著差异。然而，经阴道组

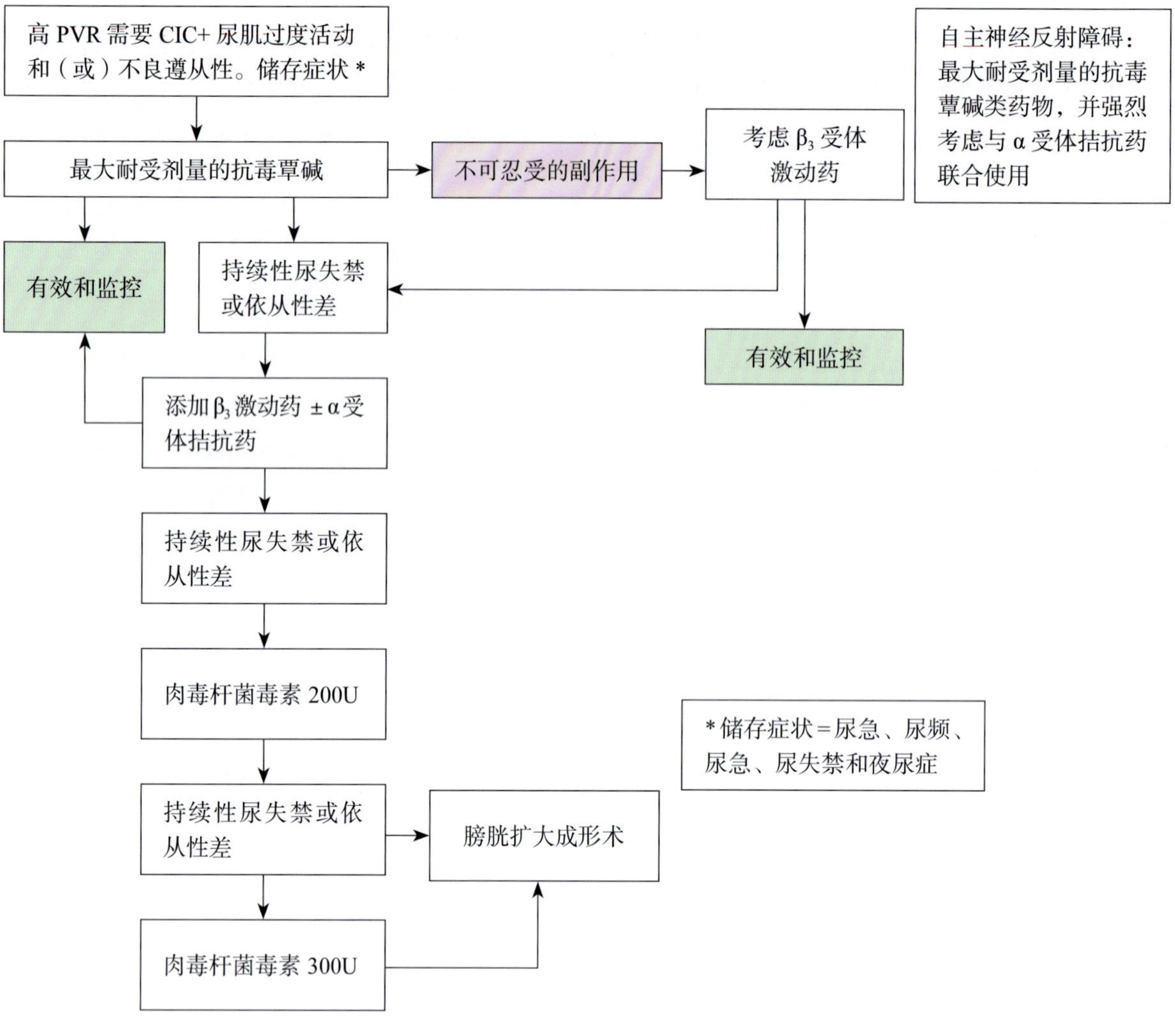

▲ 图 24-2　**NLUTD 患者膀胱顺应性差或神经源性逼尿肌过度活动的治疗流程**

的平均手术时间、住院时间和短期并发症明显缩短[34]。有关本程序的详细信息见第 13 章。

注射尿道填充术可以在门诊进行，无须全身麻醉，发病率最低。然而，它们对严重压力性尿失禁患者无效。填充剂通过膀胱镜经尿道周围或尿道内注射。由于其侵袭性最小，尿道内填塞剂是经济困难患者的一个不错的选择。以下是目前市场上 4 种 FDA 批准的药物：硅微粒（Macroplastique®）、热解碳涂层氧化锆珠（Durasphere®）、羟基磷灰石钙（Coaptite®）和聚丙烯酰胺水凝胶（Bulkamid®）[16]。大多数膨胀剂文献涉及固有括约肌缺陷人群，属于儿童神经源性下尿路功能障碍人群。然而，在一项成人研究中，它已被用作耻骨阴道吊带术后持续性低压尿失禁的辅助手术。8 年的长期随访显示，尽管重复注射，27 例患者中只有 2 例患者是大陆患者。尽管成功率较低，但由于其他出口程序失败后并发症发生率较低，填充剂可作为有用的选择[30]。

虽然在美国，在女性体内植入人工尿道括约肌（AUS）未经 FDA 批准，但法国等欧洲国家建议在先天性括约肌缺陷的女性体内植入人工尿道括约肌。在女性神经源性下尿路功能障碍患者群体中，人工尿道括约肌安置仅适用于具有良好手动灵活性且通常不需要导管插入术的患者。一项此类研究表明，女性神经源性压力性尿失禁的感染率和侵蚀率较低，结果令人满意[35]。

七、尿流改道补救治疗

对于膀胱顺应性差和（或）持续性尿失禁的患者，如保守治疗无效或严重并发症，如尿道糜烂或无法修复的瘘管，可能需要使用尿流改道进行补救治疗。对于上肢功能有限、认知障碍或肾功能差的患者，回肠导管是最佳选择。对于肾功能良好、手部灵巧的患者来说，大陆转移术（如印第安纳袋）是一个很好的选择。印第安纳袋对于膀胱出口受损的患者来说是一个特别好的选择。

手术时，可进行简单的膀胱切除术或 Spence-Allen 手术（医源性膀胱阴道瘘）以预防脓囊炎。

总结

虽然大多数神经源性下尿路功能障碍的治疗与性别无关，但女性神经源性尿失禁的治疗可能与男性不同。根据解剖结构，耻骨阴道吊带等治疗方法通常更适合女性神经源性下尿路功能障碍患者。此外，评估这些女性排尿功能障碍的其他非神经源性原因，如盆腔器官脱垂或尿瘘，也是至关重要的。了解神经源性下尿路功能障碍患者，特别是女性神经源性下尿路功能障碍患者的独特检查和管理，对于在该人群中提供出色的泌尿外科护理至关重要。

参考文献

[1] Clanet B. Management of multiple sclerosis patients. Curr Opin Neurol. 2000;13:263–70.

[2] Hicken BL, Putzke JD, et al. Bladder management and quality of life after spinal cord injury. Am J Phys Med Rehabil. 2001;80:916–22.

[3] Westgren N, Levi R. Quality of life and traumatic spinal cord injury. Arch Phys Med Rehabil. 1998;79:1433–9.

[4] Tang DH, Colayco D, Piercy J, et al. Impact of urinary incontinence on health-related quality of life, daily activities, and healthcare resource utilization in patients with neurogenic detrusor overactivity. BMC Neurol. 2014;14:74. https://doi.org/10.1186/1471-2377- 14- 74.

[5] Blaivas JG. The neurophyisiology of micturition: a clinical study of 550 patients. J Urol. 1982;127:958.

[6] Unger CA, Tunitsky-Bitton E, Muffly T, et al. Neuroanatomy, neurophysiology and dysfunction of the female lower urinary tract: a review. Female Pelvic Med Reconstr Surg. 2014;20(2):65–75. https://doi.org/10.1097/spv.0000000000000058.

[7] Abrams P, Cardozo L, Fall M, et al. The standardization of terminology of lower urinary tract function: report from the standardization subcommittee of the international continence society. Neurol Urodyn. 2002;21:167–78.

[8] Blaivas JG, Chancellor M, Weiss J, Verhaaren M. Atlas of Urodynamics. 2nd ed. Blackwell Publishing; 2007.

[9] Wein A. Lower urinary tract dysfunction in neurologic injury and disease. In: Wein A, Kavoussi L, Novick A, et al., editors. Campbell-Walsh urology. New York: Saunders; 2007. p. 2011–45.

[10] Chancellor M, Blaivas J. Spinal cord injury. In: Chancellor M, Blaivas J, editors. Practical neurourology. Boston: Butterworth-Heinemann; 1995. p. 99–118.

[11] Nitti VW. Evaluation of the female with neurogenic voiding dysfunction. Int Urogynecol J. 1999;10:119–29. https://doi.org/10.1007/s001920050031.

[12] Komatsu H, et al. Long-term evaluation of renal function and neurogenic bladder following radical hysterectomy in patients with uterine cervical cancer. J Obstet Gynaecol Res. 2020;46(10):2108–14. https://doi.org/10.1111/job/14394.

[13] Chancellor MB, Erhard MJ, Kiiholma PJ, et al. Functional urethral closure with pubovaginal sling for destroyed female urethra after long-term urethral catheterization. Urology. 1994;43:499–505. https://doi.org/10.1016/0090-4295(94)90241-0.

[14] Kreydin E, Welk B, Chung D, et al. Surveillance and management of urologic complications after spinal cord injury. World J Urol. 2018;36:1545–53.

[15] McGuire EJ, Woodside JR, Borden TA. Prognostic value of urodynamic testing in myelodysplasia patients. J Urol. 1981;126:205–9.

[16] Cameron AP, Gupta P. Surgery for female stress urinary incontinence. AUA Core Curriculum; 2021.

[17] Danfort TL, Ginsberg DA. Neurogenic lower urinary tract dysfunction: how, when and with which patients do we use urodynamics? Urol Clin North Am. 2014;41(3):445–52.

[18] Consortium for Spinal Cord Medicine. Bladder management for adults with spinal cord injury: a clinical practice guideline. Washington, DC: Paralyzed Veterans of America; 2016. Urologic evaluation. p. 16–7.

[19] Greenwell MW, et al. Kidney disease as a predictor of mortality in chronic spinal cord injury. Am J Kidney Dis. 2007;49(3):383–93.

[20] Cameron AP, Rodriguez GM, Schomer KG. Systematic review of urological followup after spinal cord injury. J Urol. 2012;187(2):391–7.

[21] Dharnidharka VR, Kwon C, Stevens G. Serum cystatin C is superior to serum creatinine as a marker of kidney function: a meta-analysis. Am J Kidney Dis. 2002;40(2):221–6.

[22] Broecker BH, Klein FA, Hackler RA. Cancer of the bladder in spinal cord injury patients. J Urol. 1981;125(2):196–7.

[23] Barboglio Romo PG, Cameron AP. Neurogenic lower urinary tract dysfunction. AUA Core Curriculum; 2021.

[24] Welk B, McArther E. Increased risk of dementia among patients with overactive bladder treated with an anticholinergic medication compared to a beta-3 agonist: a population-based cohort study. BJU Int. 2020;126(10):183–90. https://doi.org/10.1111/bju.15040.

[25] Nitti VW, et al. Results of a randomized phase III trial of mirabegraon in patients with overactive bladder. J Urol. 2013;189:1388–95.

[26] Staskin D, Frankel J, Varano S, et al. International phase III, randomized, double-blind, placebo and active controlled study to evaluate the safety and efficacy of Vibegron in patients with symptoms of overactive bladder: EMPOWUR. J Urol. 2020;204(2):316–24.

[27] Zachariou A, Filiponi M, Baltogiannis D, et al. Effective treatment of neurogenic detrusor overactivity in multiple sclerosis patients using desmopressin and mirabegron. Can J Urol. 2017;24:9107–13.

[28] Ginsberg D, Gousse A, Keppenne V, Sievert KD, et al. Phase 3 efficacy and tolerability study of onobotulinumtoxin a for urinary incontinence

from neurogenic detrusor overactivity. J Urol. 2021;187(6):2131–9.
[29] Engeler DS, Meyer D, Abt D, Muller S, et al. Sacral neuromodulation for the treatment of neurogenic lower urinary tract dysfunction caused by multiple sclerosis: a single-centre prospective series. BMC Urol. 2015;15:105. https://doi.org/10.1186/s12894–015– 0102– x.
[30] Myers JB, Mayer EN, Lenherr S, et al. Management options for sphincteric deficiency in adults with neurogenic bladder. Transl Androl Urol. 2016;5(1):145–57. https://doi.org/10.3978/j. issn.2223–4683.2015.12.11.
[31] Athanasopoulos A, Gyftopoulos K, McGuire EJ. Treating stress urinary incontinence in female patients with neuropathic bladder: the value of autologous fascia rectus sling. Int Urol Nephrol. 2012;44:1363–7.
[32] Chancellor MB, et al. Functional urethral closure with pubovaginal sling for destroyed female urethra after long-term urethral catheterization. Urology. 1994;43(4):499–505.
[33] Zimmern PE, et al. Transvaginal closure of the bladder neck and placement of a suprapubic catheter for destroyed urethra after long-term indwelling catheterization. J Urol. 1985;134(3):554–7.
[34] Willis H, Safiano N, Lloyd LK. Comparison of transvaginal and retropubic bladder neck closure with suprapubic catheter in women. J Urol. 2015;193(1):196–02. https://doi.org/10.1016/j. juro.2014.07.091.
[35] Peyronnet B, Greenwell T, Gray G, et al. Current use of the artificial urinary sphincter in adult females. Curr Urol Rep. 2020;21:53. https://doi.org/10.1007/s11934–020– 01001– 1.

第 25 章　老年性尿失禁

Urinary Incontinence in the Elderly

Casey G. Kowalik　Lara S. MacLachlan　著

尿失禁的患病率随着年龄的增长而增加，影响多达 30% 的 60 岁以上的女性[1]。随着人口老龄化，患尿失禁的女性人数将会增加。除第 3 章提到的评估标准外，了解老年人提出的需要解决的特殊情况也至关重要。老年人尿失禁的发病率与入住疗养院呈独立且显著相关性[2]。至关重要的是，不仅要了解患者的病情，而且要综合考虑所有的并发症、困扰程度、护理目标以及所有的护理人员。此外，衰弱程度与不良结果相关，与之相比，年龄本身可能并不重要。随着年龄的增长，身体会愈加衰弱，因为衰弱与患者的护理有关，所以这个概念显得越来越重要。例如，一个健壮的 75 岁女性和一个衰弱的 65 岁女性会有不同的注意事项。同样需要强调尿失禁是一种慢性疾病，治疗的目标是改善症状和生活质量，而不一定是治愈尿失禁。

一、老年性尿失禁的相关因素

女性尿失禁的发生在很大程度上是多因素造成的，但其中许多因素在老年人中更常见。首先，年龄本身就是下尿路功能障碍的危险因素（表 25-1）。随着年龄的增长及其他合并症的影响，会发生很多解剖、生理、代谢和激素变化。在对没有神经系统疾病、盆腔手术史或糖尿病病史的健康女性进行的研究中，随着年龄增长，逼尿肌收缩力、膀胱充盈感和最大尿道闭合压（MUCP）都会下降[3, 4]。一项与年龄相关的尿流动力学变化的研究发现，年龄与尿流率减慢、膀胱容量降低和排尿后残余尿增加有关[5]。研究膀胱功能正常的患者逼尿肌 M 受体发现，M3 受体的 mRNA 表达随年龄增长而降低，这可以解释逼尿肌收缩能力随年龄增长而降低的原因[6]。膀胱收缩功能减弱会导致残余尿量增多，从而导致充溢性尿失禁。此外，排空不全和最大尿道闭合压降低可能会加重压力性尿失禁（SUI）的症状。

表 25-1　年龄对下尿路的影响

- 膀胱收缩性降低[3, 6]
- 膀胱容量减少[5]
- 最大尿道闭合压降低[3, 4]
- 尿流率降低[5]
- 残余尿增加[5]

除了下尿路病变，可能还有其他因素会增加老年人尿失禁的可能性[7]。一些合并症会加重尿失禁。例如，任何伴有慢性咳嗽的情况（如肺气肿），都会加重压力性尿失禁症状。导致多尿的疾病，如糖尿病、尿崩症、利尿药的使用或原发性烦渴，都会导致多尿，并可能加剧尿失禁。充血性心力衰竭、静脉机能不全和肾病综合征等疾病会导致外周水肿。当睡眠期仰卧时，这些潴留在外周组织中的液体会回流至循环系统中，并可能导致夜尿增多。导致认知障碍的疾病，如阿尔茨海默病或谵妄，可能会由于缺乏如厕意识或动力而导致尿失禁增加。在认知障碍的患者中，即便使用已经验证过有效的调查问卷，其调查结果也是无效的。严重便秘多见于老年女性，可导致排尿功能障碍。泌尿生殖器萎缩最有可能导致阴道干燥和灼热的症状，但也可能出现泌尿系统症状，包括更年期的泌尿生殖系统综合征，阴道雌激素治疗有助于缓解症状[8]。

多药联用是另一个影响老年人的主要问题，因为许多药物可以改变下尿路功能，因此可能会对控制排尿有影响。例如，α受体拮抗药与可逆性压力性尿失禁的病因有关[9]。其他药物，如利尿药，可能会增加尿液的产生。不仅是药物本身会影响泌尿系统症状，药物的不良反应也可能产生影响。血管紧张素转换酶抑制药可能会引起咳嗽并增加尿失禁。许多药物会导致口干，这可能会导致液体摄入量增加或便秘加重，这两种不良反应都有导致尿失禁的倾向。多药联用可能对尿失禁有额外的药物治疗效果，但是却可能导致出现一种复杂的情况，虽然多药联用可以治疗尿失禁症状，但是却会因为多药联用的副作用（便秘）反而会加重尿失禁的症状。

评估老年女性的活动能力和手部灵活性很重要，因为二者都会造成与膀胱无关的功能性尿失禁或漏尿。可以理解，如果有尿急和尿失禁的女性需要较长时间到达厕所，则发生尿失禁的可能性增加。有时需要他人帮助去厕所，导致患者依赖他人才能避免尿便失禁。活动能力的评估可以用计时测试（TUG）等正式的评估方法，测量从椅子中站起来、走3m、坐回椅子的时间（计秒数），这是一种经过验证的虚弱程度的衡量标准[10]。一种非正式的测量方法可以是观察患者从椅子上移到检查台上的能力。通过确保如厕通道便捷或拓宽厕所入口可改善行动不便的问题；若手的灵活性差导致脱衣服时间长，可以穿着没有纽扣的衣服。

图25-1是强调这些问题交织复杂性的示意图。

二、老年女性的一般治疗注意事项

在老年女性中，压力性尿失禁和急迫性尿失禁的治疗方案与年轻女性相同，但还有其他需要考虑的因素，如表25-2所示。

患有尿失禁的老年女性患盆底疾病的风险增加，如盆腔器官脱垂或大便失禁[11]。人们普遍认为，这些疾病的病理生理学具有共同的起源，有如遗传、年龄、种族、绝经等内在因素，也有如分娩史、盆底手术史、合并症和肥胖等外在危险因素[12, 13]。对这些因素进行评估是非常重要的，因为它们的存在可能会改变您的治疗建议。例如，对患有尿失禁和大便失禁的女性来说，骶神经调节（SNS）可能同时治疗两者，患者可以从中获得更多潜在益处。盆腔器官脱垂和膀胱功能障碍之间的关系是复杂的，脱垂的程度和尿便失禁之间可能存在关联[14]。在这些患者中，通过非手术或手术纠正脱垂可能会改善尿便失禁症状。

衰弱是一种以脆弱性增加为特征的综合征。

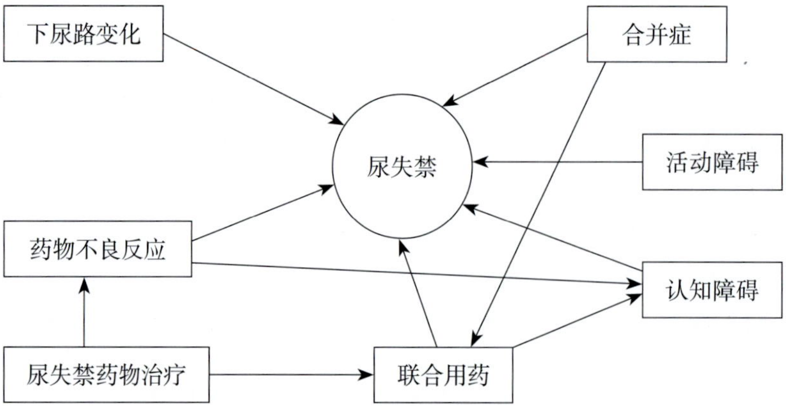

▲ 图25-1　分析与衰弱和尿失禁相关的复杂的相互作用

表 25-2 老年尿失禁患者的特殊注意事项

	评估选项
活动性	"洗手间在同一层楼吗，还是要上楼/下楼？" 计时测试，观察转移至检查台
衰弱	Fried 衰弱评估量表、计时测量
护理人员的参与	"谁帮助照顾？自理？" "你的护理人员多久能来一次"
认知	小型精神状态考试
跌倒预防	"去洗手间的路上有障碍物吗"（如地毯、楼梯）
联合用药	审查药物清单
合并症	评估每种可能导致尿失禁的原因
原发性睡眠障碍	转诊接受正式的睡眠评估
合并盆底功能障碍	体检盆腔器官脱垂，询问大便失禁情况："你曾经不小心漏出大便吗？"

衰弱与手术并发症风险增加、住院时间延长及出院到护理机构的可能性相关[15]。目前，尚无筛查和评估衰弱程度的标准方法，但有几种评估工具，如 Fried 衰弱评估量表、步态速度（如计时测试）或握力[16, 17]。衰弱与尿失禁的作用是双重的，因为盆底疾病与衰弱有关，衰弱的存在会影响治疗的选择和结局。

如果要推荐药物治疗，需注意治疗膀胱过度活动症药物与当前的药物清单之间的相互作用。例如，服用抗胆碱能药物会增加已经在服用其他抗胆碱能药物患者的抗胆碱能负担，理论上可能会增加患痴呆症的风险[18]。此外，抗胆碱能药物与跌倒风险的增加有关。

尿失禁可导致外阴皮肤破裂和皮炎，久坐（卧）导致活动能力下降，可能加剧皮肤问题。通过改善尿失禁、保持皮肤干燥、使用润肤剂隔离尿液和皮肤，可以最大限度地减少尿失禁对皮肤造成的损害。在特殊情况下，可能需要导尿，避免尿液浸湿伤口。

三、急迫性尿失禁的治疗

（一）一线治疗：行为调节

行为调节通常是治疗老年急迫性尿失禁的主要方法，对于需要在协助下进行自我护理的、存在认知和身体障碍的人，针对障碍的不同程度进行个体化治疗。

为了减少尿失禁的发生，许多老年患者自诉限制了液体的摄入。尽管违背既往认知，但一项小型随机对照试验表明，摄入充足的水分在尿失禁的治疗中是有效的[19]。老年女性被随机分为三组：分别是液体摄入量增加到 500ml，液体摄入量维持在基线水平或液体摄入量减少 300ml。尽管对液体摄取方案的依从性很差，但是在后续的随访数据显示，尿失禁症状减少的女性患者认为，增加液体的摄入量是主要的因素。

除了液体管理外，包括提示排尿技术和习惯再训练的如厕治疗计划也可用于改善急迫性尿失禁。提示个人如厕旨在增加患者对如厕和自发如厕的要求，从而减少急迫性尿失禁发作次数。当护理人员遵守协议时，对于疗养院居民和家庭护理客户来说，这是一种日间急迫性尿失禁的有效短期治疗[20]。习惯再训练首先需要确定个人的基线排尿模式与尿失禁发作节点。一旦建立了基线排尿模式，就可以创建新的排尿时间表来预防急迫性尿失禁发作。

盆底肌肉训练（PFMT）是指有意收缩盆底肌肉，抑制逼尿肌过度活动，加强尿道支持的锻炼方法。有关使用盆底肌肉训练治疗老年人急迫性尿失禁的研究表明，盆底肌肉训练可减少急迫性尿失禁发作次数，提高患者满意度[21]。行为调节疗法通常可以采取包括所有上述技术要素的综合方法。事实上，对居住在社区的老年女性进行的研究表明，包括盆底肌肉训练、习惯再训练和生活方式改变在内的行为调节的综合方法可以改善急迫性尿失禁[22]。

虽然行为调节是老年人急迫性尿失禁的有效治疗方法，但该方法需要根据个人的能力和残疾情况进行个体化设计。有认知障碍的老年患者可能需要其护理人员积极参与，以促进及时排尿或协助液体管理。功能受限的老年患者如果不能安全地转移到厕所，可能会难以如厕。为了通过行为疗法取得成功，我们必须牢记，一刀切的方法无法满足老年患者的多样化需求。

（二）二线治疗：药物治疗

药物治疗被认为是急迫性尿失禁的二线治疗方法，但由于药物治疗依从性差、联合用药和不良反应风险增加，老年人群的药物治疗面临挑战（图 25–1）。在综合评估和适当行为疗法试验后，可考虑对老年人群进行药物治疗。事实上，有人提出，对适合药物治疗的老年人的药物治疗未得到充分利用。一项针对美国疗养院居民的研究发现，只有 7% 的符合条件的居民接受了药物治疗尿失禁 [23]。

急迫性尿失禁的药物治疗包括抗毒蕈碱药和 $β_3$ 肾上腺素受体激动药。已有充分的研究证明奥昔布宁可以有效地减少老年人急迫性尿失禁发作。然而，因其已知的急性认知障碍风险，故不宜在老年人群中使用 [24, 25]。由于避免了首过效应，使用奥昔布宁的经皮制剂可能更适合老年人，这将减少其不良反应 [26]。非索罗定也在老年人群中进行了充分的研究，与年轻人群相比，具有良好的疗效和类似的不良反应 [27, 28]。曲司氯铵是唯一一种具有季胺结构的抗毒蕈碱药物，而其他的均为叔胺，具有亲水性，因此不太可能穿过血脑屏障并对中枢神经系统产生影响（如影响认知障碍）[26]。一项随机对照试验表明，与安慰剂相比，服用曲司氯铵的 50 岁以上女性的认知功能没有变化 [29]。在所有抗毒蕈碱药物中，曲司氯铵具有独特的化学结构，可能是老年急迫性尿失禁患者的首选。米拉贝隆是目前市场上唯一获批的 $β_3$ 肾上腺素受体激动药，但关于其在老年人群中的应用，目前公开数据很少；而其不良反应较轻，所以，综合分析，对于那些没有禁忌证（不受控制的 HTN 或药物相互作用）的患者来说，它可能是更好的首选。

虽然药物治疗可以成功改善老年人的急迫性尿失禁，但我们必须权衡这一弱势人群的潜在不良反应。减轻这些不良反应至关重要。例如，便秘作为抗毒蕈碱药的不良反应最终可能加重尿失禁，导致症状没有显著改善。研究表明，抗毒蕈碱药物累积使用越多，痴呆风险越高 [18, 30]。AUA/SUFU 关于膀胱过度活动症的指南建议，考虑到认知障碍的风险，在给虚弱的老年患者开药时要谨慎。对于那些在接受抗毒蕈碱药物治疗之前有认知障碍风险的患者，建议用简易精神状态检查对患者认知功能进行基线评估，以评估其导致认知能力进一步下降的风险 [31]。在给老年人开药之前要考虑的其他因素是与年龄相关的变化，这些变化可能会影响药物的药代动力学和代谢。随着年龄的增长，胃排空缓慢，可能会降低药物的吸收。此外，老年患者的血清白蛋白可能会降低，从而导致血浆游离药物水平升高 [32]。鉴于急迫性尿失禁药物治疗的风险，建议对老年人进行药物治疗时积极主动、密切监测。

（三）三线治疗：逼尿肌内注射肉毒杆菌毒素 A 和神经调节

对于一线和二线治疗方法无效的患者，AUA/SUFU 指南建议考虑三线治疗，如逼尿肌内注射肉毒杆菌毒素 A（BoNT-A）、胫后神经刺激（PTNS）或骶神经调节。

肉毒杆菌毒素 A 对于一、二线治疗无效的老年患者，经过仔细选择和充分咨询的情况下，可以选择进行肉毒杆菌毒素 A 注射。一项研究表明，接受肉毒杆菌毒素 A 注射的老年患者和年轻患者在减少平均每日急迫性尿失禁发作方面没有差异。然而，老年患者有较高的尿路感染率 [33]。另一项研究调查将肉毒杆菌毒素 A 注射分为三组：虚弱的老年患者、不虚弱的老年患者和年轻患者。结果显示，在注射肉毒杆菌毒素 A 3 个月和 6 个月后，三组的成功率相似。然而，虚弱的老年人组在 12 个月时的长期成功率显著降低。此外，虚弱的老年组的残余尿量增加，尿潴留患者恢复自主排尿的速度较慢[34]。

指南建议胫后神经刺激适用于因药物的潜在不良反应或费用因素不愿意接受药物治疗的患者，因为它本质上是微创且可逆的[31]。一项关于胫后神经刺激对老年人群有效性的回顾性研究表明，主观成功率为 70%，与已发表的胫后神经刺激对年轻人群的成功率相当[35]。老年人接受胫后神经刺激治疗的潜在障碍之一是需要每周进行 30min 的治疗，持续 12 周，然后每月进行 1 次维持治疗。这一要求可能会给那些需要他人协助交通的老年患者进行预约带来问题。

骶神经调节对于精心挑选的老年患者，如果备选方案为手术，可以考虑采用骶骨神经调节治疗难治性急迫性尿失禁。既往研究报道，与年轻患者相比，老年患者接受骶神经调节的成功率较低[36, 37]。然而，最近一项关于年龄对骶神经调节结局影响的研究对现有文献提出了挑战。这项特定研究表明，与年轻患者相比，老年患者对骶神经调节测试刺激试验的反应或置入率没有差异[38]。在考虑使用骶神经调节治疗老年人急迫性尿失禁时，需要考虑的一个重要因素是患者的认知状态和操作神经刺激器设备的能力，因为对该设备的了解不足是该疗法的禁忌证，如果误用将会无效。

四、压力性尿失禁的治疗

（一）非手术治疗方案

盆底肌肉训练可改善盆底肌肉力量、耐力和爆发力，是女性压力性尿失禁的常用治疗方法。盆底肌肉训练已被充分研究，并已被证明可以治愈或改善所有年龄组的压力性尿失禁[39]。特别是在老年人群中，有研究表明盆底肌肉训练可显著改善压力性尿失禁症状[40, 41]。

对于倾向于非手术干预的老年压力性尿失禁患者，子宫托是一种非手术选择。阴道子宫托是最古老的医疗器械之一，几个世纪以来一直用于治疗盆腔器官脱垂。最近，阴道子宫托已被重新设计为用于治疗压力性尿失禁的尿失禁子宫托。它们旨在支撑尿道和膀胱壁，增加尿道长度，并提供尿道对耻骨的轻微压迫[42]。一项对使用子宫托治疗压力性尿失禁女性的回顾性研究表明，59% 女性的尿失禁完全缓解或减少，且高龄并不影响治疗的成功率[43]。使用子宫托的常见并发症包括阴道分泌物增多（有或无异味），新发排尿困难和尿失禁。阴道糜烂是一种罕见的并发症，通常可用外用局部雌激素乳膏治疗，同时摘除子宫托，然后重新安装子宫托。子宫托确实需要定期摘除并检查阴道上皮，因此对于那些不太可能随访的患者来说，子宫托不是一个可行的选择。

（二）手术治疗方案

注射尿道填充剂是压力性尿失禁的一种微创治疗方法，对于不适合手术的老年患者来说，这是一种选择。将填充剂注射到尿道黏膜下层，可提升尿道黏膜贴合程度，从而增加尿道阻力并改善控尿能力。一项 Meta 分析评估了填充剂在所有年龄组中的疗效和有效性，结果显示，在随访>12 个月的女性中，综合客观治疗成功率为 46%[44]。然而，对接受尿道填充剂注射治疗的老年患者的研究报告称显示，客观成功率为 73.2%～77%[45, 46]。潜在并发症包括尿潴留、尿路感染和尿失禁加重。并发症发生率很低，据报道为 0%～5.7%[44, 45]。鉴于在老年患者中观察到的高成功率和低不良事件发生率，注射尿道填充剂可以被认为是老年患者手术的有效替代方法，并且在操作前不需要麻醉或停止任何药物治疗。

外科手术治疗压力性尿失禁在老年女性中更为常见，与年轻女性相比，近期老年女性的压力性尿失禁手术显著增加[47]。在过去的 20 年里，已经从阴道悬吊术和耻骨阴道（自体筋膜）悬吊术转变为更微创的尿道中段悬吊术。在老年人群中，阴道悬吊术和耻骨阴道悬吊术可能不如年轻人群那么成功。压力性尿失禁手术治疗效果试验（SISTEr）比较了 Burch 膀胱尿道悬吊术与耻骨阴道悬吊术，结果显示，与年轻患者相比，老年女性在随访时压力测试阳性可能性更大，压力性尿失禁的主观改善较少[48]。两组术后的不良事件无差异，但老年女性需要再次手术的可能性较高。

尿道中段悬吊术的微创性增加了女性（尤其是老年女性）接受手术治疗压力性尿失禁的患者数量。对老年患者行尿道中段悬吊术的疗效进行研究，结果表明老年组和青年组之间的主观治愈率没有显著差异[49]。然而，多项研究表明老年患者围术期并发症增加，如住院时间延长、短期排尿困难发生率增加、再次入院率增加、复发性尿路感染增加以及新发膀胱过度活动症发生率增加[49-51]。总之，与年轻女性相比，老年女性尿道中段悬吊术的结局相似，但相关发病率更高。在进行尿道中段悬吊手术之前，需要根据个人情况仔细权衡风险和潜在益处。

总结

有必要继续为老年尿失禁患者制订个性化的临床护理途路径，以便在该人群的决策中获得所有额外的诊断和治疗考虑因素。关于老年尿失禁女性的理想治疗，以及不同治疗方案对该人群特定因素（如认知、护理人员）的影响，仍有许多悬而未决的问题。因此，有必要在这一领域进行进一步的研究，以减轻这一弱势群体的尿失禁造成的负担。

参考文献

[1] Hunskaar S, Lose G, Sykes D, Voss S. The prevalence of urinary incontinence in women in four European countries. BJU Int. 2004;93(3):324–30.
[2] Andel R, Hyer K, Slack A. Risk factors for nursing home placement in older adults with and without dementia. J Aging Health. 2007;19(2):213–28.
[3] Pfisterer MH-D, Griffiths DJ, PhD WS, Resnick NM. The effect of age on lower urinary tract function: a study in women. J Am Geriatr Soc. 2006;54(3):405–12.
[4] Trowbridge ER, Wei JT, Fenner DE, Ashton-Miller JA, DeLancey JOL. Effects of aging on lower urinary tract and pelvic floor function in nulliparous women. Obstet Gynecol. 2007;109(3):715–20.
[5] Madersbacher S, Pycha A, Schatzl G, Mian C, Klingler CH, Marberger M. The aging lower urinary tract: a comparative urodynamic study of men and women. Urology. 1998;51(2):206–12.
[6] Mansfield KJ, Liu L, Mitchelson FJ, Moore KH, Millard RJ, Burcher E. Muscarinic receptor subtypes in human bladder detrusor and mucosa, studied by radioligand binding and quantitative competitive RT–PCR: changes in ageing. Br J Pharmacol. 2005;144(8):1089–99.
[7] Wu JM, Vaughan CP, Goode PS, Redden DT, Burgio KL, Richter HE, et al. Prevalence and trends of symptomatic pelvic floor disorders in U.S. women. Obstet Gynecol. 2014;123(1):141–8.
[8] Gandhi J, Chen A, Dagur G, Suh Y, Smith N, Cali B, et al. Genitourinary syndrome of menopause: an overview of clinical manifestations, pathophysiology, etiology, evaluation, and management. Am J Obstet Gynecol. 2016;215(6):704–11.
[9] Marshall HJ, Beevers DG. α-Adrenoceptor blocking drugs and female urinary incontinence: prevalence and reversibility. Br J Clin Pharmacol. 1996;42(4):507–9.
[10] Ansai JH, Farche ACS, Rossi PG, de Andrade LP, Nakagawa TH, Takahashi AC de M. Performance of different timed up and go subtasks in frailty syndrome. J Geriatr Phys Ther. 2019;42(4):287–93.
[11] Nygaard I, Barber MD, Burgio KL, Kenton K, Meikle S, Schaffer J, et al. Prevalence of symptomatic pelvic floor disorders in US women. JAMA. 2008;300(11):1311–6.
[12] Heilbrun ME, Nygaard IE, Lockhart ME, Richter HE, Brown MB, Kenton KS, et al. Correlation between levator ani muscle injuries on MRI and fecal incontinence, pelvic organ prolapse, and urinary incontinence in primiparous women. Am J Obstet Gynecol. 2010;202(5):488.e1–6.
[13] Rodríguez-Mias Núria L, Martínez-Franco E, Aguado J, Sánchez E, Amat-Tardiu L. Pelvic organ prolapse and stress urinary incontinence, do they share the same risk factors? Eur J Obstet Gynecol Reprod Biol. 2015;190:52–7.
[14] Cetinkaya SE, Dokmeci F, Dai O. Correlation of pelvic organ prolapse staging with lower urinary tract symptoms, sexual dysfunction, and quality of life. Int Urogynecol J. 2013;24(10):1645–50.
[15] Makary MA, Segev DL, Pronovost PJ, Syin D, Bandeen-Roche K, Patel P, et al. Frailty as a predictor of surgical outcomes in older patients. J Am Coll Surg. 2010;210(6):901–8.
[16] Savva GM, Donoghue OA, Horgan F, O'Regan C, Cronin H, Kenny RA. Using timed up-and- go to identify frail members of the older population. J Gerontol A Biol Sci Med Sci. 2013;68(4):441–6.
[17] Abellan van Kan G, Rolland Y, Houles M, Gillette-Guyonnet S, Soto M, Vellas B. The assessment of frailty in older adults. Clin Geriatr Med. 2010;26(2):275–86.
[18] Gray SL, Anderson ML, Dublin S, Hanlon JT, Hubbard R, Walker R, et al. Cumulative use of strong anticholinergics and incident dementia: a prospective cohort study. JAMA Intern Med. 2015;175(3):401–7.
[19] Dowd TT, Campbell JM, Jones JA. Fluid intake and urinary incontinence in older community-dwelling women. J Community Health Nurs. 1996;13(3):179–86.
[20] Wagg A, Gibson W, Ostaszkiewicz J, Johnson T, Markland A, Palmer MH, et al. Urinary incontinence in frail elderly persons: report from the 5th international consultation on incontinence. Neurourol Urodyn. 2015;34(5):398–406.
[21] Burgio KL, Goode PS, Locher JL, Umlauf MG, Roth DL, Richter HE, et al. Behavioral training with and without biofeedback in the treatment of urge incontinence in older women: a randomized controlled trial. JAMA. 2002;288(18):2293–9.
[22] Diokno AC, Sampselle CM, Herzog AR, Raghunathan TE, Hines S, Messer KL, et al. Prevention of urinary incontinence by behavioral modification program: a randomized, controlled trial among older women in the community. J Urol. 2004;171(3):1165–71.
[23] Narayanan S, Cerulli A, Kahler KH, Ouslander JG. Is drug therapy for urinary incontinence used optimally in long-term care facilities? J Am

Med Dir Assoc. 2007;8(2):98–104.
[24] Aaron LE, Morris TJ, Jahshan P, Reiz JL. An evaluation of patient and physician satisfaction with controlled-release oxybutynin 15 mg as a one-step daily dose in elderly and non-elderly patients with overactive bladder: results of the STOP study. Curr Med Res Opin. 2012;28(8):1369–79.
[25] Katz IR, Sands LP, Bilker W, DiFilippo S, Boyce A, D'Angelo K. Identification of medications that cause cognitive impairment in older people: the case of oxybutynin chloride. J Am Geriatr Soc. 1998;46(1):8–13.
[26] McFerren SC, Gomelsky A. Treatment of overactive bladder in the elderly female: the case for trospium, oxybutynin, fesoterodine and darifenacin. Drugs Aging. 2015;32(10):809–19.
[27] Dubeau CE, Kraus SR, Griebling TL, Newman DK, Wyman JF, Johnson TM, et al. Effect of fesoterodine in vulnerable elderly subjects with urgency incontinence: a double-blind, placebo controlled trial. J Urol. 2014;191(2):395–404.
[28] Wagg A, Khullar V, Marschall-Kehrel D, Michel MC, Oelke M, Darekar A, et al. Flexible-dose fesoterodine in elderly adults with overactive bladder: results of the randomized, double-blind, placebo-controlled study of fesoterodine in an aging population trial. J Am Geriatr Soc. 2013;61(2):185–93.
[29] Geller EJ, Dumond JB, Bowling JM, Khandelwal CM, Wu JM, Busby-Whitehead J, et al. Effect of trospium chloride on cognitive function in women aged 50 and older: a randomized trial. Female Pelvic Med Reconstr Surg. 2017;23(2):118–23.
[30] Richardson K, Fox C, Maidment I, Steel N, Loke YK, Arthur A, et al. Anticholinergic drugs and risk of dementia: case-control study. BMJ. 2018;361:k1315.
[31] Gormley EA, Lightner DJ, Burgio KL, Chai TC, Clemens JQ, Culkin DJ, et al. Diagnosis and treatment of overactive bladder (non-neurogenic) in adults: AUA/SUFU guideline. J Urol. 2012;188(6 Suppl):2455–63.
[32] Wagg AS. Antimuscarinic treatment in overactive bladder: special considerations in elderly patients. Drugs Aging. 2012;29(7):539–48.
[33] Komesu YM, Amundsen CL, Richter HE, Erickson SW, Ackenbom MF, Andy UU, et al. Refractory urgency urinary incontinence treatment in women: impact of age on outcomes and complications. Am J Obstet Gynecol. 2018;218(1):111.e1–9.
[34] Liao C-H, Kuo H-C. Increased risk of large post-void residual urine and decreased long-term success rate after intravesical onabotulinumtoxinA injection for refractory idiopathic detrusor overactivity. J Urol. 2013;189(5):1804–10.
[35] Palmer C, Nguyen N, Ghoniem G. Clinical experience with percutaneous tibial nerve stimulation in the elderly; do outcomes differ by gender? Arab J Urol. 2019;17(1):10–3.
[36] Levin PJ, Wu JM, Siddiqui NY, Amundsen CL. Does obesity impact the success of an InterStim test phase for the treatment of refractory urge urinary incontinence in female patients? Female Pelvic Med Reconstr Surg. 2012;18(4):243–6.
[37] Amundsen CL, Webster GD. Sacral neuromodulation in an older, urge-incontinent population. Am J Obstet Gynecol. 2002;187(6):1462–5; discussion 1465.
[38] Faris AER, Gill BC, Pizarro-Berdichevsky J, Dielubanza E, Clifton MM, Okafor H, et al. Impact of age and comorbidities on use of sacral neuromodulation. J Urol. 2017;198(1):161–6.
[39] Dumoulin C, Cacciari LP, Hay-Smith EJC. Pelvic floor muscle training versus no treatment, or inactive control treatments, for urinary incontinence in women. Cochrane Database Syst Rev. 2018;04(10):CD005654.
[40] Leong BS, Mok NW. Effectiveness of a new standardised urinary continence physiotherapy programme for community-dwelling older women in Hong Kong. Hong Kong Med J Xianggang Yi Xue Za Zhi. 2015;21(1):30–7.
[41] Dumoulin C, Morin M, Danieli C, Cacciari L, Mayrand M-H, Tousignant M, et al. Group-based vs individual pelvic floor muscle training to treat urinary incontinence in older women: a randomized clinical trial. JAMA Intern Med. 2020;180(10):1284–93.
[42] Al-Shaikh G, Syed S, Osman S, Bogis A, Al-Badr A. Pessary use in stress urinary incontinence: a review of advantages, complications, patient satisfaction, and quality of life. Int J Women's Health. 2018;10:195–201.
[43] Farrell SA, Singh B, Aldakhil L. Continence pessaries in the management of urinary incontinence in women. J Obstet Gynaecol Can JOGC. 2004;26(2):113–7.
[44] Capobianco G, Saderi L, Dessole F, Petrillo M, Dessole M, Piana A, et al. Efficacy and effectiveness of bulking agents in the treatment of stress and mixed urinary incontinence: a systematic review and meta-analysis. Maturitas. 2020;133:13–31.
[45] Mohr S, Siegenthaler M, Mueller MD, Kuhn A. Bulking agents: an analysis of 500 cases and review of the literature. Int Urogynecol J. 2013;24(2):241–7.
[46] Zullo MA, Ruggiero A, Montera R, Plotti F, Muzii L, Angioli R, et al. An ultra-miniinvasive treatment for stress urinary incontinence in complicated older patients. Maturitas. 2010;65(3):292–5.
[47] Lee J, Dwyer PL. Age-related trends in female stress urinary incontinence surgery in Australia – Medicare data for 1994–2009. Aust N Z J Obstet Gynaecol. 2010;50(6):543–9.
[48] Richter HE, Goode PS, Brubaker L, Zyczynski H, Stoddard AM, Dandreo KJ, et al. Two-year outcomes after surgery for stress urinary incontinence in older compared with younger women. Obstet Gynecol. 2008;112(3):621–9.
[49] Stav K, Dwyer PL, Rosamilia A, Schierlitz L, Lim YN, Lee J. Midurethral sling procedures for stress urinary incontinence in women over 80 years. Neurourol Urodyn. 2010;29(7):1262–6.
[50] Groutz A, Cohen A, Gold R, Pauzner D, Lessing JB, Gordon D. The safety and efficacy of the "inside-out" trans-obturator TVT in elderly versus younger stress-incontinent women: a prospective study of 353 consecutive patients. Neurourol Urodyn. 2011;30(3):380–3.
[51] Cohen AJ, Packiam VT, Nottingham CU, Alberts BD, Faris SF, Bales GT. 30-day morbidity and reoperation following midurethral sling: analysis of 8772 cases using a national prospective database. Urology. 2016;95:72–9.

第 26 章 最大限度地提高尿失禁手术期间的手术效果和安全性

Maximizing Intraoperative Performance and Safety During Incontinence Surgery

Kristin Chrouser Keow Mei Goh 著

一、患者在手术室中的安全

在过去数十年中，医疗机构广泛采用了诸如会诊、听取术前简报和术前讨论在内的多种方式来保障手术中患者的安全。这些基于团队的合作方式就是为了最好地沟通，并预防出现不良事件（如错误的手术部位、手术部位感染和术中失误），从而提高手术效果。各种外科协会中的操作指南和白皮书中也提供了很多保护患者安全的方式[1, 2]。在此，我们将重点关注与尿失禁手术强相关的特定患者及其安全考虑因素。

（一）患者的安全体位

在手术中，正确的体位对于防止患者受伤至关重要。一旦处于麻醉状态，患者将无法表达不适或调整姿势。有很多影响体位的风险因素，其中包括外科手术的类型、时长、手术部位，以及患者的身高、体重、年龄、营养状况、活动度和合并症等[3]。这个过程应遵循患者定位的一般指南[4]。手术人员需要熟练地使用先进的定位工具和器材。定位所需的所有器材（如支架、衬垫和臂托）应在患者到达之前准备好。同时，手术床的承重和宽度均要合适。

1. 仰卧位

尺神经病变是与仰卧位相关的最常见损伤。仰卧位的目的是将尺骨沟的压力降至最低，并避免手臂过度伸展和弯曲（>90°）[5]。另外，肩部过度外展、手臂外旋和背伸，以及头部向对侧屈曲，都会增加臂丛神经损伤的风险。为了避免这种情况，头部应处于中线并且位置端正。手臂应处于自然状态，置于中间位置并固定在铺单下面，或者手臂也可以横向放置在臂板上，并外展<90°，以防止背侧过度伸展[6]。如果翻转的手臂无意中搭在桌子上或血压袖带上，则可能发生桡神经损伤。如果手臂内旋在桌子上，则可能损伤正中神经。肘部过度伸展也会有损伤正中神经的风险。当然根据记载，即便手术中采取了以上的安全预防措施，也有发生神经损伤的情况[6]。

2. 头低足高仰卧体位

头低足高仰卧体位是阴道手术和腹腔镜/机器人盆腔手术的常见体位，但它会引起致中心静脉、颅内、肺静脉和眼内压的升高[7]。除了功能残气量和肺顺应性降低外，用胶带固定患者胸部的做法也可导致肺功能受损[8]。严重的头颈部水肿会导致喉水肿从而需要重新插管，而后部缺血性视神经病变会导致机器人前列腺切除术后视力丧失[9, 10]。过去，肩托被用来防止患者在手术台上头向移动。然而，使用肩托也可导致臂丛神经损伤[6]。

据估计，在腹腔镜妇科手术中，与错误定位相关的神经损伤案例中，上肢相关占比为0.02%～0.16%，下肢相关占比为1.5%～1.8%，在机器人辅助手术中为1%。需要注意的是，由于案例不足以及这些伤害中存在许多自限性[11]，实际发生率可能更高。增加患者神经损伤风险的因素包括：过高或过低的体重指数、年龄>60岁、吸烟或饮酒史、低血容量、低血压、手术时电解质失衡或营养不良，以及较高的 ASA 分数[12, 13]。回顾病例，手术时长被认为是影响截石位后的神经损伤的主要因素，但从最近的数据看这一推测似乎不太具有说服力[11]。为了避免神经损伤，患者的体位至关重要。当患者的腿放在支撑中或将手臂靠在手术台上时，存在神经受压迫的风险，应注意另外增加衬垫。髋部过度屈曲（＞80°～90°）、截石位中的极度外展和外旋以及患者大腿内侧的压力都会使股神经有受压损伤的风险[14]。

在陡峭的头低足高仰卧体位时是否应避免患者的头部运动一直是一个具有争议的话题。然而，由于缺乏直接的对比，没有明确的证据表明哪种技术是最好的[15]。除肩带外，其他用于稳定患者在床上位置的技术包括豆袋垫、球形气垫床或泡沫床垫，以及粉红垫®系统[15, 16]。建议使用上肢体感诱发电位这种新方法对术中神经进行实时监测，以避免对神经的伤害[17]。当进行正确的定位时，团队应注意填充所有压力点，以避免肢体过度屈曲、旋转或外展。此外，应使用便于观察所需的最小头低足高仰卧量[11]。

3. 截石位

截石位通常用于尿失禁手术中。根据髋部角度和腿部高度的不同——从低截石位（腿部相对于床轴约 35°）到高截石位（小腿＞90°），截石位可分为多级[18]。在标准截石位姿势中，腿从中线向外展 30°～45°，髋部固定在 80°～100°，小腿要平行于躯干[5]。应注意限制腿部抬高和外展，以便在不影响下肢循环或影响患者血流动力学的情况下提供足够的手术显露[19]。关于截石位造成的下肢损伤也有详细的记录。腓神经在腓骨头和支架之间有受压的危险。同样地，隐静脉也会在胫骨内侧髁处受压。髋部过度屈曲和膝盖伸展也有损伤坐骨神经的风险[5]。对在梅奥诊所接受截石位手术的患者进行回顾分析后，Warner 等发现，3608 例持续时间超过 3 个月的运动神经病变中，78% 的病例涉及腓总神经[20]。受伤的风险因素包括极端的体型和较长的手术时间（超过 2h）。在手术时长超过 4.5h 的病例中，也有需要筋膜切开术的筋膜室综合征和横纹肌溶解症的病例[5, 19]。在一项对使用过度截石位的 177 例患者进行的研究中，28 例患者出现了腓神经损伤（其中 27 例患者最终痊愈）[21]。

在截石位中，腿可以支撑在糖罐形支架、拐杖式支架或靴形支架上（图 26–1）。当使用糖罐形支架时，不应让患者的腿直接靠在垂直的支持杆上。可以在支持杆和患者腿部之间放置衬垫，但这不能确保安全。应避免患者的臀部因拐杖的旋转而过度扭转。穿上胶靴和（或）罐形支架上较宽的束带，有助于减轻脚踝和脚部的压力[22]。拐杖式支架将下肢的重量放在后膝的腘间隙上，增加了损伤后腓总神经和腘动脉的风险[23]。同样的，靴形支架可以使腿部重量分布在腿部和足部，同时允许术中调整髋关节和腿部外展角度[22]。如果需要极限截石位，会阴几乎平行于地面时，应使用垫子支撑下背部[5]。在截石位中，为了确保在靴形支架中定位，应将患者放在合适的位置，以确保在移除手术台后骶骨得到良好支撑，并且手术台导轨夹应与患者的髋部对齐。鞋跟应该放在靴形支架的底部。膝盖角度应保持＜90°，以避免过度屈曲（腿伸直时为 0°）。靴形支架的长轴应朝向对侧肩部[5]。同样在仰卧位时，也应注意上肢收起或横向伸展。此外，在拆卸或更换床脚时，注意避免伤到手指。

（二）困难情况下的体位

1. 肥胖患者

美国人的肥胖率和程度每年都在持续增加。2020 年，美国疾病控制与预防中心估计，9.8% 的美国人口被视为严重肥胖（BMI＞40kg/m^2），这个数字将继续上升[24]。这些患者给手术室带来了特殊的挑战。除了解决上述所有定位问题外，还必须注意确保患者不要躺在在起皱的床单上，并确保弹力袜、血压袖带和手术床等设备尺寸适当。在将患者移动到手术台时，使用诸如 HoverMatt®

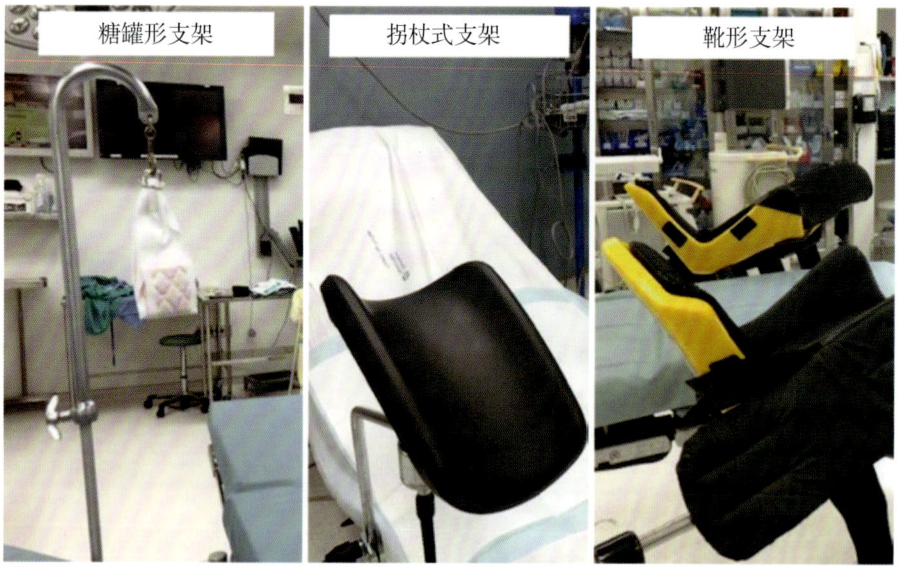

◀ 图 26-1 截石位的支架类型

的转移装置是一种有用的辅助工具，可降低患者皮肤割伤和工作人员肌肉骨骼损伤的风险。对于严重肥胖患者，应缓慢地从支架上提起和放下患者的腿，以防止腰骶部劳损，并避免循环系统的快速变化[4]。用于治疗肥胖过程的靴型支架，能承受更高的重量、具有更宽的靴形支架和升降辅助。也有报道使用气动霍耶升降机来支撑患者的腿部[22]。

2. 挛缩或截肢患者

当安置因关节收缩而活动受限的患者时，考虑在实施麻醉前将患者放置在手术所需的位置，以确认患者能够舒适地躺在该位置。有时，挛缩会使某些手术方式（如俯卧位和截石位）在身体上不可行。将截肢患者置于截石位手术需要特别考虑支撑单个截肢肢体。对于低位截肢，带额外衬垫的靴形支撑通常是足够的。如果不需要抬腿，一种策略是使用带支撑的分腿手术台来支撑断端[25]（图 26-2）。

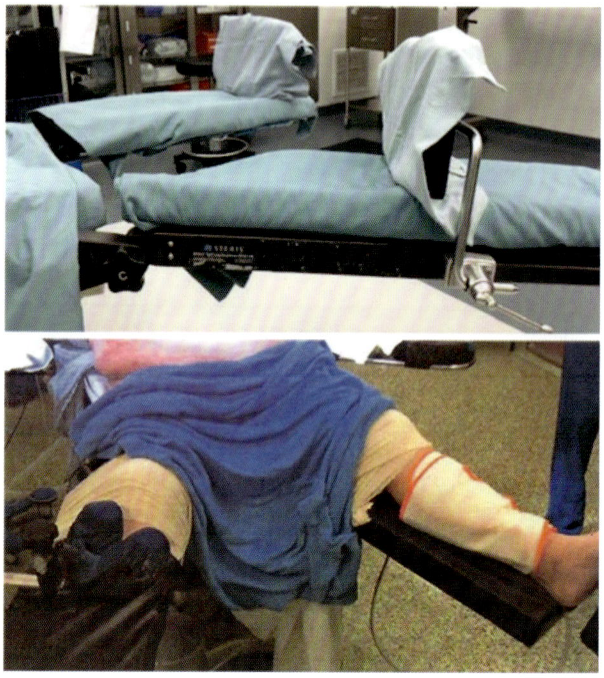

▲ 图 26-2 使用分腿手术台和支撑定位截肢者

经许可转载，由 Keow Goh（top）and James Williamson（bottom）提供

（三）术中放射线的安全使用

骶神经调节常用于难治性急迫性尿失禁的治疗。尽管该手术本身的风险很低，但它需要透视，使患者和手术团队都显露于电离辐射。可以实现准确的导线放置，可以减少患者和手术人员的辐射显露。许多研究证实，人们对辐射显露的风险（如癌症、不孕症和白内障）缺乏认识[26, 27]。应尽一切努力减少剂量和显露时间，同时最大限度地屏蔽（表 26-1）[1]。外科医生应通过使用脉冲辐射、降低脉冲率和剂量、图像保持 / 透视存储和图像准直来优化透视设置[28]。

1. 患者保护

患者的位置应该离影像增强器最近，离 X 线管一侧较远。手术团队的指定成员（护士或放射技师）应监测剂量，并报告何时达到最大剂量[29]。医疗机构应制定政策，对女性患者进行可能怀孕的筛查。如果孕妇必须显露于电离辐射，则应在腹部和骨盆上放置适当的防护，以保护胎儿[30]。

表 26-1　最小化患者和手术团队辐射显露的策略[1]

减少剂量和显露时间

- 限制透视时间
- 低剂量设置（设置为默认值）
- 最低设置下的脉冲荧光透视（例如，每秒 1 个脉冲）
- 使用点透视图像，而不是连续透视
- 使用“最后图像保持”和“保存和交换”技术
- 如果不需要看到整个图像，则准直至局部区域
- 最大化与能源的距离，最小化与像增强器的距离（减少散射）
- 尽量减少使用图像放大率（放大率增加剂量）
- 使用医生脚踏控制（避免混淆何时需要透视以及是否需要连续透视）
- 使用熟悉病例解剖结构的专业外科放射技师

屏蔽

- 使用个人防护设备（铅围裙、甲状腺护罩、铅眼镜和铅手套）
- 屏蔽患者（例如，妊娠患者的甲状腺、骨盆等放射敏感区域）

2. 工作人员保护

围术期团队成员应限制显露时间，并最大限度地远离辐射源。辐射显露量与辐射源的距离的平方成反比。此外，激活放射设备的人员应为房间内的人员提供穿戴防护设备的机会[31]。人员可以使用固定屏蔽、移动屏蔽、设备安装屏蔽或个人防护装置，如铅衣防护围裙和甲状腺防护罩。如果可能受到 X 线照射，应注意在人员背部提供覆盖。如果人员的手可能位于辐射束的路径中，则应提供防护手套和手指剂量计[31]。手术室工作人员在使用剂量计监测显露时，需要始终穿戴铅衣防护围裙和甲状腺防护罩。在一项研究中，学术培训中心只有 50%～56% 的人员使用了剂量计，而私营机构的这一比例甚至更低[32]。值得注意的是，团队领导采用辐射防护做法会影响员工的合规性[33]。妊娠人员需要遵守当地、州和联邦监管机构制订的预防措施。妊娠的团队成员应在腰罩下佩戴辐射监测器，并每月读取 1 次。应鼓励使用孕妇专用或双层铅防护服[30]。如果可能，她应尽量减少参与需要辐射的程序。

二、外科医生的安全和职业健康

外科文化鼓励外科医生为患者服务而奉献，包括严格的训练、长时间的工作，以及无视个人身体需求。手术中，外科医生通常不休息进食或排空膀胱。如果外科医生认为符合患者的最佳利益，他们愿意使用需要不符合人体工程学定位（会导致肌肉骨骼不适）的手术技术。同时，许多医生在没有进行人体工程学优化的电脑工作站上长时间的处理电子病历。不幸的是，在漫长的职业生涯中，长时间的重复性工作导致的相关肌肉骨骼损伤可能造成慢性残疾，导致他们改变病例模式 / 数量或考虑提前退休[34, 35]。尽管人们越来越关注，但很少有住院医师项目提供人体工程学原理的指导，以帮助年轻外科医生最大限度地降低其职业活动对身体的负面影响[36]。

在最近的一次评估中，68% 的外科医生报告了肌肉骨骼疼痛，61% 的外科医生指出他们的疼痛因手术而加剧，而不到 1/3 的外科医生因其症状寻求医疗救治。疼痛的发生率因外科亚专业和手术方式（如开放式、腔镜、机器人和内镜）而有所不同。41%～80% 的泌尿科医生和 54%～87% 的阴道外科医生报告了与工作相关的肌肉骨骼疼痛[35, 37, 38]。外科医生承认，为了控制疼痛，他们调整了手术时间、病例组合和手术技术[35, 37]。在一项结合了所有子专业外科医生的研究中，可穿戴技术被用于监测术中外科医生的体位，并发现 65% 的手术时间用于高危颈部姿势[39]。毫无疑问，高危姿势、放大镜和头灯都与主观疼痛评分增加相关。

虽然普遍报道外科医生与工作相关的肌肉

骨骼疾病发生率很高，但是有人认为这个较高的比例很大程度是受女性外科医生的影响。美国泌尿学协会2017年人口普查发现，女性外科医生报告工作相关疼痛的频率高于男性同行[35]，与工效学特定调查相比，女性外科医生较少出现反应偏差。45岁以下的年轻外科医生中的差异更大，65%的女性感到不适，而男性的这一比例为42%。平均而言，女外科医生比男外科医生矮，手也小。达·芬奇机器人控制台没有为身高5英尺4英寸以下的外科医生进行人体工程学优化[40]。小尺寸的手激发缝合器有困难[41]。目前的医疗设备设计不能适应当前外科医生群体中手部尺寸和握力的范围，尤其是随着越来越多的女性进入该行业[42]。不幸的是，缺乏严格的仪器可用性测试会增加女性外科医生的人体工程学压力和受伤风险。许多公司（在仪器设计时）使用的都是以男性主导外科手术时期的过时数据[43]。外科医生应鼓励公司设计能够适应各种手的大小和力量的装置和设备，因为这有助于确保所有人都能公平地进入安全的工作场所。值得注意的是，并非所有疼痛发生率的差异都与身高和手的大小有关。即使在控制了手套的尺寸，一些需要特定治疗的伤害在女性外科医生身上的发生比例（相对男性）也更高[44]。类似地，即使在控制了手术时间的长短和外科医生身高后，女性腹腔镜手术期间肌肉激活的肌电图测量值也高于男性外科医生[45]。需要更多的研究来评估开放式阴道手术或机器人手术是否也需要女外科医生更多的体力来完成同样的手术。

由于大多数尿失禁的外科治疗都是在阴道进行的，因此我们将重点关注对患者在截石位进行手术的特殊挑战，尽管其中的一些原理也适用于开放式、腹腔镜和机器人方法。肌肉骨骼疼痛的主要高危因素包括别扭的姿势、高强度活动、静态姿势和长时间不间断手术[46, 47]。截石位固有的狭窄工作空间几乎不可能保持合适的姿势。桌子高度不当会导致躯干和头部过度弯曲[48]。在观察一系列案例中，67%的阴道手术引起颈部、肩背部或臀部疼痛[49]。经客观评估，这与外科医生在手术期间肩部、躯干、颈部的高危姿势有关[50]。此外，对于教学机构中的外科医生，在阴道手术期间，主治医生通常以助手的姿势站在住院医生旁边，这会导致躯干过度侧向旋转和弯曲，以及因牵拉导致上肢的持续性紧绷[38]。

（一）充分利用人体工程学和预防损伤的策略

减少外科医生职业性肌肉骨骼损伤有多种方式，它包括调整物理环境（床和设备布置）、外科医生进行特殊活动以及在手术室外进行的预防方法等。

（二）优化物理环境的策略

保持正确的姿势对于优化手术过程中的人体工程学至关重要，且有充分的资源可以保障这一点[51, 52]。应调整手术台高度，以适应最高的外科医生（患者处于医生肘部位置），如有需要，其他人可以使用踏脚凳或垫子等[48]。颈部、肩部、背部和臀部不要过度旋转，同时确保即便不是双腿站立，身体重量也要均匀分布[53]。颈部的轴向旋转不要超过15°[51]。条件允许时，阴道外科医生最好坐着进行手术，同时在手术中根据需要调整桌子/凳子高度，以便直视前方[48]。及时调整灯光位置，从而避免别扭的姿势，并在可能的情况下收起患者的手臂，以免妨碍外科医生/助手的自由移动[53]。助手适当的旋转，或者使用自持式牵开器可以减轻压力[48]。脚踏板应直接放在工作脚的正前面[52]。显示器应放置在距离屏幕中心3～4英尺的位置，距离眼睛水平面约10°～20°[52]。屏幕上部位置的高度设计和人眼高度相近较为合理。一些研究发现，缓冲垫可以改善外科医生的不适，并且被广泛用在外科手术[54]。有人提出了一种可能的方法，是将台式阴道牵开器与嵌入式摄像机结合使用，这样在进行阴道手术时方便观察并有良好的人体工程学环境[55]。带胸部和四肢支撑的椅子以及外骨骼装备都是具有创新性的方法，这些都有望改善外科医生术中的疼痛和疲劳，但是，这些方法迄今为止还未被广泛应用[56, 57]。

（三）改善外科医生人体工程学环境和减少疼痛的策略

对于习惯危险姿势的外科医生来说，改变习惯可能很困难。可以利用换姿势时进行重新调整[53]。在长时间的手术中，穿戴带有足弓支撑和气垫的鞋子可能会有帮助，特别是对患有慢性下肢或背部不适的外科医生[48]。

术中休息 / 拉伸

术中小休息包括在非关键时刻暂停手术（每 20～40 分钟 1 次），并进行一系列短暂的 90s 的定向拉伸 / 运动。这些小休息是在不破坏手术服的情况下完成的，并且已经证明，在不增加手术时间的情况下，减少了外科医生的不适感并能使医生更加专注[58]。全神贯注在外科手术的外科医生不太可能记得休息，因此 Abdelall 等设计了一个具有自动提醒功能的应用程序，并将其有效地应用到一小群外科医生手术过程中[59]。有关访问此资源的信息，请访问 ORstretch.mayoclinic.org。

（四）手术室外的预防策略

1. 工作站的优化

在手术室外，外科医生花通常在电脑工作站上长时间工作，由于大多数桌子太高，这也会导致肌肉骨骼疼痛。可以通过使用可调节式的座椅，让下背部紧贴椅子或枕头，双脚放在地板上（或踏脚板上），膝盖成 90°，背部略微倾斜。肘部应以 90°～100° 的角度张开，手腕应保持笔直，而不是放在桌子上。不要将键盘向使用者倾斜。显示器的顶部应位于眼睛水平面或略低于眼睛水平面，因此计算机屏幕的中心位于眼睛水平面的下方约 20°，屏幕到眼睛的距离至少 20 英寸（约一个臂长）。双焦镜佩戴者应将显示器再降低 1～2 英寸。使用电脑工作时，每 20 分钟休息 20s，看下 20 英尺外的远处，以减少眼睛疲劳。当使用没有独立显示器或键盘的笔记本电脑时，要想达到好的人体工程学要求几乎不可能。

2. 运动、理疗、按摩

一项研究表明，在手术室外运动似乎对避免泌尿科医生产生工作相关疼痛具有“剂量依赖性”的作用[60]。虽然关于外科医生进行预防性运动的报道还很少，但是已经证明，针对性的运动可以改善非外科医生工作相关的颈肩疼痛[61]。对于患有工作相关的肌肉骨骼疼痛的外科医生，理疗或定期按摩也有助于改善疼痛（治疗）和保持灵活（预防）。

3. 人机工程教育

针对外科医生工作日益增加的肌肉骨骼疼痛问题，许多研究也注意到，在外科培训或继续教育期间都缺乏人体工程学方面的指导。越来越多的共识是，应该对当前的外科医生进行人体工程学方面的指导，以免下一代医生依然不能更健康地工作[36]。

三、实现外科医生和的团队最好的绩效

手术结果受外科医生多个方面因素的影响，这包括其心理因素 / 技能，以及其他各种诸如认知水平、团队沟通等称为“非技术性能力”的因素[62, 63]。非技术技能包括沟通、决策、情境意识、团队合作和领导力[64]。沟通需要以其他人能够理解的方式进行接收和传递信息。情势感知是外科医生对团队情况及现场的及时感知。当外科医生在手术过程中遇到棘手的情况，要选择并实施一种方案时，就需要做出决策。团队合作就包括与他人共同努力来达成目标。领导技能包括以身作则，同时具有激励他人的能力[65]。虽然总能很容易地单从技术方面找到导致并发症的原因，但其实很多医疗事故都可以追溯到非技术因素上[66, 67]。因此，个人绩效水平的提升活动不能仅仅局限于提升技能的速度和准度，还要涉及更广泛的技能提升。

（一）优化外科医生个人绩效的策略

1. 外科指导或教学培训

研究发现，通过各种方式（面对面、视频、模拟），专家和同行的指导能从主观上提高外科医生的水平[68]。大多数指导和 QI 项目都比较关注技术方面，但也有一些涉及非技术能力方面[69]。一

位研究者指出，虽然外科医生对其技能力的自我评估与专家的评估基本一致，但对自身非技术能力评估却很差，这就说明存在一定的认知盲区[70]。有一些教学和模拟项目，除了必要的辅导外，还能帮助获得这些关键的技能[65]。一些住院医师项目设计比较全面，涉及了广泛的技能提升，包括沟通技能和专业的提升[71]。

2. 倡导心理健康

外科医生应发挥其领导作用，通过在手术室营造健康的心理环境来提高团队绩效。从过往看，手术室并不是一个包容的环境，比如可以直言不讳或寻求帮助。然而，心理健康就鼓励学习并使团队的绩效最大化[72]。特别是在紧急情况下，这样的环境尤其重要，它能使团队高度配合并防止因外科医生失误导致严重的安全事故。

3. 心理训练

在过去的一个世纪里，心理想象/心理练习训练一直是用作提高心理素质的一种方法[73]。已经证明心理训练对受训者的手术表现有积极的影响[74]。当采用新技术，以及准备复杂或不熟悉的手术时，即便对于经验丰富的外科医生，这些心理训练方法也有助于延缓水平下降并加快学习曲线[75]。

4. 压力、情绪、冲突管理

紧急性压力在手术室是不可避免的，但如果管理不善，会让患者、外科医生和团队处于危险之中。缺乏情绪管理和破坏性的行为会使人员感到痛苦，破坏团队活力，增加紧张感，影响心理健康[76, 77]。外科医生的长期压力会导致倦怠和消耗，这也会对患者和助理人员产生负面影响。外科医生压力管理干预包括指导其应对的策略、心理彩排和放松方法[78]。术前心理练习也被证明可以减轻新手外科医生的压力[79]。心理韧性是一种衡量个人韧性和自信的指标，通常用于对在运动人员和军事人员的评价，最近才看到应用到外科医生身上[80]。士兵用来提高/保持心理韧性的技术包括可视化、自言自语、肯定、集中注意力技能和呼吸调整方法[81]。这些有助于控制与压力情境相关的反应，并改善身体和心理表现。外科医生还将发现，在手术室中锻炼冲突管理能力可以提高个人和团队绩效[82]。

5. 提升生理条件

提升外科医生生理条件包括预防低血糖、脱水、疲劳和肌肉骨骼疼痛。手术的快节奏和不可预测性，常导致医生液体摄入不足和来不及吃饭。血糖水平会与认知能力下降和易怒有关系[83, 84]。实验发现，当受试者禁食时，环境中的挫折感会导致受试者更多的负面反应[85]。易怒和消极情绪会影响非技术技能，并影响团队合作[86]。来自非外科文献的证据表明，当外科医生处于低血糖状态时，技术和非技术方面的表现可能存在风险。虽然目前还未对外科医生进行相关评估，但已发现脱水会抑制待命的医生和护士的情绪和认知功能[87]。来自非手术文献的证据表明，睡眠被剥夺对情绪的影响最大，其次是认知，最后是精神水平[88]。关注外科医生精神运动表现的研究，研究结果虽然混入了多种因素，但还是表明有一定的负面影响[89]。相比之下，大多数外科医生和护士却认为他们在手术中的表现不受疲劳的影响[90]。即使技术水平保持不变，外科医生非技术能力的下降也会对手术团队产生不利影响。

外科医生的肌肉骨骼疼痛可以从几个方面影响手术效果。疼痛会限制运动范围、力量和运动控制，从而对精神运动/技术表现产生负面影响[91, 92]。疼痛会降低精神集中度，并对术中决策和认知产生不利影响[93]。疼痛还会更容易对他人动怒，并影响个人心理健康及团队状态[94, 95]。外科医生的非技术性表现不佳可能导致团队沟通和协作减少，从而产生不良事件。显然，前面列出的人体工程学策略不仅对外科医生的职业健康很重要，而且当它们有效预防或减少与工作相关的疼痛时，也有助于提升外科医生/团队绩效并改善患者手术结果。

（二）优化外科团队绩效的策略

1. 团队训练

提高外科团队绩效的策略在一定程度上与已

经针对外科医生提出的策略重叠，特别是在非技术技能获取、培训和实践方面。说教式培训很有帮助，但可能不够，因为这些技能中有很多需要练习才能养成习惯，尤其是在团队处于压力下时。使用模拟的团队培训和指导可以帮助建立和加强这些技能的使用[96]。团队模拟在帮助成员更好地理解他人的角色和责任方面特别有效，行动后回顾提供了反思和学习的机会，这在现实世界中是罕见的。

2. 应急准备

一些机构已经开发了典型项目（如外科火灾）、特定设备（如机器人脱离）或特定专业的危机模拟（如旁路期间的代码）[97, 98]。团队模拟对于涉及执行不熟悉的程序或使用不熟悉设备的危机培训特别有用。危机放大了非技术技能的重要性，因为在危机中需要清楚地了解团队成员的角色，加强对环境的了解，以及团队成员之间更高水平的沟通和协调。这种训练可以释放压力，并提高外科急诊的表现[99]。

3. 制度文化和政策

医疗机构的文化和政策影响着手术室里的日常活动。部门 / 工会政策影响团队成员术中休息的时间安排（理想情况下，不允许安排在手术的关键点），遵守安全规定，定期提供员工教育，以及掌握和安全推广新技术的程序。需要机构的资源支持来建立复杂程序的专业团队，提高团队对病例的熟悉度，进行应急演习或模拟（手术室火灾、快速拆卸机器人好手术指令），辅导 / 训练表现出破坏性行为的个人，并简化与影响手术室日常工作或功能的“隐形团队成员”（生物医学工程 / 无菌供应 / 公司代表 / 手术日程安排）的协调过程。

总之，患者取得良好的手术效果不仅取决于一名技术熟练的外科医生，还取决于一个致力于患者健康和不断学习的可靠团队。本章提供了各种实用策略，以最大限度地提高术中患者和外科医生的安全，并提升外科医生和团队的绩效。

参考文献

[1] Chrouser K, Foley F, Goldenberg M, Hyder J, Maranchie JK, Moore JM, et al. Optimizing outcomes in urological surgery: intraoperative patient safety and physiological considerations. Urol Pract. 2020;7(4):309–18.

[2] Chrouser K, Kim FJ, Smith A, Stoffel JT, Goldenberg M. Optimizing outcomes in urologic surgery: intraoperative environmental, behavioral, and performance considerations. Urol Pract. 2020;7(5):405–12.

[3] Davis SS. The key to safety: proactive prevention. Wiley Online Library; 2018.

[4] Guideline for positioning the patient. In: Guidelines for perioperative practice. Association of periOperative Registered Nurses; 2018. p. 673–744.

[5] Akhavan A, Gainsburg DM, Stock JA. Complications associated with patient positioning in urologic surgery. Urology. 2010;76(6):1309–16.

[6] Winfree CJ, Kline DG. Intraoperative positioning nerve injuries. Surg Neurol. 2005;63(1):5–18.

[7] Wilcox S, Vandam LD. Alas, poor Trendelenburg and his position! A critique of its uses and effectiveness. Anesth Analg. 1988;67(6):574–8.

[8] Gainsburg DM, Wax D, Reich DL, Carlucci JR, Samadi DB. Intraoperative management of robotic-assisted versus open radical prostatectomy. JSLS: J Soc Laparoendosc Surg. 2010;14(1):1.

[9] Phong S, Koh L. Anaesthesia for robotic-assisted radical prostatectomy: considerations for laparoscopy in the Trendelenburg position. Anaesth Intensive Care. 2007;35(2):281–5.

[10] Weber ED, Colyer MH, Lesser RL, Subramanian PS. Posterior ischemic optic neuropathy after minimally invasive prostatectomy. J Neuroophthalmol. 2007;27(4):285–7.

[11] Han ES, Advincula AP. Safety in minimally invasive surgery. Obstet Gynecol Clin N Am. 2019;46(2):389–98.

[12] Abdalmageed OS, Bedaiwy MA, Falcone T. Nerve injuries in gynecologic laparoscopy. J Minim Invasive Gynecol. 2017;24(1):16–27.

[13] Bjøro B, Mykkeltveit I, Rustøen T, Candas Altinbas B, Røise O, Bentsen SB. Intraoperative peripheral nerve injury related to lithotomy positioning with steep Trendelenburg in patients undergoing robotic-assisted laparoscopic surgery–a systematic review. J Adv Nurs. 2020;76(2):490–503.

[14] Bradshaw AD, Advincula AP. Postoperative neuropathy in gynecologic surgery. Obstet Gynecol Clin N Am. 2010;37(3):451–9.

[15] Das D, Propst K, Wechter ME, Kho RM. Evaluation of positioning devices for optimization of outcomes in laparoscopic and robotic-assisted gynecologic surgery. J Minim Invasive Gynecol. 2019;26(2):244–52.e1.

[16] Steck-Bayat KP, Henderson S, Aguirre AG, Smith RB, Mahnert NM, Gerkin RD, et al. Prospective randomized controlled trial comparing cephalad migration in robotic gynecologic surgery using egg-crate foam versus the Pink Pad? J Robot Surg. 2019:1–5.

[17] Watson MJ, Koch B, Tonzi M, Xu R, Heath G, Lute B, et al. Decreasing the prospect of upper extremity neuropraxia during robotic assisted laparoscopic prostatectomy: a novel technique. J Robot Surg. 2020;14(5):733–8.

[18] AORN bariatric surgery guideline. Perioperative standards and recommended practices. Association of periOperative Registered Nurses; 2010. p. 481–499.

[19] Warner ME, LaMaster LM, Thoeming AK, Shirk Marienau ME, Warner MA. Compartment syndrome in surgical patients. J Am Soc Anesthesiol. 2001;94(4):705–8.

[20] Warner MA, Martin JT, Schroeder DR, Offord KP, Chute CG. Lower-extremity motor neuropathy associated with surgery performed on

patients in a lithotomy position. J Am Soc Anesthesiol. 1994;81(1):6–12.
[21] Angermeier K, Jordan G. Complications of the exaggerated lithotomy position: a review of 177 cases. J Urol. 1994;151(4):866–8.
[22] Bennicoff G. Perioperative care of the morbidly obese patient in the lithotomy position. AORN J. 2010;92(3):297–312.
[23] Graling PR, Colvin DB. The lithotomy position in colon surgery. Postoperative complications. AORN J. 1992;55(4):1029–39.
[24] Hales CM, Carroll MD, Fryar C, Ogden CL. Prevalence of obesity and severe obesity among adults. United States, 2017–2018. NCHS Data Brief. 2020;288:1–8.
[25] Williamson J, Mahon D. Shouldering responsibility for intraoperative bariatric amputees. Ann R Coll Surg Engl. 2016;98(1):71.
[26] Dauer L, Miller D, Schueler B, Silberzweig J, Balter S, Bartal G, et al. Society of Interventional Radiology Safety and Health Committee. Cardiovascular and Interventional Radiological Society of Europe Standards of Practice Committee Occupational radiation protection of pregnant or potentially pregnant workers in IR: a joint guideline of the Society of Interventional Radiology and the Cardiovascular and Interventional Radiological Society of Europe. J Vasc Interv Radiol. 2015;26(2):171–81.
[27] Buisson-Valles I, Ollivier S, Gabinski P, Basse-Cathalinat B, Verdun-Esquer C, AQUITAINS MDT. Etat des lieux de la radioprotection dans les blocs opératoires des établissements privés et publics d'Aquitaine. Arch Mal Prof Environ. 2004;65(2–3):263.
[28] Galonnier F, Traxer O, Rosec M, Terrasa J-B, Gouezel P, Celier D, et al. Surgical staff radiation protection during fluoroscopy-guided urologic interventions. J Endourol. 2016;30(6):638–43.
[29] Spruce L. Back to basics: radiation safety. AORN J. 2017;106(1):42–9.
[30] ACR-SPR practice parameter for imaging pregnant or potentially pregnant adolescents and women with ionizing radiation. 2018. https://www.acr.org/–/ media/ACR/Files/Practice-Parameters/ Pregnant-Pts.pdf. Accessed 4/11/2021.
[31] Guidelines for radiation safety. Guidelines for perioperative practice. Denver: Association of PeriOperative Registered Nurses; 2017. p. 339–74.
[32] Tok A, Akbas A, Aytan N, Aliskan T, Cicekbilek I, Kaba M, et al. Are the urology operating room personnel aware about the ionizing radiation? Int Braz J Urol. 2015;41(5):982–9.
[33] Kuon E, Weitmann K, Hoffmann W, Dörr M, Hummel A, Busch M, et al. Role of experience, leadership and individual protection in the cath lab–a multicenter questionnaire and workshop on radiation safety. RöFo-Fortschritte auf dem Gebiet der Röntgenstrahlen und der bildgebenden Verfahren: © Georg Thieme Verlag KG; 2015. p. 899–905.
[34] Tjiam IM, Goossens RH, Schout BM, Koldewijn EL, Hendrikx AJ, Muijtjens AM, et al. Ergonomics in endourology and laparoscopy: an overview of musculoskeletal problems in urology. J Endourol. 2014;28(5):605–11.
[35] The State of Urology Workforce and Practice in the United States 2017. Linthicum. Maryland: American Urological Association; 2018.
[36] Epstein S, Tran BN, Capone AC, Ruan QZ, Fukudome EY, Ricci JA, et al. The current state of surgical ergonomics education in US surgical training: a survey study. Ann Surg. 2019;269(4):778–84.
[37] Kim-Fine S, Woolley SM, Weaver AL, Killian JM, Gebhart JB. Work-related musculoskeletal disorders among vaginal surgeons. Int Urogynecol J. 2013;24(7):1191–200.
[38] Dolan L, Martin D. Backache in gynaecologists. Occup Med. 2001;51(7):433–8.
[39] Meltzer AJ, Hallbeck MS, Morrow MM, Lowndes BR, Davila VJ, Stone WM, et al. Measuring ergonomic risk in operating surgeons by using wearable technology. JAMA Surg. 2020;155(5):444–6.
[40] Lux MM, Marshall M, Erturk E, Joseph JV. Ergonomic evaluation and guidelines for use of the daVinci Robot system. J Endourol. 2010;24(3):371–5. https://doi.org/10.1089/end.2009.0197.
[41] Berguer R, Hreljac A. The relationship between hand size and difficulty using surgical instruments: a survey of 726 laparoscopic surgeons. Surg Endosc. 2004;18(3):508–12. https://doi. org/10.1007/s00464–003– 8824– 3.
[42] Stellon M, Seils D, Mauro C. Assessing the importance of surgeon hand anthropometry on the design of medical devices. J Med Devices. 2017;11(4).
[43] Meredyth N. Cute little hands. Ann Surg. 2019;270(6):964–5.
[44] Sutton E, Irvin M, Zeigler C, Lee G, Park A. The ergonomics of women in surgery. Surg Endosc. 2014;28(4):1051–5. https://doi.org/10.1007/s00464–013– 3281– 0.
[45] Armijo PR, Flores L, Pokala B, Huang C-K, Siu K-C, Oleynikov D. Gender equity in ergonomics: does muscle effort in laparoscopic surgery differ between men and women? Surg Endosc. 2021:1–6.
[46] Punnett L, Wegman DH. Work-related musculoskeletal disorders: the epidemiologic evidence and the debate. J Electromyogr Kinesiol. 2004;14(1):13–23.
[47] Reyes D, Tang B, Cuschieri A. Minimal access surgery (MAS)–related surgeon morbidity syndromes. Surg Endosc Other Interv Tech. 2006;20(1):1–13.
[48] Hullfish KL, Trowbridge ER, Bodine G. Ergonomics and gynecologic surgery: "surgeon protect thyself". Female Pelvic Med Reconstr Surg. 2009;15(6):435–9.
[49] Singh R, Leon DAC, Morrow MM, Vos-Draper TL, Mc Gree ME, Weaver AL, et al. Effect of chair types on work-related musculoskeletal discomfort during vaginal surgery. Am J Obstet Gynecol. 2016;215(5):648.e1–9.
[50] Zhu X, Yurteri-Kaplan LA, Gutman RE, Sokol AI, Iglesia CB, Park AJ, et al. Postural stress experienced by vaginal surgeons. Proceedings of the Human Factors and Ergonomics Society annual meeting. SAGE Publications Sage CA: Los Angeles; 2014. p. 763–7.
[51] Catanzarite T, Tan-Kim J, Whitcomb EL, Menefee S. Ergonomics in surgery: a review. Female Pelvic Med Reconstr Surg. 2018;24(1):1–12.
[52] Ronstrom C, Hallbeck S, Lowndes B, Chrouser KL. Surgical ergonomics. In: Surgeons as educators. Cham: Springer; 2018. p. 387–417.
[53] Rosenblatt PL, McKinney J, Adams SR. Ergonomics in the operating room: protecting the surgeon. J Minim Invasive Gynecol. 2013;20(6):744.
[54] Haramis G, Rosales JC, Palacios JM, Okhunov Z, Mues AC, Lee D, et al. Prospective randomized evaluation of FOOT gel pads for operating room staff COMFORT during laparoscopic renal surgery. Urology. 2010;76(6):1405–8.
[55] Woodburn KL, Kho RM. Vaginal surgery: don't get bent out of shape. Am J Obstet Gynecol. 2020;223(5):762–3.
[56] Gözen AS, Tokas T, Tschada A, Jalal A, Klein J, Rassweiler J. Direct comparison of the different conventional laparoscopic positions with the ethos surgical platform in a laparoscopic pelvic surgery simulation setting. J Endourol. 2015;29(1):95–9.
[57] Liu S, Hemming D, Luo RB, Reynolds J, Delong JC, Sandler BJ, et al. Solving the surgeon ergonomic crisis with surgical exosuit. Surg Endosc. 2018;32(1):236–44.
[58] Hallbeck MS, Lowndes BR, Bingener J, Abdelrahman AM, Yu D, Bartley A, et al. The impact of intraoperative microbreaks with exercises on surgeons: a multi-center cohort study. Appl Ergon. 2017;60:334–41. https://doi.org/10.1016/j.apergo.2016.12.006.
[59] Abdelall ES, Lowndes BR, Abdelrahman AM, Hawthorne HJ, Hallbeck MS. Mini breaks, many benefits: development and pilot testing of an intraoperative microbreak stretch web-application for surgeons. Proceedings of the Human Factors and Ergonomics Society annual meeting. SAGE Publications Sage CA: Los Angeles; 2018. p. 1042–6.

[60] Lloyd GL, Chung AS, Steinberg S, Sawyer M, Williams DH, Overbey D. Is your career hurting you? The ergonomic consequences of surgery in 701 urologists worldwide. J Endourol. 2019;33(12):1037–42.
[61] Zebis MK, Andersen LL, Pedersen MT, Mortensen P, Andersen CH, Pedersen MM, et al. Implementation of neck/shoulder exercises for pain relief among industrial workers: a randomized controlled trial. BMC Musculoskelet Disord. 2011;12(1):1–9.
[62] Fecso AB, Szasz P, Kerezov G, Grantcharov TP. The effect of technical performance on patient outcomes in surgery. Ann Surg. 2017;265(3):492–501.
[63] Agha RA, Fowler AJ, Sevdalis N. The role of non-technical skills in surgery. Ann Med Surg. 2015;4(4):422–7.
[64] Yule S, Flin R, Paterson-Brown S, Maran N. Non-technical skills for surgeons in the operating room: a review of the literature. Surgery. 2006;139(2):140–9.
[65] Wood TC, Raison N, Haldar S, Brunckhorst O, McIlhenny C, Dasgupta P, et al. Training tools for nontechnical skills for surgeons—a systematic review. J Surg Educ. 2017;74(4):548–78.
[66] Gawande AA, Thomas EJ, Zinner MJ, Brennan TA. The incidence and nature of surgical adverse events in Colorado and Utah in 1992. Surgery. 1999;126(1):66–75.
[67] Christian CK, Gustafson ML, Roth EM, Sheridan TB, Gandhi TK, Dwyer K, et al. A prospective study of patient safety in the operating room. Surgery. 2006;139(2):159–73.
[68] Valanci-Aroesty S, Alhassan N, Feldman LS, Landry T, Mastropietro V, Fiore J Jr, et al. Implementation and effectiveness of coaching for surgeons in practice–a mixed studies systematic review. J Surg Educ. 2020;77(4):837–53.
[69] El-Gabri D, McDow AD, Quamme SP, Hooper-Lane C, Greenberg CC, Long KL. Surgical coaching for advancement of global surgical skills and capacity: a systematic review. J Surg Res. 2020;246:499–505.
[70] Arora S, Miskovic D, Hull L, Moorthy K, Aggarwal R, Johannsson H, et al. Self vs expert assessment of technical and non-technical skills in high fidelity simulation. Am J Surg. 2011;202(4):500–6.
[71] Larkin AC, Cahan MA, Whalen G, Hatem D, Starr S, Haley H-L, et al. Human Emotion and Response in Surgery (HEARS): a simulation-based curriculum for communication skills, systems-based practice, and professionalism in surgical residency training. J Am Coll Surg. 2010;211(2):285–92.
[72] Edmondson AC, Higgins M, Singer S, Weiner J. Understanding psychological safety in health care and education organizations: a comparative perspective. Res Hum Dev. 2016;13(1):65–83.
[73] Driskell JE, Copper C, Moran A. Does mental practice enhance performance? J Appl Psychol. 1994;79(4):481.
[74] Sevdalis N, Moran A, Arora S. Mental imagery and mental practice applications in surgery: state of the art and future directions. Multisens Imagery. 2013:343–63.
[75] Hall JC. Imagery practice and the development of surgical skills. Am J Surg. 2002;184(5):465–70.
[76] Chrouser KL, Partin MR. Intraoperative disruptive behavior: the medical student's perspective. J Surg Educ. 2019;76(5):1231–40.
[77] Villafranca A, Hamlin C, Enns S, Jacobsohn E. Disruptive behaviour in the perioperative setting: a contemporary review. Can J Anesth. 2017;64(2):128–40.
[78] Wetzel CM, George A, Hanna GB, Athanasiou T, Black SA, Kneebone RL, et al. Stress management training for surgeons—a randomized, controlled, intervention study. Ann Surg. 2011;253(3):488–94.
[79] Arora S, Aggarwal R, Sirimanna P, Moran A, Grantcharov T, Kneebone R, et al. Mental practice enhances surgical technical skills: a randomized controlled study. Ann Surg. 2011;253(2):265–70.
[80] Percy DB, Streith L, Wong H, Ball CG, Widder S, Hameed M. Mental toughness in surgeons: is there room for improvement? Can J Surg. 2019;62(6):482.
[81] Asken M, Christensen LW, Grossman D. Warrior mindset. 1st ed. Human Factors Research Group. US: warrior science publications. 2010.
[82] Rogers D, Lingard L, Boehler ML, Espin S, Klingensmith M, Mellinger JD, et al. Teaching operating room conflict management to surgeons: clarifying the optimal approach. Med Educ. 2011;45(9):939–45.
[83] Feldman J, Barshi I. The effects of blood glucose levels on cognitive performance: a review of the literature. NASA Ames Research Center: Moffett Field; 2007.
[84] McCrimmon RJ, Ewing FM, Frier BM, Deary IJ. Anger state during acute insulin-induced hypoglycaemia. Physiol Behav. 1999;67(1):35–9.
[85] Benton D, Owens D. Is raised blood glucose associated with the relief of tension? J Psychosom Res. 1993;37(7):723–35.
[86] Chrouser KL, Xu J, Hallbeck S, Weinger MB, Partin MR. The influence of stress responses on surgical performance and outcomes: literature review and the development of the surgical stress effects (SSE) framework. Am J Surg. 2018;216(3):573–84.
[87] El-Sharkawy AM, Bragg D, Watson P, Neal K, Sahota O, Maughan RJ, et al. Hydration amongst nurses and doctors on-call (the HANDS on prospective cohort study). Clin Nutr. 2016;35(4):935–42.
[88] Pilcher JJ, Huffcutt AI. Effects of sleep deprivation on performance: a meta-analysis. Sleep. 1996;19(4):318–26.
[89] Hull L, Arora S, Aggarwal R, Darzi A, Vincent C, Sevdalis N. The impact of nontechnical skills on technical performance in surgery: a systematic review. J Am Coll Surg. 2012;214(2):214–30.
[90] Flin R, Yule S, McKenzie L, Paterson-Brown S, Maran N. Attitudes to teamwork and safety in the operating theatre. Surgeon. 2006;4(3):145–51.
[91] Sittikraipong K, Silsupadol P, Uthaikhup S. Slower reaction and response times and impaired hand-eye coordination in individuals with neck pain. Musculoskelet Sci Pract. 2020;50:102273.
[92] Huysmans MA, Hoozemans MJ, van der Beek AJ, de Looze MP, van Dieën JH. Position sense acuity of the upper extremity and tracking performance in subjects with non-specific neck and upper extremity pain and healthy controls. J Rehabil Med. 2010;42(9):876–83.
[93] Moriarty O, Finn DP. Cognition and pain. Curr Opin Support Palliat Care. 2014;8(2):130–6.
[94] Riskin A, Erez A, Foulk TA, Kugelman A, Gover A, Shoris I, et al. The impact of rudeness on medical team performance: a randomized trial. Pediatrics. 2015;136(3):487–95.
[95] Rosenstein AH, O'Daniel M. Impact and implications of disruptive behavior in the perioperative arena. J Am Coll Surg. 2006;203(1):96–105.
[96] Gordon M, Darbyshire D, Baker P. Non-technical skills training to enhance patient safety: a systematic review. Med Educ. 2012;46(11):1042–54.
[97] Huser A-S, Müller D, Brunkhorst V, Kannisto P, Musch M, Kröpfl D, et al. Simulated life-threatening emergency during robot-assisted surgery. J Endourol. 2014;28(6):717–21.
[98] Stevens L-M, Cooper JB, Raemer DB, Schneider RC, Frankel AS, Berry WR, et al. Educational program in crisis management for cardiac surgery teams including high realism simulation. J Thorac Cardiovasc Surg. 2012;144(1):17–24.
[99] Arora S, Sevdalis N, Nestel D, Tierney T, Woloshynowych M, Kneebone R. Managing intraoperative stress: what do surgeons want from a crisis training program? Am J Surg. 2009;197(4):537–43.

第 27 章 女性尿失禁的实验疗法和研究方向

Experimental Therapies and Research Needs for Urinary Incontinence in Women

Casey G. Kowalik　Rena D. Malik　著

缩略语

ADSC	adipose-derived stem cell	脂肪干细胞
AMDC	autologous muscle-derived cell	自体肌源细胞
OAB	overactive bladder	膀胱过度活动症
P4HB	poly-4-hydroxybutryate	聚 4- 羟基丁酸酯
PGI	patient global impression	患者总体印象量表
PRP	platelet-rich plasma	富血小板血浆
SUI	stress urinary incontinence	压力性尿失禁
TTT	tunable-tension transobturator tape	经闭孔可调节吊带手术
UMB	urinary bladder matrix	膀胱黏膜基底层
UUI	urgency urinary incontinence	急迫性尿失禁

虽然目前对于急迫性尿失禁和压力性尿失禁的治疗方案可以使患者具有较高的满意度，但探索创新或优化的方法仍在不断进行，以期获得更好的结局指标以及更少的不良反应。尿失禁是一种慢性疾病，每年会产生数十亿美元的经济影响[1]。这些成本包括但不限于：尿失禁产品的材料成本、因失业导致的收入损失、与治疗相关的医疗成本以及与尿失禁相关的抑郁、性功能障碍和低自尊等间接成本。目前对于急迫性尿失禁的管理方式包括行为矫正、抗胆碱能药或 β_3 受体激动动药治疗、膀胱注射肉毒杆菌毒素和骶神经调节。最近发现了一种新的高选择性 β_3 受体激动药批准在美国使用，在临床试验中已证实可显著减少急迫性尿失禁的临床发作且具有较少的不良反应[2]。神经调节技术的进展，包括可置入胫骨神经刺激器和 MRI 兼容骶神经刺激仪的开发，可为更广泛的人群提供额外的希望基于非手术治疗手段或需要使用磁共振兼容骶神经刺激器治疗的医疗方式。利用质粒载体的基因治疗目前正在研究中，尿微生物领域的新兴研究显示了急迫性尿失禁个体化治疗的前景。自 20 世纪 90 年代中期以来，已经使用了用于治疗压力性尿失禁的网状吊带，并不断进行改进以提高疗效且减少不良事件发生。例如，在动物模型中研究了非永久性材料或药物洗脱网状吊带。可调吊带和可调张力吊带目前正在临床研究中。经阴道探头递送的射频消融治疗和 CO_2 激光治疗目前已经获批上市，但关于压力性尿失禁改善的临床数据仍在积累。临床研究中也在探索新的概念，包括通过减少腹腔内压力的来减少压力性尿失禁发作的膀胱内装置。近年来，研

究人员一直在动物模型中寻找以干细胞为靶点的尿道括约肌再生疗法，且最近使用的自体肌源干细胞的临床研究取得了满意的结果[3]。

在本节，我们回顾了急迫性尿失禁和压力性尿失禁最新的药物治疗和医学技术进展治疗方式。最后，我们总结了当前研究的局限性，并指出了未来的研究领域。

一、紧急尿失禁的最新药物

（一）Vibegron（维贝隆）

维贝隆是高选择性 β_3 受体激动药，是急迫性尿失禁最新的补充治疗方案。与米拉贝隆类似，它附着于 β_3 肾上腺素受体，并促进膀胱壁的松弛。与其他 β 亚型相比，维贝隆对 β_3 肾上腺素受体的选择性超过 9000 倍[4]。β_3 肾上腺素受体选择性可能归因于维贝隆具有吡咯烷环的结构构型及其臂的合成构型，以激活 β_3 肾上腺素受体[4]。值得注意的是，该药物的平均半衰期为 25～38h，允许每日给药，并且不抑制 CYP2D6 酶，从而降低药物间相互作用的风险。

在日本的一项四组双盲安慰剂对照随机对照试验中分析了维贝隆的疗效[5]。出现膀胱过度活动症至少 6 个月的患者被纳入试验，并接受为期 2 周的安慰剂试运行阶段。随后，他们被随机分为四个治疗组：维贝隆（50mg 或 100mg，每日 1 次）、安慰剂或咪达那新抗胆碱能治疗（0.1mg，每日 2 次），共 12 周。评估的主要结果是从基线到研究结束每天平均排尿次数的变化。在 50mg 和 100mg 维贝格隆组中，每日排尿次数的最小二乘均值与基线相比的变化为（–2.08～2.03）在 100mg 维贝隆组，对照安慰剂组为 –1.21（$P<0.001$）。关于急迫性尿失禁，100mg 和 50mg 维贝隆组显示每日急迫性尿失禁发作减少，最小二乘均值为 –1.47～–1.35。该研究还发现，两种剂量的维贝隆在日常紧迫感、夜尿症发作、经验证的 King 健康问卷领域得分和患者总体印象（PGI）满意度方面均有显著改善。不良事件发生率低（5.6%～7.6%），最常见的包括鼻咽炎和膀胱炎。在严重急迫性尿失禁亚组中（每日≥3 次），急迫性尿失禁的减少显著改善（–2.95 和 –3.28 次急迫性尿失禁发作 / 天，分别为 50mg 和 100mg 剂量），50mg 和 100mg 剂量的排尿量和患者总体印象。试验仅在 50mg 剂量组和 100mg 剂量组中紧急情况有所改善，其记录干燥率显著增加（37.5% vs. 17.9%，P=0.020）[6]。

在全球Ⅲ期临床试验 EMPOWUR 中，1518 例膀胱过度活动症患者（其中 75% 有急迫性尿失禁）被随机分为每日 75mg 维贝隆、每日 4mg 托特罗定或安慰剂，其主要终点为急迫性尿失禁发作从基线到 12 周的变化。与安慰剂组相比，维贝隆组在 12 周时的每日急迫性尿失禁发病率显著降低，其差异具备统计学意义。与安慰剂相比，维贝隆组的不良事件包括头痛（4.0% vs. 2.4%）、鼻咽炎（2.8% vs. 1.7%）、腹泻（2.2% vs. 1.1%）和恶心（2.1% vs. 1.1%）。高血压发生率没有明显高于安慰剂组[2]。在长达 52 周的扩展试验中，发现急迫性尿失禁进一步降低，61% 的患者有急迫性尿失禁减少≥75%，第 52 周时 41% 患者为干燥状态，并报告其生活质量持续改善[7, 8]。

在对三项随机对照试验（共 2120 例膀胱过度活动症患者）的系统评价和 Meta 分析中，再次得出结论：维贝隆显著减少了急迫性尿失禁发生次数、尿急发生率且增加了每次排尿量，并在 12 周内改善了生活质量。除了鼻咽炎和膀胱炎，口干和便秘也被列为不良反应[9]。维贝隆（商品名为 Gemtesa®）于 2020 年 12 月获得美国食品药品管理局批准。

（二）基因疗法

目前正在研究利用质粒载体进行基因治疗急迫性尿失禁的方法。*Uro-902* 是表达大电导钾离子通道 α 亚基的质粒载体，该亚基通常在膀胱平滑肌细胞上高度表达，其激活降低了平滑肌细胞的兴奋性，从而降低逼尿肌过度活动[10]。Ⅰ期、双盲、安慰剂对照、序贯有效剂量试验比较了膀胱内滴注（ION-02）和直接注射（ION-03）质粒载体对逼尿肌过度活动尿流动力学改变和膀胱过度活动症对女性的影响。在膀胱灌注组中，7 例患者接受 5000μg 剂量，6 例接受 10 000μg 剂量和 5 例接受安慰剂。在直接注射组，6 例患者接受 16 000μg 剂量，3 例接受 24 000μg 剂量和 4 例接受安慰剂。就安全性而言，在 ION-02 组中，1 例患者患有莫氏Ⅱ型二度房室传导阻滞，还有 1 例患者出现疲劳、头痛、发抖和失眠。在 ION-03 组中，与安慰剂相比，大多数膀胱过度活动症参数和生活质量有显著改善，然而急迫性尿失禁并没有显著改善。治疗 24 周后，急迫性尿失禁确实从基线显著改善。与安慰剂组相比，两组的残余尿均无增加。虽然此试验仍处于早期阶段，但目前数据似乎倾向于具有更长治疗时间的治疗方案，且无尿潴留风险。

二、神经调节方面的技术进展

（一）植入式胫神经刺激器

经皮胫神经刺激器是急迫性尿失禁的可选治疗方案；然而它要求每周门诊治疗，共计 12 周，然后每 4～6 周进行 1 次维护访问。由于需要多次门诊就诊极为不便，可置入装置正在被研究（表 27–1）。BlueWind RENOVA™（BlueWind Medical, Herzliya, Israel）是一种圆柱形（直径 3.4mm，长度 25mm）无电池装置，其置入在胫神经附近，与形状为围绕脚踝袖带的外部刺激器一起使用（图 27–1）。建议每天在可获得的脉冲宽度（50～800μs）、振幅（0～9mA）和频率（5～40Hz）下使用 30min。对 34 例置入该装置的患者进行了 6 个月随访，结果显示 71% 的患者急迫性尿失禁改善率＞50%，干燥率为 27.8%[11, 12]。然而，不良事件包括 14% 的置入部位疼痛、22% 的疑似感染和 8.3% 的受试者的伤口并发症。

eCoi™（Valencia, California, the USA）是唯一一款完全置入的胫骨神经刺激器，采用无导线设计，主电池的大小和形状似美国镍币（直径 23.3mm，厚度 2.3mm）（图 27–2）。在门诊使用局部麻醉将其置入皮下的筋膜上方。该装置每周 2 次从中心阴极到最外边缘的阳极电极进行 30min 的自动刺激。它不需要持续刺激、充电、远程使用或重复门诊就诊。电池寿命平均为 3 年。在 46 例膀胱过度活动症患者中进行了试验，其中 73% 的患者急迫性尿失禁降低了 50% 或更多，30% 的患者在长达 36 周的随访中保持干燥。感染率低至 2.3%[13]。

BlueWind RENOVA™ 和 eCoin™ 的原始数据似乎有希望成为改善急迫性尿失禁的类似于目前的三线疗法。招募正在进行，正在收集长期后续数据[14, 15]。目前其他植入物的有限可用数据包括 StimGuard® 和 Bioness[16, 17]。StimGuard®（now Protect PNS）是一种无线置入式胫骨倒刺电极，可在门诊环境中完成置入，配备可充电外部电源（图 27–3）。7 次置入的原始数据表明，置入后 6 个月内急迫性尿失禁改善，急迫性尿失禁发作从 3.05 降至 1.24。3 例患者 12 个月时的数据显示，急迫性尿失禁发生率进一步改善至每天 0.66 次[18]。报道了 5 起轻微不良事件，其中包括电线隆起、缝线溃疡和刺激丧失[19]。目前，一项前瞻性、随机、对照、多中心研究正在积极招募 150 例参与者，将无线胫骨神经刺激［慢性神经传导刺激（CAN-Stim）］与标准骶骨神经刺激进行比较，主要结局指标在 3 个月是时急迫性尿失禁发作减少率≥50%[20]。

Bioness StimRouter™ 是一种带有集成接收器、锚点和 3 个电极触点的置入导线设计（图 27–4）。无线能量是使用外部脉冲发射器传送的，该外部脉冲发射器连接到外部佩戴的电极贴片。患者编程器用于更改程序和监控使用情况。该装置可在门诊就诊时在超声引导下置入。建议治疗为每周 3～7 天，每次 30min。目前正在招募 180 例患者进行前瞻性、多中心、随机、双盲临床试验，比较 StimRouter 组和假治疗组的疗效[21]。胫骨神经系统的外部组件与 MRI 不兼容，必须在行 MRI 检查前移除，但置入的导线可以保留。与目前可用的骶骨神经调节刺激器相比，置入式胫骨神经装

表 27-1　置入式胫神经刺激器设计、使用和临床试验总结

装置名称	设　计	使用方法	是否可穿戴	临床编程	患者远程控制	作者（年份）	病例数	随访时间（月）	≥ 50% 急迫性尿失禁改善	≥ 50% 严重急迫性尿失禁改善	干燥率
BlueWind RENOVA™（BlueWind Medical, Herzliya, Israel）	无导线，无电池，植入物（体积 0.3 cm^3，直径 3.4mm）	每天 30min 自我管理	√	√	√	Van Breda，2017[70]	11	3	36.4%	71%[a]	18.2%
						Heesakkers，2018[11]	29	6	51.7%	NR	27.6%
						Dorsthorst，2020[71]	16[b]	36	50%	75%～80%[b]	NR
						Dmochowski，2019[72]	20	36	75%[c]	NR	NR
eCoin™（Valencia, CA, USA）	完全置入，原电池，无导线（直径 23.3mm，2.3mm 厚），3 年电池寿命	自动刺激传递 30min 每周 2 次				MacDiarmid，2019[73]	46	6	67.4%	NR	23.9%
						MacDiarmid，2019[74]	46	12	65%	NR	26.1%
						Rogers，2020[13]	122	8.3	73%	NR	30.3%
StimGuard® now Protect PNS（Micron Medical Boca Raton, FL, USA）	无线倒刺电极，可充电外部电源	每天刺激 6h 以上	√			Sirls，2019[18]	7	12	—	—	—
Bioness StimRouter™	倒刺电极，集成接收器，外部穿戴脉冲发射器	每周 3～7 天，每次 30min	√		√	Giusto，2019[16]	—	—	—	—	—

NR. 未报道
a. 严重急迫性尿失禁：超过基线的尿失禁排尿记录
b. Heesakkers 等的扩展试验在治疗组中每协议治疗组 75%，意向治疗组 80%
c. 成功定义为在紧急排泄、渗漏或正常排泄的发生减少≥ 50%

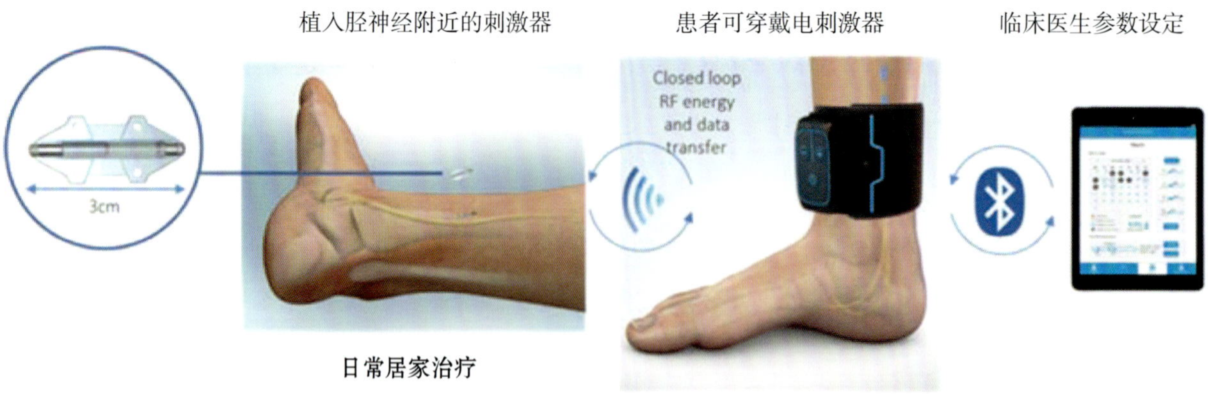

▲ 图 27-1　**BlueWind RENOVA™**
经 BlueWind Medical 许可转载

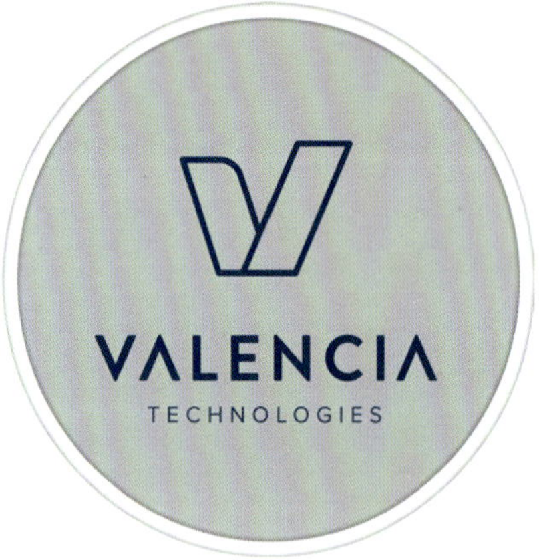

▲ 图 27-2　**eCoin™**
经 Valencia 许可转载

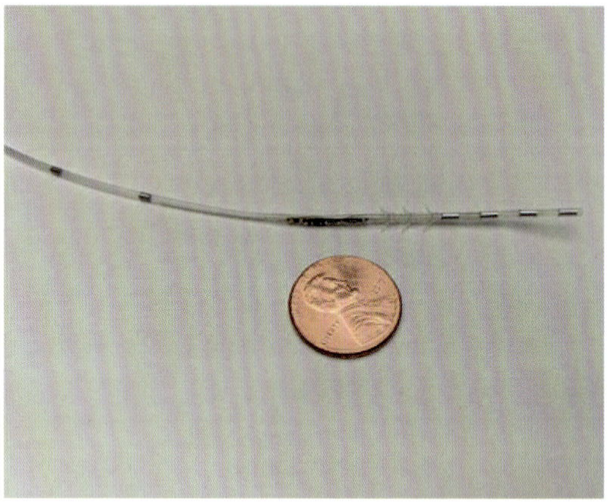

▲ 图 27-3　**StimGuard®（PNS）**
经 Micron Medical 许可转载

置提供了在基于办公室的环境中使用解剖标志进行局部麻醉的优点，无须 X 线透视检查。

（二）骶神经调节

恒定电流，可充电和 MRI 兼容的神经调节系统已成为急迫性尿失禁的治疗选择。恒定电流技术根据阻抗变化自动调整电流，以提供一致的刺激水平。初始数据表明，这可能是有益的，尤其是在置入后的前 6 个月，此时阻抗增加最为显著[22]。可充电电池具有许多优点，包括与标准置入式脉冲发生器（体积为 14cm^3）相比体积更小（Axonics 体积为 5.5cm^3，Intersim Micro 体积为 2.8cm^3），电池寿命估计可延长至 15 年。预计将继续对当前骶骨神经调节系统进行进一步修改，以继续优化和标准化导线放置，并使患者更易使用。

三、急迫性尿失禁的靶向治疗

微生物

微生物系统在维持膀胱健康方面的作用仍有待揭示，一些研究人员正在评估微生物系统对尿失禁的影响。在比较有急迫性尿失禁和无急迫性尿失禁女性的导尿样本时，每个队列的微生物组存在显著差异，表明尿液微生物参与下尿路症状复杂关系[23]。Thomas White 等的一项研究进一步证实了尿微生物群在急迫性尿失禁中的作用，可能有助于指导个体化治疗。该研究组化验了急迫性尿失禁患者的尿液，发现细菌较少且菌群单一的女性更有可能对索利那星药物的治疗产生临床疗效[24]。

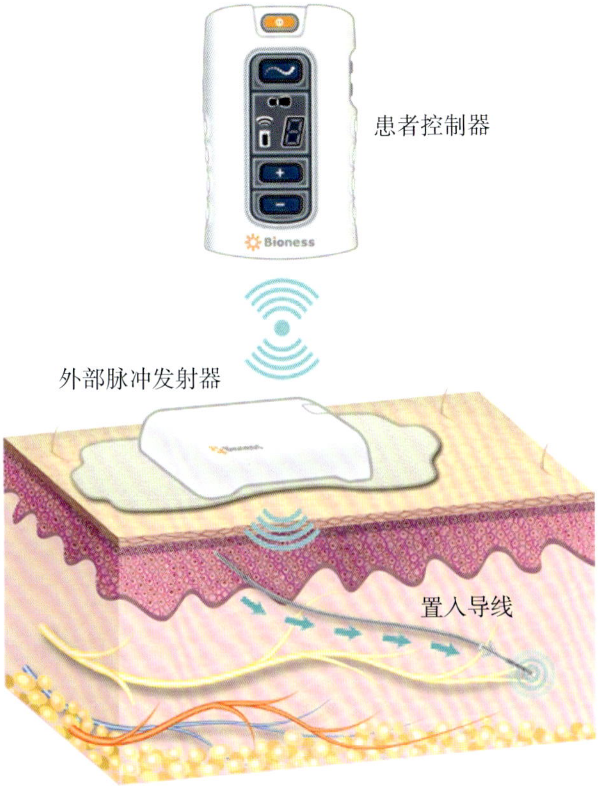

▲ 图 27-4 **Bioness StimRoute**™
经 Bioness 许可转载

四、压力性尿失禁的非手术选择

多项研究表明，通过物理治疗和生物反馈进行盆底肌肉训练不仅可以改善尿失禁，而且有助于预防尿失禁的发生。磁刺激和电刺激是两种旨在改善盆底肌肉收缩的技术。这些疗法是否会在美国获得更广泛的接受可能取决于医疗保险范围，否则其治疗费用可能会很高。

（一）磁刺激

磁刺激是一种非手术治疗方式，其治疗压力性尿失禁的成功率的报告各不相同。其提出的机制是通过产生电磁场的磁线圈刺激盆底肌肉收缩。治疗通常每周两次，每次 20min，在办公室使用类似椅子的设备进行。一项对 120 例每周接受 2 次治疗的女性进行的盲法、假对照研究的短期（2 个月）结果显示，主观尿失禁症状有所改善[25]。

（二）电刺激

电刺激的优点是治疗可以在家中进行。一项对于电刺激的 Cochrane 研究得出结论，电刺激与安慰治疗组相比有益处，但未与传统盆底物理治疗组进行充分比较[26]。在一项随机试验中，比较了电刺激的外给药和阴道内给药，结果表明，阴道外部电刺激并不劣于阴道内部电刺激，而且外部电刺激可减少尿路感染的发生[27]。

五、压力性尿失禁的悬吊术

用于治疗压力性尿失禁的中尿道网状吊带长期以来一直是外科护理的金标准，因为其微创性、快速恢复和高疗效。然而，已知合成材料会产生异物反应，并有术后网状物并发症的风险。为了尽量减少这些并发症并增加黏弹性，正在寻找替代吊带材料或非永久性材料。使用的生物材料类型包括①用富含血小板血浆（PRP）增强的合成材料或植入人成纤维细胞，可提供改善的生物相容性或减少炎性细胞反应；②单独的细胞外基质（ECM），细胞接种或增强，这提供了可生物降解和激活宿主细胞重塑和胶原沉积的额外益处。基于细胞外基质的材料包括尸体真皮、小肠黏膜下层和膀胱基质（UBM）。此外，静电纺丝材料，即通过聚合物溶液的电压驱动过程开发支架的技术，具有潜在的提高抗拉强度和紧密模拟生理微结构的潜力[28]。增强的或细胞接种的合成材料仅限于在动物模型中评估脱垂修复。在这些模型中，置入富含血小板血浆增强聚丙烯网和胶原涂层聚丙烯网导致炎症细胞浸润减少，胶原生成增加，显示生物相容性改善[29, 30]。

小规模研究已利用细胞外基质修复盆腔器官脱垂，并取得了令人鼓舞的结果；然而，由于制造、加工、材料的异质性、小样本量以及临床研究设计的局限性，细胞外基质的价值仍不清楚[31]。临床试验中对吊带材料细胞外基质的目前评估有限。目前，细胞接种的细胞外基质正在进一步研究中。膀胱基质和抗 Sca-1 和碱性成纤维细胞生长因子已交叉结合以招募宿主干细胞并导致平滑肌分化。临床前研究表明，这种独特的组合产生了一种生物相容性支架，有可能用于盆底重建[32]。

静电纺丝是一种利用电荷以随机模式随机沉积聚合物纳米颗粒的过程，以模拟人体生理结构，并随后促进细胞附着和生长[33]。与传统聚丙烯中尿道吊带材料相比，用于压力性尿失禁的电纺聚丙烯兔模型显示出更高的抗拉强度和更少的炎症反应[34]。已评估了用生物可降解材料［包括电纺聚乳酸与碳酸三亚甲酯和聚（L- 丙交酯）- 碳酸三亚甲基酯 - 乙交酯］浸渍的脂肪来源干细胞（ADSC）的体外研究，发现其可增加拉伸强度、细胞外基质沉积和血管生成[35, 36]。此外，还对含有 17-β- 雌二醇的电纺合成聚氨酯在人脂肪干细胞（ADSC）上进行了评估，并显示了具有适当拉伸强度和细胞外基质生成的血管生成潜力[37]。

（一）非永久性悬吊材料

使用可生物降解聚 -4- 羟基丁酸酯（P4HB）的单层单丝的植入物，TephaFLEX™，被认为是目前用于压力性尿失禁的永久网状材料的可能替代物。据估计，聚 -4- 羟基丁酸酯在 3 个月后逐渐失去强度，18～24 个月可完全吸收。在兔模型中，比较聚 -4- 羟基丁酸酯钩针编织、网状编织和永久性聚丙烯网，植入导致类似的组织学反应，聚 -4- 羟基丁酸酯具有更高的抗拉强度和最低的炎症反应[38]。TephaFLEX™ 吊带目前正在进行一项为期 24 个月的前瞻性单中心观察性试验，该试验估计有 25 例压力性尿失禁患者，主要结果为器械安全性和治疗后不良事件的评估[39]。

（二）药物洗脱和涂层网

已经研究了骨盆器官脱垂时通过网状物在手术部位周围局部递送药物。使用可输送抗生素的药物洗脱系统可降低术后短期感染率，同时保持网状结构的完整性[40]。虽然没有专门研究中尿道吊带，但这一概念是可以转换的。

在动物模型中研究了类固醇涂层网，理论上认为类固醇将减少局部异物反应。一项研究发现，使用涂有类固醇的网状物后，肉芽肿尺寸减小，炎细胞数量减少，胶原形成减少[41]

（三）可调节吊带

目前，可调节张力的中尿道吊带的额外优化也在研究中。Altis® 吊带是一种小型可调吊带，带有整体张力系统。最初的前瞻性行业赞助多中心试验招募了 113 例女性，90% 的患者获得了护垫重量减少≥50%，干燥率为 81%（护垫重量≤4g）。在长达 24 个月的症状困扰和生活质量问卷调查中也有显著改善[42]。在一项无赞助、前瞻性、单中心试验中，招募了 110 例女性，客观治愈率为 83%（压力诱发试验阴性），主观治愈率为 88%（ICIQ-SF=0）。并发症包括 7% 的急性尿潴留、8% 的排尿功能障碍和 7% 的疼痛[43]。一项前瞻性、观察性队列研究将 Altis® 吊带与传统的经闭孔和耻骨后吊带进行了比较，最近完成了 416 例参与者的数据累积，结果尚待确定。主要结果包括：在 6 个月的随访中护垫重量减少≥50% 的数目和 36 个月内器械和（或）手术相关不良事件发生的数目。不良事件发生率为 3.5%，与传统中尿道吊带相似[44]。此外，正在欧洲招募的正在进行的、前瞻性、上市后、单组、多中心研究[45]（Clinicaltrials.gov Identifier: NCT02049840）。

可调张力经闭孔吊带（TTT），Urosling-T（Lintex, LLC），是一种经闭孔尿道中段吊带，能够在术后早期调节张力。一项随机对照试验招募了 388 例接受可调张力经闭孔吊带或标准经闭孔尿道中段吊带治疗的参与者，目前正在进行研究，主要结果是在国际尿控制协会 - 标准压力诱发试验期间无尿漏[46]（Clinicaltrials.gov Identifier: NCT03958695）。

六、压力性尿失禁的再生治疗

（一）干细胞疗法

从几年前的动物模型开始，利用干细胞治疗压力性尿失禁的研究一直在持续。最近，在尿道括约肌内注射细胞的人体试验正在进行。干细胞有效性背后的科学依据尚未明确，但提出的原理包括①将注射的细胞并入宿主细胞；②从干细胞释放局部因子，有助于修复受损的宿主细胞；③干细胞向其他细胞类型的实际细胞分化。在压力性尿失禁患者中，尿道括约肌也可能有一些整体效应，从而改善症状[47]。

多种类型的细胞被研究，包括骨骼肌细胞（成肌细胞、祖细胞）、骨髓干细胞、脂肪来源干细胞（ADSC）和人类脐带干细胞，其中最有前景的是骨骼肌源干细胞（AMDC）（表 27–2）[3, 48-53]。在一项初步研究中，Carr 等将取自大腿肌肉的骨骼肌源干细胞注射给 8 例压力性尿失禁患者，并注意到 10 个月时护垫垫重量持续改善[48]。进一步的剂量研究和安全性试验发现，括约肌内注射骨骼肌源干细胞是安全的，38 例女性中有 3 例报告了注射部位疼痛和瘀伤。护垫重量减少差异也有统计学意义[3]。在Ⅰ期和Ⅱ期研究中，未报道归因于细胞的不良事件，与手术相关的并发症较少（瘀伤/疼痛）[53]。正在进行的Ⅲ期随机安慰剂对照试验正在招募患有压力性尿失禁的女性（ClinicalTrials.gov Identifier: NCT03104517）。

脂肪源性干细胞（ADSC）也被证明经历了细胞分化，并被注射到 5 例女性的尿道括约肌中[54]。另一个研究小组研究了给 30 例患有压力性尿失禁的女性尿道周围注射人脐带干细胞。在注射后 3 个月，80% 的患者报告主观结果改善，在 10 例术前最大尿道闭合压力（MUCP）较低的女性中，有显著增加[55]。迄今为止，还没有使用骨髓干细胞进行人体试验，这主要是由于无法获得所需的大量细胞以及无法耐受骨髓活检带来的疼痛。

（二）低强度体外冲击波治疗

动物模型已经证明，对下骨盆应用低强度体外冲击波治疗（LiSWT）可激活肌管形成并增强

表 27–2 应用间充质干细胞治疗女性压力性尿失禁的临床试验

间充质干细胞类型	研 究	细胞采集部位	研究设计	临床疗效
自体肌源细胞	Carr 等[48]	大腿	试点试验，n=8	5 例完成研究，1 项治愈，4 项在 10 个月时护垫重量减少
	Carr 等[3]	股四头肌	前瞻性队列研究，n=38	33 例完成研究
	Mitterberger 等[49]	二头肌	前瞻性队列研究，n=123	MUCP 改善 40%，主观治愈率 79%
	Gras 等[50]	股外侧肌	前瞻性队列研究，n=35	主观和客观治愈率为 14%，改善率为 37%
	Sebe 等[51]	三角肌	前瞻性队列研究，n=12	12 个月时，25% 的主观干燥率，58% 的护垫测试改善
	Blaganje 等[52]	二头肌	前瞻性队列研究，n=38，细胞注射后的电刺激	6 个月时，23% 治愈，52% 好转
	Peters 等[53]	股四头肌	来自Ⅰ/Ⅱ期试验的汇总数据，n=5	12 个月时的主观改善，更高剂量（200 × 106 AMDC-USR）护垫重量减少
脂肪干细胞	Kuismanen 等[54]	腹壁	前瞻性队列研究，n=5	患者报告结果改善，1 年尿流动力学参数无差异
人脐血干细胞	Lee 等[55]	脐带静脉	前瞻性队列研究，n=39	3 个月时主观改善 80%，10/10 女性的 MUCP 改善

细胞再生[56, 57]。假设低强度体外冲击波治疗可以将干细胞动员到损伤部位，从而减少炎症，增加盆底血供，增强膀胱干细胞激活，这可能会导致逼尿肌过度活动减少和尿道括约肌功能的改善。理论上，这种技术可以减少女性急迫性尿失禁和压力性尿失禁症状。中国台湾正在进行一项随机（低强度体外冲击波治疗与假治疗的实验组）临床试验，利用低强度体外冲击波治疗治疗尿失禁（ClinicalTrials.gov Identifier: NCT04059133）。近年来，该疗法已用于治疗勃起功能障碍，取得了一定的成功。如果成功的改进临床结果，低强度体外冲击波治疗将成为一种新的、无创的、广泛应用的女性尿失禁治疗方法。

七、压力性尿失禁的其他技术进展

（一）射频疗法

冷冻剂冷却单极射频（CMRF）装置已用于治疗压力性尿失禁。这些装置最初用于治疗女性性功能障碍和阴道松弛，其工作原理是使用阴道探头，将单极射频能量同时输送至固有层，并将冷冻剂冷却至阴道上皮的表面黏膜层。这导致成纤维细胞活化和胶原生成，并增加盆底支撑[58]。在一项针对轻度至中度压力性尿失禁女性的随机非盲试验中，35 例患者被随机分为接受 1 次或 2 次冷冻剂冷却单极射频治疗，每次治疗间隔 6 周，基于门诊环境。治疗包括 220 个 $90J/cm^2$ 的脉冲，其中 25 个脉冲在阴道口处的四个象限，保留尿道正下方的区域。在这两组中，50%～54% 的女性 1h 尿垫重量减少≥50%，75% 获得治愈，或者漏尿≤1g，在 12 个月时单冷冻剂冷却单极射频治疗组 1h 护垫重量。除 1 例患者在试验期间出现 2 次尿路感染外，未发现手术的不良事件[59]。虽然这项小型单中心研究的数据很有希望，但还需要进一步的大规模随机对照试验来证实结果。一项随机单盲对照试验比较了轻度至中度压力性尿失禁患者的冷冻剂冷却单极射频治疗与仅冷冻剂治疗和假治疗，该试验最近已完成，等待结果公布[60]。

（二）激光疗法

CO_2 激光热消融通过诱导胶原变性、重塑和新生，从而导致组织弹性增加。它被经阴道使用治疗有压力性尿失禁的更年期泌尿生殖系统综合征（GSM）症状的女性[61]。更年期泌尿生殖系统综合征的特征是阴道上皮变薄、皱襞消失、pH 改变和菌群失调。在这项研究中，161 例年龄在 45—65 岁的绝经后女性接受了 1 次 30～45min 的激光治疗，在尿道膀胱交界处使用 SmartXide2 V2LR 点阵微灼烧 CO_2 激光系统，随后每年的 12、24 和 36 个月进行治疗。根据经过验证的 ICIQ-UI-SF，患者在 1h 护垫重量测试和压力性尿失禁中表现出显著改善，组织学变化证实阴道上皮增厚，固有层组织结构改善。在对于 CO_2 和铒激光治疗女性压力性尿失禁的系统评价中（包括 13 项研究和 764 例患者），单次治疗后 6 个月和重复治疗后 24 个月，ICIQ-SF 和 1h 护垫重量显著改善。然而，需要进一步的高质量研究来确定激光治疗的类型和治疗间隔时间，以获得女性压力性尿失禁治疗的最佳结果[62]。

（三）Vesair® 膀胱内球囊

Vesair® 膀胱内球囊是一种膀胱内聚氨酯球囊，在膀胱穹顶自由浮动，旨在减弱腹部压力增加产生的膀胱内压力。这种新型装置用 30ml 空气充气，漂浮在膀胱穹顶，并吸收压力活动期膀胱内压力瞬时增加产生的压力，其通常会导致压力性尿失禁[63]。该装置已在美国完成了Ⅲ期试验，并进行了 12 个月的随访，安全性和有效性数据令人满意。在多中心、随机、假对照试验中，221 例在激发性应激试验中压力性尿失禁和护垫重量＞5g 的女性被随机分配接受膀胱内球囊装置或假手术。在膀胱镜引导使用专用尿道进入鞘插入装置，并用 30ml 空气和 0.7ml 液体氟碳充气。在 12 个月时，54.7% 接受球囊治疗的患者达到了复合终点，即衬垫重量减少＞75%，尿失禁生活质量评分增加 10 分。然而，治疗组中只有不到 50% 的患者在 12 个月时仍留在研究中，84% 的患者因器械不耐受或不良事件退出研究，其中包括刺痛、耻骨上不适、急迫感或尿路感染。虽然数据令人鼓舞，但在选定的耐受治疗的患者中，需要进一步研究，确定最佳患者群体，并对球囊进行潜在的修改，以减少不适感。

八、目前尿失禁研究的局限性

尽管尿失禁研究取得了巨大进展，但目前仍有一些因素限制了研究之间的广泛比较。在压力性尿失禁评估中，漏尿点压力（LPP）具有明确的阈值，用于定义固有括约肌缺陷（＜60cmH_2O），但研究组之间的漏尿点压力测定非标准化，使得研究之间的比较变得困难。用于激发压力性尿失禁的方法、压力记录部位（膀胱或尿道）和（或）所用压力传感器类型的差异并不一致。国际尿控制协会发布了尿流动力学性能指南，但也认可多种技术占主导地位[64]。

尿失禁动物模型的开发仍然具有挑战性。大多数情况下，这是利用急性损伤，导致盆底无力，而不是慢性过程，这是通常在女性中演变的方式。

虽然尿失禁的经济负担是巨大的，但与临床研究相关的成本也是巨大的。根据 2009—2018 年新上市治疗剂的成本数据及其相关研发支出，将药物成功上市的投资中值为 9.85 亿美元[65]。此外，NIH 拨款的减少进一步加剧了开展高质量研究以确保向患者安全提供新治疗所需的财政困难[66]。

九、未来的研究策略

旨在预防尿失禁的新疗法将是当前模式的一个受欢迎的补充，因为这些模式通常侧重于治疗而不是预防。互联网接入的日益普及，加上对社交媒体的熟练使用，使得有关尿失禁的教育内容能够接触到更广泛的受众[67]。因此，以预防为目标的内容可以针对年轻受众。此外，移动应用程序和其他基于互联网的干预措施的开发正在进行中，这些渠道可用于分发信息，并可能为研究试验招募参与者。

我们知道尿失禁可能由多种病因引起，随着我们对潜在病因的了解，尿失禁的个体亚型可能在未来发挥重要作用。根据病因、解剖学和遗传因素对尿失禁进行个性化治疗可能会改善患者的预后。随着 3D 打印技术的广泛应用，根据个体患者的解剖结构定制手术技术可能成为现实。例如，设备制造公司可以商业化生产针对尿道过度活动程度或其他变量（如抗拉强度）的患者专用的吊带。Paul 等将干细胞和 3D 打印技术结合起来，将子宫内膜中的子宫内膜间充质基质细胞生物打印到网状物上，用于骨盆器官脱垂的潜在治疗[68]。组织学工程的这一概念也可能在压力性尿失禁网状吊带的使用中发挥作用。

在确定急迫性尿失禁和压力性尿失禁中重要的生物标志物方面的进一步工作可能有助于指导基于尿液生化组成的女性个体化治疗。虽然过去对此进行了研究，但没有重大发现，但随着对不同膀胱过度活动症表型出现的理解，这可能值得进一步研究[69]。

总结

虽然目前的治疗方案是有效的，但总期望有所改进，而且针对急迫性尿失禁的药理学、基因治疗和神经调节以及针对压力性尿失禁的再生医学的研究进展寄予厚望。为了促进治疗，新技术必须经过从临床前研究到上市后分析的严格评估。这些评估应标准化，可重复，并具有可量化的结果测量，以允许对验证性数据进行多次研究。我们希望新疗法和新技术不断出现，以改善罹患尿失禁女性的生活质量。

参考文献

[1] Ward-Smith P. The cost of urinary incontinence. Urol Nurs. 2009;29(3):188–94.

[2] Staskin D, Frankel J, Varano S, Shortino D, Jankowich R, Mudd PN. International phase III, randomized, double-blind, placebo and active controlled study to evaluate the safety and efficacy of vibegron in patients with symptoms of overactive bladder: EMPOWUR. J Urol. 2020;204(2):316–24.

[3] Carr LK, Robert M, Kultgen PL, Herschorn S, Birch C, Murphy M, et al. Autologous muscle derived cell therapy for stress urinary incontinence: a prospective, dose ranging study. J Urol. 2013;189(2):595–601.

[4] Di Salvo J, Nagabukuro H, Wickham LA, Abbadie C, DeMartino JA, Fitzmaurice A, et al. Pharmacological characterization of a novel beta 3 adrenergic agonist, vibegron: evaluation of antimuscarinic receptor selectivity for combination therapy for overactive bladder. J Pharmacol Exp Ther. 2017;360(2):346–55.

[5] Yoshida M, Takeda M, Gotoh M, Nagai S, Kurose T. Vibegron, a novel potent and selective β3-adrenoreceptor a8, 16gonist, for the treatment of patients with overactive bladder: a randomized, double-blind, placebo-controlled phase 3 study. Eur Urol. 2018;73(5):783–90.

[6] Yoshida M, Takeda M, Gotoh M, Yokoyama O, Kakizaki H, Takahashi S, et al. Efficacy of vibegron, a novel β3-adrenoreceptor agonist, on severe urgency urinary incontinence related to overactive bladder: post hoc analysis of a randomized, placebo-controlled, double-blind, comparative phase 3 study. BJU Int. 2020;125(5):709–17.

[7] Staskin D, Frankel J, Varano S, Shortino D, Jankowich R, Mudd Jr PN. Once-daily vibegron 75 mg improves quality-of-life and incontinence efficacy endpoints in patients with overactive bladder: double-blind 52-week results from an extension study of the EMPOWUR international phase 3 trial. Neurourol Urodyn [Internet]. 2020 [cited 2020 Dec 20]. Available from: https://www.ics.org/2020/abstract/440.

[8] Staskin D, Frankel J, Varano S, Shortino D, Jankowich R, Mudd P. Pd21-01 once-daily vibegron 75 mg for overactive bladder (oab): double-blind 52-week results from an extension study of the international phase 3 trial (EMPOWUR). J Urol. 2020;203(Supplement 4):e453.

[9] Shi H, Chen H, Zhang Y, Cui Y. The efficacy and safety of Vibegron in treating overactive bladder: a systematic review and pooled analysis of randomized controlled trials. Neurourol Urodyn. 2020;39(5):1255–63.

[10] Rovner E, Chai TC, Jacobs S, Christ G, Andersson K-E, Efros M, et al. Evaluating the safety and potential activity of URO-902 (hMaxi-K) gene transfer by intravesical instillation or direct injection into the bladder wall in female participants with idiopathic (non-neurogenic) overactive bladder syndrome and detrusor overactivity from two double-blind, imbalanced, placebo-controlled randomized phase 1 trials. Neurourol Urodyn. 2020;39(2):744–53.

[11] Heesakkers JPFA, Digesu GA, van Breda J, Van Kerrebroeck P, Elneil S. A novel leadless, miniature implantable Tibial Nerve Neuromodulation System for the management of overactive bladder complaints. Neurourol Urodyn. 2018;37(3):1060–7.

[12] Yamashiro J, de Riese W, de Riese C. New implantable tibial nerve stimulation devices: review of published clinical results in comparison to established neuromodulation devices. Res Rep Urol. 2019;11:351–7.

[13] Rogers A, McCrery R, MacDiarmid S, Lukban J, Kaaki B, Shapiro A, et al. Pivotal study of subcutaneous tibial nerve stimulation with coin-sized implantable tibial neurostimulator (eCoin device) for urgency urinary incontinence. Neurourol Urodyn [Internet]. 2020 [cited 2020 Dec 21]. Available from: https://www.ics.org/2020/abstract/3.

[14] Valencia Technologies Corporation. Pivotal study of subcutaneous tibial nerve stimulation with eCoin for overactive bladder (OAB) with urgency urinary incontinence (UUI) [Internet]. clinicaltrials.gov. 2020 [cited 2021 Jan 5]. Report No.: NCT03556891. Available from: https://clinicaltrials.gov/ct2/show/NCT03556891.

[15] BlueWind Medical. A prospective study to assess the efficacy and safety of the BlueWind RENOVA iStim™ system in the treatment of patients diagnosed with overactive bladder (OASIS – OverActive Bladder StImulation System Study) [Internet]. clinicaltrials.gov. 2020 [cited 2021 Jan 5]. Report No.: NCT03596671. Available from: https://clinicaltrials.gov/ct2/ show/NCT03596671.

[16] Giusto L, Zahner P, Goldman H. V12-04 placement of an implantable tibial nerve stimulator under local anesthesia: step by step instructions. J Urol. 2019;201(Supplement 4):e1205.

[17] Tipton WA, de Riese WT, de Riese CS. Review of new implantable tibial nerve stimulators in comparison to established third line treatment modalities for nonneurogenic overactive bladder. Urol Pract. 2020;7(6):530–7.

[18] Sirls LT, Peters KM, Schonhoff A, Waldvogel A, Hasenau D. Early evaluation of an implanted chronic tibial nerve stimulation device versus percutaneous nerve stimulation for the treatment of urinary urge incontinence. ics.org [Internet]. 2019 [cited 2021 Jan 21]. Available from: https://www.ics.org/2019/abstract/156.

[19] Vollstedt A, Gilleran J. Update on implantable PTNS devices. Curr Urol Rep. 2020;21(7):28.

[20] Micron Medical Corporation. Multi-center, prospective, randomized, controlled, non-inferiority, clinical trial of chronic afferent nerve stimulation (CAN-Stim) of the tibial nerve versus sacral nerve stimulation (SNS) in the treatment of urinary urgency incontinence resulting from refractory overactive bladder (OAB) [Internet]. clinicaltrials.gov. 2020 [cited 2021 Jan 7]. Report No.: NCT02577302. Available from: https://clinicaltrials.gov/ct2/show/ NCT02577302.

[21] Bioness Inc. Prospective, multi-center, randomized, double-blinded trial of percutaneous tibial nerve stimulation with the Bioness StimRouter neuromodulation system versus Sham in the treatment of overactive bladder (OAB) [Internet]. clinicaltrials.gov. 2020 [cited 2021 Jan 7]. Report No.: NCT02873312. Available from:. https://clinicaltrials.gov/ct2/show/ NCT02873312.

[22] de Wachter S, McCrery R, Lane F, Benson K, Taylor C, Padron O, et al. Stimulation output and tissue impedance over 6-months of sacral neuromodulation therapy with a constant current system. Neurourol Urodyn [Internet]. 2020 [cited 2020 Dec 21]. Available from: https://www. ics.org/2020/abstract/47.

[23] Pearce MM, Hilt EE, Rosenfeld AB, Zilliox MJ, Thomas-White K, Fok C, et al. The female urinary microbiome: a comparison of women with and without urgency urinary incontinence. mBio. 2014;5(4): e01283–14.

[24] Thomas-White KJ, Hilt EE, Fok C, Pearce MM, Mueller ER, Kliethermes S, et al. Incontinence medication response relates to the female urinary microbiota. Int Urogynecol J. 2016;27(5):723–33.

[25] Lim R, Liong ML, Leong WS, Karim Khan NA, Yuen KH. Pulsed magnetic stimulation for stress urinary incontinence: 1-year Followup results. J Urol. 2017;197(5):1302–8.

[26] Stewart F, Berghmans B, B?K, Glazener CM. Electrical stimulation with non-implanted devices for stress urinary incontinence in women. Cochrane Database Syst Rev [Internet]. 2017 [cited 2021 Jan 24];2017(12). Available from: https://www.ncbi.nlm.nih.gov/pmc/ articles/PMC6486295/.

[27] Dmochowski R, Lynch CM, Efros M, Cardozo L. External electrical stimulation compared with intravaginal electrical stimulation for the treatment of stress urinary incontinence in women: a randomized controlled noninferiority trial. Neurourol Urodyn. 2019;38(7):1834–43.

[28] Whooley J, Cunnane EM, Do Amaral R, Joyce M, MacCraith

E, Flood HD, et al. Stress urinary incontinence and pelvic organ prolapse: biologic graft materials revisited. Tissue Eng Part B Rev. 2020;26(5):475–83.
[29] Darzi S, Urbankova I, Su K, White J, Lo C, Alexander D, et al. Tissue response to collagen containing polypropylene meshes in an ovine vaginal repair model. Acta Biomater. 2016;39:114–23.
[30] Parizzi NG, Rubini Oá, de Almeida SHM, Ireno LC, Tashiro RM, de Carvalho VHT. Effect of platelet-rich plasma on polypropylene meshes implanted in the rabbit vagina: histological analysis. Int Braz J Urol. 2017;43(4):746–52.
[31] D'Angelo W, Dziki J, Badylak SF. The challenge of stress incontinence and pelvic organ prolapse: revisiting biologic mesh materials. Curr Opin Urol. 2019;29(4):437–42.
[32] Li J, Chen X, Ling K, Liang Z, Xu H. Evaluation of the bioactivity about anti-sca-1/basic fibroblast growth factor-urinary bladder matrix scaffold for pelvic reconstruction. J Biomater Appl. 2019;33(6):808–18.
[33] Vashaghian M, Zaat SJ, Smit TH, Roovers J-P. Biomimetic implants for pelvic floor repair. Neurourol Urodyn. 2018;37(2):566–80.
[34] Lai K, Zhang J, Wang G, Luo X, Liu M, Zhang X, et al. A biomimetic mesh for treating female stress urinary incontinence. Biofabrication. 2017;9(1):015008.
[35] Wang X, Chen Y, Fan Z, Hua K. Comparing different tissue-engineered repair materials for the treatment of pelvic organ prolapse and urinary incontinence: which material is better? Int Urogynecol J. 2018;29(1):131–8.
[36] Mangır N, Hillary CJ, Chapple CR, MacNeil S. Oestradiol-releasing biodegradable mesh stimulates collagen production and angiogenesis: an approach to improving biomaterial integration in pelvic floor repair. Eur Urol Focus. 2019;5(2):280–9.
[37] Shafaat S, Mangir N, Regureos SR, Chapple CR, MacNeil S. Demonstration of improved tissue integration and angiogenesis with an elastic, estradiol releasing polyurethane material designed for use in pelvic floor repair. Neurourol Urodyn. 2018;37(2):716–25.
[38] El-Neemany D, O'Shaughnessy D, Grande D, Sajjan S, Jin C, Kohn N, et al. 24: histological and biomechanical characteristics of permanent and absorbable sling mesh in a rabbit model: 3–month time point. Am J Obstet Gynecol. 2019;220(3):S722.
[39] Pelvic Floor Research Foundation of South Africa. Prospective study to evaluate use of TephaFLEX™ sling implanted via a retropubic mid-urethral sling procedure for treatment of women with stress urinary incontinence [Internet]. clinicaltrials.gov. 2018 [cited 2021 Jan 7]. Report No.: NCT03673488. Available from: https://clinicaltrials.gov/ct2/show/NCT03673488.
[40] Guillaume O, Lavigne J-P, Lefranc O, Nottelet B, Coudane J, Garric X. New antibiotic-eluting mesh used for soft tissue reinforcement. Acta Biomater. 2011;7(9):3390–7.
[41] Brandt CJ, Kammer D, Fiebeler A, Klinge U. Beneficial effects of hydrocortisone or spironolactone coating on foreign body response to mesh biomaterial in a mouse model. J Biomed Mater Res A. 2011;99A(3):335–43.
[42] Kocjancic E, Erickson T, Tu L-M, Gheiler E, Drie DV. Two-year outcomes for the Altis® adjustable single incision sling system for treatment of stress urinary incontinence. Neurourol Urodyn. 2017;36(6):1582–7.
[43] Morán E, Pérez-Ardavín J, Sánchez JV, Bonillo MA, Martínez-Cuenca E, Arlandis S, et al. Mid-term safety and efficacy of the ALTIS?single-incision sling for female stress urinary incontinence: less mesh, same results. BJU Int. 2019;123(5A):E51–6.
[44] Coloplast A/S. A post-market evaluation of the Altis®single incision sling system versus transobturator or retropubic mesh sling in the treatment of female stress urinary incontinence [Internet]. clinicaltrials.gov. 2020 [cited 2021 Jan 7]. Report No.: NCT02348112. Available from: https://clinicaltrials.gov/ct2/show/NCT02348112.
[45] Coloplast A/S. The European Study of Altis single incision sling system for female stress urinary incontinence [Internet]. clinicaltrials.gov; 2018 Jan [cited 2021 Jan 7]. Report No.: NCT02049840. Available from: https://clinicaltrials.gov/ct2/show/NCT02049840.
[46] Dmitry S. A randomized clinical trial comparing a tunable-tension transobturator tape (TTT) versus standard transobturator midurethral tape (TOT) for the surgical treatment of stress urinary incontinence in women [Internet]. clinicaltrials.gov. 2019 [cited 2021 Jan 11]. Report No.: NCT03958695. Available from:. https://clinicaltrials.gov/ct2/show/NCT03958695.
[47] Gill BC, Sun DZ, Damaser MS. Stem cells for urinary incontinence: functional differentiation or cytokine effects? Urology. 2018;117:9–17.
[48] Carr LK, Steele D, Steele S, Wagner D, Pruchnic R, Jankowski R, et al. 1–year follow-up of autologous muscle-derived stem cell injection pilot study to treat stress urinary incontinence. Int Urogynecol J Pelvic Floor Dysfunct. 2008;19(6):881–3.
[49] Mitterberger M, Marksteiner R, Margreiter E, Pinggera GM, Colleselli D, Frauscher F, et al. Autologous myoblasts and fibroblasts for female stress incontinence: a 1–year follow-up in 123 patients. BJU Int. 2007;100(5):1081–5.
[50] Gräs S, Klarskov N, Lose G. Intraurethral injection of autologous minced skeletal muscle: a simple surgical treatment for stress urinary incontinence. J Urol. 2014;192(3):850–5.
[51] Sèbe P, Doucet C, Cornu J-N, Ciofu C, Costa P, de Medina SGD, et al. Intrasphincteric injections of autologous muscular cells in women with refractory stress urinary incontinence: a prospective study. Int Urogynecol J. 2011;22(2):183–9.
[52] Blaganje M, Lukanović A. Ultrasound-guided autologous myoblast injections into the extrinsic urethral sphincter: tissue engineering for the treatment of stress urinary incontinence. Int Urogynecol J. 2013;24(4):533–5.
[53] Peters KM, Dmochowski RR, Carr LK, Robert M, Kaufman MR, Sirls LT, et al. Autologous muscle derived cells for treatment of stress urinary incontinence in women. J Urol. 2014;192(2):469–76.
[54] Kuismanen K, Sartoneva R, Haimi S, Mannerström B, Tomás E, Miettinen S, et al. Autologous adipose stem cells in treatment of female stress urinary incontinence: results of a pilot study. Stem Cells Transl Med. 2014;3(8):936–41.
[55] Lee CN, Jang JB, Kim JY, Koh C, Baek JY, Lee KJ. Human cord blood stem cell therapy for treatment of stress urinary incontinence. J Korean Med Sci. 2010;25(6):813–6.
[56] Wang B, Zhou J, Banie L, Reed-Maldonado AB, Ning H, Lu Z, et al. Low-intensity extracorporeal shock wave therapy promotes myogenesis through PERK/ATF4 pathway. Neurourol Urodyn. 2018;37(2):699–707.
[57] Zhang X, Ruan Y, Wu AK, Zaid U, Villalta JD, Wang G, et al. Delayed treatment with low-intensity extracorporeal shock wave therapy in an irreversible rat model of stress urinary incontinence. Urology. 2020;141:187.e1–7.
[58] Krychman M, Rowan CG, Allan BB, Durbin S, Yacoubian A, Wilkerson D. Effect of single-session, cryogen-cooled monopolar radiofrequency therapy on sexual function in women with vaginal laxity: the VIVEVE I trial. J Women's Health. 2018;27(3):297–304.
[59] Allan BB, Bell S, Husarek K. A 12–month feasibility study to investigate the effectiveness of cryogen-cooled monopolar radiofrequency treatment for female stress urinary incontinence. Can Urol Assoc J. 2020;14(7):E313–8.
[60] Viveve Inc. Comparison of the Viveve treatment and cryogen-only treatment versus Sham treatment for stress urinary incontinence [Internet]. clinicaltrials.gov. 2020 [cited 2021 Jan 7]. Report No.: NCT04206085. Available from:. https://clinicaltrials.gov/ct2/show/NCT04206085.
[61] González Isaza P, Jaguszewska K, Cardona JL, Lukaszuk M. Long-

term effect of thermoablative fractional CO2 laser treatment as a novel approach to urinary incontinence management in women with genitourinary syndrome of menopause. Int Urogynecol J. 2018;29(2):211–5.

[62] Ni J, Gu B. Up-to-date evidences of laser therapy for female stress urinary incontinence: a systematic review and meta-analysis. ics.org [Internet]. 2020 [cited 2020 Dec 21]. Available from: https://www.ics.org/2020/abstract/98.

[63] Winkler H, Jacoby K, Kalota S, Snyder J, Cline K, Robertson K, et al. Twelve-month efficacy and safety data for the "stress incontinence control, efficacy and safety study": a phase III, multicenter, prospective, randomized, controlled study treating female stress urinary incontinence using the vesair intravesical balloon. Female Pelvic Med Reconstr Surg. 2018;24(3):222–31.

[64] Rosier PFWM, Schaefer W, Lose G, Goldman HB, Guralnick M, Eustice S, et al. International continence society good urodynamic practices and terms 2016: urodynamics, uroflowmetry, cystometry, and pressure-flow study. Neurourol Urodyn. 2017;36(5):1243–60.

[65] Wouters OJ, McKee M, Luyten J. Estimated Research and Development investment needed to bring a new medicine to market, 2009–2018. JAMA. 2020;323(9):844.

[66] 2017Factsheet_Restore NIH Funding.pdf [Internet]. [cited 2021 Jan 23]. Available from: https://faseb.org/Portals/2/PDFs/opa/2017/2017Factsheet_Restore%20NIH%20Funding.pdf.

[67] Malik RD, Kowalik CG. Patient education for overactive bladder in the digital era. Curr Bladder Dysfunct Rep. 2019;3(14):186–90.

[68] Paul K, Darzi S, McPhee G, Del Borgo MP, Werkmeister JA, Gargett CE, et al. 3D bioprinted endometrial stem cells on melt electrospun poly ε-caprolactone mesh for pelvic floor application promote anti-inflammatory responses in mice. Acta Biomater. 2019;97:162–76.

[69] Antunes-Lopes T, Cruz F. Urinary biomarkers in overactive bladder: revisiting the evidence in 2019. Eur Urol Focus. 2019;5(3):329–36.

[70] van Breda HMK, Martens FMJ, Tromp J, Heesakkers JPFA. A new implanted posterior tibial nerve stimulator for the treatment of overactive bladder syndrome: 3-month results of a novel therapy at a single center. J Urol. 2017;198(1):205–10.

[71] te Dorsthorst MJ, Digesu GA, Tailor V, Gore M, van Kerrebroeck PE, van Breda HMK, et al. 3-year followup of a new implantable tibial nerve stimulator for the treatment of overactive bladder syndrome. J Urol. 2020;204(3):545–50.

[72] Dmochowski RR, Kerrebroeck PV, Digesu GA, Elneil S, Heesakkers JP. Pd31 02 long-term results of safety, efficacy, quality of life and satisfaction of patients treated for refractory oab using an implantable tibial neurostimulation system: renova istim™system. J Urol. 2019;201(Supplement 4):e565–6.

[73] MacDiarmid S, Staskin DR, Lucente V, Kaaki B, English S, Gilling P, et al. Feasibility of a fully implanted, nickel sized and shaped tibial nerve stimulator for the treatment of overactive bladder syndrome with urgency urinary incontinence. J Urol. 2019;201(5):967–72.

[74] MacDiarmid S, Staskin DR, Lucente V, Kaaki B, English S, Gilling P, Meffan P, et al. Lba-06 12 month feasibility data of a fully-implanted, nickel-sized and shaped tibial nerve stimulator for the treatment of overactive bladder syndrome with urgency urinary incontinence. J Urol. 2019;201(Supplement 4):e994.

相　关　图　书　推　荐

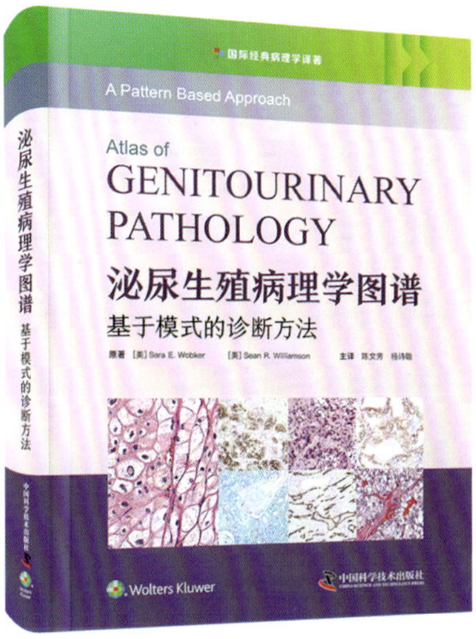

原著　[美] Sara E. Wobker
主译　陈文芳　杨诗聪
定价　280.00 元

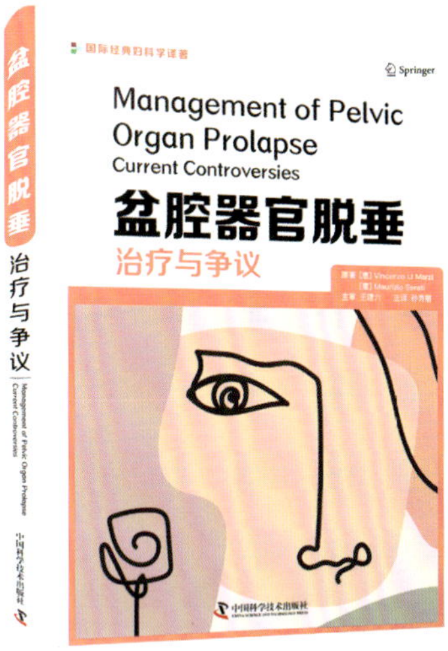

原著　[意] Vincenzo Li Marzi 等
主译　孙秀丽
定价　138.00 元

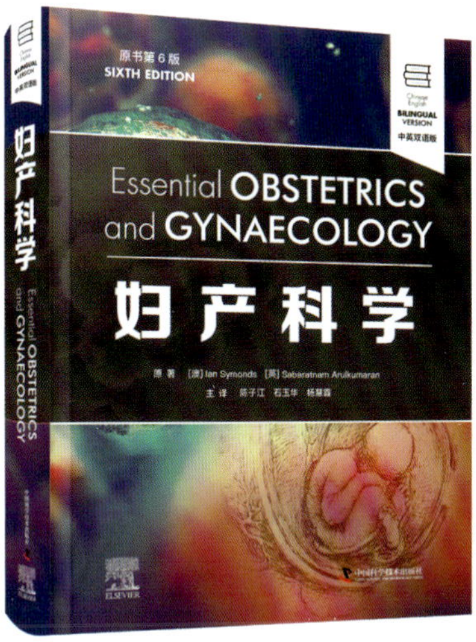

原著　[澳] Ian Symonds 等
主译　陈子江　石玉华　杨慧霞
定价　458.00 元

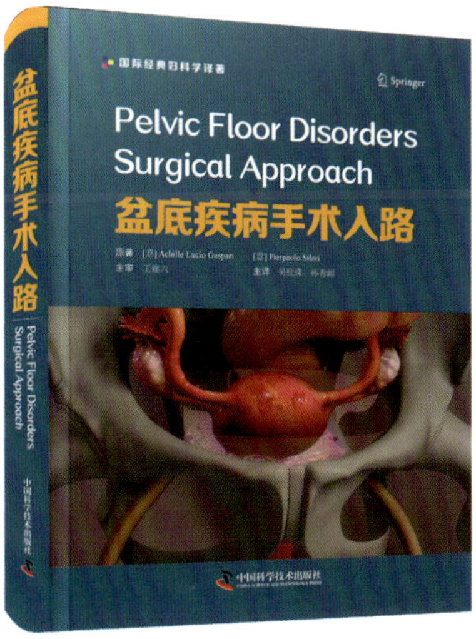

原著　[意] Achille Lucio Gaspari 等
主译　吴桂珠　孙秀丽
定价　198.00 元

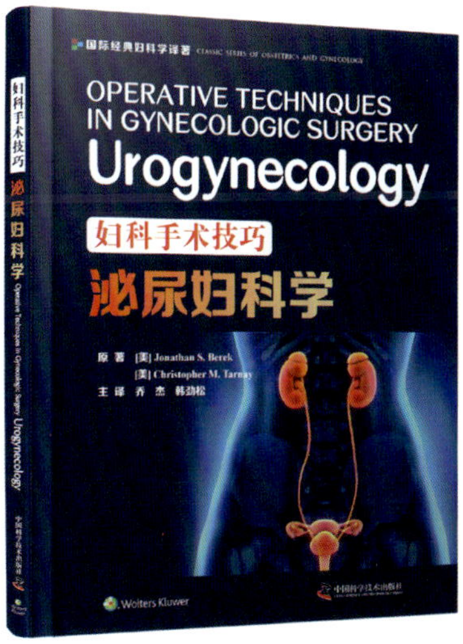

原著　[美] Jonathan S. Berek 等
主译　乔　杰　韩劲松
定价　128.00 元

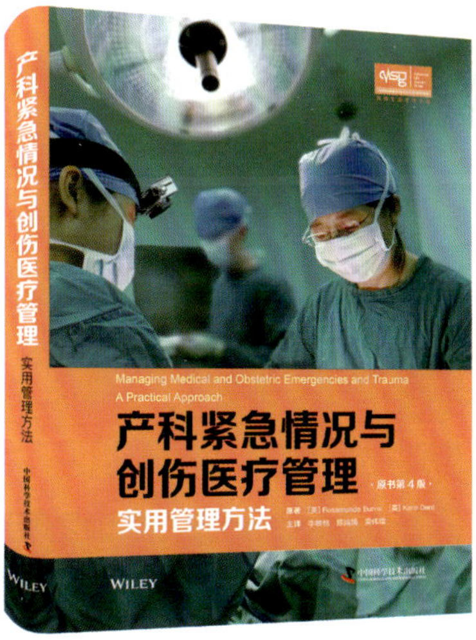

原著　[英] Rosamunde Burns 等
主译　李映桃　陈娟娟　梁伟璋
定价　258.00 元

相　关　图　书　推　荐

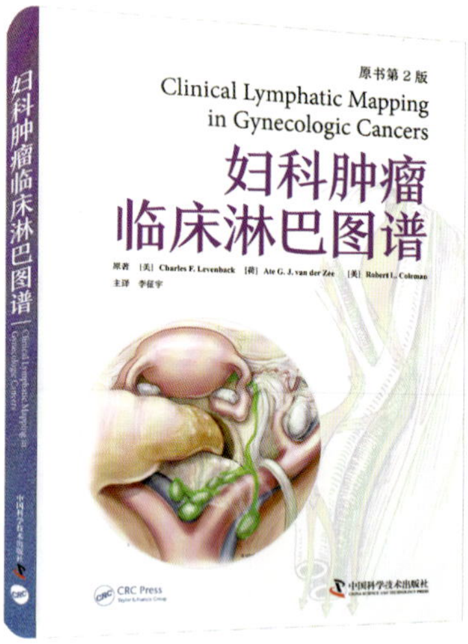

原著　[美] Charles F. Levenback 等
主译　李征宇
定价　158.00 元

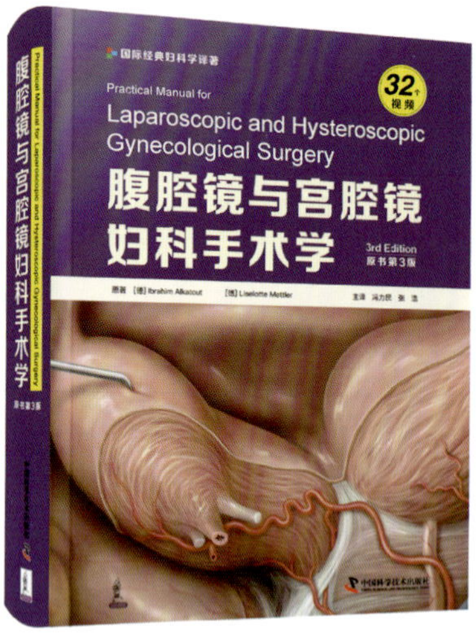

原著　[德] Ibrahim Alkatout 等
主译　冯力民　张　浩
定价　498.00 元

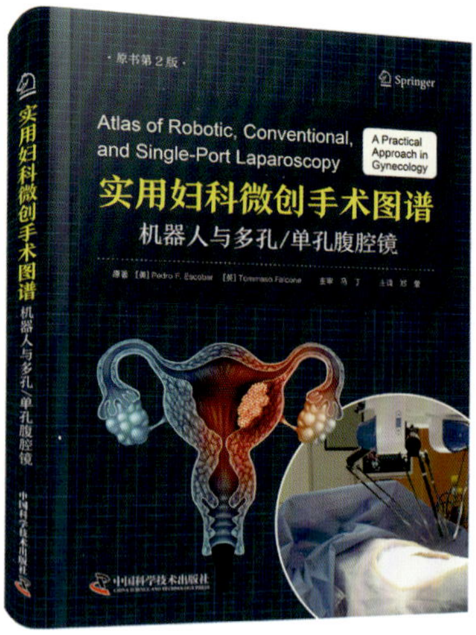

原著　[美] Pedro F. Escobar 等
主译　郑　莹
定价　188.00 元

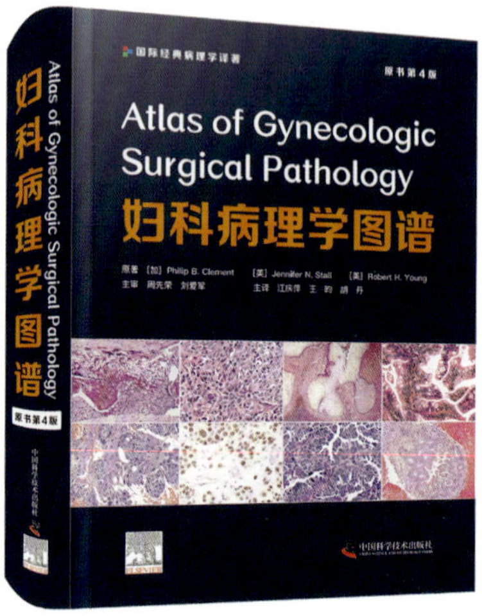

原著　[加] Philip B. Clement 等
主译　江庆萍　王　昀　胡　丹
定价　458.00 元

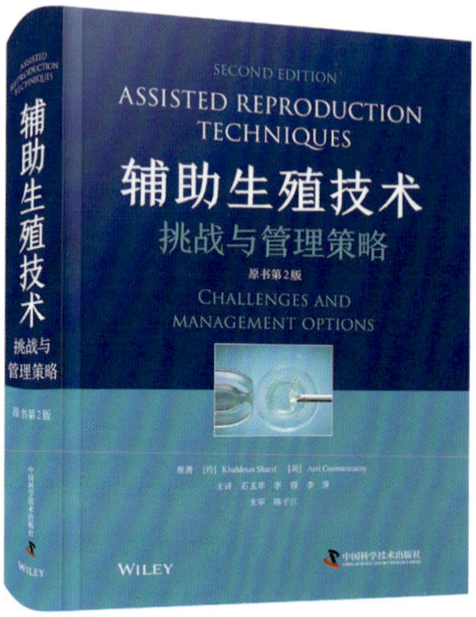

原著　[约] Khaldoun Sharif 等
主译　石玉华　李　蓉　李　萍
定价　398.00 元

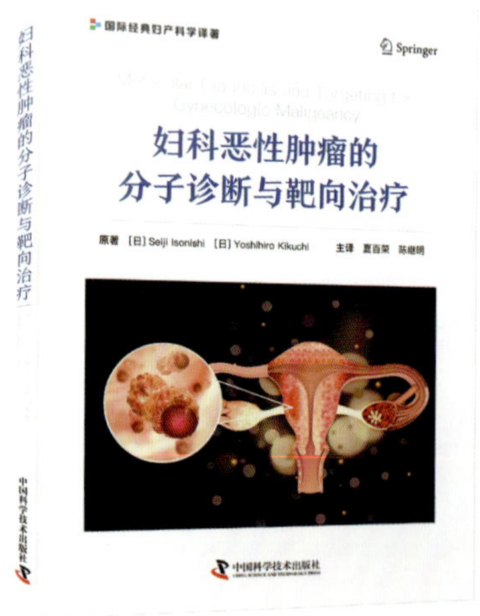

原著　[日] Seiji Isonishi 等
主译　夏百荣　陈继明
定价　138.00 元